Abernathy's
SURGICAL

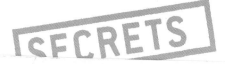

SECRETS

Abernathy's SURGICAL SECRETS

Updated Fifth Edition

Alden H. Harken, M.D.
Professor, Department of Surgery
University of California, San Francisco, School of Medicine
San Francisco, California
Chairman, Department of Surgery
University of California, San Francisco–East Bay
Oakland, California

Ernest E. Moore, M.D.
Professor and Vice-Chairman
Department of Surgery
University of Colorado Health Sciences Center
Chief of Surgery
Denver Health Medical Center
Denver, Colorado

ELSEVIER
MOSBY

ELSEVIER
MOSBY
An Affiliate of Elsevier

The Curtis Center
170 S Independence Mall W 300E
Philadelphia, Pennsylvania 19106

ABERNATHY'S SURGICAL SECRETS   ISBN: 0-323-03416-0
Updated Fifth Edition

NOTICE

Surgery is an ever-changing field. Standard safety precautions must be followed, but as new research and clinical experience broaden our knowledge, changes in treatment and drug therapy may become necessary or appropriate. Readers are advised to check the most current product information provided by the manufacturer of each drug to be administered to verify the recommended dose, the method and duration of administration, and contraindications. It is the responsibility of the licensed prescriber, relying on experience and knowledge of the patient, to determine dosages and the best treatment for each individual patient. Neither the publisher nor the author assumes any liability for any injury and/or damage to persons or property arising from this publication.

Previous editions copyrighted 2003, 2000, 1996, 1991, 1986.

Library of Congress Cataloging-in-Publication Data

Abernathy's surgical secrets/[edited by] Alden H. Harken, Ernest E. Moore.–5th ed., updated.
p.; cm
Includes bibliographical references and index.
ISBN 0-323-03416-0
1. Surgery–Examinations, questions, etc. I. Title: Surgical secrets. II. Harken, Alden H. III. Moore, Ernest Eugene. IV. Abernathy, Charles.
[DNLM: 1. Surgical Procedures, Operative–Examination Questions. WO 18.2 A146 2005]
RD37.2.S975 2005
617'.0076–dc22   2004057882

Acquisitions Editor: Linda Belfus
Developmental Editor: Stan Ward
Publishing Services Manager: Joan Sinclair
Project Manager: Cecelia Bayruns

Printed in the United States of America.

Last digit is the print number: 9   8   7   6   5   4   3   2   1

CONTENTS

III. ABDOMINAL SURGERY

IV. ENDOCRINE SURGERY

V. BREAST SURGERY

VI. OTHER CANCERS

X. TRANSPLANTATION

XI. UROLOGY

XII. HEALTH CARE

CONTRIBUTORS

Brett B. Abernathy, M.D.
Clinical Instructor, Division of Urology, Department of Surgery, University of Colorado Health Sciences Center, Denver, Colorado

Benjamin O. Anderson, M.D., FACS
Associate Professor, Department of Surgery, University of Washington School of Medicine; Clinical Medical Director, Breast Care and Cancer Research Program, University of Washington and Seattle Cancer Care Alliance, Seattle, Washington

Jyoti Arya, M.D.
Assistant Professor, Department of Surgery, University of Colorado Health Sciences Center, Denver, Colorado

Thomas E. Bak, M.D.
Assistant Professor, Division of Transplant Surgery, Department of Surgery, University of Colorado Health Sciences Center; University of Colorado Hospital, Denver, Colorado

Carlton C. Barnett, Jr., M.D.
Assistant Professor and Head, Gastrointestinal Surgical Oncology, Department of Surgery, Medical University of South Carolina, Charleston, South Carolina

James Bascom, M.D.
Professor Emeritus, Department of Surgery, University of Colorado Health Sciences Center, Denver, Colorado

Paulus C. Bauling, MBChB, M.Med., FACS
Assistant Professor, Division of Plastic and Reconstructive Surgery, Department of Surgery, University of Colorado Health Sciences Center; University of Colorado Hospital; Denver Veterans Affairs Medical Center; Denver Children's Hospital, Denver, Colorado

B. Timothy Baxter, M.D.
Professor, Department of Surgery, University of Nebraska Medical Center; Methodist Hospital, Omaha, Nebraska

Allen T. Belshaw, M.D.
Assistant Clinical Professor, Department of Surgery, University of Colorado Health Sciences Center, Denver, Colorado

Denis D. Bensard, M.D.
Associate Professor of Surgery and Pediatrics, Division of Pediatric Surgery, Department of Surgery, University of Colorado Health Sciences Center; The Children's Hospital, Denver, Colorado

Jeffrey A. Breall, M.D.
Professor of Clinical Medicine, Department of Medicine, Indiana University School of Medicine; Director of Cardiac Catheterization Laboratories and Interventional Cardiology, Krannert Institute of Cardiology, Indiana University Medical Center Indianapolis, Indiana

Elizabeth C. Brew, M.D.
Assistant Clinical Professor, Department of Surgery, University of Colorado Health Sciences Center, Denver, Colorado

Laurence H. Brinckerhoff, M.D.
Division of Cardiothoracic Surgery, Department of Surgery, University of Colorado Health Sciences Center, Denver, Colorado

Jamie M. Brown, M.D.
Associate Professor, Division of Cardiac Surgery, Department of Surgery, University of Maryland, Baltimore, Maryland

John W. Brown, M.D.
Professor and Chief of Cardiothoracic Surgery, Department of Surgery, Indiana University Medical Center; Riley Hospital for Children; Richard L. Roudebush Veterans Affairs Medical Center, Indianapolis, Indiana

Jon M. Burch, M.D.
Professor, Department of Surgery, University of Colorado Health Sciences Center; Chief, General and Vascular Surgery, Denver Health Medical Center, Denver, Colorado

Mark P. Cain, M.D.
Associate Professor, Division of Urology, Indiana University Medical Center; Riley Hospital for Children, Indianapolis, Indiana

Casey M. Calkins, M.D.
Department of Pediatric Surgery, Mercy Children's Hospital, Kansas City, Missouri

David N. Campbell, M.D.
Professor, Division of Cardiothoracic Surgery, Department of Surgery, University of Colorado Health Sciences Center, Denver, Colorado

Frank H. Chae, M.D., FACS
Assistant Professor, Department of Surgery, University of Colorado Health Sciences Center, Denver, Colorado

David J. Ciesla, M.D.
Assistant Professor, Department of Surgery, University of Colorado Health Sciences Center; Denver Health Medical Center, Denver, Colorado; Vail Valley Medical Center, Vail, Colorado

Joseph C. Cleveland, Jr., M.D.
Assistant Professor, Division of Cardiothoracic Surgery, Department of Surgery, University of Colorado Health Sciences Center; Chief, Cardiothoracic Surgery, Denver Veterans Affairs Medical Center, Denver, Colorado

Clay Cothren, M.D.
Assistant Professor, Department of Surgery, University of Colorado Health Sciences Center; Denver Health Medical Center, Denver, Colorado

Jeff Cross, M.D.
Assistant Clinical Professor, Department of Surgery, University of Colorado Health Sciences Center, Denver, Colorado

Firouz Daneshgari, M.D.
Director, Center for Female Pelvic Medicine and Surgery, Glickman Urological Institute, Cleveland Clinic Foundation, Cleveland, Ohio

J. Paul Elliott, M.D.
Clinical Assistant Professor, Department of Neurosurgery, University of Colorado Health Sciences Center, Denver, Colorado; Director of Neurotrauma, Colorado Neurological Institute, Swedish Medical Center, Englewood, Colorado

Michael E. Fenoglio, M.D.
Associate Clinical Professor, Department of Surgery, University of Colorado Health Sciences Center, Denver, Colorado

Christina A. Finlayson, M.D.
Associate Professor, Department of Surgery, University of Colorado Health Sciences Center; University of Colorado Hospital, Denver, Colorado; Director, Breast Center, Aurora, Colorado

Reginald J. Franciose, M.D.
Assistant Professor, Department of Surgery, University of Colorado Health Sciences Center; Attending Trauma Surgeon, Denver Health Medical Center, Denver, Colorado

David A. Fullerton, M.D.
Professor and Chief, Division of Cardiothoracic Surgery, Department of Surgery, University of Colorado Health Sciences Center; University of Colorado Hospital, Denver, Colorado

Glenn W. Geelhoed, M.D., M.P.H., DTMH
Professor of Surgery; Professor of International; Professor of Microbiology and Tropical Medicine; Office of the Dean and Provost, George Washington University Medical Center, Washington, District of Columbia

Doru I.E. Georgescu, M.D.
Private Practice, Thornton, Colorado

Ricardo J. Gonzalez, M.D.
Department of Surgery, University of Colorado Health Sciences Center, Denver, Colorado

Michael J.V. Gordon, M.D.
Associate Professor and Director of Hand Surgery, Division of Plastic Surgery, Department of Surgery, University of Colorado Health Sciences Center; Chief of Plastic Surgery, Denver Veterans Affairs Medical Center, Denver, Colorado

Dipin Gupta, M.D.
Division of Cardiothoracic Surgery, Department of Surgery, Temple University School of Medicine, Philadelphia, Pennsylvania

Rao Gutta, M.D.
Department of Surgery, University of Nebraska Medical Center, Omaha, Nebraska

James B. Haenel, R.R.T.
Clinical Specialist, Department of Surgery, Denver Health Medical Center, Denver, Colorado

Alden H. Harken, M.D.
Professor, Department of Surgery, University of California, San Francisco, School of Medicine, San Francisco, California; Chairman, Department of Surgery, University of California, San Francisco-East Bay, Oakland, California

Tabetha R. Harken, M.D., M.P.H.
Department of Obstetrics and Gynecology, University of Colorado Health Sciences Center, Denver, Colorado

Richard J. Hendrickson, M.D.
Instructor, Department of Surgery, University of Colorado Health Sciences Center; University of Colorado Hospital; The Children's Hospital, Denver, Colorado

Gilbert Hermann, M.D.
Clinical Professor, Department of Surgery, University of Colorado Health Sciences Center; Rose Medical Center, Denver, Colorado

Ramin Jamshidi, B.S., B.S.
Lecturer, Physics Department, University of Denver, Denver, Colorado

Jeffrey L. Johnson, M.D.
Assistant Professor, Department of Surgery, University of Colorado Health Sciences Center; Director, Surgical Intensive Care Unit, Denver Health Medical Center, Denver, Colorado

Darrell N. Jones, Ph.D.
Associate Director, Vascular Diagnostic Laboratory, Department of Surgery, University of Colorado Health Sciences Center, Denver, Colorado

Igal Kam, M.D.
Professor and Chief, Division of Transplant Surgery, Department of Surgery, University of Colorado Health Sciences Center; University of Colorado Hospital, Denver, Colorado

Frederick M. Karrer, M.D.
Professor of Surgery and Pediatrics, Department of Surgery, University of Colorado Health Sciences Center; Chairman of Pediatric Surgery, The Children's Hospital, Denver, Colorado

Lawrence L. Ketch, M.D., FAAP, FACS
Professor and Head, Division of Plastic and Reconstructive Surgery, Department of Surgery, University of Colorado Health Sciences Center, Denver, Colorado

Fernando J. Kim, M.D.
Assistant Professor, Division of Urology, Department of Surgery, University of Colorado Health Sciences Center; Chief of Urology, Denver Health Medical Center, Denver, Colorado

G. Edward Kimm, Jr., M.D., FACS
Assistant Clinical Professor, Department of Surgery, University of Colorado Health Sciences Center, Denver, Colorado; Attending Surgeon, Yampa Valley Medical Center, Steamboat Springs, Colorado

William C. Krupski, M.D.
Professor, Vascular Surgery Section, Department of Surgery, University of Colorado Health Sciences Center; University of Colorado Hospital; Denver Veterans Affairs Medical Center, Denver, Colorado

Anthony J. LaPorta, M.D.
Clinical Professor, Department of Surgery, University of Colorado Health Sciences Center; Chief, Department of Surgery, Rose Medical Center, Denver, Colorado

W. Andrew Lawrence, M.D.
Assistant Professor, Department of Surgery, University of Colorado Health Sciences Center; Denver Health Medical Center, Denver, Colorado

Kathleen Liscum, M.D.
Assistant Professor, Department of Surgery, Baylor College of Medicine; Chief of General Surgery, Ben Taub General Hospital, Houston, Texas

Joyce A. Majure, M.D., FACS
St. Joseph Regional Medical Center, Lewiston, Idaho

Robert C. McIntyre, Jr., M.D.
Associate Professor of Surgery, Division of Gastrointestinal, Tumor, and Endocrine Surgery, Department of Surgery, University of Colorado Health Sciences Center; University of Colorado Hospital; Denver Veterans Affairs Medical Center; The Children's Hospital; Denver Health Medical Center; Rose Medical Center, Denver, Colorado

Margaret M. McQuiggan, M.S., R.D., CNSD
Clinical Dietitian Specialist, Memorial Hermann Hospital, Houston, Texas

Randall B. Meacham, M.D.
Associate Professor, Division of Urology, Department of Surgery, University of Colorado Health Sciences Center, Denver, Colorado

Daniel R. Meldrum, M.D.
Assistant Professor of Surgery; Assistant Professor of Physiology; Director, Core Physiology Labs, Indiana University Medical Center; Methodist Hospital, Richard L. Roudebush Veterans Affairs Medical Center; Riley Hospital for Children, Indianapolis, Indiana

Kirstan K. Meldrum, M.D.
Assistant Professor, Division of Urology, Indiana University Medical Center; Riley Hospital for Children, Indianapolis, Indiana

Sanjay Misra, M.D.
Assistant Professor, Department of Neurosurgery, Denver Health Medical Center, Denver, Colorado

Ernest E. Moore, M.D.
Professor and Vice-Chairman, Department of Surgery, University of Colorado Health Sciences Center; Chief of Surgery, Denver Health Medical Center, Denver, Colorado

Frederick A. Moore, M.D.
James H. "Red" Duke, Jr., Professor and Vice-Chairman, Department of Surgery, University of Texas-Houston Medical School; Chief, General Surgery and Trauma and Critical Care; Medical Director, Trauma Service, Memorial Hermann Hospital, Houston, Texas

John B. Moore, M.D.
Assistant Professor, Department of Surgery, University of Colorado Health Sciences Center; Co-Director, Surgical Intensive Care Unit, Denver Health Medical Center, Denver, Colorado

Steven J. Morgan, M.D.
Assistant Professor, Department of Orthopaedics, University of Colorado Health Sciences Center; Denver Health Medical Center, Denver, Colorado

Kyle H. Mueller, M.D.
Department of Surgery, Northwestern Memorial Hospital, Chicago, Illinois

Mark Nehler, M.D.
Program Director, Department of Surgery, University of Colorado Health Sciences Center, Denver, Colorado

William R. Nelson, M.D.
Clinical Professor, Department of Surgery, University of Colorado Health Sciences Center, Denver, Colorado

Lawrence W. Norton, M.D.
Professor Emeritus, Department of Surgery, University of Colorado Health Sciences Center, Denver, Colorado

Siam Oottamasathien, M.D.
Division of Urology, Department of Surgery, University of Colorado Health Sciences Center, Denver, Colorado

Norman A. Paradis, M.D.
Associate Professor, Department of Surgery, University of Colorado Health Sciences Center; Medical Director, Emergency Medicine, University of Colorado Hospital, Denver, Colorado

David A. Partrick, M.D.
Assistant Professor, Division of Pediatric Surgery, Department of Surgery, University of Colorado Health Sciences Center; Director of Surgical Endoscopy for Infants and Children, The Children's Hospital, Denver, Colorado

William H. Pearce, M.D.
Violet R. and Charles A. Baldwin Professor of Vascular Surgery, Department of Surgery, Northwestern University Feinberg School of Medicine; Chief, Division of Vascular Surgery, Northwestern Memorial Hospital, Chicago, Illinois

Nathan W. Pearlman, M.D.
Professor, Department of Surgery, University of Colorado Health Sciences Center; University of Colorado Hospital; Denver Veterans Affairs Medical Center, Denver, Colorado

Steven L. Peterson, D.V.M., M.D.
Associate Professor, Departments of Surgery and Orthopedics, University of Colorado Health Sciences Center; Denver Health Medical Center, Denver, Colorado

Marvin Pomerantz, M.D.
Professor, Division of Cardiothoracic Surgery, Department of Surgery, University of Colorado Health Sciences Center, Denver, Colorado

Christopher D. Raeburn, M.D.
Department of Surgery, University of Colorado Health Sciences Center, Denver, Colorado

Azad Raiesdana, M.D.
Krannert Institute of Cardiology, Indiana University Medical Center, Indianapolis, Indiana

Joyesh K. Raj, M.D.
Assistant Professor, Division of Plastic and Reconstructive Surgery, Department of Surgery, University of Colorado Health Sciences Center, Denver, Colorado

Thomas F. Rehring, M.D., FACS
Clinical Assistant Professor, Division of Vascular Surgery, University of Colorado Health Sciences Center; Attending Surgeon, Colorado Permanente Medical Group; Saint Joseph Hospital, Denver, Colorado

John A. Ridge, M.D., Ph.D.
Chief, Head and Neck Surgery Section, Department of Surgical Oncology, Fox Chase Cancer Center, Philadelphia, Pennsylvania

Eric L. Sarin, M.D.
Department of Surgery, University of Colorado Health Sciences Center, Denver, Colorado

Craig H. Selzman, M.D.
Assistant Professor, Division of Cardiothoracic Surgery, Department of Surgery, University of North Carolina at Chapel Hill School of Medicine, Chapel Hill, North Carolina

J. Timothy Sherwood, M.D.
Fellow, Division of Cardiothoracic Surgery, Department of Surgery, University of Colorado Health Sciences Center, Denver, Colorado

Wade R. Smith, M.D.
Assistant Professor, Department of Orthopedics, University of Colorado Health Sciences Center; Director of Orthopedics, Denver Health Medical Center, Denver, Colorado

Gregory V. Stiegmann, M.D.
Professor of Surgery and Head, Division of Gastrointestinal, Tumor, and Endocrine Surgery, Department of Surgery, University of Colorado Health Sciences Center; University of Colorado Hospital; Denver Veterans Affairs Medical Center, Denver, Colorado

Caesar M. Ursic, M.D.
Assistant Professor, Department of Surgery, University of California, San Francisco-East Bay; Alameda County Medical Center; Highland General Hospital, Oakland, California

Alex J. Vanni
University of Colorado School of Medicine, Denver, Colorado

Gregory P. Victorino, M.D.
Assistant Professor, Department of Surgery, University of California San Francisco-East Bay; Alameda County Medical Center, Oakland, California

Michael E. Wachs, M.D.
Associate Professor, Division of Transplant Surgery, Department of Surgery, University of Colorado Health Sciences Center, Denver, Colorado

Michael B. Wallace, M.D., M.P.H.
Associate Professor of Medicine, Division of Gastroenterology and Hepatology, Department of Medicine, Mayo Medical School; Mayo Clinic, Jacksonville, Florida

Mark D. Walsh, Jr., M.D.
Department of Surgery, University of Colorado Health Sciences Center, Denver, Colorado

Thomas A. Whitehill, M.D.
Associate Professor, Vascular Surgery Section, Department of Surgery, University of Colorado Health Sciences Center; University of Colorado Hospital; Denver Veterans Affairs Medical Center, Denver, Colorado

Glenn J.R. Whitman, M.D.
Professor, Department of Surgery, Temple University School of Medicine; Temple University Hospital, Philadelphia, Pennsylvania

PREFACE TO THE FIFTH EDITION

A penetrating question is frequently more intellectually stimulating than a ponderous answer. A closed mind can be a formidable burden, and changing your mind proves that you've got one. Claude Bernarde recognized the danger of unchallenged surgical tradition when he observed: "It is what we think we know already that prevents us from learning." We must continuously assault what we think we know with questions. Alfred North Whitehead noted: "No man of science could subscribe without qualification to Galileo's beliefs or to Newton's beliefs, or to all his own scientific beliefs of ten years ago."

Indeed, our country was founded on the principle of contentious equilibrium. George Washington appointed both a Hamiltonian (Federalist) and Jeffersonian (states' rights) member to his cabinet. In our early presidential elections (up through John Quincy Adams), the "runner up" became the vice-president, thus assuring a balanced administration. The Founding Fathers recognized that when you surround yourself with "yes-men," the results are usually negative.

As surgeons, we learn both from personal experience and from the published series of others. Physical laws are predictable. When a physicist drops a brick out the window, it always goes down. The patterns in medicine are not so clear. Patients, their diseases, and our therapies are all different. The Prussian general Karl Von Clausewitz could have been describing medicine when he wrote about war: "A great part of the information obtained in war is contradictory, a still greater part is false and by far the greatest part is doubtful." Surgeons are almost unique in our ability to be self-questioning and self-critical. We must never march, like a bunch of lemmings, into a sea of intellectual acceptance.

This fifth edition of *Surgical Secrets* is again dedicated to the penetrating question. Armed with a dedication to inquiry, surgeons will happily evolve. Dinosaurs were inflexible and are extinct. Surgeons are neither.

Alden H. Harken, M.D.
Ernest E. Moore, M.D.

ACKNOWLEDGMENT

The editors gratefully acknowledge Cyrus Parsa, MD, and Andrew Luckey, MD, for contributing the Key Points, Top Secrets, and Websites for this updated edition. Both are residents in the Department of Surgery, University of California, San Francisco–East Bay, Oakland, California.

TOP 100 SECRETS

These secrets are 100 of the top board alerts. They summarize the concepts, principles, and most salient details of surgical practice.

1. Clinical determinants of brain death are the loss of the papillary, corneal, oculovestibular, oculocephalic, oropharyngeal, and respiratory reflexes for > 6 hours. The patient should also undergo an apnea test, in which the pCO_2 is allowed to rise to at least 60 mmHg without coexistent hypoxia. The patient should be observed for the absence of spontaneous breathing.

2. The estimated risks of HBV, HCV, and HIV transmission by blood transfusion in the United States are 1 in 205,000 for HBV, 1 in 1,935,000 for HCV, and 1 in 2,135,000 for HIV.

3. The most common location of an undescended testicle is the inguinal canal.

4. The most common solid renal mass in infancy is a congenital mesoblastic nephroma and in childhood a Wilms' tumor.

5. Ogilvie's syndrome is acute massive dilatation of the cecum and the ascending and transverse colon without organic obstruction.

6. The best screening method for prostate cancer is digital rectal exam combined with serum prostate-specific antigen.

7. The most common histologic type of bladder cancer is transitional cell carcinoma.

8. Carcinoma in situ of the bladder is treated with immunotherapy with intravesical bacillus Calmette-Guérin.

9. Localized renal cell carcinoma is treated with surgery (radical nephrectomy).

10. The most common cause of male infertility is varicocele.

11. The most common nonbacterial cause of pneumonia in transplant patients is cytomegalovirus.

12. Chimerism is leukocyte sharing between the graft and the recipient so that the graft becomes a genetic composite of both the donor and the recipient.

13. OKT3 is a mouse monoclonal antibody that binds to and blocks the T-cell CD3 receptor.

14. The most common disease requiring liver transplant is hepatitis C.

15. Cystic hygroma is a congenital malformation with a predilection for the neck. It is a benign lesion that usually presents as a soft mass in the lateral neck.

16. In neuroblastomas, age at presentation is the major prognostic factor. Children younger than 1 year have an overall survival rate > 70%, whereas the survival rate for children older than 1 year is < 35%.

17. The most feared complication of diaphragmatic hernia is persistent fetal circulation.

18. The three most common variants of tracheoesophageal fistula are (1) proximal esophageal atresia with distal tracheoesophageal fistula, (2) isolated esophageal atresia, and (3) tracheoesophageal fistula with esophageal atresia.

19. Atresia can occur anywhere in the GI tract: duodenal (50%), jejunoileal (45%), or colonic (5%). Duodenal atresia arises from failure of recanalization during the 8th–10th week of gestation; jejunoileal and colonic atresia are caused by an in utero mesenteric vascular accident.

20. The types of aortic dissection are ascending (type A) dissection, which involves only the ascending or both the ascending and descending aorta, and descending dissection (type B), which involves only the descending aorta.

21. A solitary pulmonary nodule is < 3 cm and is discrete on chest radiograph. It is usually surrounded by lung parenchyma.

22. Mediastinal staging is indicated in patients with apparent or documented lung cancer who have (1) known lung cancer with mediastinal nodes > 1 cm accessible by cervical mediastinal exploration, as assessed by CT scan; (2) adenocarcinoma of the lung and multiple mediastinal lymph nodes < 1 cm; (3) central or large (> 5 cm) lung cancers with mediastinal lymph nodes < 1 cm; and (4) lung cancer with risk of thoracotomy and lung resection.

23. The most common causes of aortic stenosis are now congenital anomalies and calcific (degenerative) disease.

24. In mitral regurgitation, the left ventricle ejects blood via two routes: (1) antegrade, through the aortic valve, or (2) retrograde, through the mitral valve. The amount of each stroke volume ejected retrograde into the left atrium is the regurgitant fraction. To compensate for the regurgitant fraction, the left ventricle must increase its total stroke volume. This ultimately produces volume overload of the left ventricle and leads to ventricular dysfunction.

25. The indications for CABG are (1) left main coronary artery stenosis; (2) three-vessel coronary artery disease (70% stenosis) with depressed left ventricular (LV) function or two-vessel coronary artery disease (CAD) with proximal left anterior descending (LAD) involvement; and (3) angina despite aggressive medical therapy.

26. Hibernating myocardium is improved by CABG. Myocardial hibernation refers to the reversible myocardial contractile function associated with a decrease in coronary flow in the setting of preserved myocardial viability. Some patients with global systolic dysfunction exhibit dramatic improvement in myocardial contractility after CABG.

27. The surgical treatment of ulcerative colitis is total colectomy with ileoanal pouch anastomosis.

28. Dieulafoy's ulcer is a gastric vascular malformation with an exposed submucosal artery, usually within 2–5 cm of the gastroesophageal junction. It presents with painless hematemesis, often massive.

29. The role of blind subtotal colectomy in the management of massive lower gastrointestinal bleeding is limited to a small group of patients in whom a specific bleeding source cannot be identified. The procedure is associated with a 16% mortality rate.

30. Colorectal polyps < 2 cm have a 2% risk of containing cancer, 2 cm polyps have a 10% risk, and polyps > 2 cm have a cancer risk of 40%. Sixty percent of villous polyps are > 2 cm, and 77% of tubular polyps are < 1 cm at the time of discovery.

31. Patients with colorectal cancer with lymph node involvement (Dukes' C) should receive chemotherapy postoperatively to treat micrometastases.

32. Goodsall's rule states the location of the internal opening of an anorectal fistula is based on the position of the external opening. An external opening posterior to a line drawn transversely across the perineum originates from an internal opening in the posterior midline. An external opening, anterior to this line, originates from the nearest anal crypt in a radial direction.

33. Incarcerated inguinal hernia: structures in the hernia sac still have a good blood supply but are stuck in the sac because of adhesions or a narrow neck of the hernia sac. Strangulated inguinal hernia: hernia structures have a compromised blood supply because of anatomic constriction at the neck of the hernia.

34. Chvostek's sign is spasm of the facial muscles caused by tapping the facial nerve trunk. Trousseau's sign is carpal spasm elicited by occlusion of the brachial artery for 3 minutes with a blood pressure cuff.

35. The two surgical options for Graves' disease are subtotal thyroidectomy or near-total thyroidectomy.

36. The only biochemical test that is routinely needed to identify patients with unsuspected hyperthyroidism is serum thyroid-stimulating hormone concentration.

37. The surgically correctable causes of hypertension are renovascular hypertension, pheochromocytoma, Cushing's syndrome, primary hyperaldosteronism, coarctation of the aorta, and unilateral renal parenchymal disease.

38. The "triple negative test" or "diagnostic triad" for diagnosing a palpable breast mass includes physical examination, breast imaging, and biopsy.

39. Chest wall radiation is indicated after mastectomy in patients with greater than 5 cm primary cancers, positive mastectomy margins, or more than four positive lymph nodes, all of which are associated with heightened locoregional recurrence rates.

40. Sentinel lymph nodes are the first stop for tumor cells metastasizing through lymphatics from the primary tumor.

41. The most common site of origin of subungual melanomas is the great toe. Amputation at or proximal to the metatarsal phalangeal joint and regional sentinel lymph node biopsy are advised by most authors.

42. Ramus marginalis mandibularis, the lowest branch of the nerve that innervates the depressor muscles of the lower lip, is the most commonly injured facial nerve branch during parotidectomy.

43. Waldeyer's ring is the mucosa of the posterior oropharynx covering a bed of lymphatic tissue that aggregates to form the palatine, lingual, pharyngeal, and tubal tonsils. These structures form a ring around the pharyngeal wall. This may be the site of primary or metastatic tumor.

44. A patient in whom the head and neck examination is completely normal but FNA of a cervical node reveals squamous cancer should have examination of the mouth, pharynx, larynx, esophagus, and tracheobronchial tree under anesthesia (triple endoscopy). If nothing is seen, blind biopsy of the nasopharynx, tonsils, base of tongue, and pyriform sinuses should be done at the same sitting.

45. The microorganisms implicated in atherosclerosis include *Chlamydia pneumoniae, Helicobacter pylori*, streptococci, and *Bacillus typhosus*.

46. The cumulative 10-year amputation rate for claudication is 10%.

47. The absolute reduction in risk of stroke is 6% over a 5-year period in asymptomatic patients with > 60% stenosis who undergo carotid endarterectomy plus aspirin versus patients treated with aspirin alone (5.1% versus 11%).

48. Abdominal aortic aneurysm's average expansion rate is 0.4 cm/year.

49. Heparin binds to antithrombin III, rendering it more active.

50. The patient with suspected intermittent claudication should initially be evaluated by obtaining ankle brachial index or segmental limb pressures at rest.

51. Shock is suboptimal consumption of O_2 and excretion of CO_2 at the cellular level.

52. Nitric oxide is synthesized in vascular endothelial cells by constitutive nitric oxide synthase and inducible NOS, using arginine as the substrate.

53. Saliva has the hightest potassium concentration (20 mEq), followed by gastric secretions (10 mEq), then pancreatic and duodenal secretions (5 mEq).

54. Basal caloric expenditure = 25 kcal/kg/day with a requirement of approximately 1 g protein/kg/day.

55. 6.25 g of protein contains 1 g of nitrogen.

56. Dextrose has 3.4 kcal/g, protein 4 kcal/g, fat 9 kcal/g (20% lipid solution delivers 2 kcal/mL).

57. Maximal glucose infusion rates in parenteral formulas should not exceed 5 mg/kg/min.

58. Refeeding syndrome occurs in moderately to severely malnourished patients (e.g., chronic alcoholism or anorexia nervosa) who, upon presentation with a large nutrient load, develop clinically significant decreases in serum phosphorus, potassium, calcium, and magnesium levels. Hyperglycemia is common secondary to blunted insulin secretion. ATP production is mitigated, and the classic presentation is respiratory failure.

59. Glutamine is the most common amino acid found in muscle and plasma. Levels decrease after surgery and physiologic stress. Glutamine serves as a substrate for rapidly replicating cells (interestingly, it is also the number one metabolic substrate for neoplastic cells), maintains the integrity and function of the intestinal barrier, and protects against free radical damage by maintaing GSH levels. Glutamine is unstable in IV form unless linked as a dipeptide.

60. Fever is caused by activated macrophages that release interleukin-1, tumor necrosis factor, and interferon in response to bacteria and endotoxin. The result is a resetting of the hypothalamic thermoregulatory center.

61. Cardiac output = heart rate x stroke volume; normal CO is 5–6 L/min.

62. SVR = [(MAP – CVP)/CO] x 80; normal SVR is 800–1200 dyne·sec/cm^{-5}.

63. Hypovolemic shock: low CVP and PCWP, low CO and SVO$_2$, high SVR.

64. Cardiogenic shock: high CVP and PCWP, low CO and SVO$_2$, variable SVR.

65. Septic shock: low or normal CVP and PCWP, high CO initially, high SVO$_2$, low SVR.

66. Kehr's sign is concurrent LUQ and left shoulder pain, indicating diaphragmatic irritation from a ruptured spleen or subdiaphragmatic abscess. Anatomically, the diaphragm and the back of the left shoulder enjoy parallel innervation.

67. Rebound tenderness implies peritoneal inflammation and irritation not simply abdominal tenderness.

68. The 5 Ws of post-operative fever are **w**ound (infection), **w**ater (UTI), **w**ind (atelectasis, pneumonia), **w**alking (thrombophlebitis), and **w**onder drugs (drug fevers).

69. Cricothyroidotomy should *not* be performed in patients < 12 years old or any patient with suspected direct laryngeal trauma or tracheal disruption.

70. The radial (wrist) pulse estimates SBP > 80 mmHg; femoral (groin) pulse estimates SBP > 70 mmHg; and carotid (neck) pulse estimates SBP > 60 mmHg.

71. A general rule for crystalloid infusion to replace blood loss is a 3:1 ratio of isotonic crystalloid to blood.

72. Raccoon eyes (periorbital ecchymosis) and Battle's sign (mastoid ecchymosis) are clinical indicators of basilar skull fracture.

73. CPP = MAP – ICP. Some debate exists on the minimum allowable CPP, but consensus indicates that a cerebral perfusion pressure of 50–70 mmHg is necessary.

74. Violation of the platysma defines a penetrating neck wound.

75. Tension pneumothorax is air accumulation in the pleural space eliciting increased intrathoracic pressure and resulting in a kinking of the SVC and IVC that compromises venous return to heart.

76. The most common site of thoracic aortic injury in blunt trauma is just distal to the take-off of the left subclavian artery.

77. The most common manifestation of blunt myocardial injury is arrhythmia.

78. Indications for thoracotomy in a stable patient with hemothorax include an immediate tube thoracostomy output of > 1500 mL and ongoing bleeding of 250 mL/h for 4 consecutive hours.

79. Beck's triad is hypotension, distended neck veins, and muffled heart sounds.

80. The hepatic artery supplies approximately 30% of blood flow to the liver while the portal vein supplies the remaining 70%. The oxygen delivery, however, is similar for both at 50%.

81. The Pringle maneuver is a manual occlusion of the hepatoduodenal ligament to interrupt blood flow to the liver.

82. Splenectomy significantly decreases IgM levels.

83. 90% of trauma fatalities due to pelvic fractures are due to venous bleeding and bone oozing; only 10% of fatal pelvic bleeding from blunt trauma is arterial (most common site is superior gluteal artery).

84. Intraperitoneal bladder rupture from blunt trauma: operative management; extraperitoneal rupture: observant management.

85. Pseudoaneurysm is a disruption of the arterial wall leading to a pulsatile hematoma contained by fibrous connective tissue (but not all three arterial wall layers, which defines a true aneurysm).

86. The earliest sign of lower extremity compartment syndrome is neurologic in the distribution of the peroneal nerve with numbness in the first dorsal webspace and weak dorsiflexion.

87. Posterior knee dislocations are associated with popliteal artery injuries and are an indication for angiography.

88. Management of suspected navicular fracture despite negative radiography is short-arm cast and repeat x-ray in 2 weeks; at high risk for avascular necrosis.

89. Parkland formula: lactated Ringer's at 4 mL/kg x %TBSA (second- and third-degree only) of burn. Infuse 50% of volume in first 8 hours and the remaining 50% over the subsequent 16 hours.

90. The metabolic rate peaks at 2.5 times the basal metabolic rate in severe burns > 50% TBSA.

91. Gallstones and alcohol abuse are the two main causes of acute pancreatitis.

92. Alcohol abuse accounts for 75% of cases of chronic pancreatitis.

93. Isolated gastric varices and hypersplenism indicate splenic vein thrombosis and are an indication for splenectomy.

94. The treatment for gallstone pancreatitis is cholecystectomy and intraoperative cholangiogram during the same hospital stay once the pancreatitis has subsided.

95. Proton pump inhibitors irreversibly inhibit the parietal cell hydrogen ion pump.

96. Definitive treatment of alkaline reflux gastritis after a Billroth II includes a Roux-en-Y gastro-jejunostomy from a 40-cm efferent jejunal limb.

97. Cushing's ulcer is a stress ulcer found in critically ill patients with central nervous system injury. It is typically single and deep, with a tendency to perforate.

98. Curling's ulcer is a stress ulcer found in critically ill patients with burn injuries.

99. Marginal ulcer is an ulcer found near the margin of gastroenteric anastomosis, usually on the small bowel side.

100. The most common cause of small bowel obstructions is adhesive disease; the second most common cause is hernias.

ARE YOU READY FOR YOUR SURGERY ROTATION?

Tabetha R. Harken, M.D., M.P.H., and Alden H. Harken, M.D.

CHAPTER 1

Surgery is a participatory, team, and contact sport. Present yourself to patients, residents, and attendings with enthusiasm (which covers a multitude of sins), punctuality (type A people do not like to wait), and cleanliness (you must look, act, and smell like a doctor).

1. **Why should you introduce yourself to each patient and ask about their chief complaint?**
   Symptoms are perception, and perception is more important than reality. To a patient, the chief complaint is not simply a matter of life and death—it is much more important. Patients routinely are placed into compromising, uncomfortable, embarrassing, and undignified predicaments. Patients are people, however; they have interests, concerns, anxieties, and a story. As a student, you have an opportunity to place your patient's chief complaint into the context of the rest of his or her life. This skill is important, and the patient will always be grateful. You can serve a real purpose as a listener and translator for the patient and his or her family.
   Patients want to trust and love you. This trust in surgical therapy is a formidable tool. The more a patient understands about his or her disease, the more the patient can participate in getting better. Recovery is faster if the patient helps. Similarly, the more the patient understands about his or her therapy (including its side effects and potential complications), the more effective the therapy is (this principle is not in the textbooks). You can be your patient's interpreter. This is the fun of surgery (and medicine).

2. **What is the correct answer to almost all questions?**
   Thank you. Gratitude is an invaluable tool on the wards.

3. **Are there any simple rules from the trenches?**
   1. **Getting along with the nurses.** The nurses do know more than the rest of us about the codes, routines, and rituals of making the wards run smoothly. They may not know as much about pheochromocytomas and intermediate filaments—but about the stuff that matters, they know a lot. Acknowledge that, and they will take you under their wings and teach you a ton!
   2. **Helping out.** If your residents look busy, they probably are. So, if you ask how you can help and they are too busy even to answer, asking again probably wouldn't be very high yield. Always leap at the opportunity to shag x-rays, track down lab results, and retrieve a bag of blood from the bank. The team will recognize your enthusiasm and reward your contributions.
   3. **Getting scutted.** We all would like a secretary, but one is not going to be provided on this rotation. Your residents do a lot of their own scut work without you even knowing about it. So if you feel like scut work is beneath you, perhaps you should think about another profession (maybe real estate or hair styling).
   4. **Working hard.** This rotation is an apprenticeship. If you work hard, you will get a realistic idea of what it means to be a resident (and even a practicing doc) in this specialty. (This has big advantages when you are selecting a type of internship.)
   5. **Staying in the loop.** In the beginning, you may feel like you are not a real part of the team. If you are persistent and reliable, however, soon your residents will trust you with more important jobs.

6. **Educating yourself, then educating your patients.** Here is one of the rewarding places (as indicated in question 1) where you can soar to the top of the team. Talk to your patients about everything (including their disease and therapy), and they will love you for it.

7. **Maintaining a positive attitude.** As a medical student, you may feel that you are not a crucial part of the team. Even if you are incredibly smart, you are unlikely to be making the crucial management decisions. So what does that leave? Attitude. If you are enthusiastic and interested, your residents will enjoy having you around, and they will work to keep you involved and satisfied. A dazzlingly intelligent but morose complainer is better suited for a rotation in the morgue. Remember, your resident is likely following 15 sick patients, gets paid less than $2 an hour, and hasn't slept more than 5 hours in the last 3 days. Simple things such as smiling and saying thank you (when someone teaches you) go an incredibly long way and are rewarded on all clinical rotations with experience and good grades.

8. **Having fun!** This is the most exciting, gratifying, rewarding, and fun profession—and is light years better than whatever is second best (this is not just our opinion).

4. **What is the best approach to surgical notes?**
Surgical notes should be succinct. Most surgeons still move their lips when they read. See Table 1-1.

TABLE 1-1. BEST APPROACH TO SURGICAL NOTES

Admission Orders

Admit to 5 West (attending's name)

Condition:	Stable
Diagnosis:	Abdominal pain; r/o appendicitis
Vital signs:	q 4 h
Parameters:	Please call H.O. for:
	$T > 38°C$
	$160 < BP < 90$
	$120 < HR < 60$
Diet:	NPO
Fluids:	1000 LR w 20 mEq KCl @ 100 mL/h
Med[ication]s:	ASA 650 mg PR prn for $T > 38.5°C$

Thank you.

Sign your name/leave space for resident's signature

(your beeper number)

Key: r/o = rule out, q = every, H.O. = house officer, T = temperature, BP = systolic blood pressure, HR = heart rate, NPO = nothing by mouth (this includes water and pills), ASA = aspirin, PR = per rectum, prn = as needed. Other useful abbreviations: OOB = out of bed, BRP = bathroom privileges.
Note: You cannot be too polite or too grateful to patients or nurses.

History and Physical Examination (H & P)

Mrs. O'Flaherty is a 55 y/o w ♀ [white woman] admitted with a cc [chief complaint]: "my stomach hurts." Pt [patient] was in usual state of excellent health until 2 days PTA [prior to admission] when she noted gradual onset of crampy midepigastric pain. Pain is now severe (7/10—7 on a scale of 10) and recurring q 5 minutes. Pt described + vomiting (+ bile, –blood) [with bile, without blood]. PMH [past medical history]

Hosp[italizations]:	Pneumonia (1991)
	Childbirth (1970, 1972)
	Surg[ery]—splenectomy for trauma (1967)

TABLE 1-1. BEST APPROACH TO SURGICAL NOTES *(continued)*

Allergies:	Codeine, shellfish
ETOH [alcohol]:	Social
Tobacco:	1 ppd [pack per day] x 25 years
ROS [review of systems]	
Resp[iratory]:	productive cough
Cardiac:	Ō chest pain [o = not observed, noncontributory, or not here]
	Ō MI [myocardial infarction]
Renal:	Ō dysuria
	Ō frequency
Neuro[logic]:	WNL [within normal limits]

Physical Examination (P.E.)

BP: 140/90   HR: 100 (regular)

RR [respiratory rate]: 16 breaths/min   Temp: 38.2°C

WD [well-developed], WN [well-nourished], mildly obese, 55 y/o ♀ in moderate abdominal distress

HEENT [head, eyes, ears, nose, and throat]: WNL	
Resp:	Clear lungs bilat[erally]
	Ō wheeze
Heart:	Ō m [murmur]
	RSR [regular sinus rhythm]
Abdomen:	Mildly distended, crampy, midepigastric pain
	High-pitched rushes that coincide with crampy pain
	Tender to palpation (you do not need to hurt the patient to find this out)
	Ō Rebound
Rectal:	(Always do—never defer the rectal exam on your surgical rotation)
	Hematest—negative for blood
	No masses, no tenderness
Pelvic:	No masses
	No adnexal tenderness
	No chandelier sign—if motion of cervix makes your patient hit the chandelier → pelvic inflammatory disease (PID; gonorrhea)
Extremities:	Full ROM [range of motion]
	Ō edema
	Bounding (3+) pulses
Imp[ression]:	Abdominal pain
	r/o SB [small bowel] obstruction 2° [secondary] to adhesions
Rx:	NG [nasogastric] tube
	IV fluids

(continued)

TABLE 1-1. BEST APPROACH TO SURGICAL NOTES *(continued)*

Op[erative] consent

Type and hold

[Signature]

Notes on the surgical H&P

- A surgical H&P should be succinct and focused on the patient's problem.
- Begin with the chief complaint (in the patient's words).
- Is the problem new or chronic?
- PMH: always include prior hospitalizations and medications.
- ROS: restrict review to organ systems (lung, heart, kidneys, and nervous system) that may affect this admission.
- P.E.: Always begin with vital signs (including respiration and temperature)—that is why these signs are vital.
- Rebound means inflammatory peritoneal irritation or peritonitis.

Preop[erative] note

The preoperative note is a checklist confirming that you and the patient are ready for the planned surgical procedure. Place this note in the Progress Notes:

Preop dx [diagnosis]:	SB obstruction 2° to adhesions
CXR [chest x-ray]:	Clear
ECG [electrocardiogram]:	NSR w/ST-T wave changes
Blood:	Type and crossmatch x 2 u
Consent:	In chart

Operative note

The operative note should provide anyone who encounters the patient after surgery with all the needed information:

Preop dx:	SB obstruction
Postop dx:	Same, all bowel viable
Procedure:	Exp[loratory] Lap[arotomy] with lysis of adhesions
Surgeon:	Name him/her
Assistants:	List them
Anesthesia:	GEA [general endotracheal anesthesia]
I&O [intake and output]:	In: 1200 mL Ringer's lactate (R/L)
	Out: 400 mL urine
EBL [estimated blood loss]:	50 mL
Specimen:	None
Drains:	None
	[Sign your name]

APPENDIX: REQUIRED READING

Unlike medical rounds, where in order to "keep up" you need to "one up" by quoting a current (preferably yesterday's) journal article, in surgery, you can flourish by knowing the following references—but you need to know them cold.

1. **Mangano DT, Goldman L: Pre-operative assessment of patients with known or suspected coronary disease. N Engl J Med 333:1750–1756, 1995.**
   This is an update of Goldman's original (NEJM, 1977) article in which he pioneered the concept of "risk adjusted surgical outcome." You should copy Table 2, Three Commonly Used Indexes of Cardiac Risk, and always carry it with you. Intuitively, a triathlete will weather a surgical stress better than a supreme court judge, but this article provides a point system with which you can calculate objective perioperative risk.

2. **Veronesi U, Cascinelli N, Mariani L, et al: Twenty-year follow-up of a randomized study comparing breast conserving surgery with radical mastectomy for early breast cancer. N Engl J Med 347:1227–1232, 2002.**
   Seven hundred women with less than 2 cm breast cancer were randomized to radical mastectomy or quadrantectomy and radiation therapy. After 1976, patients with positive axillary nodes also received adjuvant CMF (cyclophosphamide, methotrexate and 5-fluorouracil). After 20 years, 30 women in the conservative treatment group and 8 women in the radical mastectomy group suffered local recurrence (p , 0.01). Conversely, the incidence of deaths from all causes at 20 years was identical at 41%. The authors conclude that breast conservation therapy is the "treatment of choice" for women with "relatively small breast cancers."

3. **Fisher B, Anderson S, Bryant J, et al: Twenty-year follow-up of a randomized trial comparing total mastectomy, lumpectomy and lumpectomy plus irradiation for the treatment of invasive breast cancer. N Engl J Med 347:1223–1241, 2002.**
   Clinical investigation is hard to do. The National Surgical Adjuvant Breast and Bowel Project (NSABP) Trials, initiated 25 years ago, continue to serve as the benchmark for superb prospective, randomized investigations. In this study, 1851 women were randomized after the breast tumor was excised and the nodal status was documented. The authors conclude that lumpectomy followed by breast irradiation is appropriate therapy. In order to appreciate the huge problems in interpreting clinical trials, you must read this article carefully. Radiation did decrease death from breast cancer, but this reduction was partially offset by an increase in deaths from other causes.

4. **Barnett HJ, Taylor DW, Eliasziw M, et al: Benefit of carotid endarterectomy in patients with symptomatic moderate or severe stenosis. N Engl J Med 339:1415–1425, 1998.**
   This is the North American Symptomatic Carotid Endarterectomy Trial (NASCET) initiated in 1987. NASCET randomized patients with severe carotid stenosis (70–99%) and moderate stenosis (< 70%) into standard medical therapy or carotid endarterectomy (CEA). By 1991, the clear advantage of surgery in symptomatic patients with severe stenosis was so clear that the study was stopped for this group. This manuscript reports a 5-year reduction in ipsilateral stroke from 22.2% (medical) to 15.7% (surgical) (p = 0.045) in patients with moderate (50–69%) stenosis. Once a patient with carotid disease becomes symptomatic, that is ominous. As you witness various diseases, you subconsciously compile a list of diseases you don't want. A big burn and a big stroke are on the top of everyone's list.

5. **Endarterectomy for asymptomatic carotid artery stenosis. Executive Committee for the Asymptomatic Carotid Atherosclerosis Study. J Am Med Assoc 273:1421–1428, 1995.**
   The Asymptomatic Carotid Atherosclerosis Study (ACAS) randomized 1662 asymptomatic patients with > 60% carotid artery stenosis to medical prescription (one aspirin a day plus risk factor modification) or carotid endarterectomy. After only 2.7 years, the projected 5-year risk of ipsilateral stroke/death was 5.1% in the surgical group and 11% in the medical group. This is an aggregate (including perioperative trouble) risk reduction of 53%. This article concludes that an asymptomatic patient with a 60% or greater carotid artery lesion, who is an acceptable risk (atherosclerosis is a systemic disease) for elective surgery will enjoy a reduction in 5-year risk of ipsilateral stroke if the surgery can be accomplished with less than a 3% aggregate morbidity/mortality.

6. **Selzman CH, Miller SA, Zimmerman MA, Harken AH: The case for beta-adrenergic block-ade as prophylaxis against perioperative cardiovascular morbidity and mortality. Arch Surg 136:286–290, 2001.**
   When patients suffer perioperative morbidity and mortality, the cardiovascular system is typi-cally the culprit. Patients with coronary artery disease cannot increase coronary blood flow to meet the enhanced oxygen demand associated with surgical stress. Beta-adrenergic blockade decreases myocardial oxygen consumption, and cardioselective beta-blockers do not exacer-bate bronchospasm in patients with COPD. These authors argue that all patients over 40 years old will benefit from beta-adrenergic blockade initiated 2 weeks prior to elective surgery.

7. **Van den Berghe G, Wouters P, Weekers F, et al: Intensive insulin therapy in critically ill patients. N Engl J Med 345:1359–1367, 2001.**
   Both hyperglycemia and insulin resistance are characteristic of critically ill patients. These authors randomized 1548 SICU patients to either aggressive blood glucose control (main-tained at 80–110 mg%) or conventional therapy (give insulin only if blood glucose exceeds 215 mg%). Aggressive glucose control decreased ICU mortality from 8% to 4.6% (p , 0.04) with the largest impact in patients with multiple organ failure from a septic focus.
   In surgery, attention to detail counts big:
   ■ Keep blood sugar between 80 and 110 mg%.
   ■ Give prophylactic antibiotics 0–2 hours preop so the patient will have a good antibiotic blood level at the time of the incision.
   ■ Keep your patient warm (37°C).
   ■ Hyperoxia reduces infection.

8. **Van De Vijver MJ, He YD, van't Veer LJ, et al: A gene expression signature as a predictor of survival in breast cancer. N Engl J Med 347:1999–2009, 2002.**
   The authors postulate that 70 of our 35,000 genes dictate the character of breast cancer. So cancer, unlike cystic fibrosis and sickle cell disease, requires a constellation of genetic muta-tions—not just one. They followed 295 patients for 12 years and report that this "70 gene sig-nature" predicts survival better than the classical indicators of patient age, tumor size, tumor histology, pathologic grade, and hormone receptor status and even lymph node disease. The latter is the shocker. The authors observe that distant metastasis kills you, positive lymph nodes don't. In patients with either positive or negative lymph nodes, gene profile determines survival. Each cancer does not acquire an ability to metastasize as it grows, that capability is programmed into the very first neoplastic cell that establishes residence in your patient.

9. **Sandham JD, Hull RD, Brant RF, et al: A randomized controlled trial of the use of pul-monary artery catheters in high risk surgical patients. N Engl J Med 348:5–14, 2003.**
   This is a superb study in which 1994 surgical ICU patients were randomized to goal-directed therapy guided by a pulmonary artery catheter or standard care without a PA catheter. The patients were sick and, to be included for randomization, had to be over 60 years old, have estimated ASA class III or IV risk (major disease), and scheduled for elective or urgent sur-gery. Hospital mortality and survival at 6 and 12 months were essentially identical. Following years of impassioned debate, the utility of a PA catheter, even in sick surgical patients, can no longer be justified. Conversely, if, after you have given fluid and low-dose cardiotonic agents, your patient is not improving or still presents a confusing picture, place a PA catheter and get more information. When your patient improves, pull it out.

10. **Harken AH: Enough is enough. Arch Surg 134:1061–1063, 1999.**
    This article explores the surgeon's responsibility to assess surgical risk, to relate risk to anticipated physiologic and psychological benefit, and to develop common sense strategies to appreciate individual patient happiness. When benefits exceed anticipated operative risks—this is easy—proceed with surgery. When risks exceed benefits, this can be uncom-fortable, but sensitive recognition of this relatively common problem by the surgeon can limit extension of the patient's and family's grief, prevent the squandering of limited resources, and appropriately divert decision-making guilt from the family to the surgeon.

CHAPTER 2

CARDIOPULMONARY RESUSCITATION

Norman A. Paradis, M.D., and Alden H. Harken, M.D.

1. **Define sudden cardiac death.**

   Sudden ventricular fibrillation (VF) or pulseless electrical activity (PEA). Acute coronary ischemia and preexisting cardiac disease are the most common causes. VF is becoming less common.

2. **What is the predominant determinant of successful cardiopulmonary resuscitation (CPR)?**

   Time to restoration of spontaneous circulation, which itself is a function of the time to effective chest compression and time to defibrillation of VF. The chance of a good outcome decreases by 10% per minute. Successful outcomes are more likely if CPR is initiated promptly and if preexisting hypothermia is present.

3. **What are the ABCs?**

   Airway, **b**reathing, and **c**irculation. But things have changed. There are now three recognized phases of CPR: electrical, mechanical, and metabolic.

   1. The electrical phase lasts about 5 minutes—during that phase, only immediate electrical cardioversion may be required.
   2. The mechanical phase lasts 5 to 10 minutes after onset of arrest—during this phase, a few minutes of chest compression are required before cardioversion.
   3. The metabolic phase begins at 10 minutes postarrest. During this phase, pressor and antiarrhythmic drugs are required.

4. **How do you electrically cardiovert (shock) a patient?**

   Gel pads now are more common than hand-held paddles. If you are using paddles, place electrolyte (conductive) gel on them. Place one pad or paddle in the right subclavicular area and the other in the midaxillary line at the level of the eighth intercostal space (over the apex of the heart). If you are using a biphasic defibrillator, the fist shock should be only 100 J. With monophasic defibrillators, start at 200 J. If the patient remains in VF, rapidly increase the output to the maximum the machine allows. Take care to confirm that everyone (including you) is clear before delivering a shock.

5. **Is there an immediate need for an airway?**

   No. Defibrillation and chest compression should be initiated first. Waiting for intubation to be completed before initiation of these interventions is one of the most common mistakes in advanced life support. Children, in whom primary respiratory arrest is more common, are an exception. Restoration of ventilation in children often reveals that pulselessness was severe shock, not cardiac arrest.

6. **How do you establish an airway—even in a patient with suspected neck injury?**

   The three basic maneuvers are head tilt, chin tilt, and jaw thrust. In an unconscious patient, the jaw muscles relax. The jaw thrust subluxes the mandible, pulling the tongue and epiglottis anteriorly off the upper airway (with minimal cervical hyperextension).

7. **Is endotracheal intubation mandatory?**
   No.
   - Mouth-to-mouth ventilation delivers 16% inspired oxygen.
   - Bag-mask ventilation delivers 21% oxygen.
   - Bag-mask ventilation with an oxygen supply can deliver close to 100% oxygen.

8. **Name the advantages of endotracheal intubation.**
   A relatively secure airway. Mouth-to-mouth or bag-mask can deliver significant amounts of air to the stomach. Gastric distention impairs diaphragmatic movement and may predispose to aspiration.

9. **Does an endotracheal tube (even with the cuff up) prevent aspiration?**
   No. If you place a couple of drops of methylene blue on the tongue of an intubated patient, you can suction "blue" from the other end of the tube (beyond the cuff) within 90 seconds.

10. **Which size endotracheal tube should you use?**
    Select a tube with an internal diameter equal to the width of the patient's little finger. For a 70-kg adult, a 7.5-mm tube is fine. Do not delay ventilation trying to place a large endotracheal tube. Adequate ventilation can be achieved through smaller tubes.

11. **How do you know if the endotracheal tube is in the proper position?**
    1. Listen to both lung fields.
    2. Observe symmetric chest excursion with each tidal breath.
    3. Listen over the epigastrium (you don't want to hear gurgles from the stomach).
    These physical findings are not fully reliable, however. In patients with spontaneous circulation, it is now standard to confirm tube placement with end-tidal CO_2 (ET-CO_2) measurement. In cardiac arrest, even ET-CO_2 may be unreliable. You should confirm tube position as soon as possible by chest x-ray.

12. **Which is preferred—oral or nasal intubation?**
    Oral intubation. You can watch the tube pass directly through the vocal cords, ensuring proper placement. Nasal intubation is a blind technique, relatively contraindicated in patients with maxillofacial trauma (because of the risk of intracranial placement of the tube through an anterior fossa fracture) and in patients with known or suspected coagulopathy (because nasal mucosa is well vascularized, intubation may cause major epistaxis). Oral endotracheal intubation with "in-line" neck stabilization is preferred even in patients with suspected neck injury.

13. **What is the role of an esophageal obturator airway (EOA)?**
    None. At present, the EOA is not indicated because alternative techniques (mask or endotracheal tube) are safer and more effective.

14. **What should be your first consideration if you are unable to ventilate or intubate a patient?**
    Foreign body airway obstruction. Attempt to visualize the foreign body directly, and remove it with either suction or Magill forceps.

15. **Explain the proper method of external chest compression.**
    Place the patient on a firm surface—typically the floor or on a backboard. The rescuer should be positioned beside the patient's chest. Both hands are placed just above the xiphoid-sternal junction. Keep your arms straight and your shoulders directly over the patient's sternum. The compression depth should be 4–5 cm. Use the weight of your upper body to achieve adequate depth of compression. Perform 15 compressions followed by 2 ventilations at a rate of 100 compressions/minute.

16. **What are the essentials of external chest compressions?**
Even performed properly, external chest compression produces only a fraction of normal vital organ blood flow. Coronary blood flow occurs only during the release phase. Most providors do not use adequate force—make sure that the chest is compressed at least 2 inches in adults. Interruption in chest compression (to check the ECG rhythm or pulse) significantly reduces the efficacy of CPR.

17. **What are the complications of external chest compressions?**
Complications are common but not important. Rib and sternal fractures occur 80% of the time. Major cardiac or pericardial injuries (lacerations) are rare. Bone marrow and fat emboli are common (80% in one series). Do not let fear of complication interfere with effective chest compression.

18. **What are the indicators that effective CPR is being performed?**
Real-time indicators of vital organ perfusion are lacking. Effective CPR and pressor drugs should cause the VF waveform amplitude to increase—so called coarsening. Improved cerebral perfusion may result in gasping. During CPR, $ET-CO_2 > 15$ mmHg predicts return of spontaneous circulation. Switch chest compression providers if the $ET-CO_2$ begins to fall because this may indicate fatigue of the rescuer.

19. **Is the central line the best access to the circulation?**
Yes. Large volumes of fluid can be delivered to the venous system more quickly, however, via large-bore peripheral venous catheters. A 14G, 5-cm catheter (peripheral) can deliver twice the flow of a 16G, 20-cm catheter (central). Central line placement may be associated with significant complications, including pneumothorax, air embolus, and arterial puncture. In hypovolemic patients, in whom central veins are collapsed and peripheral veins are constricted, venous cannulation can be difficult.

20. **Does a central line offer therapeutic and diagnostic advantages?**
Yes. A central line permits bolus administration of drugs to the right side of the heart. Identification of a high central venous pressure may indicate the need to treat reversible causes of PEA, such as cardiac tamponade or tension pneumothorax.

21. **Is it necessary to monitor arterial blood gases during resuscitation?**
No. After you have an adequate airway and presumably are delivering 100% oxygen, you don't care what the arterial PO_2 is because you can do nothing about it. If possible, you may confirm the adequacy of oxygenation on the arterial side through an early arterial blood gas. Then you should focus on the adequacy of chest compression.

22. **Which is preferred—colloid or crystalloid resuscitation fluid?**
Colloid advocates claim that the big molecules remain in the intravascular space and are more effective in elevating blood volume. Crystalloid advocates state that capillaries leak albumin, especially in the shock state. Resuscitation with crystalloid is clearly safe. Given its availability, low cost, and safety, crystalloid (lactated Ringer's solution) is the choice for initial fluid resuscitation. When true cardiac arrest has occurred, however, volume is of little importance.

23. **In a patient exhibiting asystole, bradycardia, PEA, or fine fibrillation, what is your primary goal?**
Adequate vital organ perfusion, especially to the coronary arteries. Done properly, CPR may cause PEA to progress to stable hemodynamics or VF to become "coarse enough" for successful countershock.

24. **Summarize the reversible causes and treatment of PEA.**
    PEA is an orderly electrical rhythm in the absence of detectable arterial pulses. The potentially correctable situations that commonly cause electromechanical dissociation (EMD) are:
    1. Tension pneumothorax (diagnosis: hyperresonant chest, decreased breath sounds), treated by decompressing the pleural space on the side of the collapsed lung
    2. Pericardial tamponade (diagnosis: Beck's triad—distant heart sounds, distended neck veins/elevated central venous pressure, and hypotension), treated with pericardiocentesis
    3. Hypovolemia, treated with volume replacement
    4. Pulmonary embolism, treated with fibrinolysis
    5. Pump failure secondary to massive myocardial infarction, treated with fibrinolysis or mechanical assistance (intra-aortic balloon pump)
    6. Hyperkalemia, treated with calcium and bicarbonate

KEY POINTS: REVERSIBLE CAUSES OF PEA

1. Tension pneumothorax

2. Pericardial tamponade

3. Hypovolemia

4. Pulmonary embolism

5. Pump failure

6. Hyperkalemia

25. **Is clinical PEA always full cardiac arrest?**
    PEA is a heterogeneous entity with hemodynamics ranging from full cardiac arrest through normal blood pressure. Confirm true cardiac arrest as early as possible through echocardiography or placement of an arterial catheter.

26. **Name the most common cause of cardiac arrest in the perioperative period.**
    Although the incidence of VF is increased in the perioperative period, PEA secondary to potentially reversible insults is more common at this time.

27. **List the drugs commonly used during resuscitation and the appropriate dosages.**
    1. **Oxygen:** to reverse hypoxia, always provide 100% oxygen initially.
    2. **Epinephrine:** α- and β-adrenergic agonist. IV dose is 5–10 mL of 1:10,000 solution. Because of the short duration of action, a repeat dose may be necessary after 5 minutes. Epinephrine is inactivated by alkali; do not mix with bicarbonate solutions. Although it enhances myocardial performance, epinephrine greatly increases myocardial oxygen demand. Ventilate!
    3. **Vasopressin:** antidiuretic hormone—a new first-line pressor during cardiac arrest. Administer one time as a bolus of 40 U.
    4. **Amiodarone:** first-line, broad-spectrum antidysrhythmic possibly useful in treating VF/ventricular tachycardia (VT) cardiac arrest and atrial arrhythmias. It is active at cardiac sodium, potassium, and calcium channels and has a- and b-adrenergic blocking properties. In cardiac arrest, it is administered as a 300-mg rapid IV infusion. Amiodarone may cause hypotension and bradycardia; a pressor drug, such as epinephrine or dopamine, should be readily available or already administered.

5. **Atropine:** parasympatholytic (vagolytic) agent that increases the discharge rate of the sinus node. Atropine is useful in treating sinus bradycardia associated with hemodynamic compromise. An IV dose of 0.5 mg is repeated at 5-minute intervals until a desirable rate is achieved (at least 60 beats/min). Increased heart rate increases myocardial oxygen demand; atropine should be used only if the bradycardia causes hemodynamic compromise (heart rate , 60 beats/min).

6. **Dopamine:** catecholamine precursor of norepinephrine active at dopaminergic receptors. Stimulates the heart and vasoconstricts (high dose) the periphery. Use as a vasopressor to treat hypotension secondary to bradycardia or decreased peripheral vasomotor tone. Dosage should be adjusted based on clinical end points starting at 2–5 µg/kg/min up to 20 µg/kg/min. The principal toxicity, seen with prolonged dosages > 10 µg/kg/min, is splanchnic and systemic vasoconstriction with resultant injury.

7. **Dobutamine:** synthetic catecholamine that is a cardiac b-receptor agonist used to treat cardiogenic shock. It increases cardiac contractility. Reflex peripheral vasodilation may require combination with a pressor drug, such as dopamine. Dosage should be adjusted based on clinical end points starting at 5 µg/kg/min up to 20 µg/kg/min.

8. **Sodium bicarbonate (NaHCO$_3$):** no longer commonly used in cardiac arrest; in shock, it is used to reverse acidosis (hypoxia-induced anaerobic metabolism leads to acid accumulation). The initial dose is 1 mEq/kg. One ampule (50 mL) contains 50 mEq of sodium bicarbonate. Bicarbonate combines with hydrogen ions to form CO_2 and water; adequate ventilation is required for bicarbonate therapy to be fully effective. Overzealous use of bicarbonate may result in hypernatremia/hyperosmolality (each HCO_3^- is accompanied by a sodium ion).

9. **Magnesium:** effective in treating drug-induced torsades de pointes or VT. Administer 1–2 g IV over 3–5 minutes. May cause hypotension.

10. **Calcium chloride or gluconate:** positive inotropic agent. Calcium ions bind to troponin (the cardiomyocyte-specific calcium regulatory protein used to diagnose an acute myocardial infarction), which enhances the formation of cross-bridges between muscle contractile filaments with resultant fiber shortening. Dose is calcium chloride (or gluconate), 500 mg IV push. Do not mix with bicarbonate because it will precipitate.

11. **Lidocaine:** local anesthetic that suppresses ventricular arrhythmias (automatic and reentrant; see Chapter 3). An IV bolus of 1 mg/kg is followed by IV infusion at 2–4 mg/min. An additional IV bolus can be given at 10 minutes after initial dose if arrhythmias persist. Amiodarone is accepted as a preferred agent for treatment of arrhythmias.

12. **Adenosine:** a naturally occurring vasodilating hormone that is synthesized by vascular endothelial cells and dramatically slows artrioventricular (AV) nodal conduction. It is useful in the therapy of supraventricular tachyarrhythmias. Dose is 6 mg or 12 mg injected in a rapid IV bolus (which may be repeated several times). The half-life of IV adenosine is only 12 seconds. Measurable systemic hypotension occurs in < 2% of patients because adenosine is metabolized before it reaches the systemic vessels.

13. **Verapamil:** slow-channel calcium blocker used to block the AV node and to treat paroxysmal supraventricular tachycardia that causes hemodynamic compromise. Dose is 0.1 mg/kg. Dilute drug with 10 mL of saline, and infuse 1 mL/min until the supraventricular tachycardia either breaks or blocks. Repeat dose after 30 minutes if not effective. The drug reduces systemic vascular resistance and may cause hypotension.

28. **What measures should be considered postresuscitation to improve the chances of a good outcome?**
Laboratory and clinical data support use of mild hypothermia (34°C for 24 hours)in patients who remain comatose after resuscitation from cardiac arrest. Hypotension or causes of increased cerebral oxygen use (e.g., as seizures or fever) should be treated aggressively.

WEB SITES

1. http://www.emedicine.com/med/topic2963.htm

2. http://www.fpnotebook.com/CV16.htm

3. http://www.mc.vanderbilt.edu/resuscitation/docs/pea/pdf

BIBLIOGRAPHY

1. Kudenchuk PJ, Cobb LA, Copass MK, et al: Amiodarone for resuscitation after out-of-hospital cardiac arrest due to ventricular fibrillation. N Engl J Med 341:871–878, 1999.

2. Lindner KH, Dirks B, Strohmenger HU, et al: Randomised comparison of epinephrine and vasopressin in patients with out-of-hospital ventricular fibrillation. Lancet 349:535–537, 1997.

3. Mild therapeutic hypothermia to improve the neurologic outcome after cardiac arrest. N Engl J Med 346:549–556, 2002.

4. Paradis NA, et al (eds): Cardiac Arrest: The Science and Practice of Resuscitation Medicine. Baltimore, Williams & Wilkins, 1996.

5. Paradis NA, Martin GB, Rivers EP, et al: Coronary perfusion pressure and the return of spontaneous circulation in human cardiopulmonary resuscitation. JAMA 263:1106–1113, 1990.

6. Sanders AB, Kern KB, Otto CW, et al: End-tidal carbon dioxide monitoring during cardiopulmonary resuscitation: A prognostic indicator for survival. JAMA 262:1347–1351, 1989.

CHAPTER 3

EVALUATION AND TREATMENT OF CARDIAC DYSRHYTHMIAS

Alden H. Harken, M.D.

1. **Are cardiac dysrhythmias and cardiac arrhythmias the same?**
   Yes. Some purists will tell you that an arrhythmia can be only the absence of a cardiac rhythm. But these are the same purists who use the word iatrogenic to mean "caused by a physician," when, of course, the only thing that can truly be "iatrogenic" is a physician's parents.

2. **Are all cardiac dysrhythmias clinically important?**
   Most are not. Many of us have isolated premature ventricular contractions (PVCs) or premature ventricular depolarizations (PVDs) all the time. Superbly conditioned athletes frequently exhibit resting heart rates in the 30s. A clinically important cardiac dysrhythmia is a rhythm that bothers the patient. As a rule, if the patient's ventricular rate is 60–100 beats/min (regardless of mechanism), cardiac rhythm is not a problem.

3. **State the goals in the treatment of cardiac dysrhythmias.**
   Primary goal: to control ventricular rate between 60 and 100 beats/min
   Secondary goal: to maintain sinus rhythm

4. **How important is sinus rhythm?**
   It depends on the patient's ventricular function. Induction of atrial fibrillation in a medical student volunteer causes no measurable hemodynamic effect. Your ventricular compliance is so good that you do not need an atrial "kick" to fill the ventricle completely. Conversely, the worse (the stiffer) the patient's heart, the more you should try to maintain sinus rhythm. We observed a patient with a 7% left ventricular ejection fraction whose cardiac output decreased by 40% when he spontaneously developed atrial fibrillation.

5. **Do you need to be ankle-deep in ECG paper and personally acquainted with Drs. Mobitz, Lown, and Ganong to treat cardiac dysrhythmias in the intensive care unit (ICU)?**
   No.

6. **When you are called by the ICU nurse to see a patient with an "arrhythmia," what questions do you ask yourself?**
   1. *Does the patient really exhibit an arrhythmia?* What is the patient doing? Is the stuff that looks like ventricular fibrillation (VF) really just the patient brushing his teeth? Or is the rhythm strip that looks like asystole really just a loose lead? If the patient does exhibit an arrhythmia, ask yourself the following questions.
   2. *Does the arrhythmia require intervention?* Isolated PVCs usually can be ignored safely. Similarly a resting bradycardia in a triathlete is normal. This is the occasion to launch into your "2-second physical exam"—is the patient sweaty and confused or alert and happy?
   3. *What is a 2-second physical exam?* You look into the patient's eyes, hoping to determine whether he or she is perfusing his or her brain. If the patient looks back at you, you have some time. If the patient requires therapy, ask yourself the following questions.
   4. *How soon is therapy required?* At this point, the patient becomes (paradoxically) irrelevant. The most robust indicator dictating velocity of intervention is not how sick the patient is, but

how frightened you are. The dean may have had his carotid arteries firmly ligated years ago. Conversely, to match the surgical residency of your choice, you need to be firing on a lot more cylinders than the dean. You must determine rapidly whether delay in therapy is likely to put the patient at risk. If the cardiac arrhythmia is likely to inflict psychopathologic (hypoxemic) consequences not only on the patient but also, by extension, on his or her extended (societal) family, you should be frightened. If you are frightened, you must ask yourself:

5. *What is the safest and most effective therapy?*

7. **If the patient requires antiarrhythmic therapy, what is the safest and most effective strategy?**
   Therapy for cardiac arrhythmias is simple and comprises three comprehensible concepts:
   1. If the patient is hemodynamically unstable (the sole determinant of instability is whether you are frightened), cardiovert with 360 J. (For lower energy, see Chapter 2.)
   2. If the patient has a wide-complex tachycardia, cardiovert with 360 J.
   3. If the patient has a narrow-complex tachycardia, infuse an atrioventricular (AV) nodal blocker IV. If at any time the patient becomes unstable, proceed with cardioversion.

8. **In assessing a cardiac impulse, how do you distinguish supraventricular from ventricular origin?**
   Supraventricular origin: When an impulse originates above the AV node (supraventricular), it can access the ventricles only through the AV node. The AV node connects with the endocardial Purkinje system, which conducts impulses rapidly (2–3 m/sec). A supraventricular impulse activates the ventricles rapidly (< 0.08 sec, 80 msec, or two little boxes on the ECG paper), producing a narrow-complex beat.
   Ventricular origin: When an impulse originates directly from an ectopic site on the ventricle, it takes longer to access the high-speed Purkinje system. A ventricular impulse activates the entire ventricular mass slowly (< 0.08 sec, 80 msec, or two little boxes on the ECG paper), producing a wide-complex beat. (See Figure 3-1.)

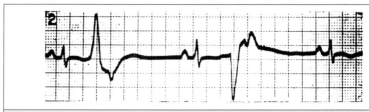

Figure 3-1. Wide complex beats are of ventricular origin. Narrow complex beats are of supraventricular origin.

9. **Extra credit: Correlate the ECG with cardiomyocyte membrane ion flux.**
   See Figure 3-2.

10. **Do all wide-complex beats derive from the ventricles?**
    No, but most do. An impulse of supraventricular origin that is conducted with aberrancy through the ventricle can take enough time to make it a wide-complex beat. In one study, 89% of 100 patients presenting to an emergency department with a wide-complex tachycardia eventually proved to exhibit ventricular tachycardia, whereas 11% were diagnosed with supraventricular tachycardia with aberrancy.

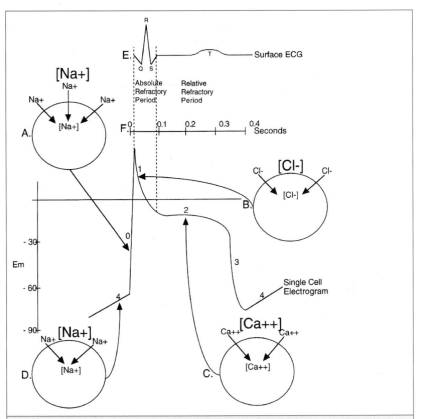

Figure 3-2. Typical action potential of a cardiac myocyte, the ionic shifts responsible for each phase, and correlation with the surface ECG. A, Phase 0 = rapid depolarization, characterized by rapid influx of sodium (Na^+) through the voltage-gated Na^+ channels. B, Phase 1 = brief repolarization, characterized by transient influx of chloride (Cl^-). C, Phase 2 = plateau phase, characterized by a rapid rise in calcium (Ca^{2+}) permeability through L-type Ca^{2+} channels. Phase 3 = repolarization with potassium (K^+) exiting the cell. D, Slow depolarization of pacemaker cells caused by slow influx of Na^+ (From Meldrum DR, Cleveland JC, Sheridan BC, et al: Cardiac surgical implications of calcium dyshomeostasis in the heart. Ann Thorac Surg 61:1273–1280, 1996, with permission.)

11. **What do you do if you cannot tell whether a ventricular complex is wide or narrow?**
    Acutely and transiently (for 5 seconds) block the AV node by giving 6 mg of adenosine IV; if the ventricular complex persists, it is ventricular. If the ventricular complex stops, it was supraventricular.

12. **To prevent lots of supraventricular impulses from getting to the ventricles, how do you block the AV node pharmacologically?**
    In **seconds:** give 6 mg adenosine IV push.
    In **minutes:** draw up 10 mg verapamil (calcium channel blocker) in 10 mL of saline and give 1 mL/min IV.
    In **hours:** put 0.5 mg digoxin in 100 mL of Ringer's lactate and infuse by IV drip over 30 minutes.

KEY POINTS: CHARACTERIZATION OF CARDIAC DYSRHYTHMIAS

1. Supraventricular origin: when an impulse originates above the AV node, it can access the ventricles only through the AV node to reach the Purkinje system, which conducts and activates the ventricles rapidly, producing a narrow-complex beat (< 2 small boxes on ECG).

2. Ventricular origin: when an impulse originates from an ectopic site on the ventricle, it takes longer to access the high-speed Purkinje system. A ventricular impulse activates the entire mass, slowly producing a wide-complex beat (> 2 small boxes on ECG).

3. Not all wide-complex beats are ventricular in origin.

4. To distinguish ventricular from supraventricular tachycardia, transiently block AV node with adenosine IVP. If ventricular complex persists, it is ventricular tachycardia; if the complex stops, it is supraventricular tachycardia.

13. **Why give digoxin?**
Digoxin is an effective AV nodal blocker, but it makes cardiomyocytes more excitable. By giving digoxin, you make supraventricular impulses more likely; but by blocking the AV node, you render these impulses less dangerous.

14. **Why infuse digoxin over 30–60 minutes IV?**
Studies indicate that a big pulse of digoxin (IV push) concentrates in the myocardium, making the myocytes hyperexcitable. Digoxin infused more slowly avoids this problem.

15. **List the steps in calling a dysrhythmia by name.**
Bradycardia: < 60 beats/min
Tachycardia: 100–250 beats/min
Flutter: atrial or ventricular rate 250–400 beats/min
Fibrillation: atrial or ventricular rate > 400 beats/min

WEB SITE

http://www.americanheart.org/presenter.jhtml?identifier=10000056#P

BIBLIOGRAPHY

Harken AH: Cardiac dysrhythmias. In Wilmore DW, Cheung L, Harken AH, et al (eds): Scientific American Surgery. New York, Scientific American, 1999.

CHAPTER 4

HOW TO THINK ABOUT SHOCK

Alden H. Harken, M.D.

1. **Define shock.**
   Shock is:
   - Not just low blood pressure
   - Not just decreased peripheral perfusion
   - Not just limited systemic oxygen delivery

   Ultimately, shock is decreased tissue respiration. Shock is suboptimal consumption of oxygen and excretion of CO_2 at the cellular level.

2. **Is shock related to cardiac output?**
   Yes. A healthy medical student can redistribute blood flow preferentially to vital organs. After a 3–4-U bleed, your typical young gunslinger can still think: "four dudes jumped me."

3. **Is organ perfusion democratic?**
   No. Limited blood flow always is redirected toward the carotid and coronary arteries. Peripheral vasoconstriction steals blood initially from the mesentery, then skeletal muscle, then kidneys and liver.

4. **Is this vascular autoregulatory capacity uniform in all patients?**
   No. With age and atherosclerosis, patients lose their ability to redistribute limited blood flow. A 20% decrease in cardiac output (or a fall in blood pressure to 90 mmHg) can be life-threatening to a Supreme Court justice, whereas it may be undetectable in a triathlete.

5. **For diagnostic and practical therapeutic purposes, can shock be classified?**
   Yes.
   1. **Hypovolemic shock** mandates volume resuscitation.
   2. **Cardiogenic shock** mandates cardiac stimulation (pharmacologic and eventually mechanical).
   3. **Peripheral vascular collapse shock** mandates pharmacologic manipulation of the peripheral vascular tone (and direct attention to the cause of the vasodilation—typically sepsis).

6. **Is it advisable to treat all shock in the same sequential fashion?**
   Ultimately, yes. Whether a cigar-chomping banker presents with a big gastrointestinal bleed (hypovolemic shock) or crushing substernal chest pain (cardiogenic shock), the surgeon should take, the following steps in order:
   1. **Optimize volume status;** give volume until further increase in right-sided (central venous pressure [CVP]) and left-sided (pulmonary capillary wedge pressure[PCWP]) preload confers no additional benefit for cardiac output or blood pressure. (This step is Starling's law—place the patient's heart at the top of the Starling curve.)
   2. If cardiac output, blood pressure, and tissue perfusion remain inadequate despite adequate preload, the patient has a pump (cardiogenic shock) problem. **Infuse cardiac inotropic drugs** (β-agonist) to the point of toxicity (typically cardiac ectopy)—lots of frightening premature ventricular contractions. For pharmacologically refractory cardiogenic shock, insert an intra-aortic balloon pump (IABP).

3. If the patient exhibits a surprisingly high cardiac output and a paradoxically low blood pressure (such unusual loss of vascular autoregulatory control is associated typically, but not always, with sepsis), **infuse a peripheral vasoconstrictor drug** (α-agonist).

7. **What is the preferred access route for volume infusion?**
Flow depends on catheter length and radius. Volume may be infused at twice the rate through a 5-cm, 14-gauge peripheral catheter as through a 20-cm, 16-gauge central line (see Chapter 2). Assessment of central venous pressure (and left-sided filling pressure) is necessary if the patient fails to respond to initial volume resuscitation.

8. **Should one infuse crystalloid, colloid, or blood?**
If the goal is only to improve preload and to repair cardiac output and blood pressure, crystalloid solution should be sufficient. It is controversial whether infused colloid remains in the vascular compartment. If the goal is to augment systemic oxygen delivery, red blood cells bind much more oxygen than plasma (see Chapter 6). Crystalloid should enhance flow, and blood should augment oxygen delivery.

9. **When cardiac preload is adequate, which inotropic agents are useful?**
Dobutamine, epinephrine, and norepinephrine are the chocolate, vanilla, and strawberry of the 32 flavors of cardiogenic drugs. These three drugs are all that the surgeon really needs.

10. **Is dopamine the same as dobutamine?**
No. Dopamine stimulates renal dopaminergic receptors and may be useful in low doses (2 mg/kg/min) to counteract the renal arteriolar vasoconstriction that accompanies shock. Dopamine has no place as a primary cardiac inotropic agent.

11. **Discuss the use of dobutamine, epinephrine, and norepinephrine.**
See Table 4-1.

12. **When is an IABP indicated?**
Mechanical circulatory support is indicated when the preload to both ventricles (CVP and PCWP) has been optimized and further cardiac stimulatory drugs are limited by frightening runs of premature ventricular contractions. Do not be afraid to resort to mechanical support.

KEY POINTS: SUMMARY OF ADRENERGIC AGENTS

1. Dobutamine: β_1 agonist (cardiac inotrope) with mild-to-moderate β_2 effects (peripheral vasodilation).

2. Epinephrine: combined β- and α-adrenergic agent, with the β effects predominating at lower doses and progressive vasoconstriction accompanying increased doses.

3. Norepinephrine: combined β- and α-adrenergic agonist, with the α effects predominating at all doses.

13. **What does an IABP do?**
Diastolic augmentation and systolic unloading.

TABLE 4-1. USE OF DOBUTAMINE, EPINEPHRINE, AND NOREPINEPHRINE

Dobutamine is a β_1-agonist (cardiac inotrope), but also has some β_2 effects (peripheral vasodilation).

Start at:	5 µg/kg/min and increase to point of toxicity (cardiac ectopy).
Note:	Infuse to desired effect (do not stick rigidly to a preconceived dose). Because dobutamine has some vasodilating effects, it may be frightening to infuse into typically hypotensive patients in shock.

Epinephrine is a combined β- and α-adrenergic agonist, with the β effects predominating at lower doses and progressive vasoconstriction accompanying increased doses.

Start at:	0.05 µg/kg/min and increase to point of toxicity (cardiac ectopy).
Note:	As with dobutamine, infuse to desired effect.

Norepinephrine is a combined α- and β-adrenergic agonist, with the α effects predominating at all doses.

Start at:	0.05 µg/kg/min and increase to point of toxicity (cardiac ectopy).
Note:	Relatively pure peripheral vasoconstriction rarely is indicated and should be used only to modulate the peripheral vascular tone in peripheral vascular collapse shock.

14. **What is diastolic augmentation?**

A soft 40-mL balloon is inserted percutaneously through the common femoral artery into the descending thoracic aorta. The balloon is not occlusive (it should not touch the aortic walls). When it is inflated, it displaces 40 mL of blood and is exactly like acutely transfusing 40 mL of blood into the aorta, augmenting each left ventricular stroke volume by 40 mL. Balloon infusion is triggered off the QRS complex from a surface ECG (any lead). The balloon always is inflated during diastole to increase diastolic blood pressure and augment coronary blood flow (CBF). Eighty percent of CBF occurs during diastole.

KEY POINTS: INTRA-AORTIC BALLOON PUMP

1. Indicated for cardiogenic shock refractory to pharmacologic manipulation.

2. Triggered by QRS complex of surface ECG; inflates during diastole (T wave) and deflates on systole (R wave or at dicrotic notch on aortic pressure curve).

3. 80% of coronary blood flow occurs during diastole.

4. Mechanistically results in diastolic augmentation and systolic unloading (afterload reduction).

15. **What is systolic unloading?**
Balloon deflation is an active (not a passive) process. Helium abruptly is sucked out of the balloon, leaving a 40-mL empty space in the aorta. The left ventricle can eject the first 40 mL of its stroke volume into this empty space—at dramatically reduced workload. An intra-aortic balloon increases coronary oxygen delivery (CBF) during diastole, while decreasing cardiac oxygen consumption just presystole.

16. **Name the contraindications to IABP.**
Aortic insufficiency: diastolic augmentation distends and injures the left ventricle.
Atrial fibrillation: balloon inflation and deflation cannot be appropriately timed.

WEB SITE

http://www.aic.cuhk.edu.hk/web8/IABP.htm

BIBLIOGRAPHY

1. Harken AH: Cardiac dysrhythmias. In Wilmore DW, Cheung L, Harken AH, et al (eds): Scientific American Surgery. New York, Scientific American, 1999.
2. Holcroft JW: Shock. In Wilmore DW, Cheung L, Harken AH, et al (eds): American College of Surgeons Surgery. New York, WebMD Corporation, 2002.

CHAPTER 5

WHAT IS PULMONARY INSUFFICIENCY?

Alden H. Harken, M.D.

1. **What is pulmonary insufficiency?**
   The alveolar-capillary surface of the lung is the size of a singles tennis court. The purpose of the lung is to match alveolar ventilation (Va) to blood flow (Q). Mismatching leads to pulmonary insufficiency.

2. **How is Va/Q mismatching characterized?**
   Shunt: decreased ventilation relative to regional blood flow; pulmonary arterial (unoxygenated) blood "shunts" by hypoventilated alveoli
   Dead space: decreased pulmonary regional blood flow relative to ventilation

3. **How much energy is expended in the work of breathing?**
   A healthy medical student expends about 3% of total oxygen consumption (energy use) on work of breathing. After injury, particularly a big burn, patients may increase fractional energy expenditure of breathing to 20% of their total energy use.

4. **Which surgical incisions most significantly compromise a patient's vital capacity?**
   Intuitively an extremity incision or injury influences vital capacity least, followed sequentially by a lower abdominal incision, median sternotomy, thoracotomy, and upper abdominal incision. An upper abdominal incision is worse than a thoracotomy!

5. **Is a chest radiograph helpful in assessing respiratory failure?**
   Yes but the radiograph must be interpreted carefully. It can be difficult to standardize x-ray technique, especially in an intensive care unit.

6. **What should you look for on the chest radiograph of a patient with impending respiratory failure?**
   1. Are both lungs fully expanded?
   2. Are there localized areas of infiltrate, atelectasis, or consolidation?
   3. Are there generalized areas of infiltrate, atelectasis, or consolidation?
   4. Are the endotracheal and other tubes in proper position?

7. **Why is the local versus generalized distinction important in assessing respiratory failure?**
   A local process may be produced by tumor or aspiration, and both are diagnosed and treated by bronchoscopy. Generalized multilobar infiltrates are more likely to represent a diffuse alveolar-capillary leak syndrome, such as adult respiratory distress syndrome (ARDS).

8. **What is ARDS?**
   A diffuse, multilobar capillary transudation of fluid into the pulmonary interstitium that dissociates the normal concordance of ventilation (Va) with lung perfusion (Q).

9. **What governs fluid flux across pulmonary capillaries into the interstitium of the lung?**
Starling initially described the balance between intravascular hydrostatic pressure (Pc), which tends to push fluid out of the capillaries, and colloid oncotic pressure (COP), which sucks fluid back in across the capillary endothelial barrier (K):

$$\text{Fluid flux} = 5\,K(Pc - COP)$$

10. **What causes ARDS?**
Anything that increases lung dysfunction by promoting wet lung:
   1. **Heart failure** backs up pulmonary intravascular Pc, forcing fluid into the pulmonary interstitium.
   2. **Malnutrition and liver failure** decrease plasma protein and COP. Fluid is not sucked back out of the lung (if the total protein and albumin are low).
   3. **Sepsis** may break down the capillary endothelial barrier (K), permitting water and protein to leak into the lung.

KEY POINTS: CLINICAL FEATURES OF ARDS

1. Severe hypoxemia refractory to increased inspired oxygen concentration

2. Diffuse pulmonary infiltrates

3. Low lung compliance

4. Large V/Q mismatch

11. **Explain high-pressure versus low-pressure ARDS.**
Purists appropriately note that lung congestion resulting from high intravascular hydrostatic pressure secondary to heart failure is really not primary respiratory distress syndrome. If the pulmonary capillary wedge pressure (PCWP) is > 18 mmHg, the diagnosis is high-pressure pulmonary edema (not ARDS). A patient with pure mitral stenosis may have (high-pressure) lung congestion, whereas a malnourished patient may develop (low-pressure) lung congestion; neither of these is, strictly speaking, ARDS, although patients with ARDS frequently have components of both.

12. **What is a normal COP?**
22 mmHg.

13. **How is COP calculated?**
Of COP, 75% normally is created by serum albumin along with globulins and fibrinogen:

$$COP = 2.1\ (\text{total protein})$$

If an osmotically active molecule such as hetastarch is infused, this calculation is fouled up.

14. **Define low-pressure ARDS.**
Low-pressure ARDS is a redundant term. To make the diagnosis of ARDS, the PCWP must be <18 mmHg. Pure ARDS exists only if the PCWP is > 4 mmHg less than the COP.

15. **How can the pulmonary capillaries leak if the COP exceeds the PCWP?**
The current concept involves a septic expression of neutrophil CD11 and CD18 adhesion receptors, which stick to pulmonary vascular endothelial intercellular adhesion molecules. Septic

stimuli provoke the adherent neutrophils to release intravascular proteases and oxygen radicals. Resultant endovascular damage breaks down the capillary endothelial barrier, permitting the lung leak—even at low hydrostatic pressure.

16. **What is a Lasix sandwich?**
Many surgeons, when their backs are against the wall, give 25 g of albumin followed in 20 minutes by 20 mg of furosemide (Lasix) IV. They reason that the albumin pulls fluid out of the water-logged lung and the Lasix promotes diuresis to rid the patient of extra water. This therapeutic concept probably works only in patients who are not very sick. The sicker the patient, the faster the infused albumin leaks and equilibrates across the damaged endovascular endothelial barrier. Little water is sucked out of the sick lung in preparation for diuresis.

17. **List the goals of therapy for ARDS.**
    1. Reduce lung edema (typically with a diuretic).
    2. Reduce oxygen toxicity (inspired oxygen concentration < 60% is safe).
    3. Limit lung barotrauma (avoid peak inspiratory pressure in > 40 cm H_2O).
    4. Promote matching of Va and Q; frequently positive end-expiratory pressure (PEEP) is useful.
    5. Maintain systemic oxygen delivery (arterial oxygen content x cardiac output).

18. **What governs the distribution of lung perfusion (Q)?**
Mostly gravity. The dependent portions of the lung always are better perfused.

19. **Discuss hypoxic pulmonary vasoconstriction (HPV).**
Most students believe that after dedicating the entire second year of medical school to pheochromocytoma and HPV, both entities may be safely forgotten. At least in the case of HPV, this is not true. A patient who has just undergone carotid endarterectomy illustrates the relevance of HPV. As the patient awakens from anesthesia, the blood pressure is 220/120 mmHg and arterial PO_2 with 100% oxygen is 500 mmHg. So that the patient will not blow the carotid anastomosis, the surgeon urgently infuses nitroprusside. In 20 minutes, the blood pressure is 120/80 mmHg, but PO_2 (still with 100% oxygen) has dropped to 125 mmHg!
    Did the lab technician screw up the blood gas analysis? No—this is an example of the clinical significance of HPV, which directs pulmonary arteriolar delivery of deoxygenated blood toward ventilated alveoli and away from poorly ventilated lung regions. The patient was using HPV to attain a PO_2 of 500 mmHg. All antihypertensive agents (e.g., nitroprusside) and most general anesthetics block HPV. The PO_2 increment from 125 to 500 mmHg is due to HPV. HPV steered perfusion toward ventilated areas of the lung.

20. **What governs the distribution of ventilation in lung?**
A large pleural pressure gradient (more negative at the top of the lung by 20 cm H_2O) squeezes gas primarily out of the dependent lung during each exhaled breath. The regional compliance of dependent lung is much better than that of lung apex, which still is distended

KEY POINTS: THERAPEUTIC GOALS IN ARDS

1. Reduce lung edema

2. Reduce oxygen toxicity (FiO_2 < 60%)

3. Minimize barotraumas (keep peak inspiratory pressure < 40 cm H_2O)

4. PEEP to promote V/Q matching

5. Maintain systemic oxygen delivery (arterial oxygen content x cardiac output)

with gas at the end of exhalation. The usual approach is to perfuse and ventilate dependent lung preferentially.

21. **How does ARDS compromise lung function?**
The trachea is held open with cartilaginous rings, but terminal bronchioles are not. Wet lung collapses the terminal bronchioles, trapping distal alveolar gas. Persistent perfusion of these poorly ventilated regions is a shunt that results in hypoxia.

22. **How long does it take for pulmonary arterial (deoxygenated) blood to equilibrate completely with trapped (poorly oxygenated) alveolar gas?**
About three fourths of a second. After that, no more oxygen is added, and no more CO_2 is eliminated from the perfusing blood. Terminal bronchiolar closure producing trapped alveolar gas is bad.

23. **What is the therapy for terminal airways closure and resultant shunt secondary to the wet lung of ARDS?**
PEEP should hold open terminal bronchioles, promoting ventilation of previously trapped alveoli and minimizing the shunt.

24. **When may the patient come off mechanical ventilation and be extubated safely?**
The patient should be sufficiently alert to protect his or her airway, require an inspired oxygen concentration no greater than $FiO_2 = 0.4$, and be comfortable breathing on a T-piece (without mechanical ventilation) for 60 minutes at a respiratory rate < 20 and a minute ventilation < 10 L/min. The patient should be able to generate a negative inspiratory force > −20 cm H_2O. Finally, after 1 hour on the T-piece, oxygenation should provide a hemoglobin saturation > 85% without respiratory acidosis (see Chapter 6).

25. **What is nitric oxide (NO)?**
NO is synthesized in vascular endothelial cells by constitutive nitric oxide synthase (cNOS) and inducible NOS (iNOS). Intuitively, inhaled NO should diffuse across ventilated alveoli to increase regional perfusion and improve matching of Va/Q.

26. **Does inhaled NO work in ARDS?**
Almost 24 randomized controlled clinical trials have assessed the therapeutic efficacy of inhaled NO. Although systemic oxygenation and pulmonary hypertension improve transiently, ventilator time and ultimate survival are not influenced. Just say NO.

WEB SITES

1. http://www.ardsnet.org

2. http://www.nlm.nih.gov/medlineplus/ency/article/000103.htm

BIBLIOGRAPHY

1. Bartlett R: Pulmonary Insufficiency. New York, American College of Surgeons, Surgery WebMd Corporation, 2002.

2. Davidson TA, Caldwell ES, Curtis JR, et al: Reduced quality of life in survivors of acute respiratory distress syndrome compared with critically ill control patients. JAMA 281:354–360, 1999.

3. Gust R, McCarthy TJ, Kozlowski J, et al: Response to inhaled nitric oxide in acute lung injury depends on distribution of pulmonary blood flow prior to its administration. Am J Respir Crit Care Med 159:563–570, 1999.
4. Pesenti A, Fumagalli R: PEEP: Blood gas cosmetics or a therapy for ARDS? Crit Care Med 27:253–254, 1999.

CHAPTER 6

WHY GET ARTERIAL BLOOD GASES?

Alden H. Harken, M.D.

1. **Is breathing really overrated?**
   It may be. A Japanese yoga master survived just fine breathing once per minute for an hour (see reference 1)!

2. **Mr. O'Flaherty has just undergone an inguinal herniorrhaphy under local anesthesia. The recovery room nurse asks permission to sedate him. She says that he is confused and unruly and keeps trying to get out of bed. Is it safe to sedate Mr. O'Flaherty?**
   No. A confused, agitated patient in the recovery room or surgical intensive care unit (SICU) must be recognized as acutely hypoxemic until proved otherwise.

3. **Mr. O'Flaherty is moved to the SICU, and at 2:00 A.M. the SICU nurse calls to report that he has a Po_2 of 148 mmHg on facemask oxygen. Is it okay to roll over and go back to sleep?**
   No. More information is needed.

4. **You glance at the abandoned cup of coffee sitting on your well-worn copy of *Surgical Secrets*. What is the Po_2 of that cup of coffee?**
   148 mmHg.

5. **How can Mr. O'Flaherty and the coffee have the same Po_2?**
   The abandoned coffee presumably has had time to equilibrate completely with atmospheric gas. At sea level, the barometric pressure is 760 mmHg. To obtain the partial pressure of oxygen in the coffee, subtract water vapor pressure (47 mmHg) and multiply by the concentration of oxygen (20.8%) in the atmosphere:

$$Po_2 = (760 - 47) \times 20.8\% = 148 \text{ mmHg}$$

6. **What is the difference between Mr. O'Flaherty's and the coffee's Po_2?**
   Nothing. Both represent the partial pressure of oxygen in fluid. A complete set of blood gases is necessary.

7. **What constitutes a complete set of blood gases?**
   Po_2
   Pco_2
   pH
   Hemoglobin saturation
   Hemoglobin concentration

8. **If Mr. O'Flaherty and the coffee have the same Po_2, how would Mr. O'Flaherty do if he were exchange-transfused with coffee?**
   Badly.

9. **Why?**
   Although the oxygen tensions are the same, the **amount** of oxygen in blood is vastly greater.

10. **How does one quantitate the amount of oxygen in blood?**
    Arterial oxygen content (CaO_2) is quantitated as mL of oxygen/100 mL of blood. (*Watch out:* Almost all other concentrations traditionally are provided per mL or per L—*not* per 100 mL.) Because mL of oxygen is a volume in 100 mL of blood, these units frequently are abbreviated as vol %.

11. **Why is blood thicker than coffee (or wine)?**
    Because hemoglobin binds a huge amount of oxygen. A total of 10 g of fully saturated hemoglobin (hematocrit about 30%) binds 13.4 mL of oxygen, whereas 100 mL of plasma at a Po_2 of 100 mmHg contains only 0.3 mL of oxygen.

12. **Does the position of the oxyhemoglobin dissociation curve make any difference?**
    - An increase in Pco_2
    - An increase in hydrogen ion concentrations **(not pH)**
    - An increase in temperature
    All shift the oxyhemoglobin curve to the right; that is, oxygen is released more easily in the tissues. Within physiologic limits, however, Mae West probably said it best: "There is less to this than meets the eye."

KEY POINTS: MEDIATORS OF OXYHEMOGLOBIN DISSOCIATION CURVE

Right Shift	Left Shift
1. Increase in Pco_2	1. Decrease in [H^+], higher pH
2. Increase in [H^+], lower pH	2. Higher altitudes/elevation
3. Increase in temperature stored	3. Decrease in 2,3-DPG (e.g., at 4 wk blood maintains *no* DPG)
4. Increase in 2,3-DPG	

---

13. **If Cao_2 or ultimately systemic oxygen delivery (cardiac output x Cao_2) is what the surgeon really wants to know, why does the nurse report Mr. O'Flaherty's Po_2 instead of his Cao_2 at 2:00 A.M.?**
    No one knows.

14. **What is the fastest and most practical method of increasing Mr. O'Flaherty's Cao_2?**
    Transfusion of red blood cells. The patient's Cao_2 is increased by 25% with transfusion from a hemoglobin concentration of 8 to 10 g/dL. The patient's arterial oxygen content is affected negligibly by an increase in arterial Po_2 from 100 to 200 mmHg (hemoglobin is fully saturated in both instances).

15. **What is a transfusion trigger?**
    The hematocrit at which a patient is automatically transfused. This is **not** a useful concept. The NIH Consensus Conference, drawing data from Jehovah's Witnesses, patients with renal failure, and monkeys concluded that it is not necessary to transfuse a patient until the hematocrit is

21%. Traditional surgical dogma mandates a hematocrit >30%. When the patient is in trouble, however, authorities in surgical critical care encourage transfusion to a hematocrit of 45% to optimize systemic oxygen delivery.

16. **What governs respiratory drive?**
Pco_2 and pH are inextricably intertwined by the Henderson-Hasselbalch equation. By juggling this equation in the cerebrospinal fluid (CSF) of goats, it is clear that CSF hydrogen ion concentration (not Pco_2) controls respiratory drive. This distinction is not clinically important, however. What is important is that if a person becomes acidotic either with diabetic ketoacidosis or by running up a flight of stairs, minute ventilation (V_E) is increased.

17. **How tight is respiratory control? Or, if you hold your breath for 1 minute, how much do you want to breathe?**
A lot (unless you are a yoga master approaching nirvana).

18. **After 60 seconds of apnea, what happens to $Paco_2$?**
It increases only from 40 to 47 mmHg. Tiny changes in Pco_2 (and pH) translate into a huge respiratory stimulus. Normally, respiratory compensation for metabolic acidosis is tight.

19. **Define base excess.**
Base excess is a poor man's indicator of the metabolic component of acid-base disorders. After correcting the Pco_2 to 40 mmHg, the base excess or base deficit is touted as an indirect measure of serum lactate. Although many parameters directing volume resuscitation in shock are more practical and direct (see Chapter 3), base deficit has been advertised as helpful. The base excess or deficit is calculated from the Sigaard-Anderson nomogram in the blood gas laboratory. Normally; there is no base excess or deficit. Acid-base status is "just right."

BIBLIOGRAPHY

1. Dekerle J, Baron B, Dupont L, et al: Maximal lactate steady state, respiratory compensation threshold, and critical power. Eur J Appl Physiol 89:280–288, 2003.
2. Miyamura M, Nishimura K, Ishida K, et al: Is a man able to breathe once a minute for an hour? The effect of yoga exercises on blood gases. Jpn J Physiol 52:313, 2002.
3. Tada T, Hashimoto F, Matsushita Y, et al: Study of life satisfaction and quality of life of patients receiving home oxygen therapy. J Med Invest 50:55–63, 2003.

CHAPTER 7

FLUIDS, ELECTROLYTES, GATORADE, AND SWEAT

Alden H. Harken, M.D.

1. **What is hypertonic saline?**
   Normal saline is 0.9% sodium chloride. Hypertonic saline is 7.5% sodium chloride (eight times as concentrated as normal saline).

KEY POINTS: ION CONCENTRATIONS IN CRYSTALLOID SOLUTIONS

1. ½ NS or 0.45% NaCl: 77 mEq of Na^+, 77 mEq of Cl^-

2. NS or 0.9% NaCl: 154 mEq of Na^+, 154 mEq of Cl^-

3. Hypertonic NS or 7.5% NaCl: 1283 mEq of Na^+, 1283 mEq of Cl^-

4. Lactated Ringer's: 130 mEq of Na^+, 110 mEq of Cl^-, 38 mEq of lactate, 4 mEq of K^+, and 3 mEq Ca^+

2. **What is hypertonic saline good for?**
   Resuscitation. The initial hypothesis was that a little hypertonic saline would pull extravascular water into the intravascular compartment, rapidly restoring volume. It now appears that an osmotic jolt (even a transient jump from 140 to 180 mOsm) would pacify circulating neutrophils so that they do not stick to the endovasculature and provoke posttraumatic inflammation.

3. **Is hypertonic saline good for anything else?**
   Pacification of "primed" neutrophils should decrease the risk of posttraumatic multiple organ failure.

4. **How do you convert 1 g of sodium into milliequivalents (mEq)?**
   Divide by the atomic weight of sodium:

   $$1g \ (1000 \ mg) \ of \ sodium \div 23 = 43.5 \ mEq$$

5. **How many mEq of sodium are in 1 teaspoon of salt?**
   104 mEq (or 2400 mg).

6. **How many mEq of sodium are in an 8-oz bottle of Gatorade?**
   5 mEq.

7. **How much does a 40-lb block of salt cost?**
   $3.40 at the feed store.

8. **What is the electrolyte content of IV fluids?**
   See Table 7-1.

TABLE 7-1. ELECTROLYTE CONTENT OF INTRAVENOUS FLUIDS

Solution (mEq/L)	Sodium	Potassium	Chloride	Bicarbonate/ Lactate
Normal saline (0.9% NaCl)	154	—	154	—
Ringer's lactate solution	130	4	109	28*
5% dextrose/ ½ normal saline	77	—	77	—

*Lactate is converted immediately to bicarbonate.

9. How do these concentrations relate to body fluid and electrolyte compartments?
   See Table 7-2.

TABLE 7-2. ELECTROLYTE CONCENTRATIONS IN BODY FLUIDS

Compartment (mEq/L)	Sodium	Potassium	Chloride	Bicarbonate/ Lactate
Plasma	142	4	103	27
Interstitial fluid	144	4	114	30
Intracellular fluid	10	150		10

10. What are the daily volumes (mL/24 h) and electrolyte contents (mEq/L) of body secretions for a 70-kg medical student?
    See Table 7-3.

TABLE 7-3. DAILY VOLUMES AND ELECTROLYTE CONTENTS OF BODY SECRETIONS

	mL/24 h	Sodium	Potassium	Chloride	Bicarbonate
Saliva	+1500	10	25	10	30
Stomach	+1500	50	10	130	—
Duodenum	+1000	140	5	80	—
Ileum	+3000	140	5	104	30
Colon	−6000	60	30	40	—
Pancreas	+500	140	5	75	100
Biliary	+500	140	5	100	30
Sweat*	+1000	50	—	—	—
Gatorade		21	—	21	—

*See question 6.

11. **Are sweat glands responsive to aldosterone? Can they be trained?**
Yes and yes. Archie Bunker's sweat contains 100 mEq/L sodium, whereas an Olympic marathon runner retains sodium (sweat sodium may be as low as 25 mEq/L).

12. **Is Gatorade really just flavored athlete's sweat?**
Yes.

13. **What are the daily maintenance fluid and electrolyte requirements for a 70-kg medical student?**

Total fluid volume	2500 mL
Sodium	70 mEq (1 mEq/kg)
Potassium	35 mEq (0.5 mEq/kg)

14. **Does the routine postoperative patient require IV sodium or potassium supplementation? Routine serum electrolyte testing?**
No and no.

15. **Can a patient with a good heart and kidneys overcome all but the most woefully incompetent fluid and electrolyte management?**
Yes.

16. **Can one throw a healthy medical student into congestive heart failure by IV infusion of 100 mL of 5% dextrose in saline solution per kg per hour?**
No. One will simply be ankle-deep in urine.

17. **What is subtraction alkalosis?**
Vigorous nasogastric suction of a patient with a lot of gastric acid eliminates hydrochloric acid, leaving the patient alkalotic.

18. **Which electrolyte is most useful in repairing a hypokalemic metabolic alkalosis?**
Chloride.

19. **List the best indicators of a patient's volume status.**
Heart rate
Blood pressure
Urine output
Big-toe temperature

20. **Does a warm big toe indicate a hemodynamically stable patient?**
Most likely. The vascular autoregulatory ability of a young healthy patient is huge. The carotid and coronary circulations are maintained until the bitter end. Conversely, if the patient's big toe is warm and perfused, the patient is stable.

21. **What is the minimal adequate postoperative urine output?**
0.5 mL/kg/h.

22. **What is a typical postoperative urine sodium?**
< 20 mEq/L.

23. **Why?**
Surgical stress prompts mineralocorticoid (aldosterone) secretion so that the normal kidney retains sodium.

24. **Explain paradoxical aciduria.**

Postoperative patients, by virtue of nasogastric suction (loss of gastric acid), blood transfusions (the citrate in blood is converted to bicarbonate), and hyperventilation (decreased Pco_2), are typically alkalotic. Patients also are stressed, and their kidneys retain sodium and water. The renal tubules must exchange some other cations for the retained sodium. The kidney chooses to exchange potassium and hydrogen ions. Even in the face of systemic alkalosis, the postoperative kidney absorbs sodium and excretes hydrogen ions, producing a paradoxical aciduria.

KEY POINTS: MECHANISMS OF PARADOXICAL ACIDURIA

1. Nasogastric suction or refractory vomiting results in loss of gastric acid.

2. Physiologic stress promotes renal retention of sodium and water.

3. To hold on to sodium, the kidney must release other cations (potassium and hydrogen).

4. Counterintuitively, the kidney will release hydrogen ions to keep sodium, resulting in acidic urine.

25. **What is third spacing?**

Hypotension and infection prime neutrophils (CD11 and CD18 receptor complexes), promoting adherence to vascular endothelial cells. Subsequent activation of adherent neutrophils spews out proteases and toxic superoxide radicals, blowing big holes in the vascular lining. Water and plasma albumin leak through the holes. The volume pulled out of the vascular space into the third space of the interstitial and hollow viscus (gut) creates relative hypovolemia and requires additional fluid replacement.

26. **What is a Lasix sandwich?**

25% albumin followed by 20 mg of furosemide (Lasix) IV. If the patient is edematous, the IV albumin theoretically sucks water osmotically out of the interstitial third space. As the excessive water enters the vascular compartment, Lasix produces a healthy diuresis. In most intensive care unit patients, however, the infused albumin rapidly equilibrates across the damaged vascular endothelium. No additional water is pulled into the blood volume. Although surgeons often order Lasix sandwiches, they probably work only in healthy patients who do not need them.

BIBLIOGRAPHY

1. Brown MD: Evidence-based emergency medicine: Hypertonic versus isotonic crystalloid for fluid resuscitation in critically ill patients. Ann Emerg Med 40:113–114, 2002.

2. Bunn F, Roberts I, Tasker R, Akpa E: Hypertonic versus isotonic crystalloid for fluid resuscitation in critically ill patients. Cochrane Database Syst Rev (1):CD002045, 2002.

3. Greaves I, Porter KM, Revell MP: Fluid resuscitation in pre-hospital trauma care: A consensus view. J R Coll Surg Edinb 47:451–457, 2002.

4. Traber DL: Fluid resuscitation after hypovolemia. Crit Care Med 30:1922, 2002.

CHAPTER 8

NUTRITIONAL ASSESSMENT AND ENTERAL NUTRITION

Margaret M. McQuiggan, M.S., R.D., CNSD, and Frederick A. Moore, M.D.

NUTRITIONAL ASSESSMENT

1. **What does a nutritional assessment include?**
   1. The **medical and surgical history** is used to establish preexisting (comorbid) conditions, metabolic stress, and alterations in organ function.
   2. The **physical examination** focuses on the muscle mass, adipose stores, skin integrity, and hydrational state.
   3. **Laboratory data** include the chemistry profile (Na, K, CO_2, Cl, BUN, creatinine, glucose), ionized Ca, serum PO_4, and Mg, complete blood count (CBC) with differential, arterial blood gases (ABGs; to assess acid-base status and CO_2 retention), albumin, transferrin, prealbumin, and urinary nitrogen.
   4. The **drug profile** can reveal agents that affect the metabolism of nutrients (insulin, levothyroxine, corticosteroids) or alter energy expenditure (beta-blockers, Diprivan).
   5. **Anthropometric data** include height and weight; skinfold testing with calipers is only useful once edema has resolved but is rarely used in the acute care setting. Although information on adipose reserve, body cell mass, intra- and extracellular water, and third space fluid may be elucidated, standards for **bioelectrical impedance analysis (BIA)** have yet to be determined.
   6. A **nutrition history** reveals preexisting nutritional practices.
   7. The **social history** explores economic data or substance abuse behaviors and may predict the likelihood of adequate home care for the patient upon discharge.

2. **What are primary and secondary malnutrition?**
   Primary malnutrition is the consumption of inadequate kilocalories, protein, vitamins, or minerals. It may occur because of poor food choices, anorexia, poverty, alcoholism, suboptimal support regimens, or after bariatric surgery. Secondary malnutrition may occur even when adequate food is infused or consumed. It results from organ dysfunction (hypoalbuminemia with cirrhosis), malabsorption (Crohn's disease), immobility (muscle wasting), drug therapy (insulin resistance with corticosteroids), or the inflammatory response (reprioritization of hepatic synthesis of acute phase instead of constitutive proteins).

3. **What is the significance of serum proteins in nutritional assessment?**
   The most readily available proteins for nutritional assessment are albumin, transferrin, and prealbumin, which are all constitutively produced in the liver. Their half-lives are 20–21 days, 10–12 days, and 2–4 days, respectively. The level of all three plummets shortly after injury or surgery as the liver reprioritizes the production of acute phase proteins. Then, as inflammation, infection, and stress begin to resolve, the liver resumes production of constitutive proteins. Adequate kilocalories and protein facilitate this process. Because of their shorter half-lives, prealbumin and transferrin are most useful in the intensive care unit (ICU) setting and should be limited to patients with creatinine clearance > 50 mL/min. Levels of both proteins may be depleted in patients with hepatic failure or cirrhosis because of decreased synthetic function. Prealbumin travels in the circulation bound to retinol-binding protein (RBP) and vitamin A. Levels of prealbumin may be elevated in renal failure despite nutritional

TABLE 8-1.   SERUM PROTEINS

Protein	Synthetic Site	Clinical Significance	Half-life	Limitations	Interpretation
Albumin	Liver	Relates to outcomes; relates to edema	20–21 days	Best-case scenario for hepatic production: 12–25 g/24 h; dilutional effects; long half-life; used alone, sensitivity poor	Normal < 3.5 g/dL Mild depletion 2.8–3.5 g/dL Moderate 2.2–2.8 g/dL Severe < 2.2 g/dL
Prealbumin	Liver	Indicates nutritional deficits before albumin	2–4 days	Short half-life	Normal > 18 mg/dL Mild depletion 10–18 mg/dL Moderate 5–10 mg/dL Severe < 5 mg/dL
Transferrin	Liver	More sensitive than albumin; relatively useful parameter in liver disease compared with albumin; can calculate from TIBC	8–10 days	Poor marker of early repletion; sensitive to changes in body iron	Mild depletion 150–200 mg/dL Moderate 100–150 mg/dL Severe < 100 mg/dL
C-reactive protein	Liver	Increases abruptly after injury; earlier and reliable indicator of disease or injury severity	48–72 hr	—	Baseline normal < 3 mg/dL Bacterial infection 30–35 mg/dL Viral infection < 20 mg/dL Posttrauma ≤ 20–35 mg/dL

TIBC = total iron-binding capacity.

KEY POINTS: HALF-LIVES OF SERUM PROTEINS USED AS NUTRITIONAL MARKERS

1. Pre-albumin: 2–4 days
2. Transferrin: 8–10 days
3. Albumin: 20–21 days

compromise, because of decreased catabolism and decreased excretion of RBP. Transferrin is elevated with iron depletion, independent of the effects of nutrition. (See Table 8-1.)

4. **What is the significance of urinary nitrogen in nutritional assessment?**
Total urinary nitrogen (TUN) is the most reliable indicator of nitrogen utilization and excretion in surgical ICU patients. However, urinary urea nitrogen (UUN) is more readily available in most hospital laboratories. Although TUN and UUN are nearly equal in healthy ambulatory patients, critically ill patients exhibit a poor correlation between the two. Optimal nutrition support should place a patient in 13 to 15 nitrogen balance. One may estimate the protein needs of the patient by adding:

$$[24 \text{ h UUN (g)} + 2 \text{ g N insensible losses} + 3] \times 6.25 = \text{required amount of protein (g)}$$

The total in brackets is multiplied by 6.25 to convert nitrogen grams to protein grams. Thus, if the laboratory reported a 13-g UUN/24 hours and a 2-g N insensible loss (skin, hair, feces) + 3 g for optimal anabolism, the patient would require 18 g N × 6.25 = 112.5 g of protein for anabolism. Urinary nitrogen is not useful as a guide for nutritional prescription in hepatic failure, renal dysfunction (< 50 mL/min creatinine clearance), or recent spinal cord injury.

5. **How are protein requirements determined?**
Protein need is determined based on the weight of the patient, current stress factors, extraordinary skin losses, and organ function. Although the recommended daily allowance (RDA) for protein for healthy individuals is only 0.8 g protein/ kg body weight, the following guidelines may be used in surgical patients. (See Table 8-2.)

TABLE 8-2. PROTEIN REQUIREMENTS IN RELATION TO INJURY LEVEL	
Injury Level	Protein Requirement
Mild stress or injury	1.2–1.4 g/kg
Moderate stress or injury	1.5–1.7 g/kg
Severe stress or injury	1.8–2.5 g/kg

6. **Should protein be severely restricted in surgical patients with hepatic failure or renal failure?**
Protein should be restricted to 0.7 g/kg in patients with encephalopathy, only if the hepatic encephalopathy produces significant clinical consequences. Only 10% of chronic liver disease patients are protein sensitive; thus, other causes of encephalopathy such as infection, constipation, and electrolyte disturbance should be explored. Otherwise, a more typical postsurgical protein load may be adopted (1.4 g/kg). In injured patients with **renal failure**, one must balance the need for increased protein with the need for increased dialysis. One should provide the amount of protein required and dialyze more frequently.

7. **How are kilocalorie needs determined?**

   There are several methods for setting kilocalorie targets in the surgical patient: standard prediction equations, kilocalorie per kilogram estimations, and indirect calorimetry. One common **prediction equation**, the Harris Benedict (HBE), was developed in 1919 for use on ambulatory, fasted, healthy people. Basal energy expenditure (BEE), the number of kilocalories required at rest daily, is calculated using the following equations:

Female	BEE = 655 + 9.6 (kg) + 1.8 (cm) − 4.7 (age)
Male	BEE = 67 + 14 (kg) + 5 (cm) − 6.7 (age)

   Subsequently, the above sums are multiplied by stress factors to determine total kilocalorie goals. (See Table 8-3).

   Many clinicians use a total **kcal/kg goal** as shown in Table 8-4.

TABLE 8-3. KCAL NEEDS IN RELATION TO STRESS LEVELS

Stress Level	Example	Kcal Needs
Mild	Closed fracture, pneumonia, or splenic laceration	BEE × 1.2
Moderate	Bowel resection, hepatorrhaphy, or thoracotomy	BEE × 1.4
Severe	Major bowel perforation with resection, major open wounds, intraabdominal abscess	BEE × 1.6

TABLE 8-4. KCAL/KG GOALS

Patient	Feeding Level (kcal/kg)	Level by Indirect Calorimetry
Normal weight patients	25–30	REE[†] × 1.0
Underweight patients	35–40	REE × 1.2
Obese patients	20–25*	REE × 0.85
Morbidly obese	10–20*	REE × 0.75

*Use adjusted weight.
[†]Resting energy expenditure (REE) is the measure of energy expenditure in a fed state and is generally 10% higher than BEE.

8. **What is indirect calorimetry?**

   It is a bedside test in which the patient's production of carbon dioxide and consumption of oxygen are measured for approximately 30 minutes until steady state is achieved. Results are inserted into the modified Weir equation:

   $$REE = [(3.796 \times VO_2) + (1.214 \times VCO_2)] \times 1440 \text{ min/day}$$

   where REE = resting energy expenditure (kcal/day), VO_2 = oxygen consumption (L/min), and VCO_2 = CO_2 exhaled (L/min).

The chart reports the number of kilocalories the patient is predicted to consume in 24 hours and the respiratory quotient (RQ). $RQ = VCO_2/VO_2$ and provides information on the type of substrate being used. The RQs for the metabolism of fat, protein, and carbohydrate are 0.7, 0.83, and 1.0, respectively. Overfeeding results in an RQ > 1.0.

KEY POINTS: RESPIRATORY QUOTIENT

1. Defined as ratio of CO_2 produced to O_2 consumed

2. Easy to perform on mechanically ventilated patients

3. Identifies principal metabolic substrate used by the patient

4. Ratio for fat (0.7), protein (0.83), and carbohydrates (1.0)

5. Ratio < 1 indicates starvation or underfeeding; ratio > 1 indicates overfeeding, lipogenic status

6. Increased CO_2 production linked to difficulty with ventilator weaning and impaired immune response

9. **When is indirect calorimetry useful?**
   The test may be performed on mechanically ventilated patients as soon as they are relatively stable, with a fractional concentration of oxygen in inspired gas (FiO_2) < 60% and peak end-expiratory pressure (PEEP) < 10. Studies are helpful:
   - When overfeeding (e.g., in diabetes mellitus, chronic obstructive pulmonary disease [COPD]) would be undesirable
   - When underfeeding (e.g., renal failure, large wounds) would be especially detrimental
   - In patients whose physical or clinical factors promote energy expenditure deviant from normal
   - When drugs are used that might alter energy expenditure (e.g., paralytic agents, beta blockers)
   - In patients who do not respond as expected to calculated regimens

ENTERAL NUTRITION

10. **When should enteral nutrition be considered?**
    Always, but especially when a patient is unlikely to meet > 70% of nutritional needs by mouth. Patients who have sustained major head injury (Glasgow Coma Scale score < 8), major torso trauma, major trauma to the pelvis and long bones, or major chest trauma benefit from enteral nutrition. Approximately 85% of postoperative patients (even those undergoing gastrointestinal [GI] surgery) tolerate early enteral feeding (within 24 hours).

11. **How do you access the GI tract for feeding?**
    By blind placement of a nasogastric (NG) tube or duodenal placement of a nasoduodenal tube. More distal placement may be achieved endoscopically with a nasojejunal tube (NJ). Gastric decompression and nasojejunal feeds may be accomplished concurrently after endoscopic percutaneous endoscopic gastrostomy or jejunostomy (PEG or PEJ). Alternatively, a gastrostomy or feeding jejunostomy may be placed intraoperatively.

12. **What types of enteral formulas are available?**
    Polymeric enteral feedings are soy-based, lactose-free products that contain intact protein, carbohydrates, and fat. Most offer 1 kcal/mL and 37–62 g of protein per liter. Some have additional

insoluble or soluble fiber. Special modifications of the standard formulas include **"immune-enhancing"** agents such as fish oil, arginine, glutamine, and nucleotides. **"Elemental"** formulas contain amino acids, di-, tri- and quatra-peptides, dextrose, and minimal fat. Several concentrated formulas (2 kcal/mL) are available for use in patients with congestive heart failure (CHF), renal failure, and hepatic failure. In general, products that are **disease specific** or contain nutrients in elemental form are more expensive than standard products.

13. **Are specialized formulas necessary for critically ill patients with diabetes mellitus?**
    No. Formulas with reduced carbohydrates and increased fat loads are marketed as being superior in maintaining glycemic control. These products have not undergone prospective, randomized, controlled trials (PRCTs) to demonstrate superior outcome in ICU patients. The use of standard high-protein formulas in an isocaloric or hypocaloric load combined with appropriate insulin therapy may be the most effective treatment for insulin resistance in stressed type 2 diabetic patients. Glycemic control associated with enhanced outcome is best achieved with insulin, as opposed to carbohydrate restriction. Furthermore, gastric feedings with high-fat formulas in diabetic patients with gastroparesis may be associated with delayed gastric emptying and increased risk of aspiration.

14. **Should specialized "pulmonary" formulas be used on all patients on ventilators?**
    No. Specialized high omega-6 fat formulas have been marketed to reduce CO_2 production in COPD patients who are CO_2 retainers. In theory, these minimize CO_2 retention and facilitate weaning. However, avoidance of overfeeding is more beneficial than provision of a high-fat formula.

15. **What complications are related to enteral support?**
    Electrolyte abnormalities, hyperglycemia, GI intolerance, pulmonary aspiration, and nasopharyngeal erosions.

16. **Should one wait for bowel sounds or flatus before beginning enteral feedings?**
    No.

17. **Should one delay nutrition support longer in obese patients, assuming they have increased reserves?**
    No. Obese patients have more fat, but during stress, all patients become hypermetabolic and break down endogenous protein stores to mobilize amino acids for gluconeogenesis, protein production, and energy production. So, even obese individuals "auto-cannabalize." As with normal-weight patients, obese patients require high-protein nutritional supplementation to meet increased amino acid demands. Theoretically, by providing nutritional support, protein breakdown is minimized.

18. **Should enteral formulas be diluted for initial presentation?**
    No. Dilution delays the attainment of feeding goals. Manipulation of the formula increases the likelihood of bacterial contamination. Furthermore, solution osmolarity is a relatively minor culprit in the incidence of diarrhea.

19. **How should enteral feeding–related diarrhea be managed?**
    Mild diarrhea usually requires no treatment. Moderate to severe diarrhea may require feeding reduction, antidiarrheal agents, and stool studies for *Clostridium difficile*. The medication profile should be evaluated for sorbitol-containing elixirs, laxatives, stool softeners, and prokinetic agents. Sanitation issues related to formula handling must be monitored. Some success has been reported with lactobacillus (yogurt) in antibiotic-associated diarrhea or with soluble fiber.

20. **Do enteral feedings contain enough water to meet all fluid needs?**
Most 1-kcal/mL formulas (standard) contain 85% water by volume, and 2-kcal/mL formulas contain 70% water. Water is generally not an issue in ICU patients receiving multiple intravenous (IV) fluids and drugs. However, on the wards or in patients bound for home or postcare facilities, it is essential to write a water prescription with the tube feeding order. General guidelines for the total water needs of patients are shown in Table 8-5.
   Thus, if the total calculated need for fluid is 2400 mL for a 60-kg patient and the tube feeding provided 2000 mL of free water, an order should be written to deliver 200 mL of water to the patient twice daily.

TABLE 8-5. DAILY WATER NEEDS IN RELATION TO AGE		
Patient	Age	Daily Water Needs
Average adult	25–55 years	35 mL/kg
Young, active adult	16–25 years	40 mL/kg
Adult	> 55–65 years	30 mL/kg
Elderly	> 65 years	25 mL/kg

21. **How is enteral nutrition infused?**
Enteral nutrition is generally infused continuously, in bolus form, or cyclically. Continuous infusion is preferred in critically ill patients who require postpyloric feedings. Bolus feedings are generally used in more stable patients with gastric feedings. Cyclic feedings or nocturnal feedings benefit patients who are on concurrent oral intake and in transition to full oral support.

22. **Is enteral nutrition better than total parenteral nutrition (TPN)?**
Yes. Substrates delivered enterally are better tolerated, are associated with fewer metabolic and hepatic complications, and help preserve normal mucosal ("barrier") integrity. A review of five studies contrasting TPN with no nutrition or early enteral nutrition concluded that TPN is associated with a greater incidence of septic morbidity.

CONTROVERSIES

23. **How fat is fat?**
Lean body mass is three times more metabolically active than adipose tissue. Multiple definitions of clinical obesity exist: > 120% ideal body weight (IBW), > 130% IBW, body mass index (BMI) > 30, body fat > 24–28% of body weight in men and > 30–35% in women. Measured weight is a poor indicator of relative adiposity. Self-reported weights or weights reported by family members are often erroneous in the ICU setting. Fluid resuscitation and edema make visual assessment challenging and limit the usefulness of noninvasive technology such as bioelectrical impedance (BIA) for measuring body composition. Although measured energy expenditure in kcal/kg of actual weight may sometimes approach that of normal-weight patients, feeding at the measured body weight level may be associated with profound hyperglycemia, hypercapnea, and the inability to clear triglycerides.

24. **Should actual, ideal, or adjusted body weight be used in nutrition calculations for obese patients?**
Studies using an obesity-adjusted weight in kilocalorie calculations (IBW + 0.25 [actual IBW]) report greater correlation with measured energy expenditure than when using actual weight.

25. **Which is more important, nitrogen or caloric balance?**
    Ultimately, maintaining a positive nitrogen balance may be more important than achieving a positive kilocaloric balance.

26. **Are postpyloric feedings superior to gastric feedings?**
    After major surgery or injury, the stomach exhibits decreased motility for several days. Early enteral feeding, with its known benefits, may not be accomplished through a gastric feeding in the early stages of injury. Jejunostomy feedings have been associated with higher kilocalorie intake, more timely return to anabolism, and a lower pneumonia (aspiration) rate than continuous gastric feeding.

27. **When should immune-enhancing formulas be used?**
    Rarely. PRCTs have demonstrated that immune-enhancing diets (IEDs) improve outcome and reduce septic morbidity in patients prone to intraabdominal sepsis after major torso trauma and after major operative resection of upper GI cancers. The use of IEDs should be restricted to these patients, and the duration of use should be limited because of the increased expense. The IEDs have not been adequately tested in other types of patients and, when tested in mixed ICU patients, some evidence suggests that they might even be harmful in addition to being expensive.

28. **Are arginine-containing formulas contraindicated in patients with sepsis?**
    Arginine is thought to be a semi-essential amino acid in critically ill patients. It is a metabolic fuel for lymphocytes and fibroblasts. It is also a secretagogue for a variety of hormones (most notably growth hormone). PRTs have shown that supplemental arginine improves wound healing and immune responsiveness in high-risk surgical patients. Arginine is also one of the key ingredients of the newer IEDs. The other key ingredients include glutamine, omega-3 fatty acids, and nucleotides. A large number of PRTs have compared IEDs with standard enteral formula and have shown that IEDs reduce infections and decrease hospital length of stay. The most convincing data come from PRTs that have enrolled patients undergoing major upper GI cancer resections. PRTs that have enrolled less homogenous ICU patients have had a difficult time demonstrating improved outcome, and subset analysis suggest that IEDs may be harmful in ICU patients with sepsis. Reviewing the potential immunomodulating effects of the key ingredients in IEDs has led some authorities to hypothesize that arginine supplementation is harmful in the patients with sepsis. These patients exhibit increased levels of inducible nitric oxide synthase (iNOS). Arginine is a substrate for iNOS and, in its presence, arginine combines the molecular oxygen to produce citrulline and nitric oxide (NO). The resulting NO may have numerous adverse effects in sepsis, including vasodilation, cardiac dysfunction, and direct cytotoxic injury by generating potent reactive oxygen (peroxynitrite) species. Unfortunately, little data support or refute this hypothesis.

29. **Should formula with increased fish oil be used in patients at risk for acute respiratory distress syndrome (ARDS)?**
    One industry-funded PRCT demonstrated superior outcome in patients with ARDS when provided a high omega-3 fatty acid enteral product versus a high-omega-6 "pulmonary" formula. Unfortunately, the control diet is not the standard of care and may worsen ARDS. High omega-6 fatty acids increase inflammation and production of lipid mediators, which worsen V/Q mismatch in the lung, which worsen oxygenation in ARDS. Duplication of the results and comparison with standard, moderate-fat polymeric formula is needed.

WEB SITE

http://www.gpnotebook.co.uk/simplepage.cfm?ID=516948028

BIBLIOGRAPHY

1. ASPEN Board of Directors and the Clinical Guidelines Task Force: Guidelines for the use of enteral and parenteral nutrition in adult and pediatric patients. J Parent Enter Nutr 26(suppl 1):1SA–138SA, 2002.

2. Cutts ME, Dowdy RP, Ellersieck MR, Edes TE: Predicting energy needs in ventilator dependent critically ill patients: Effect of adjusting weight for edema or adiposity. Am J Clin Nutr 66:1250–1256, 1997.

3. Gadek JE, DeMichele SJ, Karlstad MD, et al: Effect of enteral feeding with eicopentaenoic acid, gamma-linolenic acid, and antioxidants in patients with acute respiratory distress syndrome. Crit Care Med 27:1409–1420, 1999.

4. Konstantinides FN, Konstantinides NN, Li JC, et al: Urinary urea nitrogen: Too sensitive for calculating nitrogen balance studies in surgical clinical nutrition. J Parent Ent Nutr 15:189–193, 1991.

5. Kozar R, McQuiggan M, Moore F: Nutritional support of trauma patients. In Shikora S, Martindale RG, Schwaitzburg S (eds): Nutritional Considerations in the Intensive Care Unit. Silver Spring, MD, Aspen, 2002, pp 229–244.

6. Malone AM: Is a pulmonary formula warranted for patients with pulmonary dysfunction? Nutr Clin Practice 11:189–191, 1997.

7. McClave SA, Snider HL: Understanding the metabolic response to critical illness: Factors that cause patients to deviate from the expected pattern of hypermetabolism. New Horizons 2:139–146, 1994.

8. Montecalvo MA, Steger KA, Farber HW, et al: Nutritional outcome and pneumonia in critical care patients randomized to gastric versus jejunal tube feedings. Crit Care Med 20:1377–1387, 1992.

9. Moore FA, Feliciano DV, Andrassy R, et al: Enteral feeding reduces post operative septic complications: A meta analysis. Ann Surg 216:62–71, 1992.

10. Talpers SS, Romberger DJ, Pingleton SK: Nutritionally associated increased carbon dioxide production: Excess total kilocalories vs high proportion of carbohydrate kilocalories. Chest 102:551–555. 1992.

11. Van den Berghe G, Wouters P, Weekers F, et al: Intensive insulin therapy in critically ill patients. N Engl J Med 345:1359–1367, 2001.

CHAPTER 9

PARENTERAL NUTRITION

Margaret M. McQuiggan, M.S., R.D., CNSD, and Frederick A. Moore, M.D.

1. **What is parenteral nutrition?**
   Parenteral nutrition is the provision of protein as amino acids (4 kcal/g), dextrose (3.4 kcal/g), and fat (lipid 20% solution delivers 2 kcal/mL), vitamins, minerals, trace elements, fluid, and sometimes insulin through an intravenous (IV) infusion. Acid-base status may be influenced by the amount of chloride and acetate used in providing sodium and potassium. The concentrations of calcium and phosphorus are limited to avoid precipitation of a calcium phosphate salt.

2. **What are the indications for parenteral nutrition?**
   Parenteral nutrition should be used when the gastrointestinal (GI) tract is totally nonfunctional, such as in major bowel resection, "short gut," peritonitis, intestinal hemorrhage, paralytic ileus, high-volume enterocutaneous fistulas, ileus, and severe intractable diarrhea (> 1 L/day).

3. **What types of access are available for the delivery of parenteral nutrition?**
   Central parenteral solutions are highly concentrated hyperosmolar solutions with osmolarities up to 3000 mOsm/L. These should be delivered into a large lumen vein (e.g., subclavian) or, less commonly, a femoral vein. If a multiple-port catheter is used, a "virgin port" should be reserved exclusively for nutrient infusion. When long-term parenteral nutrition infusion is planned in the postacute setting, a long-term access device (e.g., Hickman or Broviac catheter) may be used. This may not be necessary, however, when the central venous catheter is placed under sterile conditions and the patient or family is taught meticulous care.

4. **What is peripheral parenteral nutrition (PPN)?**
   Although used infrequently, PPN may be used when the need for parenteral nutrition is < 7–10 days and central line placement is not desired. Solutions are low osmolarity (< 900 mOsm/L) to prevent thrombosis at the entry site. The inclusion of fat emulsion, which has a near-isotonic osmolarity, helps decrease the overall solution osmolarity while increasing total kilocalories. Because of the dilute nature of the solution, a large volume is required to provide ample nutrition to the patient. Thus, PPN may not be desirable in fluid-restricted individuals, such as patients with congestive heart failure (CHF).

5. **Should patients with pancreatitis be exclusively fed parenterally?**
   Although patients with pancreatitis have traditionally been given "gut rest" and total parenteral nutrition (TPN), some studies demonstrate improved outcome with enteral feeding past the ligament of Treitz. The type of formula and level of the GI tract into which nutrients are infused determine the degree to which pancreatic exocrine stimulation is stimulated. TPN is not superior to enteral nutrition in patients with pancreatitis who require nutritional support.

6. **Are IV lipids contraindicated in patients with pancreatitis?**
   In instances of pancreatitis caused by congenital hyperlipidemia, lipids should be withheld. This cause is rare in clinical practice.

7. **When should concentrated amino acid and dextrose solutions be used?**
   Standard amino acids are generally in an 8.5% (8.5 g/100 mL) or 10% concentration. Concentrated solutions are 15% amino acid. Dextrose is maximally concentrated at 70% solution, although D50% is more commonly used in standard TPN solutions. Maximally concentrated TPN may be desirable in patients with CHF, hepatic failure, or acute renal failure with hemodialysis. Because of increased expense, concentrated amino acids should be used judiciously.

8. **Should iron be included in parenteral nutrition?**
   Iron deficiency is rarely an acute intensive care unit (ICU) issue. Blood transfusion delivers 250 mg of elemental iron per unit. In longer-term TPN, iron supplementation may become necessary. Ideally, this should be by the enteral route because of the high anaphylactic potential of IV and intramuscular iron.

9. **What complications are associated with parenteral nutrition?**
   Fluid and electrolyte imbalance, altered glucose metabolism, increased liver function tests (LFTs), hepatic steatosis, systemic candidiasis, site infections, and gut atrophy are associated with TPN. Hemothorax or pneumothorax may occur during central line placement. Although rare, air emboli or extravascular placement of central lines have been reported. The reported incidence of catheter-related sepsis (CRS) is variable.

10. **What factors play a role in CRS?**
    Preventative measures can be divided into three categories:
    1. Catheter insertion
    2. Catheter maintenance
    3. Catheter removal
    During insertion, the skin should be prepared with chlorhexadine rather than alcohol or povidone iodine, and maximal sterile barriers should be used. Although it is commonly thought that multiple lumen catheters have a higher rate of CRS compared with single lumen catheters, randomized studies using rigorous central venous catheter protocols demonstrate comparable rates of CRS. Catheter care should entail scheduled dressing and tubing change every 48–72 hours; antibiotic ointment is of questionable merit (but is commonly used), and gauze is superior to transparent occlusive dressing. Finally, removing the catheter at set intervals effectively reduces CRS, but the benefits must be weighed against the risks of mechanical complications associated with a new catheter placement at a different site. Guidewire changes at set intervals are of debatable value but may be an effective method for early diagnosis of local catheter colonization or infection. Antimicrobial and antiseptic-bonded catheters are now available, and studies indicate that their use reduces the incidence of CRS. These devices cost substantially more than standard catheters and should therefore be limited to usage in high-risk patients.

11. **Why do parenterally fed patients often develop hyperglycemia?**
    Parenterally fed patients may develop hyperglycemia because of increased stress and the inflammatory response, limited mobility, concurrent steroid therapy, and excessive kilocalorie intake. Glucose infusion rates should not exceed 5 mg/kg/min.

12. **How should hyperglycemia be managed?**
    Information on the home glucose control regimen should be taken from the medication history. Regular insulin may be required in the initial TPN in patients with baseline hyperglycemia, insulin resistance, or insulinopoenia. Supplemental insulin needs should be evaluated daily before reordering TPN. Maintaining the blood glucose < 110 mg/dL has been shown to significantly improve patient outcome. Tight control may merit the usage of continuous IV regular insulin (i.e., insulin drip). NPH insulin is geared toward patients consuming meals at regular intervals and, thus, is not appropriate with continuous IV feedings.

KEY POINTS: HYPERGLYCEMIA SECONDARY TO PARENTERAL NUTRITION

1. Cause: increased stress and inflammatory response, limited mobility, concurrent steroid therapy, overfeeding.

2. Glucose infusion should **not** exceed 5 mg/kg/min.

3. Supplemental insulin may be required in the parenteral formula.

4. Maintaining blood glucose < 110 mg/dl improves patient outcome.

13. **Why are IV fat emulsions used, and when are they contraindicated?**
Theoretically, fat emulsions are used to prevent essential fatty acid deficiency. In reality, this condition is rare, takes several weeks to develop, and requires only 3–4% of kilocalories as linoleic acid (or 10% of kilocalories as a standard fat emulsion). Fat emulsions are also used to provide additional kilocalories after glucose infusion has reached 5 kcal/kg/min. Practically speaking, lipids are packaged and billed in 100-cc, 250-cc, and 500-cc units; therefore, they are generally included in TPN formulations in these standard volumes. Fat emulsions should be avoided with hyperlipidemia-induced pancreatitis (a small percentage of most pancreatitis) and when serum triglycerides are significantly elevated (e.g., < 500 mg/dL). When delivered in total-nutrient admixtures (three-in-one solutions), lipid emulsions are stable for 24 hours. When infused as a sole nutrient, hang times should not exceed 12 hours because of the potential for bacterial growth.

14. **What is refeeding syndrome?**
Refeeding syndrome occurs when a patient is moderately to severely malnourished and has limited substrate reserves. Patients typically present with chronic alcoholism or anorexia nervosa, after bariatric surgery, or as a result of chronic starvation. When presented with a large nutrient load, the patient rapidly develops clinically significant decreases in serum potassium, phosphorus, calcium, and magnesium levels because of compartment shifts of these elements. Hyperglycemia is commonly caused by blunted basal insulin secretion.

15. **How is refeeding syndrome best managed?**
Ample quantities of potassium, phosphorus, calcium, and magnesium should be provided with the initial parenteral mixtures within the solubility limits of the solution. The initial kilocaloric provision should be reduced by 25% of goal by reducing dextrose kilocalories. Blood glucose is monitored three to four times daily, and serum K, PO_4, Ca, and Mg should be evaluated daily for 5 days after initiating feeding while the kilocalories are advanced to goal levels.

16. **How should parenteral nutrition be monitored?**
Parenteral nutrition should be monitored daily with a chemistry profile (Na, K, Cl, CO_2, glucose), Mg, phosphorus, and Ca during the first several days of initial therapy in the critical care setting. Accucheck blood glucose determinations are needed every 6 hours. As the fluid and electrolyte balance achieves stability, frequency may be reduced to 1–2 times weekly. The adequacy of the regimen may be assessed by evidence of proper wound healing, maintenance of hydrational status, preservation of body cell mass, and a timely repletion of constitutive protein levels. Overfeeding may be evidenced by insulin resistance, hypertriglyceridemia, increased LFTs, and hypercapnia.

17. **What infusion schedules are used for TPN?**
TPN is most often delivered by continuous infusion. In more ambulatory patients and those on home therapy, a cyclic or nighttime infusion schedule may be adopted as long as adequate hydration can be maintained. This dictates a 12- to 18-hour infusion period.

18. **How should TPN be discontinued?**
When TPN is no longer needed, the infusion rate should be reduced by half for 2 hours, halved again for 2 hours, and then discontinued. This "ramp down" prevents reactive hypoglycemia.

19. **What is the cost of parenteral nutrition?**
Parenteral solution costs may vary widely depending on the constituents. The cost of TPN solution components, preparation, access devices, and laboratory monitoring costs approximately 10 times that of a standard enteral feeding. Many third-party payers do not provide more reimbursement for parenteral therapy than enteral in the hospital setting.

CONTROVERSIES

20. **Does preoperative TPN enhance surgical outcome?**
It is well documented that malnourished patients are at an increased risk for septic complications, problems with wound healing, longer hospital stays, and increased mortality. However, nutritional status may be a reflection of the severity of disease. Results of studies evaluating preoperative TPN and outcome are variable. Preoperative TPN may decrease the rate of postoperative complications, but not mortality, in moderately malnourished patients with GI cancers. When malnourished GI cancer patients were fed high-kilocalorie TPN only after surgery, complication rates increased. Perioperative enteral nutrition may lower postoperative complications in patients with a variety of cancers. Provision of immune-enhancing diets, when adequately tolerated, may decrease complications and reduce length of hospital stays after surgical resection of upper GI cancer. In elderly, underweight women with hip fractures, supplemental enteral feedings increase functional status, reduce complications, and decrease length of stay. After major abdominal surgery, early enteral nutrition reduces complications, especially wound infection. Further research is needed in homogenous patient populations using current level of feeding practice and glycemic control in order to determine the impact on outcome of perioperative nutritional support.

21. **Should TPN solutions contain the same percentage of fat kilocalories that are recommended in the diet of healthy Americans (i.e., 30% of total kilocalories)?**
The American Heart Association's (AHA) recommendations for 30% of total kilocalories as fat are geared toward cardiovascular disease prevention in healthy people and were never intended for IV feeding in critically ill individuals. Furthermore, the AHA suggests that those kilocalories should be divided almost equally between saturated; monounsaturated; and polyunsaturated fat, including omega-3 series fatty acids. Current lipid formulations available in the United States are made from either soybean oil or a mixture of soybean and safflower oil; thus, they are predominately polyunsaturated (i.e., omega-6) fat. Glucose kilocalories are the most cost-effective kilocalories, followed by standard amino acid kilocalories, and then lipid calories. Lipid infusions 1 g/kg of body weight have been associated with decreased immunocompetence and oxygenation in critically ill patients.

22. **Does supplemental glutamine enhance outcome in surgical patients?**
Glutamine is the amino acid found in greatest concentration in muscle and plasma; it decreases after surgery and injury and with stress. Thus, it is considered a conditionally essential amino acid. It plays a role as a metabolic substrate for rapidly replicating cells, is thought to maintain the integrity and function of the intestinal barrier, and protects against free radical damage because of its role in maintaining GSH levels.

Glutamine is not included in standard amino acid solutions because of limited solubility and stability; in its dipeptide form bound to alanine or glycine, glutamine is more stable and soluble. Supplementation may reduce infectious complication rates and decrease length of hospital stays in surgical patients.

WEB SITE

http://www.acssurgery.com/abstracts/acs/acs0623.htm

BIBLIOGRAPHY

1. Al-Omran M, Groof A, Wilke D: Enteral versus parenteral nutrition for acute pancreatitis. Cochrane Database Syst Rev (2):CD002837, 2001.

2. ASPEN Board of Directors and the Clinical Guidelines Task Force: Guidelines for the use of enteral and parenteral nutrition in adult and pediatric patients. J Parent Ent Nutr 26(suppl):1SA-26SA, 2002.

3. Havala T, Shronts E: Managing the complications associated with refeeding. Nutr Clin Practice 5:23–29, 1990.

4. McClave SA, Snider H, Owens N, Sexton LK: Clinical nutrition in pancreatitis. Digest Dis Sci 42:2035–2044, 1997.

5. Novak F, Heyland DK, Avenell A, et al: Glutamine supplementation in serious illness: A systematic review of the evidence. Crit Care Med 30:2022–2029, 2002.

6. Satanarayana R, Klein S: Clinical efficacy of perioperative nutrition support. Curr Opin Clin Nutr Metab 198:51–58, 1997.

7. Van den Berghe G, Wouters P, Weekers F, et al: Intensive insulin therapy in critically ill patients. N Engl J Med 345:1359–1367, 2001.

CHAPTER 10

WHAT DOES POSTOPERATIVE FEVER MEAN?

Alden H. Harken, M.D.

1. **What is a fever?**
   Normal core temperature varies between 36°C and 38°C. Because we hibernate a little at night, we are cool (36°C) just before rising in the morning; after revving our engines all day, we are hot at night (38°C). A fever is a pathologic state reflecting a systemic inflammatory process. The core temperature is > 38°C but rarely > 40°C.

2. **What is malignant hyperthermia?**
   A rare, life-threatening response to inhaled anesthetics or some muscle relaxants. Core temperature rises > 40°C. Abnormal calcium metabolism in skeletal muscle produces heat, acidosis, hypokalemia, muscle rigidity, coagulopathy, and circulatory collapse.

3. **How is malignant hyperthermia treated?**
   - Stop the anesthetic.
   - Give sodium bicarbonate (2 mEq/kg IV).
   - Give dantrolene (calcium channel blocker at 2.5 mg/kg IV).
   - Continue dantrolene (1 mg/kg every 6 hours for 48 hours).
   - Cool patient with alcohol sponges and ice.

KEY POINTS: MALIGNANT HYPERTHERMIA

1. Rare, familial (autosomal dominant with variable penetrance) catastrophic response to inhaled anesthetics or muscle relaxants.

2. Mechanism: abnormal calcium metabolism in skeletal muscle.

3. Clinical manifestations: core temperature > 40°C, trismus, hypercapnia, tachycardia, tachypnea, hypertension, cardiac dysrhythmias, metabolic acidosis, hypoxemia, myoglobinuria, coagulopathy.

4. Management: halt anesthetic; administer dantrolene over 48 hours, supplemental sodium bicarbonate; actively cool patient.

4. **What causes fever?**
   Macrophages are activated by bacteria and endotoxin. Activated macrophages release interleukin-1, tumor necrosis factor, and interferon, which reset the hypothalamic thermoregulatory center.

5. **Can fever be treated?**
   Yes. Aspirin, acetaminophen, and ibuprofen are cyclooxygenase inhibitors that block the formation of prostaglandin E_2 in the hypothalamus and effectively control fever.

6. **Should fever be treated?**
   This is controversial. No evidence suggests that suppression of fever improves patient outcome. Patients are more comfortable, however, and the surgeon receives fewer calls from the nurses.

7. **Should fever be investigated?**
   Yes. Fever indicates that something (frequently treatable) is going on. The threshold for inquiry depends on the patient. A transplant patient with a temperature of 38°C requires scrutiny, whereas a healthy medical student with an identical temperature of 38°C 24 hours after an appendectomy can be ignored.

8. **Summarize a fever work-up.**
   - Order blood cultures, urine Gram stain and culture, and sputum Gram stain and culture.
   - Look at the surgical incisions.
   - Look at old and current IV sites for evidence of septic thrombophlebitis.
   - If breath sounds are worrisome, obtain a chest x-ray.

9. **What is the most common cause of fever during the early postoperative period (1–3 days)?**
   The traditional answer is atelectasis. A total pneumothorax does not cause fever, however. Why does a little atelectasis cause fever, whereas a lot of atelectasis (pneumothorax) does not? The most likely explanation is that sterile atelectasis (and early postoperative lung collapse typically is not infected) has nothing to do with fever.

10. **Do surgical incisions compromise spontaneous breathing patterns?**
    Yes. Vital capacity was measured in a large group of patients 24 hours after various surgical procedures. An upper abdominal incision was the worst, followed by lower abdominal incision, then (counterintuitively) thoracotomy, median sternotomy, and extremity incision.

11. **Should atelectasis be treated with incentive spirometry?**
    Yes—but not to avoid fever.

12. **Define a wound infection.**
    A wound infection contains > 10^5 organisms per gram of tissue. An infected incision appears erythematous (red), edematous (swollen), and tender.

13. **Are certain wounds prone to infection?**
    Each milliliter of human saliva contains 10^8 aerobic and anaerobic, gram-positive and gram-negative bacteria. All human bite wounds must be considered as contaminated. Animal bite wounds typically are less contaminated. (It is safer to kiss your dog than your fiancé[e].)

14. **Do incisions become infected early after surgery?**
    The incision must be examined in a patient with a fever (39°C) < 12 hours after surgery. Look for a foul-smelling, serous discharge in a particularly painful wound (all incisions hurt) with or without crepitus. Gram stain of the serous discharge for gram-positive rods confirms or excludes the diagnosis of clostridial infection.

15. **Summarize the therapy for clostridial gas gangrene.**
    - The wound should be opened immediately, with fluid resuscitation of the patient. The mainstay of therapy is aggressive surgical debridement of necrotic tissue (skin, muscle, fascia). Make a big hole, and do not worry about closing it.
    - Give penicillin, 12 million U/day IV for 1 week.
    - Hyperbaric oxygen is not helpful.

16. **Are nonclostridial necrotizing wound infections a cause of concern?**
Hemolytic streptococcal gangrene, idiopathic scrotal gangrene, and gram-negative synergistic necrotizing cellulitis are distinct entities but have been lumped into the single category of necrotizing fasciitis. All require the same initial approach:
1. Fluid and electrolyte resuscitation
2. Broad-spectrum antibiotics ("triples")
3. Aggressive surgical debridement of all necrotic tissue

17. **What are triple antibiotics?**
A shotgun approach to potentially life-threatening infections when the patient is seriously ill and the surgeon is seriously concerned:
1. Gram-positive coverage (e.g., ampicillin)
2. Gram-negative coverage (e.g., gentamicin)
3. Anaerobic coverage (e.g., metronidazole [Flagyl])
To avoid overgrowth of yeast and resistant bacteria, focus on the culprit bacteria as soon as the cultures define it.

KEY POINTS: CLOSTRIDIAL VERSUS NONCLOSTRIDIAL NECROTIZING WOUND INFECTIONS

1. Clostridial infection involves underlying muscle resulting in myonecrosis or gas gangrene.

2. Nonclostridial infection involves subcutaneous fascia (also known as necrotizing fasciitis).

3. Similar management: fluid and electrolyte resuscitation, antibiotics (high-dose penicillin for clostridial infection, broad-spectrum triples for necrotizing fasciitis), and aggressive surgical debridement of necrotic tissue.

18. **Give the doses for triple antibiotics.**

Ampicillin	1 g every 6 hours IV in adults
	40 mg/kg every 6 hours IV in children
Gentamicin	7 mg/kg IV every 24 hours (this single daily dose is less nephrotoxic than 2 mg/kg IV every 8 hours)
Metronidazole	500 mg IV every 6 hours in adults
	7.5 mg/kg IV every 6 hours in children

19. **Which surgical procedures predispose to wound infections?**
Gastrointestinal procedures, especially when the colon is opened.

20. **When do wound infections typically occur?**
12 hours to 7 days postoperatively.

21. **How is a wound infection treated?**
The wound should be opened and completely drained.

22. **Is it necessary to irrigate an infected wound?**
Tap water irrigation decreases the bacterial load and promotes healing. Alcohol is toxic to tissues. Sodium hydrochlorite (Dakin solution) and hydrogen peroxide kill fibroblasts and slow epithelialization. As a rule of thumb, put nothing into a wound that you would not put in your eye.

23. **When do urinary tract infections (UTIs) occur?**
The longer the urethral (Foley) catheter is in place, the more likely the infection. Urologic instrumentation at the time of surgery may accelerate the process considerably. Germs crawl up the outside of the urethral catheter, and by 5–7 days after surgery most patients harbor infected urine.

24. **How is a UTI diagnosed?**
Urine culture with > 10^5 bacteria/mL defines a UTI. White blood cells on urinalysis are highly suspicious.

25. **Name the most common late causes of postoperative fever.**
Septic thrombophlebitis (from an IV line) and occult (usually intraabdominal) abscesses tend to present ≥ 2 weeks after surgery.

WEB SITES

1. http://www.mhacanada.org

2. http://www.anes.ucla.edu/dept/mh.html

BIBLIOGRAPHY

1. Bansal BC, Wiebe RA, Perkins SD, Abramo TJ: Tap water for irrigation of lacerations. Am J Emerg Med 20:469–472, 2002.
2. Helmer KS, Robinson EK, Lally KP, et al: Standardized patient care guidelines reduce infectious morbidity in appendectomy patients. Am J Surg 183:608–613, 2002.
3. Lewis RT: Oral versus systemic antibiotic prophylaxis in elective colon surgery: A randomized study and meta-analysis send a message from the 1990's. Can J Surg 45:173–180, 2002.
4. Singer AJ, Quinn JV, Thode HC Jr, Hollander JE, TraumaSeal Study Group: Determinants of poor outcome after laceration and surgical incision repair. Plast Reconstr Surg 110:429–435, 2002.

CHAPTER 11

OXYGEN MONITORING AND ASSESSMENT

James B. Haenel, R.R.T., and Jeffrey L. Johnson, M.D.

1. **How does a pulse oximeter work?**
   Light-absorption characteristics differ for the four most common circulating species of hemoglobin in adults:
   1. Reduced hemoglobin (RHb)
   2. Oxygenated hemoglobin (O_2Hb)
   3. Methemoglobin (Met Hb)
   4. Carboxyhemoglobin (CO Hb)
   Current pulse oximeters transmit two wavelengths of light, red (680 nm) and infrared (940 nm), and these differentiate O_2Hb from RHb. Using optical plethysmography, the pulse oximeter measures hemoglobin saturation only during arterial **pulsation.**

2. **How accurate is pulse oximetry?**
   The device is highly accurate at saturations > 80%. This results in an overall accuracy of ± 5%.

3. **Are clinicians accurate in determining arterial desaturation by "visual oximetry" (how red is the blood)?**
   No. Pulse oximetry should be regarded as the fifth vital sign.

4. **How does the pulse oximeter respond to an abnormal species of hemoglobin?**
   In carbon monoxide or cyanide poisoning, the oximeter interprets an abnormal hemoglobin as a combination of O_2Hb and RHb, which results in an erroneously high saturation. Based on the light absorption of Met Hb, the pulse oximeter may display a saturation of 85%.

5. **Can any other environmental or clinical conditions result in inaccurate pulse oximetry values?**
   Reliability depends on a strong arterial pulse plus good light transmission. Inaccuracy results with hypotension (mean arterial pressure < 50 mmHg), hypothermia (< 35°C), vascular disease (poor peripheral perfusion), and vasopressor therapy (vasoconstriction). Bright lights, intravenous dyes, nail polish, and excessive motion each may produce bad information.

6. **What is the relationship between oxyhemoglobin saturation (Sao_2) and partial pressure of oxygen (Pao_2)?**
   Proper interpretation of pulse oximetry requires recall of the oxyhemoglobin dissociation curve. A rightward shift (decreased hemoglobin affinity for oxygen) facilitates oxygen unloading at the tissue level. Increasing temperature, increasing $Paco_2$, increasing 2,3-diphosphoglycerate, and increasing hydrogen ion concentration—all "increases"—shift the curve to the right. When the Pao_2 is > 100 mmHg, however, the curve is virtually flat. Consequently a large drop in Pao_2 (e.g., from 200 to 100 mmHg) may occur with no discernible change in Sao_2. (See Figure 11-1.)

7. **What are the indications for continuous pulse oximetry?**
   Any patient who either is or might get sick. Pulse oximetry should be considered standard monitoring in critical care units. Pulse oximetry is uniquely valuable during patient transport, when

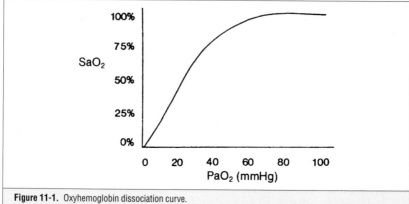

Figure 11-1. Oxyhemoglobin dissociation curve.

weaning from the ventilator, and after major ventilator changes. Critically ill patients who are outside the intensive care unit (ICU) (emergency department or radiology suite) also should be monitored by pulse oximetry.

8. **How does a continuous mixed venous oximeter work?**
Mixed venous oximetry uses reflective spectrophotometry. Narrow wavebands of light are transmitted via a fiberoptic bundle to the blood flowing past the tip of the catheter and are reflected by a separate fiberoptic bundle to a photodetector that determines relative absorption of the specific wavelength. A microprocessor calculates mixed venous hemoglobin saturation (Svo_2).

9. **What is the normal value for mixed venous oxygen saturation?**
The normal oxygen tension in mixed venous blood (Pvo_2) is 40 mmHg. Under physiologic conditions, this is equivalent to an Svo_2 of 75%, which is on the steep portion of the oxyhemoglobin dissociation curve. Three fourths of the oxygen (see Chapters 4, 5, and 6) delivered out of the aorta (Do_2) returns to the right heart unused.

10. **Using a pulmonary artery catheter, how can oxygen delivery and consumption be determined?**
The Fick equation shows the relationship between systemic oxygen delivery (Do_2) and oxygen consumption (Vo_2):

$$Vo_2 = CO \times (Cao_2 - Cvo_2)$$

where Cao_2 is arterial oxygen content, Cvo_2 is mixed venous oxygen content, and CO is cardiac output. Oxygen delivery is determined by the following equation:

$$Do_2 = Cao_2 \times CO$$

where Cao_2 is ($1.36 \times$ [hemoglobin concentration] $\times$ [arterial oxygen saturation] $+ Pao_2 \times 0.003$) and Cvo_2 is ($1.36 \times$ [hemoglobin concentration] $\times$ [venous oxygen saturation] $+ Pao_2 \times 0.003$).

11. **Describe the four primary causes of a sudden fall in Svo_2.**
A stable, normal Svo_2 ensures a balance of Do_2 and Vo_2, whereas a sudden fall in Svo_2 provides an early warning of (1) low CO, (2) arterial oxygen desaturation, (3) drop in hemoglobin, or (4) increased Vo_2.

12. **Why does Svo$_2$ rise during general anesthesia?**
General anesthesia suppresses metabolic demands; vo$_2$ decreases (extracting less oxygen peripherally), and Svo$_2$ rises.

13. **Why does Svo$_2$ rise with septic shock?**
During sepsis, large peripheral shunts, high cardiac output, and poor oxygen extraction contribute to an elevated Svo$_2$.

14. **State the advantages of continuous monitoring of Svo$_2$.**
Svo$_2$ provides prompt feedback about therapeutic interventions and disease progression. Svo$_2$ trends are more important, however, than absolute values. With time, the catheter tip gets progressively gummed up with tissue proteins; the catheter should be recalibrated every 12–24 hours.

15. **Are there any disadvantages to computer-generated hemodynamic profiling?**
Yes—even when it is wrong, we tend to believe it. Comprehensive hemodynamic profiling includes a constellation of parameters: cardiac output, Pao$_2$, Svo$_2$, urine output, serum lactate level, and great-toe temperature.

16. **What is dual oximetry?**
Dual oximetry consists of simultaneous monitoring of arterial (Sao$_2$) and mixed venous (Svo$_2$) hemoglobin saturation to provide real-time, continuous information about pulmonary function, oxygen transport, and oxygen extraction ratio. Dual oximetry is particularly useful for real-time assessment during a best trial of positive end-expiratory pressure.

17. **What is transcutaneous oxygen monitoring (TCM)?**
TCM is a method of continuously recording skin Po$_2$ (Ptco$_2$), which is not equal to arterial Po$_2$. In 1975, Van Duzee observed that the lipid component of the stratum corneum melts as skin temperature increases, and gas diffusion can increase by 1000-fold. The Ptco$_2$ electrode is designed to heat the skin to 44°C. The elevated temperature also increases dermal blood flow and "arterializes" the capillary blood. The interpretation of pulse oximetry and TCM are the same, however.

18. **If the skin beneath the sensor is arterialized, why is the Ptco$_2$ not equal to the Pao$_2$?**
Four factors contribute to the difference between Ptco$_2$ and Pao$_2$:
1. The rightward shift of the oxygen-hemoglobin dissociation curve with heating
2. Variations in the skin oxygen permeability
3. Metabolic consumption of oxygen by the dermal tissue
4. Cutaneous blood flow
Because factors 1 and 3 tend to cancel each other, the relationship between Ptco$_2$ and Pao$_2$ is effectively linear and depends only on oxygen permeability and skin blood flow.

19. **What is an oxygen debt?**
An oxygen debt is the net cumulative difference between oxygen consumption measured at baseline and during any pathologic state. It is the amount of oxygen needed by the cells to compensate for the mismatch between oxygen delivery and oxygen demand.

20. **Name the five physiologic mechanisms responsible for causing hypoxemia. Do they all result in a widened alveolar-arterial gradient (A-a gradient)?**
1. Low inspired oxygen fraction (e.g., high altitude)
2. Alveolar hypoventilation (physiologic dead space)
3. Diffusion limitation
4. Ventilation/perfusion mismatch (most common cause for hypoxemia—this really includes both mechanism 2 and 5)

5. Shunt (adult respiratory distress syndrome, severe pneumonia)

Alveolar hypoventilation and a low FiO_2 may result in hypoxemia with a normal A-a gradient.

KEY POINTS: PHYSIOLOGIC CAUSES OF HYPOXEMIA

1. Low FiO_2: normal A-a gradient

2. Alveolar hypoventilation or dead space: normal A-a gradient

3. Diffusion defect: abnormal A-a gradient

4. Ventilation/perfusion mismatch: most important cause with abnormal gradient

5. Shunt: abnormal A-a gradient; does not correct with oxygen therapy alone

---

21. **How should a hypoxic event be managed?**

Before you even start trying to make the diagnosis, give oxygen. The first maneuver for intubated patients is to hand-ventilate with an ambu-bag. A ruptured endotracheal tube cuff is self-evident, whereas difficult bagging implies airway obstruction, bronchospasm, or tension pneumothorax. Inability to pass a suction catheter confirms endotracheal tube obstruction. If the obstruction is not reversible by changing head position or by cuff deflation, the endotracheal tube must be replaced immediately. If there is difficulty with bagging and no evidence of airway obstruction, listen to the chest for breath sounds to exclude a tension pneumothorax. The mechanical ventilator and breathing circuit must be examined for malfunction. Send arterial blood gases to confirm hypoxia (low PO_2) and rule out hypoventilation (high PCO_2).

Next, get a chest x-ray (to rule out a pneumothorax and to confirm the correct position of the endotracheal tube) and review recent medications, interventions (e.g., suctioning, position changes, nursing care), and changes in clinical status. Most acute hypoxic events in the ICU are due to easily identified and reversible mechanical problems, such as disconnects from oxygen delivery systems or mucus plugging that requires suctioning. (See Figure 11-2).

EXTRA-CREDIT QUESTIONS

22. **Four hours after your patient undergoes an exploratory laparotomy following a motor vehicle accident, the nurse reports that the patient's vital signs, urine output, and oxygen transport numbers are normal. Can the patient still be in trouble?**

The Advanced Trauma Life Support Program defines shock as an abnormality of the circulatory system that results in inadequate organ perfusion and tissue oxygenation. This definition is easy to understand with uncompensated shock. Critically injured patients rarely make the transition from uncompensated shock to normal physiology, however, without some evidence of continued suboptimal tissue perfusion. This altered physiologic state may exist in 85% of patients who exhibit normal blood pressure, heart rate, and urine output. Assessing the sufficiency of blood flow to vital organs based on normal oxygen transport indices offers incomplete information about the adequacy of flow distribution and whether cellular oxygen use is appropriate. To correct fully an oxygen debt in a high-risk patient, oxygen transport variables should be maximized with simultaneous monitoring of indirect biochemical indices of perfusion, such as lactate, base deficit, and gastric mucosal pHi. (Good urine output and a warm big toe are reassuring.)

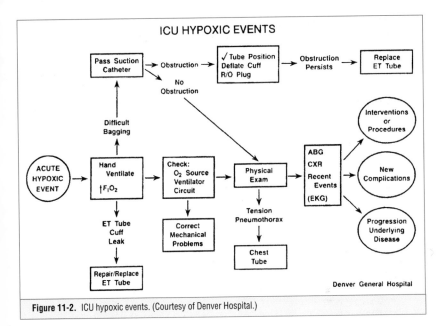

Figure 11-2. ICU hypoxic events. (Courtesy of Denver Hospital.)

23. **Do supranormal oxygen transport indices (Do_2, Vo_2, cardiac index) serve as useful resuscitation end points?**

Probably, but this is controversial. In a meta-analysis of severely ill patients who received early resuscitation (8–12 hours postoperatively or *before* organ failure), there was a 23% decrease in mortality with early goal-oriented (supranormal oxygen delivery) resuscitation. The supranormal oxygen delivery targets are a cardiac index of 4.5 L/min/m², oxygen delivery index > 600 mL/min/m², and oxygen consumption index > 170 mL/min/m². Most young, otherwise healthy patients achieve these objectives with little extra assistance. Conversely, cardiovascular disease may place the older patient at higher risk, and attempts to achieve supranormal oxygen transport goals (by whipping an old heart) may increase mortality. Although the final answer about the efficacy of supranormal resuscitation is unknown, the message is clear: All patients should be rewarmed promptly, mechanical ventilation must be optimized, adequate sedation and pain control must be achieved, and the patient must be volume-resuscitated appropriately.

24. **Are there any organ-specific indicators of the adequacy of blood flow?**

ECG and urine output assess cardiac and renal perfusion. Cerebral perfusion is probably adequate if the patient can recall "how many dudes jumped me." Gastric tonometry is a method of assessing the adequacy of the splanchnic circulation. Splanchnic hypoperfusion occurs early in the course of shock (see Chapter 4) and may precede changes in systemic hemodynamic indices, oxygen transport variables, and acid-base balance.

25. **How is gastric tonometry performed?**

The gastric tonometer consists of a CO_2-permeable balloon secured to the distal end of a nasogastric tube. CO_2 in the adjacent gastric mucosa is allowed to equilibrate with the saline-filled balloon. After 60 minutes of equilibration, the saline is aspirated as a measure of the gastric mucosal Pco_2, and arterial blood gases are obtained for bicarbonate concentration [HCO_3^2]. Gastric intramucosal pH is calculated from the Henderson-Hasselbach equation:

$$pHi = 6.1 + \log_{10} \frac{\text{arterial } [HCO_3^-]}{\text{NG tube } PCO_2 \times 0.03}$$

Normal pHi is approximately 7.38 (range = 7.35–7.41). Survival benefits in critically ill patients have been shown if admission pHi can be corrected and maintained at values > 7.32 within the initial 24 hours.

WEB SITES

1. http://www.acssurgery.com/abstracts/acs/acs0606.htm

2. http://www.acpmedicine.com/abstracts/sam/med1401.htm

BIBLIOGRAPHY

1. Comroe JH, Botello S: Unreliability of cyanosis in recognition of arterial anoxemia. Am J Surg 214:1, 1947.
2. Elliott DC: An evaluation of the end points of resuscitation. J Am Coll Surg 187:536–547, 1998.
3. Hess D: Detection and monitoring of hypoxemia and oxygen therapy. Respir Care 45:65–80, 2000.
4. Ivatury RR, Simon RJ, Islam S, et al: A prospective randomized study of end points of resuscitation after major trauma: Global oxygen transport indices versus organ-specific gastric mucosal pH. J Am Coll Surg 183:145–154, 1996.
5. Kern JW, Shoemaker WC: Meta-analysis of hemodynamic optimization in high-risk patients. Crit Care Med 30:1686–1692, 2002.
6. Moore FA, Haenel JB, Moore EE, Whitehill TA: Incommensurate oxygen consumption in response to maximal oxygen availability predicts postinjury multiple organ failure. J Trauma 33:58–67, 1992.

CHAPTER 12

CENTRAL VENOUS AND PULMONARY ARTERY PRESSURE MONITORING

Dipin Gupta, M.D., Glenn J.R. Whitman, M.D., and Alden H. Harken, M.D.

1. **What does a catheter in the central venous circulation measure?**
   All intrathoracic veins have nearly the same pressure. A catheter in the central venous circulation (anywhere) measures this central venous pressure (CVP) (or right atrial pressure). CVP, plus a little right atrial "kick," pushes blood into the right ventricle. This right ventricular "filling pressure" is also termed *preload*.

2. **What does a pulmonary artery (PA) catheter measure?**
   A PA catheter (Swan-Ganz catheter) is threaded through the central venous circulation out into the PA. The catheter has three ports—one at the tip and side ports at 4 cm from the tip (the "VIP port") and 29 cm from the tip (the "CVP port"). With inflation of the balloon at the distal catheter tip and subsequent occlusion of a pulmonary capillary vessel, the transducer at the tip of the catheter "sees" only a static column of blood between it and the left atrium. This pulmonary capillary wedge pressure approximates left atrial pressure or left ventricular filling pressure or LV preload.

   When pulmonary vascular resistance is normal, PA diastolic pressure can be used as a substitute for wedge or left atrial pressure. It is not necessary in this circumstance to inflate the balloon to estimate the wedge pressure. This spares the patient the risk of PA rupture from balloon inflation (another advantage is that you do not need to get up to replace the Swan-Ganz catheter when the balloon breaks—usually at 2 A.M.).
   A PA catheter can measure blood pressure at three points:
   1. The level of the superior vena cava (CVP)
   2. The PA (with the balloon deflated)
   3. The pulmonary venous pressure/left atrial pressure (with the balloon inflated)

      Other important parameters, most importantly cardiac output and mixed venous oxygen saturation, can be measured or calculated based on numbers derived from the PA catheter (see questions 9 and 10).

3. **Discuss the complications of central venous catheters and PA catheters.**
   Immediate complications are pneumothorax (2%); inadvertent arterial cannulation (2%); catheter malposition (7%); and, more rarely, air embolism, hemothorax, chylothorax, arrhythmia, brachial plexus injury, vocal cord paralysis, and death (each substantially less frequent than 1%).[4] Additionally, "floating" a hard PA catheter across the tricuspid valve and through the right ventricular outflow tract holds the potential for ventricular tachycardia (and if you "nudge" the atrioventricular node, you can provoke complete heart block).

   Delayed complications are thrombosis (33% by radiographic studies) and less commonly bacteremia, endocarditis, or clavicular osteomyelitis. Fibrin forms on the catheter within hours of insertion, and the incidence of vessel thrombosis increases with time. PA-related bloodstream infections occur in 4.8 cases per 1000 catheter-days.[2] This is roughly equivalent to one bloodstream infection among 100 patients with a catheter in place for 2 days. In autopsy series (clearly not healthy patients), the incidence of infective endocarditis is usually < 2% but increases dramatically with increasing insertion duration.[2]

4. **What are the relative contraindications to percutaneous subclavian or internal jugular venous catheterization?**
   In a patient who is anticoagulated or who has a platelet count < 50,000, it is typically safer to place a central venous line by peripheral cutdown. Inadvertent arterial puncture is tolerated fairly well unless the patient is coagulopathic. A patient with hyperinflated lungs (chronic obstructive pulmonary disease) is more likely to have a pneumothorax during catheter placement.

5. **How do you percutaneously place a sheath for PA catheter placement?**
   1. Place the patient in mild head-down (Trendelenburg) position and turn the head toward the contralateral side.
   2. Using sterile technique and after administering local anesthesia, insert an 18-G needle on a 10-mL syringe at the point where the deltopectoral groove abuts the clavicle and pointing just north of the suprasternal notch. Hugging the undersurface of the clavicle, apply gentle suction with the syringe. When you hit the vein, dark (nonpulsatile) blood easily flows back into the syringe.
   3. Remove the syringe, and insert a soft, flexible wire through the 18-G needle.
   4. Remove the needle, leaving the flexible wire in place.
   5. Slide a plastic sheath (with the dilator inside) over the guidewire. Remove the wire and the dilator, leaving the sheath in place (if the sheath bleeds profusely, you are in the right place). Aspirate the catheter fully to evacuate all air and flush with saline (Figure 12-1).
   6. A chest x-ray must be obtained to confirm proper position and exclude pneumothorax and hemothorax.

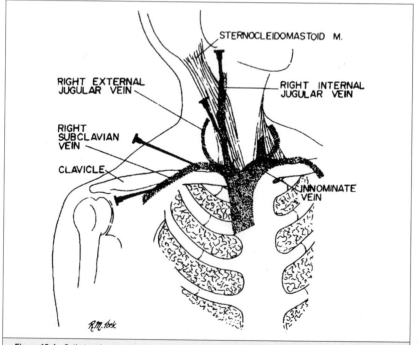

Figure 12-1. Catheter placement by percutaneous subclavian vein puncture.

6. **As a PA catheter passes through the central venous circulation, what do the pressure waveforms look like?**
    See Figure 12-2.

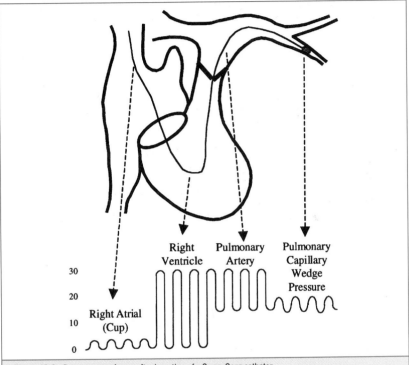

Figure 12-2. Pressure waveforms after insertion of a Swan-Ganz catheter.

7. **What is the value of the CVP and PA pressure?**
    Starling's law states that (up to a point) increasing end-diastolic volume (preload) increases stroke volume (volume of blood ejected during systole, which is multiplied by heart rate to yield cardiac output). Clinically, we cannot measure end-diastolic volume, so filling pressures are used as a surrogate.
    CVP is an estimate of the pressure with which blood flows into the *right side* of the heart. This number does not reflect left-sided filling pressures. As stated earlier, PA diastolic or wedge pressures allow a better estimate of *left-sided* filling pressure.

8. **Name other parameters that can be measured or calculated with use of a PA catheter.**
    Cardiac output, venous oxygen saturation, pulmonary and systemic vascular resistance.

9. **How is cardiac output measured?**
    There are two ways to use a PA catheter to calculate cardiac output:
    1. The technique of **thermodilution**, in which a volume (10 mL) of saline with known temperature (108°C) is injected into the proximal port of a PA catheter. A temperature probe at the distal catheter tip measures the change in temperature of blood from the time when the cold saline was injected and the time that it passes by the probe. The precise volume and temperature of the injectate allow calculation of the amount of blood passing by the probe, which is a measure

of cardiac output. Because cardiac output changes by 15% during the respiratory cycle, injection should be synchronized with end-expiration. A left-to-right intracardiac shunt adds warm blood to the cold saline bolus, giving a falsely elevated measurement of cardiac output.

2. The **Fick principle**, which relates cardiac output to venous oxygen saturation (see question 11).

10. How is the oxygen content of blood calculated?

An oximetric PA catheter has a fiberoptic monitor at its distal tip that continuously measures hemoglobin saturation $[So_2 (\%)]$. The catheter tip in the PA measures mixed venous blood (Svo_2) oxygenation. After 24 hours of placement, the catheter becomes covered with fibrin, and measurements become less reliable.

The amount of oxygen in blood (Cao_2) comprises that portion dissolved in blood (almost nothing) and that portion attached to hemoglobin (lots).

The amount dissolved is calculated by:

$$O_2 \text{ dissolved} = 0.003 \times Pao_2$$

The amount attached to hemoglobin is calculated by:

$$O_2 \text{ attached} = 1.38 \times [Hb] \times Sao_2$$

For example, if hemoglobin = 12 g/dL, Pao_2 = 60 mmHg, and Sao_2 = 90%, then Cao_2 = (0.003 × 60) + (1.38 × 12 × 0.90) = 15.08 mL oxygen/100 mL blood. Dissolved oxygen usually comprises only a small percentage of Cao_2 (< 1% in this example). Clinically, it is excluded from calculations (see Chapter 6).

11. How is the oxygen content of the blood used?

Assuming normal parameters of hemoglobin = 15 g/dL, Sao_2 = 96%, and Svo_2 = 75%, the difference in oxygen content between the arterial circulation and the venous circulation $(A-Vo_2)$ is 4.35 vol%. For every 100 mL of blood that travels around the body, the tissues extract 4.35 mL of oxygen. The normal range for the $A-Vo_2$ is 3–5 vol%.

The Fick principle uses this $A-Vo_2$ to determine cardiac output. Nonstressed patients typically consume oxygen at the rate of 125 mL/min/m². This is really a "wild guess" because we do not usually determine $A-VO_2$ unless a patient is stressed. By measuring the $A-Vo_2$, we can determine the oxygen contribution for each 100 mL of blood that travels around the body. If the measured $A-Vo_2$ difference = 4.35 mL of oxygen, every 100 mL of cardiac output contributes 4.35 mL to the Vo_2 of 250 mL (for a person who is 2 m², or 2 × 125 mL/min/m²). A total of 5.75 L of blood must travel around the patient's body each minute to meet the oxygen requirement. By "assuming" Vo_2 (typically a big assumption) and by calculating the $A-VO_2$, one can approximate cardiac output.

12. Explain the significance of the Svo_2.

This is a "poor man's" cardiac output measure. In a patient with a fixed metabolic rate (or stable oxygen consumption), as cardiac output increases (delivering more blood/min and more oxygen/min), the patient extracts less oxygen per 100 mL of blood peripherally, and more oxygen per 100 mL returns to the right side of the heart (as your patient gets healthier, Svo_2 rises). Conversely, as cardiac output decreases (delivering less oxygen/min peripherally to meet fixed demand), the patient extracts more oxygen per 100 mL of blood. Returning venous blood contains less oxygen, and Svo_2 decreases. Knowing the the differential diagnosis of a **falling Svo_2** is important: (1) progressive anemia, (2) cardiac failure, (3) decreasing arterial saturation, and (4) increased basal metabolic rate. The differential diagnosis of a **rising Svo_2** is (1) sepsis, (2) left-to-right intracardiac shunt, (3) left-to-right peripheral shunt (dialysis access), and (4) inadvertent wedging of the pulmonary artery catheter. The other more gratifying possibility is that your patient is improving in response to your therapy!

KEY POINTS: Svo$_2$ TRENDS

1. "Poor man's" estimation of cardic output

2. Decreased Svo$_2$: progressive anemia, cardiac failure, decreasing arterial saturation, increased basal metabolic rate

3. Increased Svo$_2$: sepsis, cyanide toxicity, left-to-right intracardiac shunt, left-to-right peripheral shunt, inadvertent wedging of PA catheter

13. **How do you determine the systemic (peripheral) vascular resistance (SVR)?**

$$SVR = [(MAP - CVP)/CO] \times 80$$

where SVR = systemic vascular resistance (dyne • sec/cm^{-5}), MAP = mean arterial blood pressure (mmHg), CVP = central venous pressure (mmHg), and CO = cardiac output (L/min).
Normal SVR is 800–1200 dyne • sec/cm^{-5}. Multiplying by 80 corrects SVR values from Wood units (mmHg/L/min) to standard metric units (dyne • sec/cm^{-5}).

14. **How is a PA catheter used to evaluate shock?**
Management of the patient in shock requires knowledge of intracardiac "filling" pressures (CVP, PA pressure), cardiac ouput, SVR, and Svo$_2$. Prompt PA catheter placement guides therapy (see Chapter 4 and Table 12-1).
Hypovolemic shock. Right and left filling pressures (CVP and wedge/PA pressures) are low, as are cardiac output and Svo$_2$. SVR is high. The diagnosis is confirmed when volume repletion with rising filling pressure is associated with increased cardiac output, normalization of system pressure, and decreased SVR.
Cardiogenic shock. Shock despite adequate filling pressures means that the pump is failing. Cardiac output and SvO$_2$ are low. If SVR is high, infuse dobutamine, 5 µg/kg/min, to stimulate

TABLE 12-1. PA CATHETER EVALUATION OF SHOCK						
	CVP	PA	Wedge	CN	SVR	Svo$_2$	Therapy
Hypovolemic shock	↓	↓	↓	↓	↑	↓	Increase intravascular volume
Cardiogenic shock	↑	↑	↑	↓	↓/↑	↓	Optimize filling pressures, minimize afterload, inotropes
Septic shock	–/↓	–/↓	–/↓	↑	↓	↑	Increase intravascular volume, increase afterload

the heart and reduce SVR. If SVR is low, infuse epinephrine, 0.05 µg/kg/min, to stimulate the heart and increase SVR.

Septic shock. The hallmarks of septic shock are normal or low-normal filling pressure, supranormal cardiac output, high Svo_2, and low SVR (< 600 dyne • sec/cm^{-5}). Treatment requires fluid resuscitation and systemic vasoconstriction while the underlying cause (e.g., abdominal abscess) is treated.

15. **What is the evidence supporting the use of a PA catheter?**
There is no definitive evidence in support of PA catheterization. A prospective trial of > 5700 patients with various disease processes (mostly medical patients) revealed that patients who underwent PA catheterization had *higher* 30-day mortality, *higher* hospital costs, and *longer* intensive care unit length of stay.[1]

Regardless, we recommend PA catheterization[3] for patients with cardiogenic shock, unexplained shock, or unexplained acidosis; all patients undergoing peripheral vascular surgery; and high-risk patients undergoing aortic surgery. Traumatically injured patients, patients with respiratory failure, and critically ill pediatric patients may benefit as well. If you cannot determine what the patient's volume status is, insert a PA catheter.

16. **Do central venous catheters or PA catheters need to be changed on a regular basis?**
In accordance with Centers for Disease Control guidelines, central venous catheters do not need to be replaced routinely if the exit wounds are dressed properly and sterilized routinely. PA catheters should be changed every 5 days to minimize risks of thrombus and infection.

When catheter-related infection is documented, a new catheter must be placed at a different location. Removed catheters in the setting of bacteremia are always sent for culture.

WEB SITES

1. http://www.acssurgery.com/abstracts/acs/acs0606.htm

2. http://www.acpmedicine.com/abstracts/sam/med1401.htm

BIBLIOGRAPHY

1. Connors AF, Speroff T, Dawson NV, et al: The effectiveness of right heart catheterization in the initial care of critically ill patients. JAMA 276:889–897, 1996.

2. Mermel LA, Maki DG: Infectious complications of Swan-Ganz pulmonary artery catheters. Am J Respir Crit Care Med 149:1020–1036, 1994.

3. Pulmonary Artery Consensus Conference Participants: Pulmonary artery consensus conference: Consensus statement. Crit Care Med 25:910–925, 1997.

4. Ruesch S, Walder B, Tramer MR: Complications of central venous catheters: Internal jugular versus subclavian access: A systematic review. Crit Care Med 30:454–460, 2002.

CHAPTER 13

SURGICAL WOUND INFECTION

Steven L. Peterson, D.V.M., M.D.

1. **Why should we worry about surgical wound infection?**

   Approximately 30 million patients undergo surgery each year in the United States, and 20% of these patients acquire at least one nosocomial infection in the postoperative period. Infections at surgical sites are the third most common form of these infections and complicate 1–12% of all operations. The risk of death is four times higher in patients who develop wound infections, and each infection costs $12,000–30,000 to treat.

   Commonly reported rates for specific operations are:

Cholecystectomy	3%	Inguinal herniorrhaphy	2%
Appendectomy	5%	Thoracotomy	6%
Colectomy	12%		

2. **What comprises a surgical wound infection?**

   Surgical wound infections more appropriately are called surgical site infections (SSIs) and must occur within 30 days of surgery unless a foreign body is left in situ. In the case of implanted foreign material, 1 year must elapse before surgery can be excluded as causative. SSIs are subdivided based on depth of tissue involvement into three clinically relevant categories.
   1. Superficial incisional SSIs—involving only the skin and subcutaneous tissue
   2. Deep incisional SSIs—involving deep soft tissue layers, such as fascial or muscle layers of the incision
   3. Organ space SSIs—involving any anatomic structure opened or manipulated during the operative procedure

3. **List the classic signs of superficial incisional, deep incisional, and organ space SSIs.**

   Superficial and deep incisional SSIs:
   - Calor (heat)
   - Rubor (redness)
   - Tumor (swelling)
   - Dolor (pain)
   - Purulent drainage

   Organ space SSIs should be suspected in the presence of systemic signs and symptoms:
   - Fever
   - Ileus
   - Shock

   Definitive diagnosis of organ space SSIs may require imaging studies.

4. **Why do these infections occur?**

   Many factors contribute; however, the fundamental principle is that traumatic and surgical wounds violate the normal protective layer of skin. The importance of an intact integument has been shown experimentally in which it was determined that an inoculum of 8 million bacteria is required for infection of intact skin, 1 million are required for violated skin, and only 100 are required when foreign material is present.

5. **Surgery always violates the skin and we often leave foreign material. How can we avoid SSIs?**

Although it is true that the basic act of surgery compromises the patients' defenses, we can take steps to prevent wound infection. These steps involve the surgeon and the patient.

6. **What can the surgeon do to decrease SSIs?**

The first step the surgeon can take is appropriate hand washing. The classic surgical scrub consists of 3 minutes of brushing with povidone-iodine or chlorhexidine gluconate. This protocol has been shown to have a high rate of noncompliance, which may contribute to SSIs. Data indicate improved compliance with comparable SSI rates using a much simpler protocol consisting of a 1-minute hand wash with nonantiseptic soap followed by hand-rubbing with a liquid aqueous alcoholic solution. Whether such simpler scrub protocols also can be applied in the future to the preparation of the patient is unknown.

7. **What else can the surgeon do to control SSIs?**

The surgeon may limit the duration of surgery and follow good surgical principles by eliminating dead space, controlling hemorrhage, minimizing placement of foreign material (including excessive suture), and exhibiting gentle tissue handling. The surgeon should ensure that the patient remains warm during the perioperative period. This simple act of warming was shown in two prospective studies to decrease significantly the incidence of SSIs.

8. **Can't the surgeon predict who is going to get infected and just give them lots of antibiotics to stop infection from happening?**

To a degree SSIs can be anticipated. Factors that have been shown to have some predictive value to the surgeon are the physical status of the patient as classified by the American Society of Anesthesiologists, results of intraoperative cultures, and duration of preoperative hospital stay. Adequacy of regional blood supply also is important, as evidenced by the low infection rate in facial wounds. The classic description of wounds based on degree of gross contamination also may be of value. This scheme places wounds into one of four categories:

1. **Clean wounds** are atraumatic wounds in which no inflammation is encountered, no breaks in sterile technique occur, and no hollow viscus is entered.
2. **Clean-contaminated wounds** are identical except that a hollow viscus is entered.
3. **Contaminated wounds** are caused by trauma from a clean source or by minor spillage of infected materials.
4. **Dirty-infected wounds** are caused by trauma from a contaminated source or gross spillage of infected material into an incision.

Reported infection rates for each category are 2.1%, 3.3%, 6.4%, and 7.1%. Antibiotics can help but only when used appropriately.

9. **How do I use antibiotics correctly to prevent SSIs?**

First by knowing what organism you are targeting, then choosing an appropriate antibiotic and delivering it at the appropriate time via the appropriate route. Because you usually will not have a preoperative culture to guide therapy, you need to base your choice of antibiotic on predicted organisms. Staphylococci are the most common skin organism and the most common etiologic agent in SSIs. Cefazolin, a first-generation cephalosporin, is usually the recommended antibiotic for prophylaxis in clean surgical procedures. In circumstances in which known contamination has occurred, initial antibiotics should be tailored based on the violated organ's common flora. If the gut was entered, enterobacteriaceae and anaerobes are common; biliary tract and esophageal incisions yield these organisms plus enterococci. The urinary tract or vagina may contain group D streptococci, *Pseudomonas*, and *Proteus* spp.

10. **If antibiotics are used, how and when should they be administered?**

Maximal benefit is obtained when tissue concentrations are therapeutic at the time of contamination. Efficacy is enhanced when prophylactic antibiotics are administered IV 20–30 minutes before surgical incision; late administration is similar to no administration. Multiple-dose regimens have no proven benefit over single-dose regimens. Indiscriminate antibiotic selection outside recommended hospital protocols may increase the incidence of SSIs. In special circumstances, administration routes other than IV may be indicated.

KEY POINTS: WOUND CLASSIFICATION AND INFECTION RATE (%)

1. Clean: atraumatic, no breaks in sterile technique, no entry into respiratory, alimentary, or genitourinary tract (2.1%)

2. Clean-contaminated: same as above except entry into respiratory, alimentary, or genitourinary tract (3.3%)

3. Contaminated: trauma from a clean source or minor spillage of infected materials (6.4%)

4. Dirty: trauma from a contaminated source or spillage of infected materials (7.1%)

11. **Name other routes that you would use for prophylactic antibiotic administration.**
In patients with nasal carriage of *Staphylococcus aureus*, intranasal administration of mupirocin ointment may have some efficacy in decreasing nosocomial and surgical site infections. In elective colon surgery, a meta-analysis of published studies indicated that orally administered antibiotics combined with IV antibiotics are superior to IV antibiotics alone in preventing surgical site infections.

12. **Does all that pulsatile lavage the surgeon uses in the operating room really do any good?**
Yes. High-pressure pulsatile lavage has been evaluated extensively in soft tissue contamination and shown to be seven times more effective in reducing bacterial load than bulb syringe lavage. The inherent elastic recoil of the soft tissues allows particulate matter to escape between pulses of fluid. The optimal pressure and pulse frequency seems to be 50–70 lb/in.^{2} and 800 pulses/min. Adding antibiotics to lavage solutions, although commonly practiced, has not been shown definitively to improve outcome.

13. **What can the patient do to help decrease SSIs?**
Stop smoking. Although obesity, poor nutritional status, advanced age, and diabetes are risk factors for SSIs, cigarette smoking is probably the leading preventable patient factor for SSIs just like it is the leading preventable cause of death and disability in the United States. Half of all people who smoke eventually die from a smoking-related illness. Smoking not only kills, but also more than triples that risk of incisional wound breakdown; in one study, smoking increased the incidence of SSIs in clean operative procedures sixfold, from 0.6% to 3.6%. Tobacco use results in decreased blood flow and decreased oxygen delivery to the wound. Toxic tobacco by-products also directly impede all stages of wound healing. Despite this knowledge, surgeons continue to operate electively on smokers, and most smokers continue to smoke up until the day of surgery.

14. **When prevention fails, what do you do for SSIs?**
The first line of therapy in SSIs is drainage. This is established by reopening the wound or, in the case of deep space infections, using computed tomography-guided or ultrasound-guided

techniques for drain placement or presurgical planning. Antibiotic therapy is used to control associated cellulitis and generalized sepsis.

15. **What may happen with untreated superficial or deep incisional SSIs?**
Locally the wound breaks down, and infection dissects through the tissue planes and continues to advance. If the infection progresses rapidly, necrotizing fasciitis may develop. Finally, the strength layers of the wound closure break open (dehisce).

16. **Define wound dehiscence.**
The partial or total disruption of any or all layers of the operative wound.

17. **Define evisceration.**
Rupture of the abdominal wall and extrusion of the abdominal viscera.

18. **What factors predispose to dehiscence?**
Age > 60 years, obesity and increased intra-abdominal pressure, malnutrition, renal or hepatic insufficiency, diabetes mellitus, use of corticosteroids or cytotoxic drugs, and radiation have been implicated in wound dehiscence. Infection also plays an important role; an infective agent is identified in more than half of wounds that undergo dehiscence. Despite these excuses, the most important factor in wound dehiscence is the adequacy of closure. Fascial edges should not be devitalized. Ideally the linea alba sutures should be placed neither too laterally nor too medially. Excessive lateral placement may incorporate the variable blood supply of the rectus abdominis muscle and compromise fascial circulation. Excessive medial placement misses the point of maximal strength at the transition zone between the linea alba and rectus abdominis sheath. In addition, sutures should be tied correctly without excessive tension, and suture material of adequate tensile strength should be chosen.

19. **When does wound dehiscence occur?**
It may occur at any time after surgery; however, it is most common between the 5th and 10th postoperative days, when wound strength is at a minimum.

20. **What are the signs and symptoms of wound dehiscence?**
Normally a ridge of palpable thickening (healing ridge) extends about 0.5 cm on each side of the incision within 1 week. Absence of this ridge may be a strong predictor of impending wound breakdown. More commonly, leakage of serosanguineous fluid from the wound is the first sign. In some instances, sudden evisceration may be the first indication of abdominal wound dehiscence. The patient also may describe a sensation of tearing or popping associated with coughing or retching.

21. **Describe the proper management of wound dehiscence.**
If the dehiscence is not associated with infection, elective reclosure may be the appropriate therapeutic course. If the condition of the patient or wound makes reclosure unacceptable, however, the wound should be allowed to heal by second intention. An unstable scar or incisional hernia may be dealt with at a later, safer time. Dehiscense of a laparotomy wound with evisceration is a surgical emergency with a reported mortality of 10–20%. Initial treatment in this instance consists of appropriate resuscitation while protecting the eviscerated organs with moist towels; the next step is prompt surgical closure. Exposed bowel or omentum should be lavaged thoroughly and returned to the abdomen; the abdominal wall should be closed; and the skin wound should be packed open. Vacuum-assisted wound closure may be valuable in select cases.

http://www.acssurgery.com/abstracts/acs/acs0102.htm

BIBLIOGRAPHY

1. Barie PS: Modern surgical antibiotic prophylaxis and therapy: Less is more. Surg Infect 1:23–29, 2000.

2. Garner GB, Ware DN, Cocanour CS, et al: Vacuum-assisted wound closure provides early fascial reapproximation in trauma patients with open abdomens. Am J Surg 182:630–638, 2001.

3. Kluytmans J, Voss A: Prevention of postsurgical infections: Some like it hot. Curr Opin Infect Dis 15:427–432, 2002.

4. Krueger JK, Rohrich RJ: Clearing the smoke: The scientific rationale for tobacco abstention with plastic surgery. Plast Reconstr Surg 108:1063–1073, 2001.

5. Myles PS, Iacono GA, Hunt JO, et al: Risk of respiratory complications and wound infection in patients undergoing ambulatory service. Anethesiology 97:842–847, 2002.

6. Parienti JJ, Thibon P, Heller R, et al: Hand-rubbing with an aqueous alcoholic solution vs traditional sugical hand scrubbing and 30-day surgical site infection rates: A randomized equivalence study. JAMA 288:722–727, 2002.

7. Perl TM, Cullen JJ, Wenzel RP, et al: Intranasal mupirocin to prevent postoperative Staphylococcus aureus infections. N Engl J Med 346:1871–1877, 2002.

8. Seltzer J, McGraw K, Horsman A, Korniewicz DM: Awareness of surgical site infections for advanced practice nurses. ACCN Clin Iss 13:398–409, 2002.

CHAPTER 14

PRIORITIES IN EVALUATION OF THE ACUTE ABDOMEN

Alden H. Harken, M.D.

1. **What is the surgeon's responsibility when confronted by a patient with an acute abdomen?**
   1. To identify how sick the patient is
   2. To determine whether the patient (a) needs to go directly to the operating room, (b) should be admitted for resuscitation or observation, or (c) can be sent safely home

2. **Which is the most dangerous course?**
   To send the patient home.

3. **Is it important to make the diagnosis in the emergency department?**
   No. Frequently time spent confirming a diagnosis in the emergency department is lost to inhospital resuscitation or treatment in the operating room. The only patient who needs a relatively firm diagnosis is a patient who is to be sent home.

4. **If the essential goal is not to make the diagnosis, what should the surgeon do?**
   1. Resuscitate the patient. Most patients do not eat or drink when they are getting sick. Most patients are depleted of at least several liters of fluid. Fluid depletion is worse in patients with diarrhea or vomiting.
   2. Start a big IV line.
   3. Replace lost electrolytes (see Chapter 7).
   4. Insert a Foley catheter.
   5. Examine the patient (frequently).

5. **Are symptoms and signs uniquely misleading in any groups of patients?**
   Yes. Watch out for the following groups:
   - The very young, who cannot talk.
   - Diabetics, because of visceral neuropathy.
   - The very old, in whom, much as in diabetics, abdominal innervation is dulled.
   - Patients taking steroids, which depress inflammation and mask everything.
   - Patients with immunosuppression (a heart or kidney transplant patient may act cheerful even with dead or gangrenous bowel).

6. **Summarize the history needed.**
   1. **The patient's age.** Neonates present with intussusception; young women present with ectopic pregnancy, pelvic inflammatory disease, and appendicitis; the elderly present with colon cancer, diverticulitis, and appendicitis.
   2. **Associated problems.** Previous hospitalizations, prior abdominal surgery, medications, heart and lung disease? An extensive gynecologic history is valuable; however, it is probably safer to assume that all women between 12 and 40 years old are pregnant.
   3. **Location of abdominal pain.** *Right upper quadrant:* gallbladder or biliary disease, duodenal ulcer. *Right flank:* pyelonephritis, hepatitis. *Midepigastrium:* duodenal or gastric ulcer, pancreatitis, gastritis. *Left upper quadrant:* ruptured spleen, subdiaphragmatic abscess.

Right lower quadrant: appendicitis (see Chapter 37), ectopic pregnancy, incarcerated hernia, rectus hematoma. *Left lower quadrant:* diverticulitis, incarcerated hernia, rectus hematoma. ***Note:*** Cancer, unless it obstructs (colon cancer), and bleeding (diverticulosis) typically do not hurt.

4. **Duration of pain.** The pain of a perforated duodenal ulcer or perforated sigmoid diverticulum is sudden, whereas the pain of pyelonephritis is gradual and persistent. The pain of intestinal obstruction is intermittent and crampy. Note: Although the surgeon is rotating through a gastrointestinal service, the patient may not know this and may present with urologic, gynecologic, or vascular pathology.

PHYSICAL EXAMINATION

7. **Are vital signs important?**
   Yes. They are vital. If heart rate and blood pressure are on the wrong side of 100 (heart rate > 100 beats/min, systolic blood pressure < 100 mmHg), watch out! Tachypnea (respiratory rate >16) reflects either pain or systemic acidosis. Fever may develop late, particularly in the immunosuppressed patient who may be afebrile in the face of florid peritonitis.

8. **What is rebound?**
   The peritoneum is well innervated and exquisitely sensitive. It is not necessary to hurt the patient to elicit peritoneal signs. Depress the abdomen gently and release. If the patient winces, the peritoneum is inflamed (**rebound tenderness**).

9. **What is mittelschmerz?**
   Mittelschmerz is pain in the middle of the menstrual cycle. Ovulation frequently is associated with intraperitoneal bleeding. Blood irritates the sensitive peritoneum and hurts.

10. **What do bowel sounds mean?**
    If something hurts (e.g., a sprained ankle), the patient tends not to use it. Inflamed bowel is quiet. Bowel contents squeezed through a partial obstruction produce high-pitched tinkles. Bowel sounds are notoriously unreliable, however.

11. **Explain the significance of abdominal distention.**
    Distention may derive from either intraenteric or extraenteric gas or fluid (worst of all, blood). Abdominal distention is always significant and bad.

12. **Is abdominal palpation important?**
    Yes. Remember, the patient is (or should be) the surgeon's friend. There is no need to cause pain. Palpation guides the surgeon to the anatomic zone of most tenderness (usually the diseased area). It is best to start palpation in an area that does not hurt. Rectal (test stool for blood) and pelvic examinations localize pathology further.

13. **What is Kehr's sign?**
    The diaphragm and the back of the left shoulder enjoy parallel innervation. Concurrent left upper quadrant and left shoulder pain indicate diaphragmatic irritation from a ruptured spleen or subdiaphragmatic abscess.

14. **What is a psoas sign?**
    Irritation of the retroperitoneal psoas muscle by an inflamed retrocecal appendix causes pain on flexion of the right hip or extension of the thigh.

LABORATORY STUDIES

15. **How is a complete blood count helpful?**
    1. **Hematocrit.** If the hematocrit is high (> 45%), the patient is most likely dry or may have chronic obstructive pulmonary disease. If it is low (< 30%), the patient probably has a more chronic disease (associated with blood loss—always do a rectal and test the stool for blood).
    2. **White blood cell count.** It takes hours for inflammation to release cytokines and elevate the white blood cell count. A normal white blood cell count is entirely consistent with significant abdominal trouble.

16. **Is urinalysis necessary?**
    Yes. White blood cells in the urine may redirect attention to the diagnosis of pyelonephritis or cystitis. Hematuria points to renal or ureteral stones. Because an inflamed appendix may lie directly on the right ureter, red and white blood cells may be found in the urine of patients with appendicitis.

17. **What is a "three-way of the abdomen"?**
    1. **Upright chest radiograph.** Look for free air under the diaphragm (perforated viscus) and pneumonia or pneumothorax.
    2. **Upright abdomen.** Look for free air under the diaphragm and air-fluid levels (intestinal obstruction). Remember to look for sigmoid or rectal air (partial obstruction).
    3. **Supine abdomen.** This radiograph tells nothing.
    Most ureteral stones can be visualized. Only 10% of gallstones are radiopaque, and appendiceal fecaliths are rarely noted.
    Honors: Air in the biliary system indicates a biliary-enteric fistula; this in association with intestinal air-fluid levels makes the diagnosis of gallstone ileus.

KEY POINTS: RADIOGRAPHIC EVALUATION FOR THE ACUTE ✔ ADBOMEN

1. May assist in diagnostic evaluation but should not supplant physical exam in evaluaton of an acute abdomen.

2. Three-way of the abdomen: look for free air under the diaphragm, intrathoracic pathology, air-fluid levels, dilated alimentary canal, distal air in rectum.

3. Ultrasound: useful for biliary, ob-gyn, and vascular assessments; may note intraperitoneal or retroperitoneal fluid collections.

4. Computed tomography: increasing use in clinical arena, with excellent visualization of abdominal structures. Drawbacks: cost, radiation exposure.

18. **What is a sentinel loop?**
    Except in children (who swallow everything, including air), small bowel gas is always pathologic. A single loop of small bowel gas adjacent to an inflamed organ (e.g., the pancreas) may point to the diseased organ.

19. **Is ultrasound valuable?**
    Yes, if the working diagnosis is cholecystitis, gallstones, ectopic pregnancy, ovarian cyst, abdominal aortic aneurysm, or intraperitoneal/retroperitoneal fluid.

20. Is abdominal computed tomography (CT) valuable?
Yes, if the working diagnosis is an intra-abdominal abscess (sigmoid diverticulitis), pancreatitis, retroperitoneal bleeding (leaking abdominal aortic aneurysm; this patient should have gone straight to the operating room), or intrahepatic or splenic pathology.

21. What is a double-contrast CT scan?
The bowel is delineated with barium or Gastrografin. The blood vessels are delineated with an iodinated vascular dye. The CT scan precisely displays the abdominal contents relative to vascular and intestinal landmarks. Contrast CT of pancreatitis is valuable to assess zones of perfusion or necrosis.

SURGICAL TREATMENT

22. If the patient is sick (and not getting better), what should be done?
After fluid resuscitation, the patient's abdomen should be explored. An exploratory laparotomy has been touted as the logical conclusion of a complete physical examination.

23. Is a negative laparotomy harmful?
Yes, but patients can uncomfortably survive a negative laparotomy, whereas missed bowel infarction (or appendicitis) can be life-threatening.

24. Name the most challenging problem in all of medicine.
An acute abdomen.

WEB SITE

http://www.acssurgery.com/abstracts/acs/acs0301.htm

BIBLIOGRAPHY

1. D'Agostino J: Common abdominal emergencies in children. Emerg Med Clin N Am 20:139–153, 2002.
2. Dhillon S, Halligan S, Goh V, et al: The therapeutic impact of abdominal ultrasound in patients with acute abdominal symptoms. Clin Radiol 57:268–271, 2002.
3. Gajic O, Urrutia LE, Sewani H, et al: Acute abdomen in the medical intensive care unit. Crit Care Med 30:1187–1190, 2002.
4. Rozycki GS, Tremblay L, Feliciano DV, et al: Three hundred consecutive emergent celiotomies in general surgery patients: Influence of advanced diagnostic imaging techniques and procedures on diagnosis. Ann Surg 235:681–689, 2002.

CHAPTER 15

SURGICAL INFECTIOUS DISEASE

Glenn W. Geelhoed, M.D., M.P.H., DTMH

1. **Have modern antibiotic developments controlled many, if not most, of the problems of surgical infection?**

   No. In seriously ill surgical patients in intensive care unit (ICU) settings, the problems of sepsis have increased and remain among the principal causes of death in ICU patients, especially those with multiple organ failure and impairments of host defense. Antibiotic treatment may change the biographical sketch of the flora associated with patients' deaths but cannot overcome the multiple causes of failing host resistance to infection that accompany barrier breeches to microbial invasion and the inflammatory and immunologic responses to the "usual suspects."

2. **What kinds of barrier breech allow microbial invasion that may set up surgical infection?**

   The skin and mucosal linings of the body maintain a barrier between the multifloral outside world and the sterile interior milieu of the tissues and organs (even when the outside world is a tube of heavily populated flora through the middle of usually sterile body cavities, such as the gastrointestinal [GI] tract). It is easy to see the barrier breech when a knife penetrates the skin, carrying exterior flora beneath the skin, or when that knife perforates and spills the contaminated contents of the gut into the abdomen. It is less obvious when the breech is caused by a low-flow state or when inadequate nutrition or toxins impair mucosal immunoglobulins, making the "bug–body barrier" permeable. These polymicrobial communities of organisms may begin to invade through the breech in such barriers, particularly if there are further failures in the third line of defense in humoral and cellular resistance.

3. **What is the difference between contamination and infection?**

   The presence of microorganisms does not an infection make!

   Resident communities of flora on body surfaces do little harm, and gut flora are even beneficial when contained in the gut. It is even possible for bacteria to be transiently present outside their usual commensal residences without constituting an infection in the normally intact host. For example, in vigorously brushing one's teeth, gram-negative bacteria of various kinds that are resident in the oral cavity are introduced into the bloodstream but probably quickly were eliminated by normal defense mechanisms—unless they met lowered host resistance or seeded a prosthetic heart valve.

4. **How can the enormous load of bacteria in the lower GI tract be beneficial?**

   Bugs can be beautiful. These are the same bacteria that have lived with and in humans symbiotically for millennia. They synthesize vitamin K—something we literally cannot do without—or crowd out pathogenic organisms by their overwhelming numbers. They also help to metabolize bile salts and play a role in detoxifying some environmental hazards, similar to septic systems.

5. **Whenever intraabdominal bowel spillage is encountered, is it mandatory to culture the fecal contamination and obtain sensitivities of all identified organisms?**

   No. There is a difference between contamination and infection. Therefore, cultures of fecal spillage into the peritoneum will not provide useful information. The contaminant, just because of its change in position with reference to the bowel wall, is not likely to be sterile. When would you like the laboratory to quit? Will you be content to hear a report of *Escherichia coli* and bacteroides, two of the more than 800 species that even the most compulsive laboratory can hardly be competent to identify, given the exposure to air and time lapse until processing on different media? How will information from a sampling error of mixed, community-acquired contaminants change your therapy? If, for instance, no anaerobes are identified from the fecal specimen, will you be so confident that they are not present as to exclude these species from coverage?

The lesson to be learned is that culture of community-acquired **contaminants** is expensive, incomplete, and unedifying; the culture of invading microbes in **infections**, particularly hospital-acquired microbes that persist after treatment, may give critical information and is a more appropriate use of microbiologic resources.

6. **What are preps (e.g., bowel preps)?**
    Preps are decontamination procedures, designed to reduce resident flora before an elective invasive procedure. Preps may take the form of a simple process such as an alcohol swab smeared over the skin before a quick prick of the subcutaneous injection or may involve preparation of a larger area of the skin surface for the surgical field of incision (see question 7).

    A bowel prep is similarly designed to reduce the resident flora in the gut through (1) mechanical catharsis (i.e., purge); (2) osmotic or volume dilution with large volumes of saline, other electrolyte solutions, or mannitol; or (3) oral administration of nonabsorbed antibiotics. Of these methods, the most important is clearly mechanical catharsis because it purges huge amounts of flora, which may account for up to two thirds the dry weight of colon contents. One of the most cogent reasons for the choice of certain oral antibiotics in bowel preps (see question 9) is their vigorous cathartic action.

7. **How is the skin or mucosal cavities of a patient sterilized to prepare a sterile field for operative incision?**
    There is one way, hardly recommended, by which patients can be "sterilized": similar to instruments and drapes, they can be placed in an autoclave. But short of this absurd example, the skin is never sterile. Decontamination processes are never perfect, particularly in so complex a tissue with crevices and accessory skin structures in which bacteria reside. Resting gloved hands on a "sterile field" does not include the skin or mucosal surfaces.

    At best, we simply reduce the flora to the low-level inoculum that can be handled by most intact host defense systems—as in the example of brushing your teeth—but living tissue surfaces are never "sterile." A method that kills all microbial organisms from such surfaces would also devitalize mammalian cells and render them more susceptible to lower-level microbial inocula.

8. **What means can be used to reduce surface resident flora without further injuring the skin or mucosa?**
    - **Volume lavage** (for mnemonic value only: dilution is the solution to pollution)
    - **Defatting**, which solubilizes the sebaceous oils that may trap flora
    - **Microbicidal killing** with a bacteriostatic agent

    To an amazing extent, one cheap, simple fluid that may serve as a diluent, fat solvent, and antimicrobial is alcohol. Alcohol is nearly ideal as prepping solution, with the minor disadvantages that it is dehydrating and minimally flammable. Because it vaporizes and disappears, flora may spread from interstices, outside the field, or even via aerosolized fallout onto the field, thus requiring the addition of extended-duration bacteriostasis to the alcohol prep.

    Iodine also kills bacteria but with a greater hazard to sensitive mammalian cells (it oxidizes the cell walls of small plants). A lower initial concentration of iodine and a longer duration of action can be achieved by incorporation of an iodophor, a substance in nearly universal use in preps. The application of moisture- and vapor-permeable "incise drapes" or desiccation preventing "ring drapes" may further retard repopulation of flora over the prepped (but still not sterile) field.

9. **What are "pipe cleaner" antibiotics?**
   Pipe cleaners are orally administered antibiotic regimens that reduce the flora in the GI tract, from which they are not well absorbed. They are an almost ideal component of bowel preps because they are potent cathartic agents and accomplish the vast majority of their "pipe cleaning" by mechanical purgative action. The most popular pipe cleaners include a neomycin or erythromycin base.

10. **What is selective gut decontamination? How does it work?**
    It does not work. This method used pipe cleaners in patients at high risk for the development of sepsis from multiple organ failure with the theoretic aim of reducing the risk involved in barrier breech of the GI tract and inoculation with gut flora. Good experimental evidence indicated that this method should reduce the high mortality rate in seriously ill patients at high risk of surgical sepsis. After prolonged clinical trials, however, it failed to demonstrate a benefit in patient survival. The likely reason is that whereas the laboratory studies were done in intact animal models with functioning host defense systems, failures of defense beyond the barrier breech may explain why selective gut decontamination failed to benefit seriously ill patients. Furthermore, resident hospital flora repopulated the purged gut over time, but with virulent forms of microbes selected by their resistance to the broad-spectrum antibiotics. The method still has some use in patients undergoing procedures such as high-dose chemotherapy or bone marrow transplantation and in some patients isolated in "life islands" (e.g., patients with immunodeficiency diseases or burns).

ANTIBIOTICS

11. **Are antibiotics the classic wonder drugs?**
    Only because you wonder if they are going to work, if they are going to cause more harm than good, and if the next generation will be unaffordable or toxic.
    Skepticism is healthy with regard to any procedure or agent in heath care but especially with regard to antibiotics, which are embraced almost universally as agents that both prevent and cure infections. The primacy of the host defense in this vital process and the potential interference by the very drugs given credit for infection control are overlooked. We must look critically at the limited role that antibiotics should play in health care and restrain their overuse, which generates even more harm than unnecessary expense.

12. **What is meant by generations of antibiotics, as in third-generation cephalosporins?**
    The earliest antibiotics were bacteriostatic, largely through interference in protein synthesis, so that they might keep a microorganism from reproducing even if they did not kill it. The difference between **infestation** (presence of living microbes in the host) and **infection** (replication and spread of microorganisms in the host) may be useful in understanding how earlier drugs possibly controlled infection but were less capable of eliminating organisms in any brief period of therapy.
    Penicillin changed all that. It may be the first antibiotic with a legitimate claim to the title "wonder drug" because it has the microbicidal capability of eradicating sensitive organisms. Penicillin was the first generation of the beta-lactam antibiotics, joined by the congener first-generation cephalosporins (e.g., cefazolin). They shared beta-lactam structure and had good gram-positive coverage with less range in any effect over gram-negative microbes.
    The second-generation beta-lactam antibiotics (e.g., cefoxitin) covered new classes of microbes beyond gram-positive aerobes, such as many of the Bacteroides species, but had little effect on gram-negative aerobic microbes. Because the third-generation cephalosporins covered some of the latter microbes, they were touted as single-agent therapy for all principal-risk flora.

As with penicillin, the original wonder drug, the wonderment waned with failures of the new agents because of rapidly induced antimicrobial resistance. The most easily measured and calculated difference in the generations is cost: wholesale values are about $2.00/g for the first generation, $5.00/g for the second, and $30.00/g for the third. Despite this bracket creep in cost, the higher generations lose some of their potency against the original gram-positive organisms for which the first-generation agents were truly wonderful. Therefore, it takes 2 g of moxalactam to be half as good as 1 g of cefazolin for gram-positive coverage. It does not take a pharmacoeconomist to ask, "What have I got in return for this 60-fold surcharge?"

13. **What is the role of third-generation cephalosporins in surgical prophylaxis?**
None (no more wondering here!). If the principal-risk flora are gram-positive, the first generation is better; if the anaerobic risk is sizable, the second generation is better. And either class is cheaper by far and seems to have generated less resistance than the third-generation cephalosporins, which are unconscionably expensive for use in prophylaxis and rarely as effective as other single-agent therapy for established surgical infection. Specific indications, such as pediatric meningitis, hospital-acquired pneumonia, or other specific infections outside the indications of surgical predominance, might use or exclude these agents.

14. **How do enzyme inhibitors combined with antibiotics enhance their antimicrobial spectrum?**
Microorganisms have defense mechanisms of their own, and the strains that have the capacity to make antibiotic-degrading enzymes achieve an unnatural selection advantage with the widespread use of antibiotics. This is what happened to penicillin: penicillinases emerged. But clever pharmaceutical manufacturers closed that loophole for bacterial ingenuity in degrading penicillin by strategic placement of a methyl group to ruin the survival fitness of penicillinase producers. Methicillin was the result, but the persistence of the microbes means that we now have a plague of methicillin-resistant *Staphylococcus aureus* (MRSA). Besides, microbes outnumber pharmaceutical manufacturers and have a shorter turnaround time than the approval process of the Food and Drug Administration (FDA). Microbes will always be ahead of us in ingenuity if only because of their numbers.

Newer strategies by the bacteria included the production of beta-lactamases. The response of the pharmaceutical industry was a group of inhibitors of beta-lactamase, such as clavulanic acid or sulbactam. The combination of a beta-lactamase inhibitor with a modified penicillin such as ampicillin should have enhanced activity against bacteria that produce beta-lactamase, provided that they were ampicillin-sensitive in the first place. Higher doses of the original agent for a shorter time may accomplish the same effect, often at lower cost, because the combined drugs were developed much more recently and are under patent protection.

15. **What are the most expensive kinds of antibiotic therapy?**
- Drugs that are given when they are not needed.
- Drugs that are badly needed but do not work.
- Drugs that cause more harm than good because of host toxicity, whatever their antibiotic potential.

16. **Can oral antibiotics be given in place of intravenous antibiotics in seriously ill surgical patients?**
Yes, if only they could take them! These patients almost invariably can take nothing by mouth (NPO), are often unconscious, and are as likely as not to be on a ventilator. In addition, the gut has been put out of commission by nasogastric suction tubes, laparotomy, and ileus, and primary intraabdominal problems often associated with the need for the antibiotics, such as intraabdominal sepsis and pancreatitis. Usually such patients are on complete gut rest and are likely to be on parenteral nutrition as well.

The attempt to use some form of gut-delivered antibiotic is based on the favorable pharmacokinetics and spectrum of quinolones, which can be started intravenously and switched as soon as possible to the oral form when feeding has resumed. Nearly all such patients begin on some form of intravenous (IV) antibiotic program and the start-up of the antibiotic regimen is more important than the form to which patients are tapered before treatment is discontinued.

PROPHYLAXIS

17. Should systemic antibiotic prophylaxis be used in elective colon resection?
Yes, beyond any statistical shadow of a doubt. At least two dozen clinical trials have been carried out using placebo controls against a variety of antibiotics, principally those active against at least the anaerobic-predominant flora, and nearly all have shown a reduction in infectious complications in the antibiotic group. Never again should this point need repeating, and no patient should be placed at risk when systemic antibiotic prophylaxis has been established as the standard of care. No new clinical trials against placebo in this group of patients with known risk can be performed ethically given the confirmed risk reduction.

Other risk groups (e.g., cesarean section after membrane rupture) besides patients undergoing colon resection have been standardized by trials in large patient populations and have shown similar risk reduction. The benefit of prophylaxis has been demonstrated. In other groups of patients that cannot be standardized because of unusual contamination factors or unique factors of host resistance impairment, guidelines for rational prophylaxis should follow similar principles.

18. Are two prophylactic doses better than one in preventing infection? Are three doses better still?
Only one dose of prophylactic antibiotic can be proved, beyond statistical or clinical doubt, to be efficacious—the dose in systemic circulation at the time of the inoculum. Whether the dose needs to be repeated one or more times during the 24 hours after the inoculum depends on the blood levels of the drug, which are largely a function of protein binding and clearance rate. We also know for sure that 10 days of the same prophylactic drug that is efficacious if given immediately before the inoculum results in a higher risk of infection than no antibiotic at all.

KEY POINTS: PREOPERATIVE ANTIBIOTIC PROPHYLAXIS

1. Timing of administration is the most important factor.

2. Dose 30 minutes before incision so that antibiotic is circulating before the inoculum.

3. No evidence supports continuation of prophylaxis beyond 24 hours.

19. What factors determine the timing of antibiotic administration under the criteria of prophylaxis?
The one immutable principle has been set out above—the most important element in timing of prophylaxis is that the drug be circulating before the inoculum. When should it stop? When the reduction in infection risk is no longer provable and before continued use will defeat the prophylactic purpose (as explained above). To summarize with an arbitrary rule of thumb: *there is no justification for prophylactic antibiotic 24 hours after the inoculum of an invasive procedure.*

What does this rule imply? Should we not continue prophylaxis for weeks to cover the presence of a prosthetic hip joint? Presumably, the prosthetic hip will be in the patient for many years—but surely you do not argue that the antibiotic should continue on a daily basis as long as the hip is in place! What is "prophylaxed" is not the prosthetic hip but the procedure of implantation. And it is not only implantation that poses a risk to the patient with a prosthesis—so does hemorrhoidectomy done years later, for which prophylaxis is made mandatory by the presence of the hip prosthesis.

The prosthetic or rheumatic heart valve is a risk, but the indication for the use of prophylactic antibiotics is an invasive procedure—a root canal is an example in which an inoculum is unavoidable. *Operations are covered by prophylactic antibiotics; the conditions that are risk factors during the operation are not.*

20. **To be safe, why not administer prophylactic antibiotics to all patients undergoing any kind of operation?**
Can you give me the indication for a prophylactic antibiotic in a patient undergoing a clean elective surgical procedure that implants no prosthesis, such as hernia repair?

"Sure," one of my brighter students once responded, "the patient who has a serious impairment in host response, such as acute granulocytic leukemia in blast crisis."

I responded, "Why on earth are you fixing his hernia? That is a clean error [hopefully not a clean kill] in surgical judgment that has nothing to do with antibiotics at all. A patient with that degree of host impairment does not undergo an elective surgical procedure."

Rule of thumb: *If you can provide the indication for a prophylactic antibiotic to cover a clean elective nonprosthetic operation for a patient, you have provided the contraindication for the operation.*

MANAGEMENT OF SURGICAL INFECTIONS

21. **What is the drug of choice for the treatment of an abscess?**
A knife. Surgically drain the abscess. Abscesses have no circulation of blood within them to deliver an antibiotic. The antibiotic, even if injected directly into the abscess, would be worthless because the abscess contains a soup of dead microorganisms and white blood cells (WBCs). Even if the organisms were barely alive, they would not be reproducing and incorporating the antibiotic. The drug most likely would not work at all at the pH and pKa conditions of the abscess environment.

If there is an indication for an antibiotic, it would be in the circulation around the compressed inflammatory edge of the abscess and the cellulitis (at the vascularized "peel of the orange") and uncontaminated tissue planes through which the necessary drainage must be carried out. A *focal* infection is managed by a *local* treatment, which is both *necessary* in all abscesses and *sufficient* treatment in many. Adjunctive systemic antibiotics are occasionally indicated for protection of the tissues through which drainage is carried out. If it helps to make this fundamental surgical principle clear, here is the rule of thumb for management of abscesses: *Where there is pus, let there be steel.* Perhaps one of the most gratifying procedures in all of medicine is the drainage of pus with immediate relief of local and systemic symptoms (e.g., a perirectal abscess).

22. **Which abscess treatment is the important one in determining the outcome of a patient with intraabdominal sepsis?**
It is the drainage of the *last* abscess that counts. There should be little applause for drainage of a pelvic abscess in the patient who retains a subphrenic abscess. The patient responds dramatically when the *last* pus is drained.

This has been an area of significant advance in managing surgical infections because noninvasive scanning capability has facilitated the finding of multiple pockets of pus. Furthermore, such modalities as the computed tomography (CT) scan not only *find* but also percutaneously *direct the fixing* of the last abscess. What might have been an indication for an exploratory return trip to the operating room only a decade before (i e , a failing patient on appropriate therapy should trigger the first response, "Where's the pus?") is now a good indication for a CT scan to find and drain the focal infection.

23. **Which is preferred for draining an intraabdominal abscess, a needle or a knife?**
Which can be done most expeditiously? The patient with intraabdominal sepsis is very ill, and the earliest, safe drainage is the procedure of choice. There may be advantages to the less invasive CT scanning, which can be repeated and has less morbidity if the results are negative. Surgery, on the other hand, can fix associated conditions that may have caused the abscess, such as the devitalized loop of bowel or the leak in the anastomosis that can be exteriorized. Each method is likely to find multiple collections, and each can leave external drains for lavage and continuing drainage. Whether by needle or by knife, the urgency and adequacy of local treatment of focal infection determine which methods takes precedence.

24. **What is the role of gallium scintiscanning in early finding of abscesses in the abdomen?**
There is none. Ordering a gallium scan is a temporizing means of self-deception that some progress is being made in finding out what is wrong with the patient. In fact, it merely postpones decisions about intervention in critical illness for several days, often to a point beyond salvage. Gallium scanning involves bowel prepping, a vigorous WBC response from an active bone marrow, and false-positive test results at the sites of tubes and incisions. It is a time-consuming and unreliable test that is the obverse of the principles of *early* and *definitive* management. Do not order a gallium scan to satisfy a consultant that "something is being done for this patient."

EXTRA-CREDIT QUESTIONS

25. **Should all patients undergoing elective laparotomy receive prophylactic antibiotic coverage?**
No. Doing so would contribute to driving up the cost of antibiotics and their complication rate and devaluing formerly good drugs by rendering them useless against common flora against which they were once highly potent. Operating room nurses have always classified the kind of operation by its status with respect to microbial exposure: clean, contaminated, or septic. These categories are approximation of the microbial risk exposure, and if additionally are superimposed categories of patient resistance (higher risk associated with aging, obesity or other malnutrition, concomitant drugs, or viral or mycobacterial or neoplastic disease immune compromise), these same strata are called class I, II, and III.

26. **Which abscess is the most important one to be drained?**
It is the *last* abscess that counts in drainage because the patient's dramatic response is often only achieved when the last pus is drained. Draining a pelvic abscess, for example, but leaving behind a subphrenic abscess, would not result in the quenching of the inflammatory mediators of the sepsis syndrome.

27. **Is postoperative fever the earliest and most frequent sign of an incisional infection?**
Postoperative fevers are much more frequent than are wound infections, and the typical wound infection presents far later. The principal sources of postoperative fever are:
   Wind (atelectasis or pneumonia)
   Water (urinary tract infection)
   Walk (get your patient up and around; thrombophlebitis)
   Wound

28. **Should you begin amphotericin at the first isolation of *Candida* species drawn from any intravenous catheter line?**
No. Again, remember the distinction between colonization and infection, as well as the source from which the specimen is taken. The IV lines through which hyperalimentation solutions are

infused make colonization possible. The presence of a fungus such as *Candida* species is frequent in patients who do not have an invasive fungal infection or a true candidemia. The latter might be distinguished from catheter colonization by a blood culture drawn from another source, such as a venopuncture. If evidence of any invasive fungal infection is also present (e.g., as endoscopic biopsy of inflammatory mucositis), a choice of antifungal therapies is now indicated.

Topical fungal solutions (e.g., mycostatin mouthwashes or lavage) may control the local fungal infection and may sometimes be instituted as prophylaxis in high-risk patients (e.g., patients on antirejection therapy for bone marrow or solid organ transplantation).

Systemic antifungal agents include fluconazole, caspifungin, and amphotericin.

29. Are antibiotic drug combinations always superior to a single antibiotic agent?
Monotherapy is superior to combination antibiotic treatment regimens, but this is provable probably only in the highest-risk patients. With the carbapenem class antibiotic agents, a large multicenter clinical trial proved imipenem therapy superior to aminoglycoside and a macrolide antibiotic, with survival demonstrably superior only in the patients with the highest APACHE scores. Ertapenem monotherapy was the equivalent of ceftriaxone and metronidazole in a smaller, more recent trial.

More is not always better, and the R and S on culture reports does not translate directly to the M and M (morbidity and mortality) at the Death and Complications Conference reports. It is not just important that the effective antibiotic regimen kills the bacteria; also important are *how* this microbicidal effect is carried out and what effect it may have on the patient in quenching or prolonging the systemic inflammatory response.

30. Is antibody treatment of circulating endotoxin a clinically important tool?
Not yet. The neutralization of circulating endotoxin might give a theoretic benefit to patients with sepsis, and animal studies looked promising. But antigen/antibody complexes initiate complement cascade and release of activate leukocyte products such as leukotrienes that may further augment the inflammatory process. The complexes are also filtered in the kidney where they may further impair renal function. To date, no clinical therapeutic benefit has been demonstrated for such monoclonal antibody therapy.

31. What is the role of human recombinant activated protein C in patients with sepsis?
Of the multiple clinical trials of mediator neutralization or receptor blockade, the evidence to date seems marginally favorable only for a few, and the major response to treatment comes from early and complete control of the focus of sepsis (not the cytokine sequelae).

WEB SITES

1. http://www.acssurgery.com/abstracts/acs/acs0102.htm

2. http://www.medscape.com
    Search: preoperative antibiotics

BIBLIOGRAPHY

1. Bartlett JG: Intra-abdominal sepsis. Med Clin North Am 79:599–617, 1995.
2. Bernard GR, Vincent JL, Laterre PF, et al: Efficacy and safety of recombinant human activated protein C for severe sepsis. N Engl J Med 344:699, 2001.

3. Bilik R, Burnweit C, Shandling B: Is abdominal cavity culture of any value in appendicitis? Am J Surg 175:267–270, 1998.

4. Christou NV, Turgeon P, Wassef R, et al: Management of intra-abdominal infections. The case for intraoperative cultures and comprehensive broad-spectrum antibiotic coverage. The Canadian Intra-abdominal Infection Study Group. Arch Surg 131:1193–1201, 1996.

5. Ciftci AO, Tanyei FC, Buyukpamukcu N, Hicsonmea A: Comparative trial of four antibiotic combinations for perforated appendicitis in children. Eur J Surg 163:591–596, 1997.

6. Falagas ME, Barefoot L, Griffith J, et al: Risk factors leading to clinical failure in the treatment of intra-abdominal or skin/soft tissue infections. Eur J Clin Microbiol Infect Dis 15:913–921, 1996.

7. Geelhoed GW: Preoperative skin preparation: Evaluation of efficacy, timing, convenience, and cost. Infect Surg 85:648–669, 1985.

II. TRAUMA

INITIAL ASSESSMENT

Eric L. Sarin, M.D., and John B. Moore, M.D.

CHAPTER 16

1. **What is the "golden hour"?**
   The first hour after injury provides a unique opportunity to provide life-saving interventions. Because more than half of trauma deaths occur early due to bleeding or brain injury, rapid transport, appropriate triage, evaluation, resuscitation, and intervention can affect outcomes. The "golden hour" concept needs to be extended to several hours in the rural setting, but with the same structured approach. Trauma surgeons harbor the unique idea that an injured patient is their responsibility *before* they reach the hospital.

2. **Name the major components of the initial assessment of the trauma patient.**
   Primary survey, resuscitation, secondary survey, reevaluation, and definitive care.

3. **What is the purpose of the primary survey?**
   To identify life-threatening injuries in a prioritized time frame.

4. **Define the ABCDE mnemonic of the primary survey that reinforces the fact that life-threatening injuries kill in a predictable order.**
   A **A**irway control with cervical spine (C-spine) protection
   B **B**reathing with oxygenation and ventilation
   C **C**irculation with hemorrhage control
   D **D**isability or neurologic status
   E **E**xposure of patient with temperature control

5. **What are the adjuncts to the primary survey?**
   All trauma patients should receive high-flow supplemental oxygen by nasal cannula or face-mask. Continuous monitoring should include pulse oximetry, cardiac ECG monitor, and a cycled blood pressure cuff. Two large-bore IV lines are placed as blood is drawn for screening tests, including blood type and crossmatch. Nasogastric or orogastric tubes are placed for gastric decompression and to prevent aspiration. A Foley catheter is inserted to assess urine flow and character of urine. Radiographs should include the "big three" for major trauma "mechanism": cervical spine, chest x-ray, and pelvic x-ray.

6. **Identify the one concept that can prevent unexpected acute deterioration of the trauma patient during initial assessment.**
   Re-evaluation. If deterioration occurs, proceed back to the ABCs and start over again.

7. **Name the two major causes of death during the first 24 hours after injury.**
   Exsanguination and central nervous system injury.

8. **How is the airway assessed?**
   Ask the patient a question. A response in a normal voice suggests that the airway is not in immediate danger. A hoarse, weak, or stridorous response may imply airway compromise. An agitated or combative response indicates hypoxia (agitation or confusion in any surgical

patient always means hypoxia)—until proved otherwise. No response indicates the need for a "definitive airway"(a cuffed tube in the trachea).

9. **Name the most common causes of upper airway obstruction in the trauma patient.**
The tongue, followed by blood, loose teeth or dentures, vomit, and soft tissue edema.

10. **What are the initial maneuvers used to restore an open airway?**
The chin lift and jaw thrust physically displace the mandible and the tongue anteriorly to open the airway, and manual clearance of debris and suctioning of the oropharynx optimize patency. Oropharyngeal and nasopharyngeal airways (trumpets) are useful adjuncts in maintaining an open airway in obtunded patients. All of these maneuvers must be accomplished with in-line stabilization of the cervical spine.

11. **What are the indications for a definitive airway?**
Apnea, inability to maintain or protect the airway (compromised consciousness), inability to maintain oxygenation, hemodynamic instability, need for muscle relaxation or sedation, and need for hyperventilation.

12. **List the types of definitive airway that are available.**
- Orotracheal intubation
- Nasotracheal intubation
- Surgical airway (cricothyroidotomy or tracheostomy)

13. **When should a surgical airway be performed?**
In any circumstance in which the patient requires a definitive airway but neither orotracheal nor nasotracheal intubation can be accomplished safely, such as in patients with extensive maxillo-facial trauma or high-risk anterior neck trauma. Cricothyroidotomy should not be performed in patients with direct laryngeal trauma, patients with tracheal disruption, or patients < 12 years old. Tracheostomy and transtracheal ventilation are the preferred alternatives under these circumstances.

14. **How does one "clear the C-spine"?**
Injury to the cervical spine (C-spine) must be excluded before moving the head or neck of the trauma patient. Alert patients without other significant injuries may be moved without x-rays if they are asymptomatic and have no cervical spine tenderness to direct palpation. Patients with symptoms or other major (distracting) injury require a three-view cervical spine series (anteroposterior, lateral, and odontoid) to evaluate the cervical spine. Visualization to the level of C7–T1 is mandatory because 10% of unstable cervical spine fractures occur at this level. If the standard three-view series is inadequate, a "swimmer's view" (patient's arm extended above the head with the x-ray focused through the axilla) can be performed. In high-risk patients with symptoms and equivocal films or sedated/intubated intensive care unit patients, computed tomography (CT) scan of the neck may be necessary to rule out unstable bony injury. Persistent symptoms in the absence of bony injury may require evaluation of potential ligamentous injury with flexion-extension films, CT, or magnetic-resonance imaging.

15. **Do cervical spine collars adequately immobilize the cervical spine?**
No. Soft collars allow for almost 100% of normal flexion, extension, and rotation. A semi-rigid (Philadelphia) collar allows 30% normal flexion and extension, > 40% normal rotation, and > 60% lateral movement. Proper immobilization of the cervical spine is achieved with the patient on a backboard in a semirigid collar, lateral sandbags, and anterior 3-inch adhesive taping.

KEY POINTS: CERVICAL SPINE CLEARANCE

1. Alert patients without other significant potentially distracting injuries can be cleared without radiographic evaluation in the absence of neck pain and midline cervical tenderness on palpation.

2. Obtunded, comatose, or alert patients with distracting injuries (e.g., long bone fractures) require maintenance of C-spine precautions and radiographic evaluation of the C-spine with three-view cervical spine series.

3. C7-T1 must be visualized; otherwise the "swimmer's view" is required.

4. If there is no radiographic evidence of injury but midline tenderness persists, obtain flexion-extension films to evaluate for ligamentous injury.

5. Spinal cord injury without radiographic abnormality is more common in children and usually can be detected with CT or MRI.

16. **What technique can help increase the success of oral tracheal intubation?**
Rapid sequence intubation with manual in-line stabilization.

17. **Discuss nonairway conditions that pose an immediate threat to breathing.**
Tension pneumothorax occurs from air in the pleural space under pressure. The most common culprit is an iatrogenic pneumothorax caused by overenthusiastic positive-pressure ventilation (watch out, it's easy to get excited when you are "bagging" a recently intubated patient). Treatment consists of needle decompression of the chest followed by tube thoracostomy (36 tube midaxillary line at the fourth to fifth intercostal space). An **open pneumothorax** results from an open wound of the chest wall causing free communication of the pleural space with the atmosphere interfering with the thoracic bellows mechanism. The ineffective ventilation responds to coverage of the opening and insertion of a chest tube. **Flail chest** results from multiple rib fractures of contiguous ribs creating a free-floating segment that limits breathing. A small flail chest in a healthy patient responds to oxygen supplementation and adequate analgesia. Large flail chest in less healthy patients requires prompt endotracheal intubation and mechanical ventilation.

18. **What are the preferred sites of emergent IV access?**
Peripheral venous access in the upper extremities (i.e., antecubital fossa) with a large-bore 14G or 16G catheter. Percutaneous or cutdown alternatives include the ankle or groin saphenous vein. Central venous access is indicated for measurement of central venous pressure after the initial fluid boluses and can help explain ongoing hemodynamic instability. Good flow rates can be achieved by using the shorter, larger introducing catheters during aggressive fluid infusion. In children < 6 years old, the interosseous route at the distal femur or proximal tibia provides a surprisingly effective alternative.

19. **What are the key elements in assessing hemodynamic stability?**
Mental status (**a**lert, **v**erbal, **p**ain, and **u**nresponsive), skin perfusion (pink/warm versus pale/cool), and hemodynamic parameters (blood pressure, heart rate, respiratory rate). Remember the gross estimates of systolic blood pressure (SBP) by palpable pulses. The radial (wrist) pulse estimates SBP > 80 mmHg; femoral (groin) pulse, SBP > 70 mmHg; and carotid (neck) pulse, SBP > 60 mmHg. The urine flow rates assist in estimating end-organ perfusion.

20. **Identify the three components to the minineurologic examination during the primary survey.**
    Mental status (when you look the patient in the eye, does he look back?), pupillary status, and best motor activity. This brief interaction assists in differentiating a toxic metabolic insult versus mass lesion. The pupils should be examined for size, symmetry, and reactivity.

21. **List the three main components of the Glasgow Coma Scale (GCS).**
    1. Best eye-opening response, scored 1–4.
    2. Best verbal response, scored 1–5.
    3. Best motor response, scored 1–6.
    Points from each component are added up. An overall score of 13–15 indicates a mild closed head injury, a score of 9–12 indicates a moderate head injury, and a score < 8 indicates a severe head injury. **A general rule:** A GCS score of ≤ 8 mandates endotracheal intubation.

22. **What is the most common cause of shock in the trauma patient?**
    Hypovolemia from acute blood loss. The other less common causes of shock include cardiogenic, neurogenic, or septic.

23. **What fluids should be used for initial resuscitation?**
    The mainstay of fluid resuscitation is rapid crystalloid infusion (lactated Ringer's or normal saline). Colloid infusions are more expensive, show no proven advantages, and have no role in acute trauma resuscitation. Blood should be administered to optimize oxygen-carrying capacity when crystalloid infusion is > 50 mL/kg or if the patient presents with class IV hemorrhage. The general rule for crystalloid infusion to replace blood loss is a 3:1 ratio of crystalloid to blood.

24. **Discuss the most common causes of cardiogenic shock after injury and how they are differentiated and treated.**
    Acute pericardial tamponade is caused by the accumulation of blood or air within the pericardial sac under pressure. This accumulation results in impairment of venous return and right ventricular filling/emptying. Treatment is directed toward temporary pericardial sac decompression and movement to the operating room for definitive therapy. **Tension pneumothorax**, associated with increased intrathoracic pressure, likewise results in impaired venous return. Treatment should be urgent chest decompression by needle followed by chest tube. **Air embolism** results in cardiac dysfunction from the air within the coronary arteries. Treatment should include cross-clamping of the pulmonary hilum, aspiration of the left ventricle, and massaging of the coronary arteries (to milk out any air). **Cardiac contusion** rarely leads to shock. Treatment includes invasive cardiac monitoring with judicious fluid restoration and appropriate cardiotropic medications.

25. **How can I learn proficiency at an initial assessment?**
    Take the Advanced Trauma Life Support course promulgated by the American College of Surgeons, which emphasizes the skills of providing a definitive airway, a competent chest tube, and proper IV access.

26. **Which diagnostic technique has expedited the localization of major blood loss, assisted in diagnosing pericardial tamponade, and replaced diagnostic peritoneal lavage?**
    Ultrasound. This technique is rapid, noninvasive, user-friendly, portable, compact, and reproducible.

27. **What does FAST mean with respect to evaluation of the trauma patient?**
    *F*ocused *a*ssessment for the *s*onographic examination of the *t*rauma patient. The four areas examined in this sequence are pericardial area, right upper quadrant, left upper quadrant, and the pelvis.

CONTROVERSIES

28. **What is the role of the pneumatic antishock garment?**
The military antishock trouser (MAST) has fallen out of favor in most instances. The MAST suit is valuable for patients requiring long-distance transfer who have major bleeding from pelvic fractures. The MAST suit should be avoided in the presence of major thoracoabdominal trauma, especially if a diaphragmatic injury is suspected. The traction splints still are preferred for femur fracture transfer; they decrease bleeding and assist with pain control.

29. **In a patient in shock with an obvious head injury, grossly positive peritoneal aspirate, and suggestion of a thoracic aortic injury on chest x-ray, what are the priorities after initial resuscitation?**
An exploratory laparotomy is indicated based on the hemodynamic instability in the face of a grossly positive peritoneal tap (even if the patient has torn his aorta, you should fix active intra-abdominal bleeding first). The patient should have a CT scan of the head and chest immediately thereafter. Intraoperative intracranial pressure monitoring may be diagnostic and therapeutic.

WEB SITES

1. http://www.east.org/tpg/chap3.pdf

2. http://www.east.org/tpg/chap3u.pdf

3. http://www.east.org/tpg/bluntabd.pdf

4. http://www.surgery.ucsf.edu/eastbaytrauma/Protocols/ER%20protocol%20pages/c-spine_eval.htm

5. http://www.surgery.ucsf.edu/eastbaytrauma/Protocols/ER%20protocol%20pages/FAST-files/FAST.htm

BIBLIOGRAPHY

1. American College of Surgeons, Committee on Trauma: Advanced Trauma Life Support Course, 6th ed. Chicago, American College of Surgeons, 1997.

2. Bell RM, Krantz BE: Initial assessment. In Mattox KL, Feliciano DV, Moore EE (eds): Trauma, 4th ed. Norwalk, CT, Appleton & Lange, 2000.

3. Biffl WL, Moore EE, Harken AH: Emergency department thoracotomy. In Mattox KL, Feliciano DV, Moore EE (eds): Trauma, 4th ed. Norwalk, CT, Appleton & Lange, 2000.

4. Rozycki GS, Ballard RB: Ultrasound in the initial trauma evaluation. In Trunkey DD, Lewis FR (eds): Current Therapy of Trauma, 4th ed. St. Louis, Mosby, 1999.

CHAPTER 17

POSTTRAUMATIC HEMORRHAGIC SHOCK

John B. Moore, M.D., and Ernest E. Moore, M.D.

1. **Are hemorrhagic shock and hypovolemic shock the same?**
Yes.

2. **What is hemorrhagic shock?**
Shock exists when the cardiovascular system is no longer able to meet the body's metabolic and oxygen needs—inadequate tissue perfusion.

    Hemorrhage is the most common cause of shock after injury. Depletion of the vascular volume results in decrease of the driving pressure returning blood to the heart, decrease of the end-diastolic ventricular volume, and decrease in stroke volume; all result in decrease in cardiac output.

3. **What is the initial management of hemorrhagic/hypovolemic shock?**
Prompt and aggressive fluid resuscitation.

4. **Describe the cellular manifestations of hemorrhagic shock.**
Inadequately perfused and oxygenated cells are unable to perform normal aerobic metabolism. This inability results in the production of lactic acid, creating a "gap" metabolic acidosis. The production of adenosine triphosphate (ATP) is decreased, and the cell no longer can maintain membrane polarization/integrity. The first evidence of this is swelling of the endoplasmic reticulum, followed by mitochondrial damage, lysozyme rupture, and the entry of sodium and water into the cell. The loss of interstitial water into cells exacerbates the extracellular and the intravascular volume deficit.

5. **List the clinical manifestations of hemorrhagic shock.**
   - Hemodynamic instability with rapid pulse > 100 beats/min and blood pressure < 90 mmHg.
   - Altered mental status with lethargy and confusion.
   - Decreases in urine output < 0.5 mL/kg/h, central venous pressure, pulmonary capillary wedge pressure, cardiac output, and mixed venous oxygenation saturation (revealed by invasive monitoring).

6. **How can blood volume be estimated in adults and children?**
In adults, multiply the ideal weight in kg × 7% (70 cc/kg).
In children, multiply ideal weight in kg × 9% (90 cc/kg).

7. **State the first physiologic response to hypovolemia.**
The patient tries to compensate for the decrease in stroke volume by increasing heart rate (tachycardia).

8. **What are the skin manifestations?**
The skin becomes cool, clammy, and pale. The subcutaneous veins collapse (making it hard to start an IV line). Capillary refill is delayed ≥ 2–3 seconds.

9. **Can the neck veins tell you anything?**
Lack of pulsations or collapsed external jugular veins indicate low right heart filling pressure (i.e., hypovolemia); conversely, distended veins indicate heart failure or cardiogenic shock.

10. **Is the hematocrit a reliable guide for estimating acute blood loss?**
    No. A decrease in the hematocrit occurs with refill of the intravascular space from the interstitial space or during administration of exogenous crystalloid resuscitation fluid. This process is not immediate, and serial hematocrits do reflect blood loss.

11. **What is the appropriate choice for IV solution during resuscitation?**
    Lactated Ringer's or normal saline. Isotonic crystalloid fluid requirements in hemorrhagic shock are estimated at three times the blood loss (3:1 rule). The initial volume replacement should be directed by the response to therapy rather than relying on estimated blood loss (the amount of blood on the pavement is a guess). Don't add dextrose to the initial fluids; this just exacerbates the physiologic hyperglycemia and provokes an osmotic diuresis. Dextrose 5% is added to IV solutions after initial resuscitation for its protein-sparing effect in the fasting trauma patient.

12. **What is base deficit, and how is it useful during resuscitation?**
    Base deficit depends on the hematocrit, pH, and Pco_2 and provides information on the metabolic component of acidosis. If you correct the Pco_2 back to 40 mmHg, the pH should be 7.40. If your patient is still acidotic, he or she has a base deficit. The worse the base deficit, the lower (less adequate) is your patient's peripheral perfusion.

13. **What are the clinical classifications of shock and the associated clinical manifestations?**
    See Table 17-1. But watch out—these estimates are not nearly as accurate or valuable as determining your patient's response to therapy/resuscitation.

TABLE 17-1.	CLINICAL CLASSIFICATIONS OF SHOCK	
Class	Description	Clinical Manifestations
Class 1	Blood volume loss ≤ 15% Can compare this with a blood donor	Occasional mild tachycardia, headache, and postural dizziness
Class 2	Blood volume loss ≤ 30%	Tachycardia, tachypnea, and decreased pulse pressure
Class 3	Blood volume loss ≤ 40%	Marked tachycardia, tachypnea, decreased mental status, hypotension, and decreased urine output
Class 4	Blood volume loss > 40%	Marked tachycardia, marked tachypnea, significantly decreased systolic blood pressure, obtundation to unconscious mental status, and no urine output

14. **What are the other types of shock, and how do they differ from hemorrhagic shock?**
    In addition to **hemorrhagic/hypovolemic shock**, there are neurogenic, cardiogenic, and septic shock. **Neurogenic shock** (this is uncommon) is caused by sudden loss of autonomic vascular tone, resulting in vasodilation. The systolic blood pressure is low, the pulse pressure is low, but the skin remains warm. **Cardiogenic shock** (less common in young gunslingers and frequent in the country club set) results from pump failure secondary to intrinsic heart muscle damage (myocardial infarction) or mechanical compression (cardiac tamponade). **Septic shock**

(more common in surgical intensive care unit patients) is characterized by hypotension and low systemic vascular resistance.

15. **When should fluid resuscitation be initiated on the multiply traumatized patient?**
Immediately! Begin therapy (fluid through big IV lines) while you are doing the primary survey directed at life-threatening injuries. It is inappropriate to wait until the trauma patient fits a precise physiologic classification of shock before starting aggressive volume restoration.

KEY POINTS: CLASSIFICATIONS OF SHOCK

1. Hemorrhagic: most common cause of posttraumatic shock; low filling pressures and cardiac output, low SVO_2, high SVR.

2. Neurogenic: uncommon; low SVR with bradycardia; skin remains warm.

3. Cardiogenic: pump failure secondary to intrinsic myocardial damage (infarction) or mechanical compression (tamponade); high filling pressures, low cardiac output, low SVO_2.

4. Septic: more common in surgical intensive care unit than in trauma bay; initially high cardiac output, low SVR, high SVO_2.

16. **What are the potential sources of occult blood loss when trying to figure out a patient's hemodynamic status?**
The pleural spaces, abdominal cavity, retroperitoneal/pelvic space (pelvic fractures), major long bone fractures, and at the scene externally ("on the sidewalk"). Femur fractures can hide > 1 L of blood, whereas each rib fracture can account for 150 mL.

17. **What is the patient called who becomes unstable after the initial resuscitation, and why is it important to recognize this phenomenon?**
This guy is a "transient responder." This indicates ongoing blood loss! Look for it (more aggressive work-up) or transfer to a trauma center.

18. **When is blood transfusion indicated during initial resuscitation?**
If the patient arrives who is not responding to aggressive ("wide open") crysalloid infusion, the patient should receive uncrossed, O-negative packed red blood cells. Do not wait for type-specific blood if immediate infusion is required—the blood bank is not generally using the same clock (they are not as frightened because they cannot see the patient).

19. **How does hemorrhagic shock lead to multiple organ failure (MOF)?**
Severe hemorrhagic shock begins an inflammatory cascade that cannot be reversed in some patients despite adequate resuscitation. During the Vietnam War, the patients in hemorrhagic shock were treated rapidly, but later died as a result of pulmonary failure or adult respiratory distress syndrome (ARDS). Patients with ARDS can be mechanically ventilated but later die from a combination of liver, cardiac, and bone marrow failure or MOF. MOF is the leading cause of late postinjury mortality in 85% of these deaths. In addition to the cellular derangement in ATP synthesis; shock causes the release of platelet-activating factor, interleukin-8, and arachidonic acid metabolites that activate neutrophils to adhere to endothelial cells and release cytotoxic mediators, which blow big holes in the endovasculature, flooding the interstitial space and causing organ damage. The mesenteric circulation is

a hotbed of proinflammatory cytokine synthesis (the gut is the "motor for MOF"). In addition to directly activating neutrophils, the mesenteric circulation appears to release agents (probably phospholipases and other toxic lipids) into the mesenteric lymph that cause neutrophil activation and lung injury.

WEB SITES

1. http://www.east.org/tpg/endpoints.pdf

2. http://ww.acssurgery.com/abstracts/acs/acs0603.htm

3. http://www.acssurgery.com/abstracts/ascs/acs0501.htm

BIBLIOGRAPHY

1. American College of Surgeons: Shock. In Advanced Trauma Life Support, 6th ed. Chicago, American College of Surgeons, 1997, p 97.

2. Capone AC, Safar P, Stezoski W, et al: Improved outcome with fluid restriction in treatment of uncontrolled hemorrhagic shock. J Am Coll Surg 180:49, 1995.

3. Choi P, Yip G, Quinonez L, Cook D: Crystalloid versus colloids in fluid resuscitation: A systematic review. Crit Care Med 27:200, 1999.

4. Holcroft JW: Shock. In American College of Surgeons: Surgery: Principles and Practice. New York, Web/MD, 2002, p 63.

5. Moore EE: Blood substitutes: The future is now. J Am Coll Surg 196:1, 2003.

6. National Institutes of Health Consensus Conference: Perioperative red blood cell transfusion. JAMA 260:270, 1988.

7. Peitzman AB: Management of shock. In Moore EE, Mattox KL, Feliciano DV (eds): Trauma, 5th ed. New York, McGraw-Hill, 2003.

CHAPTER 18

TRAUMATIC BRAIN INJURY

J. Paul Elliott, M.D., and Sanjay Misra, M.D.

1. **Is traumatic brain injury (TBI) a common problem?**
   Yes. In the United States, 1 in 12 deaths is due to injury. One third of traumatic deaths are associated with TBI. Of deaths resulting from motor vehicle accidents, 60% are due to brain injury. Even more common is minor TBI, which accounts for 75% of admissions for head trauma.

2. **What is a concussion?**
   The relatively common occurrence of transient loss of neurologic function without macroscopic brain abnormality. Concussion is on one end of a spectrum that extends to coma. The Glasgow Coma Scale (GCS) score is used to categorize brain injuries as follows: mild, 14–15; moderate, 9–13; and severe, ≤ 8.

3. **How is the GCS score derived?**
   The GCS is a means of identifying change in neurologic status. Its principal strengths are ease of use and reproducibility among observers. It is a 15-point scale; 15 is the best score, and 3 is the worst. The score is derived from the addition of the three individual components: best eye-opening response (1–4 points), best verbal response (1–5 points), and best motor response (1–6 points). The GCS is insensitive to pupillary response and focality. A patient with a perfect score of 15 may have hemiparesis and a life-threatening lesion.

4. **When should a neurosurgeon be consulted?**
   For patients with loss of consciousness and subsequent neurologic abnormality or abnormality on computed tomography (CT) scan. These patients usually but not always have a GCS score ≤ 13.

5. **How does one initially assess the brain-injured patient?**
   Just like any trauma patient. The first steps are assessment of the ABCs (airway, breathing, circulation) and rapid physiologic resuscitation. The neurologic examination is crucial. The initial examination includes (1) level of consciousness, (2) pupillary examination, and (3) motor examination. Repetition of the neurologic examination is also crucial. If deterioration is missed and appropriate treatment is not initiated quickly, irreversible brain injury may result. Finally, watch for concurrent cervical spine injury.

6. **What takes priority in a hypotensive patient with TBI?**
   Hypotension in patients with head injury frequently accompanies other injuries. Do not assume that hypotension is due to the brain injury alone. Hypotension resulting from brain injury is a terminal event.

7. **What is the significance of anisocoria in a patient with a decreased level of consciousness?**
   Anisocoria (unequal pupils) is a true neurologic emergency. Commonly a mass lesion (e.g., sub-dural or epidural hematoma, contusion, or diffuse swelling of one hemisphere) leads to uncal

herniation and stretching of the ipsilateral third nerve. Time is crucial. Give mannitol, get a CT scan, and proceed with surgical decompression (if possible).

8. **What if the larger pupil is reactive?**
    If the larger pupil is reactive, the third cranial nerve is functioning. Think of Horner's syndrome (miosis, ptosis, and anhydrosis) on the other side. This syndrome may be due to injury to the sympathetic nerves traveling with the carotid artery in the neck. Consider evaluation (angiography) for a carotid dissection.

9. **Are terms such as *semicomatose* nonsense?**
    Yes. Patients are **alert** (like medical students and surgeons), **lethargic** (like internists, in whom arousal is maintained by verbal interaction), **obtunded** (like hospital administrators, who require constant mechanical stimulation to maintain arousal), or **comatose** (like most deans, in whom neither verbal nor mechanical stimulation elicits arousal). Change in level of consciousness is often the first sign of increasing intracranial pressure (ICP); it is also the most poorly documented part of the neurologic examination. Document all findings!

10. **How is motor response tested?**
    Ascertain the ability to follow commands by asking the patient to hold up fingers and move his or her arms and legs. If the patient does not follow commands (he or she may be a dean), test response to painful central stimulus. Localization of painful stimulus is confirmed by the patient's hand reaching toward a sternal rub. The patient may be in even bigger trouble if in response to pain he or she exhibits flexor posturing (decorticate), extensor posturing (decerebrate), or no response. Flexor posturing indicates a high brainstem injury, and extensor posturing is associated with low brainstem dysfunction. The patient with no motor response may have a cervical spine injury.

11. **What is the significance of periorbital ecchymosis (raccoon eyes) and ecchymosis over the mastoid (Battle's sign)?**
    In the absence of direct trauma to the eyes or mastoid regions, periorbital ecchymosis and ecchymosis over the mastoid are reliable signs of basilar skull fractures. Of patients with basilar skull fractures, 10% have cerebrospinal fluid (CSF) leaks, including rhinorrhea or otorrhea. Persistent CSF leaks are associated with meningitis.

12. **Should scalp lacerations be explored in the emergency department?**
    Yes—but gently. You want to know whether there is an underlying fracture. A laceration over a linear nondisplaced fracture can be cleaned and closed. If CSF or brain tissue is evident in the wound or if a depressed fracture is identified, surgical intervention is required to debride the wound and to close any dural tears. If you are worried, get a head CT scan.

13. **Which patients need CT scans of the head?**
    The CT scan is used partly as a triage tool with minor brain injuries and can be cost-effective compared with admission to the intensive care unit for observation. Conversely, patients with focality on examination do not proceed to the operating room without a CT scan.

14. **What are the common traumatic surgical lesions?**
    If the ventricles are large (ventriculomegaly), a ventriculostomy can drain excessive CSF. Epidural hematomas (from arterial bleeding), subdural hematomas (from venous bleeding), and intraparenchymal hematomas with significant mass effect should be surgically evacuated. A depressed skull fracture or foreign body (e.g., a bullet) also requires a trip to the operating room.

15. **When is ICP monitoring indicated?**
When the neurologic examination becomes insensitive (when the patient is unconscious) to changes in ICP. It also may be indicated when there is known brain injury and the patient will be under general anesthesia for a surgical procedure for an extended period.

16. **Describe the initial treatment of patients with a suspected increase in ICP.**
The brain, similar to every other organ, must have adequate blood flow and oxygen delivery. The ABCs come first. Systolic blood pressures < 90 mmHg and Pa_{O_2} < 60 mmHg are correlated significantly with poor outcomes in patients with TBI. Keep the systolic blood pressure > 100 mmHg and avoid hypoxia.

17. **Should all patients with elevated ICP be hyperventilated?**
Decreasing the P_{CO_2} is the most rapidly effective treatment for elevated ICP. The goal is usually a P_{CO_2} of 30–35 mmHg. Any patient with a depressed level of consciousness and inability to protect the airway should be intubated. Before a CT scan is obtained, patients thought to have a mass lesion by neurologic examination should be hyperventilated until definitive treatment is achieved. Avoid chronic hyperventilation, which can cause ischemic brain injury.

18. **In hemodynamically stable patients, how do you decrease ICP?**
Mannitol, 1 g/kg, as an IV bolus. Also be sure the cervical collar is not obstructing venous outflow through the jugular system.

KEY POINTS: INDICATIONS FOR BLOOD TRANSFUSION IN THE TRAUMA BAY

1. An unstable adult patient who does not respond to 2 L of "wide open" crystalloid infusion should receive uncrossed, O-negative packed red cells.

2. For pediatric patients, give 20 mL/kg of lactate Ringer's by bolus; then repeat if necessary.

3. If the pediatric patient does not respond to lactate Ringer's, proceed to transfuse 10 mL/kg uncrossed, O-negative packed red cells.

4. Do not wait for type-specific blood in the unstable patient who is not responding to crystalloid resuscitation.

19. **What is the end point of diuresis?**
Serum sodium of 150 mEq/L and serum osmolarity of 320 mOsm are usually the upper limits of diuresis. Blood volume should be maintained with colloids to help form an osmotic gradient between the extravascular and the intravascular spaces. Anticipate intravascular hypovolemia, and treat with colloids and blood products as necessary.

20. **What is the significance of cerebral perfusion pressure (CPP)?**
CPP is the difference between mean arterial pressure (MAP) and ICP:

$$CPP = MAP - ICP$$

CPP is important. Neurologic outcome is best in patients with CPPs in the 60s–70s. Some patients require treatment with pressors to maintain the CPP; if CPP is < 60 mmHg, you may be creating a dean.

21. **Why should all children with TBI be undressed and examined thoroughly?**
Half of children suffering nonaccidental trauma (child abuse) have TBI.

22. **Should posttraumatic seizures be treated prophylactically?**
Patients with brain parenchymal abnormalities on CT scan after head injury may benefit from
1 week of antiseizure prophylaxis. Early seizures can increase the metabolic demand of the
injured brain and adversely affect ICP. Of patients who have seizures within the first 7 days of
injury, 10% also have late seizures. Prevention of early seizures does not reduce the incidence
of late seizures, however.

23. **Which coagulopathy is associated with severe brain injury?**
Disseminated intravascular coagulation. The presumed mechanism is massive release of
thromboplastin from the injured brain into the circulation. The serum levels of fibrin degradation
products roughly correlate with the extent of brain parenchymal injury. All severely brain-injured
patients should be evaluated with prothrombin time, partial thromboplastin time, platelet
counts, and fibrinogen levels.

24. **What other medical complications may result from severe head injury?**
Diabetes insipidus (DI) secondary to the inadequate secretion of antidiuretic hormone is caused
by injury to the pituitary or hypothalamic tracts. The kidney is unable to decrease free water loss.
Usually the urine output is > 200 mL/hr, and the urine specific gravity is < 1.003. The serum
sodium may rise precipitously if DI is not treated promptly. The treatment of choice in trauma
is IV infusion of synthetic vasopressin (Pitressin), which has a 20-minute half-life and can be
titrated to produce the appropriate urine output. Because most trauma-induced DI is self-
limited, long-term 1-deamino-8-D-arginine vasopressin (DDAVP), which has a 12-hour half-life,
is not necessary.

25. **If a patient is awake with significant neurologic symptoms but no abnormality
on CT scan, what are the likely explanations?**
A spinal cord injury or carotid or vertebral artery dissection.

26. **Are gunshot wounds that cross the midline of the brain uniformly fatal?**
No (although such a wound killed Lincoln). The tract that the bullet takes is important, but so is
the energy that it imparts to the brain.

27. **What is the significance of concussion?**
In most studies of minor TBI, > 50% of patients have complaints of headache, fatigue, dizziness,
irritability, and alterations of cognition and short-term memory. It is important to alert the patient
to the likelihood of developing these symptoms. The neurobehavioral problems significantly
affect patients' lives. The symptoms usually resolve within 3–6 months after injury.

28. **Can patients with minor TBIs be discharged from the emergency department?**
Patients whose examination (including short-term memory) returns to normal and who have
a normal head CT scan can be discharged to home if they are accompanied by a responsible
person.

29. **Is brain injury permanent? Is the outcome always poor?**
No and no. Brain injury occurs in two phases. The primary injury occurs at the moment of
impact. Secondary injury is preventable and treatable. Examples include hypoxia, hypotension,
elevated ICP, and decreased perfusion to the brain secondary to ischemia, brain swelling, and
expanding mass lesions. Rapid surgical management and avoidance of secondary injury
improve outcome. Although previously it was believed that the brain was not capable of repair, it
is now clear that neuronal repair and reorganization occur after injury.

WEB SITES

1. http://www.acssurgery.com/abstracts/acs/acs0501.htm

2. http://www.surgery.ucsf.edu/eastbaytrauma/Protocols/ER%20protocol%20pages/closedhea dinjury.htm

3. http://www.ascsurgery.com/abstracts/acs/acs0612.htm

BIBLIOGRAPHY

1. Brain Trauma Foundation: Management and Prognosis of Severe Traumatic Brain Injury. New York, Brain Trauma Foundation, 2000. Available at www.braintrauma.org.

2. Mazzola CA, Adelman PD: Critical care management of head trauma in children. Crit Care Med 30:S393–S401, 2002.

3. Narayan RK, Michel ME, Ansell B, et al: Clinical trials in head injury. J Neurotrauma 19:503–557, 2002.

4. Narayan RK, Wilberger JE, Povlishock JT: Neurotrauma. New York, McGraw-Hill, 1996.

5. Shaw NA: The neurophysiology of concussion. Prog Neurobiol 67:281–344, 2002.

CHAPTER 19

SPINAL CORD INJURIES

J. Paul Elliott, M.D., and Sanjay Misra, M.D.

1. **What is the difference between a spinal injury and a spinal cord injury?**
   Spinal injuries include damage to the bone, disc, or ligaments. These injuries sometimes result in spinal instability. They also may be associated with spinal cord injury, which is damage to the neural tissue, often with clinical deficit. It is crucial to determine whether there is (1) a spinal injury, (2) a spinal cord injury, and (3) spinal instability.

2. **Describe the evaluation of a patient with a suspected spine injury.**
   First, be sure that the patient is adequately immobilized and everyone knows to maintain spinal precautions. Second, inspect and palpate the spine for external trauma and step-off. Finally, do a complete neurologic examination including all four extremities. Assess strength, sensation (light touch/proprioception and pain/temperature), muscle tone, reflexes, and rectal tone. Carefully document your results.

3. **How do you minimze the risk of additional spine injury in hospital?**
   Trauma patients should be protected with a rigid cervical collar. The thoracic and lumbar spine are protected using initial spine board immobilization. The patient should be log-rolled during initial evaluation, then removed from the board and transferred to an appropriate hospital bed to prevent decubitus ulcers. Spine precautions should be maintained until the spine is "cleared," meaning there is no spinal instability or the instability has been treated.

4. **How is the level of the spinal cord injury defined?**
   The level does not refer to the level of the injury to the spinal column (vertebrae, discs, and ligaments) but to the most caudal level in the cord with intact function. If a patient has normal function of the deltoids (C5) and little or no function of the biceps (C6) or below, the patient has a C5 motor level injury. Right and left sides should be documented separately.

5. **Which injuries commonly are associated with cervical spine injury?**
   Head injury. Forces associated with significant head and brain injury may be transmitted throug the cervical spine. Of patients with spinal cord injuries, 50% have associated head injuries. Approximately 15% of patients with one spine injury have a second injury elsewhere in the spine.

6. **How can the spinal cord be evaluated in patients with associated head injury?**
   All patients should have a rectal examination to evaluate tone. A patulous anus is a good indication of spinal cord or cauda equina injury. Flaccid motor tone and absent reflexes should raise suspicion of spinal cord injury. These findings are extremely unusual with isolated brain injury. Priapism is common with spinal cord injury but not caused by head injury. Radiographic imaging should be used liberally when a spinal cord injury is suspected.

7. **Which other significant injury may present as a high thoracic cord lesion?**
   Thoracic aortic dissection may present as a T4 region cord injury T4 is a watershed zone in the cord between the vertebral arterial distribution and the aortic radicular arteries.

8. **What is spinal shock?**

Absence of all spinal cord function below the level of the lesion results in flaccid motor tone and areflexia. Neurogenic shock refers to the hypotension that may result from cervical or upper thoracic complete spinal cord lesions. The hypotension is due to the lack of sympathetic vasomotor innervation below the lesion and is characterized by bradycardia from unbalanced vagal input to the heart. Fluid resuscitation and pressors with both α and β stimulation work best. Strictly a stimulation may result in profound bradycardia or asystole. Usually the spinal shock resolves, and vasomotor tone returns over the first few days. Occasionally, apparent complete injuries significantly improve or resolve because of resolution of diffuse cord dysfunction—the cause is not clear.

9. **Describe an adequate radiologic evaluation.**

Minimal cervical spine evaluation includes cross-table lateral, anteroposterior, and open-mouth odontoid views. The relationship between C7 and the top of T1 must be visualized. Mild traction on the shoulders with the lateral film or swimmer's views help in patients with large shoulders. If this area cannot be seen on plain films, a lateral tomogram or computed tomography (CT) scan may be needed. Oblique views are helpful in viewing the pedicles and facet joints. For the thoracic and lumbosacral spine, anteroposterior and lateral views are obtained. Patients with evidence of possible fractures should have CT scans to define the injury in greater detail. Spiral CT scans may be used for rapid screening.

10. **Describe the proper way to read a lateral cervical spine film.**

Make a habit of doing a thorough systematic review in the same way with every film. First look at the prevertebral soft tissue space, which may be the only radiographic abnormality in 40% of C1 and C2 fractures. The space anterior to C3 should not exceed one third of the body of C3. At the C6 level, the entire body of C6 generally fits into the prevertebral soft tissue space. Check the alignment of the anterior, then posterior edges of the vertebral bodies. Be sure that the intervertebral disc spaces are of relatively equal height. Assess each facet joint. Check the spinous processes for alignment and abnormal splaying. Finally, evaluate each vertebra for fracture.

11. **What about the anteroposterior (AP) film?**

Carefully inspect the alignment of the midline spinous processes. Abrupt angulations suggest unilateral facet dislocation. More subtle changes may indicate facet instability or fracture. Body fractures may be more obvious in the AP view.

12. **Can a patient have a spinal cord injury and normal plain radiographs?**

Yes, with purely ligamentous injuries between vertebrae. Spinal cord injury without radiographic abnormality (SCIWORA) is common in children; 30% of children with spinal cord injuries have no radiographic abnormality. SCIWORA is less common in adults (about 5% of spinal cord injuries). In patients with preexisting cervical stenosis, either congenital or degenerative, hyperextension or flexion may result in cord injury without spinal column disruption.

13. **Is magnetic resonance imaging (MRI) useful in the evaluation of acute spine trauma?**

Yes. If plain radiographs and CT scans do not explain adequately the extent of injury noted on the neurologic examinations, MRI should be used to evaluate the spine for herniated discs, ligamentous injuries, and evidence of spinal cord injury.

14. **Fractures of C1 and C2 are visualized best with which view?**

The **odontoid view**. Look for overhang of the lateral mass of C1 off the lateral edges of C2. This occurs in **Jefferson's fractures** (burst fractures of the C1 ring). Sum total overhang of both C1 lateral masses on C2 of ≥ 7 mm is associated with disruption of the transverse ligament and instability. If you see a C1 fracture, look carefully for a C2 fracture. The three types of odontoid fractures are:

- Type I occurs in the dens.
- Type II occurs across the base of the dens where it joins the body of C2.
- Type III extends into the body of C2.

Type II dens fracture requires a halo or operative screw fixation. Get a CT scan to investigate fully any fracture suspected on plain films.

15. **What is hangman's fracture?**
Bilateral fractures through the pedicles or pars interarticularis of C2 that are caused by a severe hyperextension injury, usually secondary to high-speed motor vehicle accidents. Think about the mechanism of injury: the C2–C3 disc space may be disrupted anteriorly. In judicial hangings, the fatal injury is the spinal cord stretch caused by the drop in combination with the C2 fracture. Most patients with hangman's fracture present neurologically intact. They are often treated with a halo.

16. **Define deficits in complete transverse myelopathy, anterior cord syndrome, central cord syndrome, and Brown-Séquard syndrome.**
Complete transverse myelopathy may result from transection, stretch, or contusion of the cord. All function below the level of the lesion—motor, sensory, and reflexive—is lost. Complete transverse myelopathy may be accompanied by spinal shock or neurogenic shock. Approximately 50% of spinal cord injuries are complete.
Anterior cord syndrome results from injury of the anterior two thirds of the spinal cord (the distribution of the anterior spinal artery), which carries motor, pain, and temperature tracts. Light touch and proprioception are intact because the posterior columns are preserved.
Central cord syndrome results from injury to the central area of the spinal cord. Often it is found in patients with preexisting cervical stenosis resulting from spondylotic changes. Characteristically, deficits are more severe in the upper extremities than in the lower extremities. Motor function usually is affected more than sensory function.
Brown-Séquard syndrome characteristically is seen in penetrating injuries, but also may be seen in blunt injury, especially with unilateral, traumatically herniated discs. The syndrome results from injury to half of the spinal cord. Clinically, motor, position, and vibration sense are affected on the side ipsilateral to the injury; these tracts cross in the brainstem. Pain and temperature sensation are abolished contralateral to the lesion; these tracts cross in the cord at or near the level of innervation.

KEY POINTS: DIAGNOSTIC PEARLS FOR TRAUMATIC SPINAL CORD INJURY

1. Complete traverse myelopathy: complete distal motor, sensory, and reflexive deficit.

2. Anterior cord syndrome: loss of motor, pain, and temperature sensation with preservation of light touch and proprioception since the posterior columns are intact.

3. Central cord syndrome: deficits more severe in upper than lower extremities and motor function affected more than sensory function.

4. Brown-Séquard syndrome: loss of ipsilateral motor, position, and vibratory senses and contralateral pain and temperature sense.

17. **What is the role of methylprednisolone in the treatment of acute cord injury?**
   The results of the Second National Acute Spinal Cord Injury Study (NASCIS II) suggest that high-dose methylprednisolone results in a statistically significant improvement in outcome. The dose is a 30-mg/kg load, followed by 5.4 mg/kg/h for 23 hours. The NASCIS III trial reported that patients dosed 3–8 hours after injury had improved outcomes when treated for 48 hours with the methylprednisolone rather than 24 hours. In patients dosed within 3 hours of injury, no further gains were documented by treating beyond 24 hours. Penetrating trauma was not evaluated in the study. Reevaluation of available data has put the value of these steroids in doubt.

18. **Do patients with spinal cord injuries ever undergo acute surgery?**
   Yes. Patients with deterioration in the neurologic examination may undergo urgent spinal cord decompression. Deterioration may be due to herniated disc material, epidural hemorrhage, or cord swelling in a narrowed canal, causing cord compression and worsening symptoms. Patients also undergo surgery for stabilization of an unstable spine to allow early mobilization and rehabilitation.

19. **How is the bony injury treated?**
   1. Prevention of further injury using spinal precautions
   2. Obtaining normal alignment using body position, traction, and bracing
   3. Open reduction, decompression, and fusion as necessary

20. **What is the outcome in patients with spinal cord injury?**
   With complete lesions (no motor or sensory function below the lesion), the chances of recovery are poor; 2% of patients recover ambulation. The prognosis is markedly better for patients with incomplete lesions—75% experience significant recovery. Appropriate treatment of bony injuries helps to prevent pain and late neurologic deterioration.

WEB SITE

http://www.acssurgery.com/abstracts/acs/acs0502.htm

BIBLIOGRAPHY

1. Blackmore CC, Mann FA, Wilson AJ: Helical CT in the primary trauma evaluation of the cervical spine: An evidence-based approach. Skeletal Radiol 29:632–639, 2000.

2. Bracken MB, Shepard MJ, Holford TR, et al: Administration of methylprednisolone for 24 or 48 hours or tirilazad mesylate for 48 hours in the treatment of acute spinal cord injury: Results of the Third National Acute Spinal Cord Injury randomized controlled trial. JAMA 277:1597–1604, 1997.

3. Crim JR, Moore K, Brodke D: Clearance of the cervical spine in multitrauma patients: The role of advanced imaging. Semin Ultrasound CT MR 22:283–305, 2001.

4. Guidelines for the management of acute cervical spine and spinal cord injuries: Initial closed reduction of cervical spine fracture-dislocation injuries. Neurosurgery 50:S44–S50, 2002.

5. Imhof H, Fuchsjager M: Traumatic injuries: Imaging of spinal injuries. Eur Radiol 12:1262–1272, 2002.

6. Rekate HL, Theodore N, Sonntag VK, Dickman CA: Pediatric spine and spinal cord trauma: State of the art for the third milennium. Childs Nerv Syst 15:743–750, 1999.

7. Takhtani D, Melhem ER: MR imaging in cervical spine trauma. Magn Reson Imaging Clin North Am 8:615–634, 2000.

CHAPTER 20

PENETRATING NECK TRAUMA

Clay Cothren, M.D., and Ernest E. Moore, M.D.

1. **Why are penetrating neck wounds unique?**
   Although comprising only a small percentage of body surface area, the neck contains a heavy concentration of vital structures.

2. **What constitutes a penetrating neck wound?**
   Violation of the platysma muscle defines a penetrating neck wound. This investing fascial layer of the neck is superficial to vital structures. If the platysma is not penetrated, the wound is managed as a simple laceration.

3. **Identify the boundaries of the three zones of the neck.**
   Zone I extends from the sternal notch to the cricoid cartilage.
   Zone II extends from the cricoid cartilage to the angle of the mandible.
   Zone III comprises the area cephalad to the angle of the mandible.
   These zones have distinct management implications.

4. **Which side of the neck is more likely to be injured?**
   The left side because most assailants are right-handed.

5. **Do gunshot wounds and knife wounds cause the same relative injuries?**
   Gunshot wounds generally tend to inflict more tissue damage (see Table 20-1).

TABLE 20-1. GUNSHOT VERSUS TAB WOUNDS		
Structure	**Gunshot Wounds**	**Stab Wounds**
Artery	20%	5%
Vein	15%	10%
Airway	10%	5%
Digestive	20%	< 5%

6. **What are the priorities in the management of penetrating neck trauma?**
   The ABCs (airway, breathing, and circulation) are the first priority in every trauma patient. Patients should be intubated orally, although cricothyrotomy may be necessary with an extensive neck wound. Although the patient may present with a patent airway, early elective airway control is advisable in patients with expanding hematomas. Pneumothoraces or hemothoraces may be associated with these injuries depending on the trajectory. While hemorrhage is being controlled with direct pressure, IV access is secured with two large-bore peripheral lines.

7. **How should bleeding be controlled at the accident scene and in the emergency department?**
Direct pressure is nearly always successful, even for major arterial lesions. Do not blindly place clamps because the risk of injury to vital structures is high.

8. **Should you explore the wound in the trauma bay?**
Only if the patient is asymptomatic and there has been no evidence of hemorrhage. Probing the wound may dislodge a clot, causing marked hemorrhage.

9. **What physical signs are consistent with significant injury?**
Ongoing hemorrhage from the wound, expanding or pulsatile hematoma, hemoptysis, hematemesis, neurologic deficits, dysphagia, dysphonia, hoarseness, and stridor mandate an early trip to the operating room.

10. **How often do patients with crepitus (in the neck) have a significant injury?**
One third of patients with crepitus have an injury of the pharynx, esophagus, larynx, or trachea. In two thirds of these patients, however, the air has been introduced through the wound entrance site, and there is no significant underlying injury.

11. **What is selective management of penetrating neck trauma?**
Previously, operative exploration was advocated for all zone II injuries violating the platysma; this approach has lost support. With 50% of penetrating neck wounds not associated with significant injury, exploration is not mandatory. Alert and asymptomatic patients are evaluated with a combination of diagnostic studies (see later) or are observed expectantly with frequent serial physical examinations.

KEY POINTS: SELECTIVE MANAGEMENT OF PENETRATING INJURIES TO ZONE II

1. Penetrating injury implies violation of the platysma.

2. Mandatory exploration of all zone II injuries is not necessary since 50% of wounds are not associated with significant injury.

3. Alert and asymptomatic patients should be observed expectantly for at least 24 hours.

4. Symptomatic patients (exsanguinations or expanding hematoma) proceed to the operating room for exploration.

5. Aerodigestive symptoms (e.g., stridor, dysphonia) mandate further diagnostic testing: laryngoscopy, bronchoscopy, and esophagram.

12. **Should arteriography be performed on all patients?**
Preoperative arteriograms generally are performed in hemodynamically stable patients with zone I injuries. Their value is to identify injuries to major vessels in the thoracic outlet that may require a thoracic operative approach. Wounds in zone III are treated best by angioembolization if there is evidence of significant bleeding.

13. **What is the value of other diagnostic studies, such as esophagography, esophagoscopy, laryngoscopy, and bronchoscopy?**
Routine use of esophagography, bronchoscopy, and laryngoscopy has been advocated in zone I and selected nonoperatively managed zone II patients. Esophagoscopy is combined with esoph-

agography if esophageal injury is suspected; if water-soluble contrast material does not show a leak, barium is used. Missed esophageal injuries can be deadly, with a 20% mortality rate if diagnosis is delayed only 12 hours. Angiography remains the gold standard for diagnosis of arterial injury, and this modality may be therapeutic for zone III injuries (zone III is tough to expose surgically). Intraoperative endoscopy with insufflation may be used provocatively to show an air leak and associated esophageal injury.

14. **What is the role of CT?**
    If patients have a high-risk trajectory (i.e., transcervical gunshot wounds), CT may identify the "line of fire" and help determine the need for angiography (see Figure 20-1).

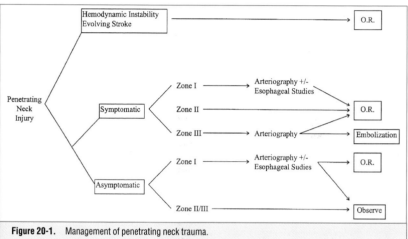

Figure 20-1. Management of penetrating neck trauma.

15. **Should an asymptomatic patient with a penetrating neck wound be sent home from the emergency department?**
    No. Life-threatening penetrating neck wounds initially may be difficult to sort out; the safest policy is to observe all patients in the hospital for at least 24 hours.

WEB SITES

1. http://www.acssurgery.com/abstracts/acs/acs0504.htm

2. http://www.surgery.ucsf.edu/eastbaytrauma/Protocols/ER%20protocol%20pages/penetrneck.htm

BIBLIOGRAPHY

1. Albuquerque FC, Javedan SP, McDougall CG: Endovascular management of penetrating vertebral artery injuries. J Trauma 53:574–580, 2002.

2. Atteberry LR, Dennis JW, Monawat SS, Frykberg ER: Physical examination alone is safe and accurate for evaluation of vascular injuries in penetrating zone II neck trauma. J Am Coll Surg 179:657–662, 1994.

3. Biffl WL, Moore EE, Rehse DH, et al: Selective management of penetrating neck trauma based on cervical level of injury. Am J Surg 174:678–682, 1997.

4. Demetriades D, Velmahos G, Asensio JA: Cervical pharygoesophageal and laryngotracheal injuries. World J Surg 25:1044–1048, 2001.

5. Gracias VH, Reilly PM, Philpott J, et al: Computed tomography in the evaluation of penetrating neck trauma: A preliminary study. Arch Surg 136:1231–1235, 2001.

6. Hirshberg A, Wall MJ, Johnston RH, et al: Transcervical gunshot injuries. Am J Surg 167:309, 1993.

7. Mazolewski PJ, Curry JD, Browder T, Fildes J: Computed tomographic scan can be used for surgical decision making in zone II penetrating neck injuries. J Trauma 51:315–319, 2001.

8. McIntyre WB, Blaard JL: Cervicothoracic vascular injuries. Semin Vasc Surg 11:232–242, 1998.

CHAPTER 21

BLUNT THORACIC TRAUMA

Jeffrey L. Johnson, M.D., and Ernest E. Moore, M.D.

1. **How often do patients with isolated blunt chest trauma need an emergent operation?**
   Rarely. In patients who arrive in the hospital alive, operative injuries to the pulmonary, vascular, and mediastinal structures are surprisingly rare; only 5% of patients with isolated blunt injury to the chest require thoracotomy.

2. **In a patient with a hemothorax after blunt chest injury, what is the most important guide for the decision to operate?**
   The hemodynamic status of the patient. Hemothorax after blunt injury is most often caused by nonoperative lesions of the lung and chest wall. In stable patients, therefore, evacuation of the hemothorax (with a chest tube); reexpansion of the lung, and correction of coagulopathy, hypothermia, and acidosis should be the initial focus. Chest tube output is helpful but is not the principal consideration.

3. **What is a tension pneumothorax?**
   Air in the pleural space under pressure caused by a one-way valve mechanism. This can be a life-threatening condition because the increase in intrathoracic pressure decreases venous return, which impaires right ventricular filling, resulting in a decrease in cardiac output.

4. **What are the clinical signs of tension pneumothorax?**
   Hypotension, tachycardia, absent breath sounds on the involved side, and distended neck veins. If the patient is doing badly and a tension pneumothorax is suspected, the chest should be decompresed without waiting for a radiograph.

5. **How are patients with tension pneumothorax treated?**
   For prehospital care, needle decompression should be done at the fifth intercostal space in the midaxillary line (never the midclavicular line). In the hospital, however, an experienced physician can completely decompress the pleural space just as rapidly with a tube thoracostomy.

6. **Does it matter how many ribs are broken?**
   Yes. Six or more fractures indicate a higher risk of pain induced hypoventilation with resultant pneumonia and acute respiratory distress syndrome (ARDS), particularly in elderly patients.

7. **What is a flail chest?**
   When multiple ribs are fractured in two or more places, the chest wall moves paradoxically (flails) with respiration.

8. **How does flail chest impact ventilation?**
   In spontaneously breathing patients, the portion of the thoracic cage that has lost bony continuity retracts inward during inspiration. This paradoxical motion (exacerbated by excruciating pain) impairs ventilation.

9. **Do all patients with a flail segment require positive pressure ventilation to avoid hypoventilation?**

No. The impact of a flail segment on ventilation is not always profound, and with good analgesia, many patients can maintain their own work of breathing. Standard indications for intubation should be used.

10. **Does flail chest affect oxygenation?**

Flail chest per se has little direct impact on oxygenation. However, virtually all patients with flail chest have an underlying pulmonary contusion. The severity of the pulmonary contusion is a more important determinant of outcome and need for intubation than the impaired mechanics of the chest wall. The pathophysiology of blunt injury to the chest with severe bony injury should be thought of as a single process (i.e., flail chest/pulmonary contusion).

11. **What is the natural history of pulmonary contusion?**

Similar to other tissues, the lung undergoes shearing of parenchyma and rupture of small blood vessels (bruise) after a direct thump or rapid deceleration. This tissue injury is followed by edema. Thus, patients with pulmonary contusion typically deteriorate in the first 48 hours. Be careful because the initial chest radiograph may appear deceptively benign.

12. **What is the most common initial presentation of blunt injury to the thoracic aorta?**

Death in the field. Eighty-five percent of patients with a torn thoracic aorta die of exsanguination before they reach the hospital. Disruption of the heart and great vessels is second only to head injury as a cause of death attributable to blunt trauma.

13. **Of patients surviving to reach the hospital, what is the most common injury to the thoracic aorta?**

A tear across the intima and media just distal to the takeoff of the left subclavian artery. Because the adventitia is intact, the patient does not immediately exsanguinate, and if the lesion is detected promptly and surgically treated, the survival rate is 85%.

14. **What are the clinical signs of a torn thoracic aorta?**

There are no definitive signs. Suspicion must be based on the mechanism of injury (i.e., rapid deceleration). The unusual physical signs associated with aortic disruption include upper extremity hypertension; unequal upper extremity pressures; loss of lower extremity pulses; and expanding hematoma in the root of the neck, which is extremely serious.

15. **What findings on chest radiograph are associated with rupture of the descending thoracic aorta?**

Similar to the physical signs in this condition, no initial radiographic signs are definitive; however, watch for an indistinct aortic knob, widened mediastinum (> 8 cm at the level of the aortic knob), apical cap, left pleural effusion, depression of the left mainstem bronchus, rightward displacement of the esophagus (look for and follow the nasogastric tube), first-rib fractures, displacement of the trachea, and loss of the aortopulmonary window. A total of 15% of patients with a torn aorta have a normal mediastinum by radiograph, and 7% have a completely normal chest radiograph.

16. **In the stable patient with a major mechanism of injury or chest radiographs consistent with aortic injury, how is the diagnosis made?**

Dynamic helical computed tomography of the chest approaches 100% sensitivity for detecting aortic injury; it is widely available and applicable to all stable patients. The definitive test remains aortography because it more precisely identifies the site (ascending or descending aorta) and extent of injury.

17. **How does one identify the patient with a myocardial contusion?**
Only two things happen to the bruised heart: arrhythmia and pump failure. By far, the most common manifestation of blunt cardiac injury is arrhythmia. Studies confirm that patients with an initial electrocardiogram (ECG) that is normal have an exceedingly small chance of developing clinically significant arrhythmias during their hospital course. Any ECG abnormality is an indication for admission and 24 hours of cardiac monitoring. Hemodynamic compromise from blunt cardiac injury is unusual and not subtle; echocardiography should be used in patients with evidence of impaired contractility. Cardiac enzymes are poor predictors of arrhythmia or pump failure and are not recommended.

KEY POINTS: CHARACTERISTICS OF BLUNT CARDIAC INJURY

1. Most common manifestation is arrhythmia, although pump failure can occur.

2. Diagnostic evaluation with ECG: if normal, no further work-up is needed; if abnormal, 24 hours of inpatient monitoring is required.

3. If any evidence of myocardial dysfunction is seen, an echocardiogram should be performed.

4. Although some controversy remains, the trauma literature suggests that cardiac enzyme levels are not useful.

18. **Where do blunt injuries to a bronchus usually occur? How do they present?**
They usually occur within a few centimeters of the carina. The mainstem bronchi are splayed apart with severe anteroposterior compression of the chest. As the lungs are displaced laterally, the mainstem bronchi may tear near the site where they are fixed at the carina. The typical presentation is a massive air leak, failure to reexpand the lung ("dropped lung"), or both after tube thoracostomy.

19. **What are the indications for emergency department thoracotomy after blunt chest injury?**
Emergency thoracotomy should be done in patients with cardiovascular collapse after arrival in the emergency department. The outcome, however, is typically dismal: fewer than 1% of patients survive neurologically intact.

20. **What is traumatic asphyxia?**
Traumatic asphyxia is the result of a protracted crush injury to the upper torso or epigastrium. In such an injury, venous hypertension is transmitted to the valveless veins of the upper body. Patients pres-

WEB SITES

1. http://www.east.org/tpg/chap8.pdf

2. http://www.east.org/tpg/chap2.pdf

3. http://www.acssurgery.com/abstracts/acs/acs0505.htm

4. http://www.acssurgery.com/abstracts/acs/acs0602.htm

5. http://www.surgery.ucsf.edu/eastbaytrauma/Protocols/ER20%20protocol%20pages/thoracic_aorta.htm

6. http://www.surgery.ucsf.edu/eastbaytrauma/Protocols/ER20%20protocol%20pages/bluntcardiac.htm

ent with altered sensorium, petechial hemorrhages, cyanosis, and edema of the upper body. Although its initial presentation can be dramatic, with supportive care, the outcome is usually good.

BIBLIOGRAPHY

1. Allen GS, Coates NE: Pulmonary contusion: A collective review. Am Surgeon 62:895–900, 1996.

2. Branney SW, Moore EE, Feldhaus KM, et al: Critical analysis of two decades of experience with postinjury emergency department thoracotomy in a regional trauma center. J Trauma 45:87–95, 1998.

3. Bulger EM, Arneson MA, Mock CN, et al: Rib fractures in the elderly. J Trauma 48:1040–1046, 2000.

4. Dyer DS, Moore EE, Ilke DN, et al: Thoracic aortic injury: How predictive is mechanism and is chest CT a reliable screening tool? A prospective study of 1500 patients. J Trauma 48:673–682, 2000.

5. Fabian TC, Richardson JD, Croce MA, et al: Prospective study of blunt aortic injury: Multicenter trial of the American Association for the Surgery of Trauma. J Trauma 42:374–383, 1997.

6. Karmy-Jones R, Jurkovich GJ, Nathens AB, et al: Timing of urgent thoracotomy for hemorrhage after trauma: A multicenter study. Arch Surg 136:513–518, 2001.

7. Kiser AC, O'Brien SM, Detterbeck FC: Blunt tracheobronchial injuries: Treatment and outcome. Ann Thorac Surg 71:2059–2065, 2001.

8. Yeong EK, Chen MT, Chu SH: Traumatic asphyxia. Plast Reconstr Surg 93:739–744, 1994.

CHAPTER 22

PENETRATING THORACIC TRAUMA

Jeffrey L. Johnson, M.D., and Ernest E. Moore, M.D.

1. **How often do patients with penetrating chest wounds need an operation?**
   Surprisingly rarely. Most civilian penetrating injuries are from knives and low-energy handguns. Consequently, although injuries to the chest wall and lung are common, the majority of patients can be treated with tube thoracostomy alone. Formal thoracotomy or median sternotomy is required in < 15% of isolated penetrating chest injuries.

2. **What are the indications for emergency department thoracotomy (EDT) after penetrating chest wounds?**
   Patients who arrive at the emergency department with cardiac activity and have suffered circulatory collapse either en route or in the resuscitation area can benefit from EDT. Unlike blunt injury, a treatable cause is more commonly found after penetrating injury (e.g., pericardial tamponade). EDT results in a survival (and walk out of the hospital) of about 20%.

3. **What is the "6-hour rule" for penetrating chest injuries?**
   In a patient with a penetrating chest injury, an upright chest radiograph with no evidence of pneumothorax after 6 hours makes the likelihood of delayed pneumothorax or occult injury to an intrathoracic organ vanishingly small. The "6-hour rule" identifies patients who can be safely discharged.

4. **How much blood in the pleural space can be reliably detected by chest radiograph?**
   250 mL, but the patient must be fully upright in order for 250 mL to blunt the costophrenic angle on radiograph.

5. **What are the indications for operation in a stable patient with hemothorax after penetrating chest injury?**
   Immediate return of > 1500 mL of blood from the pleural space or ongoing bleeding in excess of 250 mL/h for 3 consecutive hours. Obviously, this also depends on the size of the patient; for example, a football lineman can safely lose more blood than a piccolo player.

6. **What is a "clam shell" thoracotomy?**
   Bilateral anterolateral thoracotomies with extension across the sternum. This procedure allows rapid access to both pleural spaces, pulmonary hilae, and the mediastinum.

7. **What is an open pneumothorax?**
   A defect in the chest wall that connects the pleural space with the outside world. A close-range shotgun blast would cause an open pneumothorax.

8. **How is an open pneumothorax treated?**
   The defect in the chest wall should be covered with an occlusive dressing that is fixed on only three sides. This temporary fix prevents entry of air into the pleural space while allowing egress of air under pressure. A chest tube is then inserted. Formal repair of the chest wall can wait until other significant injuries are excluded.

9. **Where is "the box"?**
It is located on the anterior chest between the midclavicular lines from clavicle to costal margin. Penetrating wounds are likely to cause cardiac injury in this region. A typical penetrating cardiac injury has a wound in the box; the heart also can be reached from the root of the neck, axilla, and epigastrium.

10. **What is Beck's triad? How often is it present in patients with tamponade caused by penetrating chest injuries?**
Beck's triad is hypotension, distended neck veins, and muffled heart tones. These signs are difficult to appreciate in trauma patients (especially muffled heart sounds in a busy and noisy resuscitation room) and are present in only 40% of patients with tamponade from penetrating injuries. The absence of distended neck veins can be explained because most patients have concomitant hypovolemia.

KEY POINTS: INDICATIONS FOR THORACOTOMY WITH PENETRATING CHEST INJURY

1. Unstable patients proceed directly to the operating room after trauma survey, tube thoracostomy placement, and resuscitation.

2. Stable patients receive a tube thoracostomy and observant management; 85% of patients respond to this therapy alone.

3. 15% of patients require operative management, which is indicated if immediate pleurovac output is 1500 mL or if output remains > 250 mL/h for 4 consecutive hours.

11. **In a stable patient with suspected penetrating cardiac injury, what is the most important initial study?**
After completion of the primary survey (i.e., airway, breathing, circulation), bedside ultrasonography should be performed. This rapid, sensitive method for detecting pericardial fluid indicates cardiac injury. Initial study results may be negative with only a small effusion; therefore, serial examinations are very important.

12. **What is the initial therapeutic maneuver in a patient with a penetrating cardiac wound who is not yet hypotensive?**
Percutaneous pericardial drainage. Early pericardial tamponade does not appear immediately life threatening; however, one of the early effects of tamponade is subendocardial ischemia, which puts the patient at risk for refractory arrhythmias. Immediate decompression of the pericardium ensures safer transport to the operating room for definitive repair.

13. **In a penetrating chest wound, how is injury to the diaphragm evaluated?**
At end expiration, the dome of the diaphragm reaches the level of the nipples (surprisingly high). Any penetrating injury below the level of the nipples may have an injury to the diaphragm. Diagnostic peritoneal lavage is the preferred initial procedure. Red blood cell counts < 1000/mm^3 are negative for injury. Counts > 10,000 are positive for injury; for counts of 1000–10,000, thoracoscopy is indicated to visualize completely the hemidiaphragm at risk.

14. **Why is it important to detect a small diaphragmatic laceration?**
Abdominal viscera herniate from the positive-pressure abdominal cavity into the negative-pressure pleural space. The morbidity of a strangulated (dead bowel) diaphragmatic hernia is not trivial, often because of delay in diagnosis.

15. **Does a patient with a gunshot wound traversing the mediastinum need an operation?**
No. Surprisingly, not all wounds that pass completely through the mediastinum injure a critical structure. In fact, only one third of patients have an injury that requires exploration. Stable patients should be evaluated with history (odynophagia, hoarseness?), physical examination (deep cervical emphysema, expanding hematoma, pulseless extremity?), angiography, bronchoscopy, and esophagoscopy.

16. **Are prophylactic antibiotics warranted to prevent empyema after tube thoracostomy?**
A meta-analysis of currently published randomized studies on prophylactic antibiotics for tube thoracostomy suggests a benefit. The number of doses required is unclear; furthermore, the utility in blunt multisystem injury patients may be questioned because of the risk of emergence of resistance.

17. **What is the most important risk factor for posttraumatic empyema?**
Persistent hemothorax. Blood incubated at 37° is an excellent culture medium for bacteria; therefore, expedient evacuation of blood from the pleural space via tube thoracostomy or video-assisted thoracoscopic surgery is central in the management of traumatic hemothorax.

18. **What is a bronchovenous air embolism?**
The classic presentation of bronchovenous air embolism is a patient with a penetrating chest injury who arrests after intubation and application of positive-pressure ventilation. The underlying pathophysiology is passage of air under pressure from a lacerated bronchus to an adjacent lacerated pulmonary vein. Air then travels across the lungs to the left side of the heart and into the coronary arteries.

19. **How is bronchovenous air embolism diagnosed and treated?**
Diagnosis is based only on the typical history (see question 18). Therapy is directed toward removal of air from the left ventricle and coronary arteries. The procedure includes the Trendelenberg (head down) position with the right side down and immediate thoracotomy and aspiration of the apex of the left ventricle, the aortic root, and occasionally the coronary arteries.

20. **What is Hamman's sign?**
A crunching sound on auscultation of the chest that indicates air in the mediastinum.

21. **In a penetrating esophageal injury, where may air be evident on physical examination?**
It may be evident in the deep subcutaneous tissues of the neck. In the upright position, air in the mediastinum dissects into a plane continuous with the deep cervical fascia.

22. **How do patients with penetrating tracheobronchial injuries present?**
Patients with lacerations of the trachea and major bronchi present with subcutaneous emphysema, hemoptysis, and dyspnea. Chest radiographs reveal a pneumothorax, pneumomediastinum, or both. After tube thoracostomy, continuous air leak and failure of the lung to reexpand ("dropped lung") should prompt suspicion of a major bronchial injury.

23. **What does a blurry bullet on a chest radiograph indicate?**
It indicates a bullet lodged in the myocardium. Movement of the heart causes the bullet's image to be blurry on x-ray. Beware the blurry bullet.

WEB SITE

http://www.acssurgery.com/abstracts/acs/acs0505.htm

BIBLIOGRAPHY

1. Branney SW, Moore EE, Feldhaus KM, et al: Critical analysis of two decades of experience with postinjury emergency department thoracotomy in a regional trauma center. J Trauma 45:87–95, 1998.

2. Karmy-Jones R, Carter Y, Stern E: The impact of positive pressure ventilation on the diagnosis of traumatic diaphragmatic injury. Am Surg 68:167–172, 2002.

3. Mandal AK, Sanusi M: Penetrating chest wounds: 24 years experience. World J Surg 25:1145–1149, 2001.

4. Mattox KL, Wall MJ, Pickard LR: Thoracic trauma: General considerations and indications for thoracotomy. In Feliciano DV, Moore EE, Mattox KL (eds): Trauma. Stamford, CT, Appleton & Lange, 1996, pp 345–354.

5. Nagy KK, Lohmann C, Kim DO, et al: Role of echocardiography in the diagnosis of occult penetrating cardiac injury. J Trauma 38:859–862, 1995.

6. Rhee PM, Foy H, Kaufmann C, et al: Penetrating cardiac injuries: A population-based study. J Trauma 45:366–370, 1998.

7. Stassen AA, Lukan JK, Spain DA, et al: Reevaluation of diagnostic procedures for transmediastinal gunshot wounds. J Trauma 53:635–638, 2002.

8. Wall MJ, Granchi T, Liscum K, et al: Penetrating thoracic vascular injuries. Surg Clin North Am 76:749–761, 1996.

CHAPTER 23

BLUNT ABDOMINAL TRAUMA

David J. Ciesla, M.D., and Ernest E. Moore, M.D.

1. **What elements of the history are important in evaluating a patient with suspected blunt abdominal trauma (BAT)?**
First, the mechanism of injury (e.g., motor vehicle collision, automobile-pedestrian accident, fall) is important. In motor vehicle accidents, note the position of the victim in the car, velocity of impact (high, moderate, low), type of accident (front, lateral, or rear impact; side swipe; rollover), and type of restraint used (shoulder restraint, air-bag, lap belt). Information about damage to the vehicle, such as a broken windshield or bent steering wheel, may raise suspicion of cervical and chest injuries. In a fall, it is important to note the distance fallen and the site of anatomic impact. Vertical landing on the feet or in a sitting position causes a different pattern of injury than lateral landing on the side. Serial vital signs and mental status are always important.

2. **Is physical examination accurate in the diagnosis of intraabdominal injury?**
No. The examination results may be normal in up to 50% of patients with acute intraabdominal bleeding. Signs of intraabdominal injury include abrasions and contusions over the lower chest and abdomen; subcutaneous emphysema or palpable rib fracture; clinically evident pelvic fracture; abdominal pain, tenderness, guarding, or rigidity; blood in the urine or urethral meatus; high-riding prostate or blood on rectal examination; and microscopic hematuria.

3. **Which organs are most frequently injured in BAT?**

Liver, 50%	Colon, 5%
Spleen, 40%	Duodenum, 5%
Mesentery, 10%	Vascular, 4%
Urologic, 10%	Stomach, 2%
Pancreas, 10%	Gallbladder, 2%
Small bowel, 10%	

4. **What diagnostic studies are helpful in BAT?**
   1. **Ultrasound:** reliably identifies peritoneal fluid (blood) and pericardial fluid but may miss up to 25% of isolated solid organ injuries.
   2. **Computed tomography (CT) scan:** identifies the presence and severity of solid organ injury (liver and spleen), detects intraabdominal air and fluid (blood, mucus, urine), and aids in evaluation of pelvic fractures. CT scanning can also identify bowel, pancreatic, renal, and bladder injuries.
   3. **Diagnostic peritoneal lavage (DPL):** grossly positive DPL (> 10 mL blood returned by aspiration of the catheter) indicates significant hemoperitoneum. Positive by cell count after infusion of 1 L of crystalloid fluid (> 100,000 red blood cells/mm^3, presence of bile or fibers) indicates intraabdominal bleeding, injury to hollow viscus, or hepatobiliary system injury. Lavage fluid exiting through a chest tube or urinary catheter indicates diaphragmatic or bladder injury.

5. **How has the availability of ultrasound (US) changed the initial evaluation of BAT?**
The focused abdominal sonography for trauma (FAST) examination has largely supplanted the DPL. The FAST examination can be performed in a hemodynamically unstable patient during

the early secondary survey with immediate transfer to the operating room when hemoperitoneum is identified. CT scan is safe in the hemodynamically stable patient. DPL is still useful when US is equivocal or not available and for evaluation of hollow organ injury.

6. **How is hollow organ injury diagnosed?**
CT findings include peritoneal fluid without solid organ injury, extravasation of oral contrast into the peritoneal cavity, and free intraabdominal air. Suggestive signs include mesenteric stranding and hematoma. Peritoneal lavage results suggestive of hollow organ injury include elevated amylase, alkaline phosphatase, or biliribun levels and the presence of particulate matter.

KEY POINTS: USEFUL DIAGNOSTIC MODALITIES IN BAT

1. Primary and secondary surveys are crucial, but further diagnostic testing is required in most patients.

2. FAST: reliably identifies intraabdominal and intrapericardial fluid but is poor at hollow viscus evaluation.

3. DPL: effective for evaluation of hemoperitoneum and a useful adjunct along with FAST exam.

4. CT: excellent modality with 99.97% negative predictive value for BAT.

7. **What are the indications for urgent operation in a patient with BAT?**
Any hemodynamically unstable patient who exhibits significant hemoperitoneum (by US or DPL) requires emergency laparotomy. Other indications for urgent laparotomy include free intraabdominal air and evidence of hollow viscus injury.

8. **How does time in the emergency department (ED) impact the mortality of patients requiring emergent operation for BAT?**
The probability of death from trauma is related to both the extent of hypotension and the interval from the time of injury to definitive surgery. An estimated increase in mortality of 1% is incurred for every 3 minutes spent in the ED up to 90 minutes.

9. **What is the role of angiographic embolization?**
Angiographic embolization may be effective for hemorrhage control in hemodynamically stable patients. Favorable embolization sites include liver, spleen, and kidney injuries; lumbar arteries with retroperitoneal hemorrhage; and pelvic blood vessels associated with pelvic fracture.

10. **What is the "bloody viscus cycle"?**
The bloody viscus cycle is a syndrome of hypothermia, acidosis, and coagulopathy that occurs with profound hemorrhagic shock and massive transfusion. It represents a circular cascade of events in which severe hemorrhagic shock accompanied by metabolic failure provokes a coagulopathy that exacerbates further bleeding.

11. **What is a staged or abbreviated laparotomy (damage control surgery)?**
Staged laparotomy is terminated before all definitive procedures are completed with the intent to return to the operating room to complete the operation at a later (and safer) time. The purpose of this approach is to delay additional surgical stress until the patient is in a more favorable physiologic state. The objectives of the initial operation become to (1) arrest bleeding and correct coagulopathy; (2) limit peritoneal contamination and the secondary inflammatory response (to control gastrointestinal spillage); and (3) enclose the abdominal contents to protect viscera and limit heat, fluid, and protein loss from an open abdomen.

12. **When is staged laparotomy used in trauma patients?**
- Inability to achieve hemostasis because of recalcitrant coagulopathy (pack the bleeding)
- Inaccessible major venous injury (retrohepatic caval injury)
- Demand for control of a life-threatening extraabdominal (e.g., head or thoracic) injury
- Inability to close the abdominal incision because of extensive visceral edema
- Need to reassess the abdominal contents because of questionable viability at the time of the initial operation

WEB SITE

http://www.east.org/tpg/bluntabd.pdf

BIBLIOGRAPHY

1. Branney SW, Moore EE, Cantrill SV, et al: Ultrasound based key clinical pathway reduces the use of hosptial resources for the evaluation of blunt abdominal trauma. J Trauma 42:1086–1090, 1997.
2. Burch JM, Denton JR, Noble RD: Physiologic rationale for abbreviated laparotomy. Surg Clin North Am 77:779–782, 1997.
3. Clarke JR, Trooskin SZ, Doshi PJ, et al: Time to laparotomy for intra-abdominal bleeding from trauma does affect survival for delays up to 90 minutes. J Trauma 52:420–425, 2002.
4. Davis KA, Fabian TC, Croce MA, et al: Improved success in management of blunt splenic injuries: Embolization of splenic artery pseudoaneurysms. J Trauma 44:1008–1013, 1998.
5. Livingston DH, Lavery RF, Passannante MR, et al: Free fluid on abdominal computed tomography without solid organ injury after blunt abdominal injury does not mandate celiotomy. Am J Surg 182:6–9, 2001.
6. Miller MT, Pasquale MD, Bromberg WJ, et al: Not so fast. J Trauma 54:52–59, 2003.

CHAPTER 24

PENETRATING ABDOMINAL TRAUMA

Clay Cothren, M.D., and Ernest E. Moore, M.D.

1. **Why is there a different approach to stab and gunshot wounds?**
   Whereas one third of stab wounds to the anterior abdomen do not penetrate the peritoneum, 80% of gunshot wounds violate the peritoneum. Furthermore, penetration of the
   peritoneum by a bullet is associated with visceral or vascular injuries in > 95% of cases,
   whereas only one third of stab wounds violating the peritoneal cavity produce significant
   injury. (See Figure 24-1.)

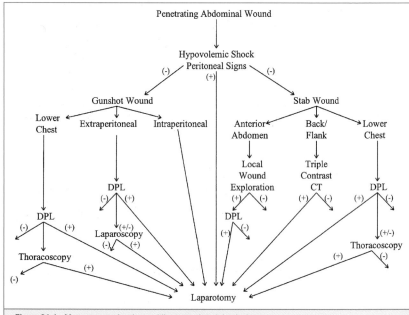

Figure 24-1. Management of patients witih penetrating abdominal trauma.

2. **What is the secondary survey for a penetrating abdominal wound?**
   The ABCs (i.e., airway, breathing, and circulation) are the first priority in every trauma patient. Look
   everywhere—watch out; it is easy to overlook synchronous injuries. This includes looking for additional entry or exit sites; evaluation for blood in the gastrointestinal (GI), genitourinary (GU), and
   gynecologic systems; and blunt mechanism injuries (e.g., some unfortunate patients are both
   stabbed and beat up). The "mechanism" of injury includes the time of injury, type of weapon, length
   or caliber of the weapon, depth of penetration, and estimated blood loss at the scene. (See Figure
   24-2.)

3. **What are the appropriate initial studies in patients with penetrating abdominal trauma?**
    In stable patients, a chest radiograph excludes hemo- or pneumothorax and determines the position of intravenous catheters (e.g., endotracheal, nasogastric, and pleural tubes). Biplanar abdominal radiographs are helpful in locating retained foreign bodies, such as bullets, and may reveal pneumoperitoneum. Entrance and exit wounds should be identified with a radiopaque marker. This may be helpful in determining the trajectory of missiles. Injuries in proximity to the rectum obligate sigmoidoscopy (see Chapter 28), whereas injuries in proximity to the urinary tract should be evaluated with computed tomography (CT) scanning (see Chapter 31).

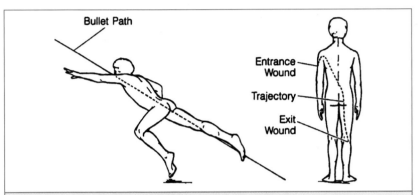

Figure 24-2. An example of how the path of a bullet through contorted body can produce confusion when the patient is examined in the emergency department. An entrance wound will be found at the left upper arm and an exit wound at the medial aspect of the right knee. The bullet could have damaged any structure that was in between these two wounds when the patient's body was contorted.

4. **What are the indications for prompt laparotomy in patients with stab wounds?**
    Abdominal distention and hypotension, overt peritonitis, and obvious signs of abdominal visceral injury (hematuria, hematemesis, proctorrhagia, evisceration; palpation of diaphragmatic defect on chest tube insertion; radiologic evidence of injury to GI or GU tracts) mandate immediate exploration.

5. **What are the indications for immediate laparotomy in patients with gunshot wounds?**
    Because of the high incidence of visceral injury, early exploration is indicated for all gunshot wounds that violate the peritoneum.

6. **When is emergency department (ED) thoracotomy indicated for a penetrating abdominal wound?**
    Almost never. But it should be considered when a patient, after penetrating trauma, presents in cardiac arrest or profound hypotension (< 60 mmHg) refractory to initial resuscitation. Thoracotomy allows open cardiac massage and access to cross clamp the descending aorta to improve coronary and cerebral perfusion as well as decrease subdiaphragmatic hemorrhage. Closed cardiac massage is ineffective when the patient is hypovolemic. (See Figure 24-3.)

7. **What is the general plan for abdominal exploration in patients with penetrating trauma?**
    A midline abdominal incision provides rapid entry and wide exposure; it may be extended as a median sternotomy to access the chest or continued inferiorly into the pelvis. The aorta should

be palpated to assess blood pressure (BP). All findings, including a low BP, should be communicated to the anesthetist. Evacuation of blood and placement of tamponade packs into areas of suspected blood loss should be followed by exploration of the wound tract. Actively bleeding areas are digitally controlled until the culprit vessel can be occluded. Hollow visceral injuries are temporarily isolated with noncrushing clamps. The entire abdomen is systematically explored before undertaking extensive repairs so that injuries can be prioritized.

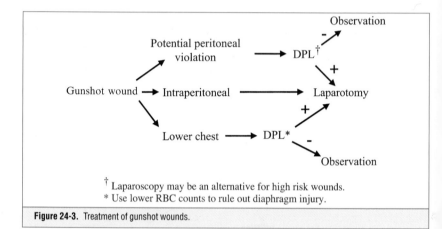

† Laparoscopy may be an alternative for high risk wounds.
* Use lower RBC counts to rule out diaphragm injury.

Figure 24-3. Treatment of gunshot wounds.

8. **How is an anterior abdominal stab wound evaluated in asymptomatic patients?**
    The first step is local exploration of the wound to determine peritoneal penetration. If the tract clearly terminates superficially, above the fascia, no further evaluation or treatment is required. If the fascia is penetrated or the peritoneum violated, diagnostic peritoneal lavage (DPL) is performed. Double-contrast (oral and intravenous) CT scanning is not routinely used because of its relative insensitivity for detecting hollow visceral injuries. Ultrasonography is useful for detecting intraperitoneal fluid but is helpful only if the results are positive. (See Figure 24-4.)

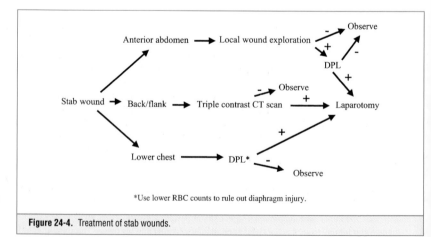

*Use lower RBC counts to rule out diaphragm injury.

Figure 24-4. Treatment of stab wounds.

9. **What constitutes a positive DPL result after penetrating trauma?**
   A grossly positive tap (aspiration of >10 mL of blood or aspiration of GI or biliary contents) mandates immediate exploration. A negative initial aspirate result is followed by the instillation of 1000 mL of saline (15 mL/kg in children) into the abdomen through a dialysis catheter, followed by gravity drainage of the fluid back into the saline bag. The finding of > 100,000/mm^3 red blood cells (RBCs), the combined elevation of amylase > 20 IU/L and alkaline phosphatase > 3 IU/L, or elevated bilirubin level are also indications for exploration.

10. **How are stab wounds to the flank and back evaluated?**
    The incidence of significant injuries is 10% for stab wounds to the back and 25% for stab wounds to the flank. However, evaluation of such wounds is problematic because the retroperitoneum is not sampled by DPL and physical examination is even less sensitive. The major concern is missed colonic perforation. At present, triple-contrast (oral, intravenous, and rectal) CT scan and serial physical examination are the two primary modes of assessment. Operative exploration is advisable if CT scanning demonstrates wound trajectory in the vicinity of the colon.

KEY POINTS: CLINICAL APPROACH TO PENETRATING ABDOMINAL TRAUMA

1. Gunshot wounds to the abdomen generally require operative exploration (> 80% violate the peritoneum).

2. Stab wounds with evisceration or hypotension are operatively explored.

3. Stab wounds in stable patients are managed with local wound exploration (66% violate the peritoneum) plus DPL, ultrasound, or CT scan. If tests are positive, the patient goes to the operating room.

4. During celiotomy, pack the upper quadrants and pelvis; then address vascular, solid organ, and alimentary tract injuries in succession.

5. Prophylactic antibiotics for the first 24 hours decrease postoperative wound infection.

11. **How is a lower chest stab wound evaluated?**
    The lower chest is defined as the area between the nipple line (fourth intercostal space) anteriorly, the tip of the scapula (seventh intercostal space) posteriorly, and the costal margins inferiorly. Because the diaphragm reaches the fourth intercostal space during expiration, the abdominal organs are at risk (even after what appears to be a clear "chest" wound). Stab wounds to the lower chest are associated with abdominal visceral injury in 15% of cases, whereas gunshot wounds to the lower chest are associated with abdominal visceral injury in nearly 50% of cases. Thus, wounds to the lower chest should also be managed as abdominal wounds to rule out intraabdominal injury. In the case of lower chest stab wounds, an RBC count of > 10,000/mm^3 warrants laparotomy to rule out a diaphragmatic injury; thoracoscopic exploration (not thoracotomy) may also be performed for counts of 1000–10,000/mm^3.

12. **Which patients with abdominal gunshot wounds are managed nonoperatively?**
    Stable patients with tangential missile tracts or equivocal peritoneal penetration are candidates for DPL. The cutoff for RBC counts is reduced to 10,000/mm^3, above which laparotomy is indicated. Patients with a negative DPL result are observed for 24 hours. For RBC counts of 100–10,000/mm^3, laparoscopy may be used to exclude intraperitoneal injury. Selective management of gunshot wounds to the back and flank are generally based on triple contrast CT.

13. **What is the role for presumptive antibiotics?**
Short courses (< 24 hours) of high-dose antibiotics are initiated only when the decision has been made to perform a laparotomy. Coverage of both anaerobic and aerobic flora is desirable. Tetanus prophylaxis should be given to all patients with penetrating injuries.

CONTROVERSY

14. **What is the role of laparoscopy and thoracoscopy after penetrating abdominal trauma?**
Although an intriguing diagnostic modality with additional therapeutic capabilities, laparoscopy thus far appears to have limited application after trauma. With the exception of suspected diaphragmatic injury, an isolated solid organ injury, or evaluation for peritoneal penetration, laparoscopy has yet to demonstrate advantages over the algorithm delineated above. The potential for missed injuries, poor evaluation of the retroperitoneum, and expense are major drawbacks. In patients with wounds to the lower chest with pneumothorax (and, thus, an indication for chest tube placement), thoracoscopy is reasonable to exclude diaphragmatic injury.

WEB SITES

1. http://www.east.org/tpg/atbpenetra.pdf

2. http://www.surgery.ucsf.edu/eastbaytrauma/Protocols/ER%20protocol%20pages/abdominal_stab.htm

BIBLIOGRAPHY

1. Chiu WC, Shanmuganathan K, Mirvis SE, Scalea TM: Determining the need for laparotomy in penetrating torso trauma: A prospective study using triple-contrast enhanced abdominopelvic computed tomography. J Trauma 51:860–868, 2001.

2. Freeman RK, Al-Dossari G, Hutcheson KA, et al: Indications for using video-assisted thoracoscopic surgery to diagnose diaphragmatic injuries after penetrating chest trauma. Ann Thorac Surg 72:342–347, 2001.

3. Henneman PL, Marx JA, Moore EE, et al: Diagnostic peritoneal lavage: accuracy in predicting necessary laparotomy following blunt and penetrating trauma. J Trauma 30:1345–1355, 1990.

4. McAlvanah MJ, Shaftan GW: Selective conservatism in penetrating abdominal wounds: A continuing reappraisal. J Trauma 18:206–212, 1978.

5. McAnena OJ, Marx JA, Moore EE: Peritoneal lavage enzyme determinations following blunt and penetrating abdominal trauma. J Trauma 31:1161–1164, 1991.

6. Moore EE, Marx JA: Penetrating abdominal wounds: A rationale for exploratory laparotomy. JAMA 253:2705–2708, 1985.

7. Reber PU, Schmied B, Seiler CA, et al: Missed diaphragmatic injuries and their long-term sequelae. J Trauma 44:183–188, 1998.

8. Simon RJ, Rabin J, Kuhls D: Impact of increased use of laparoscopy on negative laparotomy rates after penetrating trauma. J Trauma 53:297–302, 2002.

CHAPTER 25

HEPATIC AND BILIARY TRAUMA

Reginald J. Franciose, M.D., and Ernest E. Moore, M.D.

1. **How often is the liver injured in trauma?**
   The liver is both big and central, so it is an easy target.

2. **Do the liver and spleen respond similarly to injury?**
   No. The liver has a unique ability to establish spontaneous hemostasis even with extensive injuries. For this reason, the majority of liver injuries in hemodynamically stable patients can be managed nonoperatively. In contrast, many splenic fractures continue to bleed; therefore, a greater percentage require operative intervention.

3. **What are the determinants of mortality after acute liver injury?**
   The mechanism of injury and the number of associated abdominal organs injured determine mortality. The mortality for stab wounds to the liver is 2%; for gunshot wounds, 8%; and for blunt injuries, 15%. The mortality rate for isolated grade III hepatic injuries is 2%; for grade IV, 20%; and for grade V, 65%. Retrohepatic vena cava injuries carry mortality rates of 80% for penetrating trauma and 95% for blunt trauma.

4. **What history and physical signs suggest acute liver injury?**
   Any patient sustaining blunt abdominal trauma with hypotension must be assumed to have a liver injury until proven otherwise. Specific signs that increase the likelihood of hepatic injury are contusion over the right lower chest, fracture of the right lower ribs (especially posterior fractures of ribs 9–12), and penetrating injuries to the right lower chest (below the fourth intercostal space, flank, and upper abdomen). Physical signs of hemoperitoneum may be absent in as many as one third of patients with significant hepatic injury.

5. **What diagnostic tests are helpful in confirming acute liver injury?**
   A focused abdominal sonography for trauma (FAST) examination can detect or rule out hemoperitoneum and pericardial tamponade. Diagnostic peritoneal lavage (DPL) is sensitive for hemoperitoneum (99%). Ultrasound is highly sensitive in identifying > 200 mL of intraperitoneal fluid. It is noninvasive and may be repeated at frequent intervals, but it is relatively poor for staging liver injuries. Abdominal computed tomography (CT) scan currently is used only in hemodynamically stable patients who are candidates for nonoperative management. The major shortcoming of CT is the relatively poor correlation between hepatic CT staging and subsequent risk of hemorrhage.

6. **What is the role of hepatic angiography and radionuclide biliary excretion scans in the diagnosis of liver injury?**
   Selective hepatic artery embolization is effective therapy for hepatic arterial bleeding, both for avoidance of surgery and for recurrent postoperative bleeding.

SURGICAL ANATOMY OF THE LIVER

7. **How many anatomic lobes are present in the liver? What is their topographic boundary?**

   The liver is divided into two anatomic lobes, the right and the left. Their boundary lies in an oblique plane extending from the gallbladder fossa anteriorly to the inferior vena cava posteriorly. The three hepatic veins define the division between the lobar segments and the planes of surgical resection. Lobar segments are numbered I–VIII, according to Couinaud's nomenclature. (See Figure 25-1.)

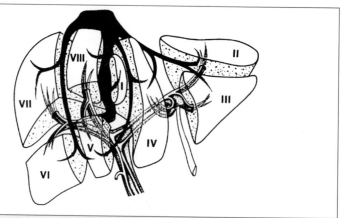

Figure 25-1. The functional division of the liver and the segments according to Couinaud's nomenclature. (From Bismuth H: Surgical anatomy and anatomical surgery of the liver. World J Surg 6:6, 1982, with permission.)

8. **What is the blood supply to the liver and the relative contribution of each structure to hepatic oxygenation?**

   The hepatic artery supplies approximately 30% of the blood flow to the liver and 50% of its oxygen supply. The portal vein provides 70% of the liver's blood flow and 50% of its oxygen. The relative significance of arterial flow in cirrhotic patients is greater; therefore, hepatic artery ligation is not recommended in patients with cirrhosis.

9. **What are the most common variations in hepatic arterial supply to the right and left lobes of the liver?**

   In most people, the common hepatic artery originates from the celiac axis and divides into right and left hepatic arterial branches within the porta hepatis. Approximately 15% of people have a replaced right hepatic artery (sole arterial supply to the right lobe) that originates from the superior mesenteric artery (SMA). A replaced right hepatic artery always supplies a cystic artery; thus, ligation should be followed by cholecystectomy. A replaced left hepatic artery (approximately 15% of people) arises from the left gastric artery; it may be the sole blood supply to the left lobe or may contribute to blood supply in conjunction with a normal left hepatic artery. In 5% of people, the hepatic arterial supply does not arise from the celiac axis. In these people, either the right and left hepatic arteries are replaced or a single main hepatic trunk derives from the SMA.

10. **What is the venous drainage of the liver?**

    The right, middle, and left hepatic veins are the major venous tributaries and enter the inferior vena cava below the right hemidiaphragm.

KEY POINTS: BLOOD SUPPLY AND DRAINAGE OF THE LIVER

1. Hepatic artery delivers 30% of blood flow.

2. Portal vein delivers 70% of blood flow.

3. In 15% of the population the right hepatic artery originates from the superior mesenteric artery.

4. In 15% of the population the left hepatic artery originates from the celiac artery.

5. In 5% of the population neither hepatic artery originates from the celiac artery.

6. Venous drainage: right, middle, and left hepatic veins drain into the inferior vena cava.

OPERATIVE MANAGEMENT OF LIVER INJURY

11. **How are acute liver injuries classified?**
Liver wounds are generally graded on a scale of I to VI according the depth of parenchymal laceration and involvement of the hepatic veins or retrohepatic portion of the inferior vena cava. Optimal methods of obtaining hemostasis vary with the severity of the injury.

12. **Do all patients with a traumatic liver injury require surgery?**
No. Nonoperative treatment is the standard for victims of blunt trauma who remain hemodynamically stable (approximately 85% of patients). One third of such patients require blood transfusions, but if the volume exceeds 6 units in the first 24 hours, angiography should be done. CT scan should be repeated in 5–7 days for grade IV and V injuries. Complications, including perihepatic infection, biloma, and hemobilia, have been reported in 10% of nonoperative patients.

13. **What are the options for temporary control of significant hemorrhage in victims of hepatic trauma?**
Ongoing hemorrhage leads to the vicious cycle of acidosis, hypothermia, and coagulopathy. Manual compression, perihepatic packing, and the Pringle maneuver are the most effective temporary strategies.

14. **What is the Pringle maneuver?**
The Pringle maneuver is a manual or vascular clamp occlusion of the hepatoduodenal ligament to interrupt blood flow into the liver. Included in the hepatoduodenal ligament are the hepatic artery, portal vein, and common bile duct. Failure of the Pringle maneuver to control liver hemorrhage suggests either (1) injury to the retrohepatic vena cava or hepatic vein or (2) arterial supply from an aberrant right or left hepatic artery (see question 9).

15. **What is the finger fracture technique?**
Finger fracture hepatotomy or tractotomy is the method of exposing bleeding points deep within liver lacerations by blunt dissection. Pushing apart the liver parenchyma enables points to be identified and ligated. This method is most commonly required for penetrating injuries.

16. **What is the role of selective hepatic artery ligation in securing hemostasis in patients with a major liver injury?**
Deep lacerations of the right or left hepatic lobe may result in bleeding that cannot be completely controlled by suture ligation of specific bleeding points within the liver parenchyma. In this

situation, either the right or left artery can be ligated for control of the bleeding with little risk of ischemic liver necrosis.

17. **Why is retrohepatic vena caval laceration lethal?**
Exposure requires either extensive hepatotomy, extensive mobilization of the right lobe, or right lobectomy, or transection of the vena cava. The large caliber and high flow of the inferior vena cava results in massive hemorrhage during surgical exposure, whereas clamping of the inferior vena cava often results in hypotension attributable to an abrupt decrease in venous return to the heart.

18. **What is the physiologic rationale for use of a shunt in attempted repair of retrohepatic vena caval injuries?**
Hemorrhage control requires maintenance of venous return to the heart while both antegrade and retrograde bleeding through the laceration is stopped. These requirements are met by shunting blood through a tube spanning the laceration between the right atrium and lower inferior vena cava.

19. **What is the intrahepatic balloon tamponading device?**
For transhepatic penetrating injuries, a 1-inch Penrose drain is sutured around a red rubber catheter. This forms a long balloon that is threaded through the bleeding liver injury and inflated with contrast media through a stopcock in the red rubber catheter. The balloon tamponades liver hemorrhage. The catheter is brought out through the abdominal wall, deflated, and removed 24–48 hours later.

20. **What are the indications for perihepatic packing?**
Liver packing with planned reoperation for definitive treatment of injuries in patients who have hypothermia, acidosis, and coagulopathies is a life-saving maneuver. Laparotomy pads (> 20) are packed around the liver to compress and control hemorrhage. The skin of the abdomen is then closed with towel clips (abbreviated laparotomy), and the patient's metabolic abnormalities are corrected with planned reoperation within 24 hours.

21. **What is the abdominal compartment syndrome?**
The abdominal compartment syndrome is a potentially lethal complication of perihepatic packing. It may occur when intraabdominal pressure exceeds 20 cmH$_2$O. Intraabdominal pressure increases because of bowel and liver edema secondary to ischemia and reperfusion injury or continued hemorrhage into the abdominal cavity. As pressure increases beyond 20 cmH$_2$O, venous return, cardiac output, and urine output decrease, but ventilatory pressures increase. Patients must return promptly to the operating room for decompression of the abdomen. A manometer attached to the Foley catheter is useful in following intraabdominal pressure.

BILIARY TRACT INJURY

22. **Why are complications associated with bile duct leaks?**
Bilomas (i.e., collections of bile) frequently become infected and may result in lethal peritonitis. Biliopleural fistula, a communication between the biliary system and pleural cavity, persists because of the relative negative pressure in the thorax and may result in a bile empyema.

23. **What is the initial management of an established bile leak?**
Endoscopic transampullary stenting frequently allows spontaneous resolution of bile duct injuries. Extensive injuries require hepaticojejunostomy for reconstruction.

WEB SITES

1. http://www.acssurgery.com/abstracts/acs/acs0506.htm

2. http://www.acssurgery.com/abstracts/acs/acs0508.htm

BIBLIOGRAPHY

1. Croce MA, Fabian TC, Menke PG, et al: Nonoperative management of blunt hepatic trauma is the treatment of choice for hemodynamically stable patients. Ann Surg 221:744–753, 1995.

2. Gaines BA, Ford HR: Abdominal and pelvic trauma in children. Crit Care Med 30(suppl):S416-S423, 2002.

3. Hiatt JR, Gabbay J, Busutill RW: Surgical anatomy of the hepatic arteries in 1000 cases. Ann Surg 220:50–52, 1994.

4. Meldrum DR, Moore FA, Moore EE, et al: Cardiopulmonary hazards of perihepatic packing for major liver injury. Am J Surg 170:537–540, 1995.

5. Meredith JW, Young JR, Bowling J, Roboussin D: Nonoperative management of adult blunt hepatic trauma: The exception or the rule? J Trauma 36:529–534, 1994.

6. Moore EE: Staged laparotomy for the hypothermia, acidosis, and coagulopathy syndrome. Am J Surg 172:405–410, 1996.

7. Moore EE, Cogbill TH, Malangoni MA, et al: Organ injury scaling. Surg Clin North Am 75:293–303, 1995.

8. Pachter HL, Hofstetter SR: The current status of nonoperative management of adult blunt hepatic injuries. Am J Surg 169:442–454, 1995.

9. Poggetti RS, Moore EE, Moore FA, et al: Balloon tamponade for bilobar transfixing hepatic gunshot wounds. J Trauma 33:694–697, 1992.

10. Sheik-Gafoor M, Singh B, Moodley J: Traumatic thoracobiliary fistula: Report of a case with an overview of current diagnostic and therapeutic options. J Trauma 45:819–821, 1998.

11. Tai NR, Boffard KD, Goosen J, Plani F: A 10-year experience of complex liver trauma. Br J Surg 89:1532–1537, 2002.

12. Verous M, Cillo U, Brolese A, et al: Blunt liver injury: From non-operative management to liver transplantation. Injury 34:181–186, 2003.

CHAPTER 26

SPLENIC TRAUMA

David J. Ciesla, M.D., and Ernest E. Moore, M.D.

1. **What is the physiologic role of the spleen?**
   In fetal development, the spleen serves as a major site for hematopoiesis. In early childhood the spleen produces immunoglobulin M (IgM) and tuftsin. The spleen also functions as a filter, allowing resident macrophages to remove abnormal red blood cells (RBCs), cellular debris, and encapsulated and poorly opsonized bacteria.

2. **What injury patterns are associated with splenic trauma?**
   Direct blunt force, deceleration, and compression to the left torso. Think **spleen** after a motor vehicle accident or fall: lower rib fractures, left side–only rib fractures, and high-energy transfer (big hits) increase the probability of splenic injury.

3. **What are the signs and symptoms of splenic injury?**
   The main sign is pain in the left upper quadrant. This is produced by stretching the splenic capsule. Peritoneal irritation (rebound tenderness) is caused by extravasated blood (blood is very irritating). Vital signs vary depending on associated blood loss and are not specific for injuries to the spleen. Unfortunately, a large number of patients with a significant splenic injury exhibit no signs or symptoms at all.

4. **What studies can help in diagnosing splenic trauma?**
   Ultrasound (US) can be performed in the emergency department and can rapidly identify as little as 200 mL fluid/blood. When US is not available, diagnostic peritoneal lavage (DPL) is an accurate and sensitive measure of intraabdominal bleeding.
   Hemodynamically stable patients permit more thorough evaluations. Although US is extremely sensitive for detecting intraabdominal bleeding, computed tomography (CT) not only can detect and quantify intraabdominal blood but also can characterize specific intraabdominal injuries.

5. **How are splenic injuries classified, and why is that important?**
   Management is governed by the hemodynamic status of the patient, but therapy is also influenced by the CT grade of splenic injury. Nonoperative management is most successful in grades I–III, whereas operative intervention is often required for grade IV injuries. Grade V injuries demand prompt operative intervention. (See Table 26-1.)

6. **Do splenic injuries require laparotomy?**
   No. Nonoperative management is successful in approximately 95% of patients with grades I–III. Hemodynamically stable patients with evidence of ongoing bleeding (requiring transfusion) may be treated by selective arterial embolization if a bleeding site is identified on angiography.

7. **What are contraindications to nonoperative management of splenic injuries?**
   - Hemodynamic instability
   - Persistent coagulopathy
   - Additional intraabdominal injury requiring operative intervention

TABLE 26-1. GRADES OF SPLENIC INJURY

Grade	Description
I	Hematoma: nonexpanding subcapsular < 10% surface area
	Laceration: nonbleeding capsular < 1 cm parenchymal depth
II	Hematoma: nonexpanding, subcapsular < 50% surface area
	Nonexpanding intraparenchymal < 5 cm diameter
	Laceration: bleeding, capsular < 3 cm parenchymal depth
III	Hematoma: subcapsular > 50% surface area, expanding, ruptured with active bleeding
	Intraparenchymal > 5 cm diameter or expanding
	Laceration: capsular > 3 cm parenchymal depth, involving trabecular vessel
IV	Hematoma: ruptured, intraparenchymal, with active bleeding
	Laceration: involves segmental or hilar vessels with > 25% splenic devascularization
V	Laceration: shattered spleen
	Vascular: hilar avulsion or complete splenic devascularization

8. **What is the failure rate of nonoperative management of splenic injury?**
    Any patient with signs of hemodynamic instability, persistent bleeding, worsening pain or tenderness, or progressive injury by CT scanning has failed nonoperative management. Approximately 60% of all splenic injuries can be managed nonoperatively with a failure rate of 12%. Factors that predict nonoperative failure include multiple injuries, grade III–V spleen injuries, age > 55 years, and blood traunsfusion.

KEY POINTS: EXPECTANT MANAGEMENT OF SPLENIC INJURIES

1. Nonoperative management is successful in 95% of grades I-III injuries.

2. 60% of all splenic injuries are managed nonoperatively, with a 12% failure/conversion rate.

3. Factors that predict failure/conversion to operative treatment include injury > grade III, age > 55 years, and blood transfusion requirements.

4. Patients with evidence of ongoing bleeding (e.g., contrast "blush" on CT or ongoing transfusion requirements) may be managed with selective arterial embolization.

9. **What is delayed rupture of the spleen?**
    This is a rare complication that occurs in < 1% of patients with a splenic injury. Delayed splenic rupture should be distinguished from a delay in diagnosis of splenic injury and rupture of a known splenic injury. True delayed splenic rupture occurs > 48 hours in a patient with a history of abdominal trauma and no overt clinical evidence of intraabdominal injury on initial presentation.

10. **What are the general principles of operative management of the injured spleen?**
The first priority is to control bleeding. This can usually be accomplished by packing and manual compression of the spleen. If successful, the abdomen is then thoroughly explored for other injuries. Complete mobilization of the spleen by division of the splenocolic, splenorenal, phrenosplenic, and gastrosplenic ligaments is required for complete assessment of the spleen. The short gastric vessels can be ligated with division of the gastrosplenic ligament. Repair of the spleen can be accomplished by application of hemostatic agents, direct pledgeted suture repair of the splenic parenchyma, partial splenectomy, and construction of a "splenic wrap" using absorbable mesh. If splenectomy is required, the splenic artery and vein should be ligated individually prior to removing the spleen.

11. **What early complications arise after splenectomy?**
Bleeding, acute gastric dilatation, gastric perforation, pancreatitis (the splenic artery courses along the top of the pancreas), and subphrenic abscess.

12. **What is splenic autotransplantation?**
Autotransplantation is accomplished by implanting splenic tissue parenchymal slices into pouches created in the gastrocolic omentum.

13. **Does splenic autotransplantation preserve splenic function?**
Autotransplantion after splenectomy is controversial. At least 30% of the original splenic mass is needed to provide normal function. After autotransplantation, IgG and IgM levels are increased in response to pneumococcal vaccine compared with patients after splenectomy alone.

14. **Does postsplenectomy leukocytosis predict infection?**
Elevations in white blood cell (WBC) count and platelet count (PC) after splenectomy are a common physiologic event. After the fourth postoperative day, however, a WBC $> 15 \times 10^3$ and a PC/WBC < 20 are highly associated with sepsis and should not be confused with the physiologic response to splenectomy.

15. **Should a follow-up CT scan be performed after nonoperative management of splenic injuries before patient discharge?**
No. Most patients who fail nonoperative management do so within 5 days and will exhibit hemodynamic evidence of ongoing hemorrhage. However, follow-up CT should be performed for grade III and IV injuries at 4–6 weeks before getting back to vigorous physical activity.

16. **What is OPSS, and how is it prevented?**
Overwhelming post splenectomy sepsis (OPSS) is a devastating bacteremia (typically encapsulated bacteria) that occurs in 2% of patients after splenectomy. The risk of OPSS is greatest when splenectomy is performed during infancy. The most common organisms are pneumococcus (50%), meningococcus, *Escherichia coli, Haemophilus influenzae*, staphylococcus, and streptococcus. Although rare, OPSS carries a mortality rate of 75% and has spurred interest in splenic preservation. OPSS is primarily prevented by postoperative vaccination. Pneumococcal, meningococcal, and *Haemophilus* flu vaccines should be given 2 weeks after splenectomy and are recommended every 5 years. Sepsis can occur despite vaccination; consequently, long-term prophylaxis with oral penicillin is recommended for children.

WEB SITES

1. http://www.east.org/tpg/bluntabd.pdf

2. http://www.acssurgery.com/abstracts/acs/acs0506.htm

BIBLIOGRAPHY

1. Cocanour CS, Moore FA, Ware DN, et al: Delayed complications of nonoperative management of blunt adult splenic trauma. Arch Surg 133:619–624, 1998.

2. Leemans R, Manson W, Snijder JA, et al: Immune response capacity after human splenic autotransplantation: Restoration of response to individual pneumococcal vaccine subtypes. Ann Surg 229:279–285, 1999.

3. Moore EE, Cogbill TH, Jurkovich GJ, et al: Organ injury scaling: Spleen and liver (1994 revision). J Trauma 38:323–324, 1995.

4. Shatz DV: Vaccination practices among North American trauma surgeons in splenectomy for trauma. J Trauma 53:950–956, 2002.

5. Toutouzas KG, Velmahos GC, Kaminski A, et al: Leukocytosis after posttraumatic splenectomy: A physiologic event or sign of sepsis? Arch Surg 137:924–928, 2002.

6. Uecker J, Pickett C, Dunn E: The role of follow-up radiographic studies in nonoperative management of spleen trauma. Am Surg 67:22–25, 2001.

CHAPTER 27

PANCREATIC AND DUODENAL INJURY

Caesar M. Ursic, M.D.

1. **How common are pancreatic injuries?**

   The pancreas is not commonly injured because of its protected retroperitoneal position, and thus accounts for only 8% of all penetrating and 2% of all blunt visceral injuries.

2. **What other injuries are typically associated with penetrating pancreatic trauma?**

   Liver injury is the most frequent concomitant injury, with a reported incidence of ≤ 50%. Other commonly associated injuries include the stomach (40%), large abdominal vessels such as the aorta and vena cava (40%), spleen (25%), kidneys (2%), and duodenum (20%).

3. **How are pancreatic injuries diagnosed and staged preoperatively?**

   Preoperatively, computed tomography with intravenous contrast enhancement may actually demonstrate a transected pancreas or major destruction of portions of the gland and has a high positive predictive value; however, it suffers from a low negative predictive value (i.e., it may miss even big injuries). Ultrasound does not consistently image the retroperitoneum adequately and is often hampered by overlying bowel gas. Elevated serum amylase concentrations are nonspecific for pancreatic injury and can be normal in a high proportion of patients shown subsequently to harbor significant injuries to the gland. Diagnostic peritoneal lavage is also unreliable. Short of mandatory exploration, there are no universally reliable methods to assure early diagnosis of significant pancreatic injuries. Surgeons must pay particular attention to the mechanism of injury and subtle signs and symptoms of the physical examination and combine them with data obtained from imaging studies.

4. **What are some of the commonly used surgical options for the treatment of pancreatic injuries?**

   Most low-grade penetrating and blunt injuries to the pancreas are adequately treated by closed suction drains placed at surgery. First, the integrity of the main pancreatic duct should be evaluated, either by direct inspection or by intraoperative pancreatography. Distal duct injuries (defined as those occurring to the left of the superior mesenteric vessels) are treated with distal pancreatectomy, with or without splenectomy, and closed drainage of the pancreatic stump. Preservation of the spleen is preferable. Injuries to the proximal portion of the gland that do not involve the main duct are treated with closed suction drainage. Injury to the pancreatic duct in the head or neck of the pancreas may require resection of significant portions of distal pancreas. If more than 80% of the gland is removed, the risk of endocrine and exocrine pancreatic insufficiency is high. Try to preserve distal glandular tissue by incorporating it into a Roux-en-Y pancreaticojejunostomy. With severe pancreatic head destruction, instances involving significant injuries to the duodenum and distal biliary structures may require a pancreaticoduodenectomy (i.e., Whipple procedure). Recent reports of successful nonoperative management of complete pancreatic transections in pediatric patients may shift the approach to these injuries away from resection, although the current standard of care remains surgical.

KEY POINTS: SURGICAL OPTIONS FOR PANCREATIC INJURIES

1. Low-grade injuries are treated with simple closed suction drainage at the time of celiotomy.

2. In unstable patients, debride, obtain hemostasis, and drain. Deal with the resultant fistula at a later time.

3. If ductal injury is suspected in a stable patient, visualize with ERCP or cholangiogram.

4. If ductal injury is present in the head or neck of the pancreas, ligate proximally and attempt to preserve pancreatic tissue with Roux-en-Y pancreaticojejunostomy.

5. Always place a jejunal feeding tube.

5. **Is an elevated serum amylase level diagnostic of pancreatic trauma?**
No. Up to 40% of patients who have sustained significant pancreatic injury do not show elevations in their initial serum amylase level. There appears to be a slightly higher positive predictive value if the elevated amylase level is obtained more than 3 hours after the patient's injury, although elevated amylase is common with trauma not involving the pancreas. Up to 40% of patients sustaining isolated head trauma can present with serum hyperamylasemia, which is unrelated to pancreatic injury.

6. **How do blunt pancreatic injuries differ in children and adults?**
Adult pancreatic injury is usually either penetrating (e.g., stab and gunshot wounds) or high-speed blunt forces (e.g., motor vehicular crashes). Children usually present after direct blows to the epigastrium, typically from bicycle handlebars, which compress the pancreas between the anterior surface of the thoracic spine and the handlebar, often resulting in complete glandular transection.

7. **What is the optimal route of nutritional supplementation after a major pancreatic injury?**
Direct feeding into the stomach is contraindicated because it stimulates pancreatic exocrine secretion and aggravates healing, potentiating secondary pancreatitis and pancreatic fistulas formation. Postpyloric enteral nutrition can be delivered safely and effectively via a feeding jejunostomy tube placed at the completion of the abdominal exploration and pancreatic repair.

8. **Describe the common complications of pancreatic injuries.**
Complications are common. The two most common are pancreatic fistulas and intraabdominal abscesses. Other problems are pancreatitis, pancreatic pseudocyst, and pancreatic hemorrhage. Most patients who die after sustaining injuries to the pancreas do so as a result of late complications and not from the pancreatic injury itself.

9. **What is the role of computed tomography (CT) scanning in diagnosing blunt duodenal injuries?**
Although CT is an excellent tool for visualizing solid organ injuries, CT is less useful with injuries to hollow organs such as the duodenum. Even the addition of an oral contrast agent to the study does not seem to improve the diagnostic yield. Subtle signs of duodenal injury on CT scans include periduodenal edema or fluid and retroduodenal air, which usually indicates a duodenal rupture and spillage of small amounts of intralumenal contents into the retroperitoneum.

10. **What is the importance of the Kocher maneuver?**
In 1903, Kocher described what has now become a routine maneuver during the exploratory celiotomy to visualize and repair injuries to the duodenum, distal common bile duct, and

pancreatic head. The avascular lateral peritoneal attachments to the duodenum are incised sharply; then the duodenal sweep is elevated and reflected medially, allowing for inspection and palpation of its posterior surface as well as of the head of the pancreas.

11. **What are the four portions of the duodenum and their surgical relationships?**
The **first portion** of the duodenum starts at the pylorus (intraperitoneally) and passes backward (retroperitoneally) toward the gallbladder (the remainder of the duodenum is retroperitoneal). The **second portion** descends 7–8 cm and is anterior to the vena cava. The left border of the duodenum is attached to the head of the pancreas, at the site where the common bile and pancreatic ducts enter; it shares a common blood supply with the head of the pancreas through the pancreaticoduodenal arcades. The **third portion** of the duodenum turns horizontally to the left, with its cranial surface in contact with the uncinate process of the pancreas, and passes posterior to the superior mesenteric artery and vein. The **fourth portion** continues to the left, ascending slightly and crossing the spine anterior to the aorta, where it is fixed to the suspensory ligament of Treitz at the duodenojejunal flexure.

12. **How are duodenal injuries classified?**
An organ injury scale has been adopted that allows for standardized descriptions of duodenal injuries, which extend from grade I (least severe) to grade V (most severe). The grading of duodenal injuries assists surgeons in selecting the appropriate surgical procedure for the repair or reconstruction of these frequently complex injuries. (See Table 27-1.)

TABLE 27-1.	GRADES OF PANCREATIC INJURY	
Grade	Injury	Description
I	Hematoma	Involving single portion of duodenum
	Laceration	Partial thickness; no perforation
II	Hematoma	Involving more than one portion
	Laceration	Disruption < 50% of circumference
III	Laceration	Disruption 50–75% circumference of D2 or disruption of 50–100% of D1, D3, D4
IV	Laceration	Disruption > 75% of D2 or involving ampulla or distal common bile duct
V	Laceration	Massive disruption of duodenopancreatic complex
	Vascular	Devascularization of duodenum

D1, D2, D3, and D4 refer to the portions of the duodenum (i.e., first through fourth).

13. **What are the main surgical options for penetrating duodenal injuries?**
Most simple lacerations can be repaired primarily. Complex lacerations with devitalized margins or lacerations that involve > 50% of the duodenal circumference require debridement of margins and re-anastomosis of the divided ends. If tension on the suture line is anticipated because of extensive tissue loss, adjunctive techniques such as Roux-en-Y duodenojejunostomy or pyloric exclusion are more appropriate. Protection of a duodenal repair is best assured by a tube duodenostomy and generous external drainage. With severe duodenal injury that involves distal biliary structures and the pancreatic head, a pancreaticoduodenectomy (i.e., Whipple procedure) may be the most appropriate option.

WEB SITE

http://www.acs.surgery.com/abstracts/acs/acs0507.htm

BIBLIOGRAPHY

1. Asensio JA, Demetriades D, Hanpeter DE, et al: Management of pancreatic injuries. Curr Probl Surg 36:325–419, 1999.

2. Ilahi O, Bochicchio GV, Scalea TM: Efficacy of computed tomography in the diagnosis of pancreatic injury in adult blunt trauma patients: A single-institutional study. Am Surg 68:704–707, 2002.

3. Ivatury RR, Nallathambi M, Gaudino J, et al: Penetrating duodenal injuries. Analysis of 100 consecutive cases. Ann Surg 202:153–158, 1985.

4. Jobst MA, Canty TG Sr, Lynch FP: Management of pancreatic injury in pediatric blunt abdominal trauma. J Pediatr Surg 34:818–823, 1999.

5. Moore EE, Cogbill T, Malangoni M, et al: Organ injury scaling II: Pancreas, duodenum, small bowel, colon, and rectum. J Trauma 30:1427, 1990.

6. Patel SV, Spencer JA, el-Hansani S, Sheridan MB: Imaging of pancreatic trauma. Br J Radiol 71:985–990, 1998.

7. Patton J, Lyden S, Croce M, et al: Pancreatic trauma: a simplified management guideline. J Trauma 43:234–239, 1997.

8. Takishima T, Sugimoto K, Hirata M, et al: Serum amylase level on admission in the diagnosis of blunt injury to the pancreas: Its significance and limitations. Ann Surg 226:70–76, 1997.

9. Vasquez JC, Coimbra R, Hoyt DB, et al: Management of penetrating pancreatic trauma: An 11-year experience of a level-1 trauma center. Injury 32:753–759, 2001.

10. Wales PW, Shuckett B, Kim PC: Long-term outcome after nonoperative management of complete traumatic pancreatic transection in children. J Pediatr Surg 36:823–827, 2001.

11. Young PR Jr, Meredith JW, Baker CC, et al: Pancreatic injuries resulting from penetrating trauma: A multi-institution review. Am Surg 64:838–843, 1998.

CHAPTER 28

TRAUMA TO THE COLON AND RECTUM

W. Andrew Lawrence, M.D., and Jon M. Burch, M.D.

COLON TRAUMA

1. **How do most colon injuries occur?**
   Nearly all (> 95%) colon injuries are caused by penetrating trauma from gunshot, stab, iatrogenic, or sexual injury. Blunt colonic trauma is rare and usually results from seat belts during motor vehicle accidents.

2. **How are colon injuries diagnosed?**
   They are usually diagnosed during laparotomy for penetrating trauma. For patients in whom the need for laparotomy has not been established, chest and upright abdominal radiographs assess free air and detect the location of penetrating objects. Triple-contrast computed tomography (CT) or soluble-contrast radiographs (followed by barium, if necessary) can diagnose retroperitoneal colon injuries. White blood cells or fecal material in diagnostic peritoneal lavage (DPL) is highly suggestive of a bowel injury.

3. **How are colon injuries graded?**
   Grade I—contusion hematoma without devascularization; or partial-thickness laceration
   Grade II—laceration < 50% circumference
   Grade III—laceration > 50% circumference
   Grade IV—transection of the colon
   Grade V—transection with segmental tissue loss

4. **What are three surgical options for managing a colon injury?**
   1. **Primary repair:** suturing of simple sidewall perforations or resection and primary anastomosis for more complex injuries
   2. **Colostomy:** injured colon is exteriorized as a loop colostomy or the injured area is resected and an end ileostomy or proximal colostomy is formed
   3. **Exteriorized repair:** a repaired perforation or anastomosis is suspended on the abdominal wall. If the suture line does not leak after 10 days, it can be returned to the abdominal cavity under local anesthesia. If the repair breaks down, it is treated like a loop colostomy.

5. **What are the advantages and disadvantages of each of these options?**
   1. **Primary repair** is desirable because definitive treatment is carried out at the initial operation and the patient is spared the morbidity of a colostomy and its reversal. The disadvantage is that suture lines are created in suboptimal conditions, so leakage may occur.
   2. **Proximal colostomy** avoids an unprotected suture line in the abdomen but requires a second operation to close the colostomy. Stomal complications, including necrosis, stenosis, obstruction, and prolapse, may occur.
   3. **Exteriorized repair** is similar to colostomy formation in that it avoids formation of an intraperitoneal suture line. Unfortunately, many patients require a colostomy closure, and stomal complications similar to those of colostomies may occur.

6. **How are most patients with colon injuries surgically managed?**
   Primary repair is safe and effective in essentially all patients with colon trauma. Handsewn and stapled anastomoses have equal complication rates.

KEY POINTS: SURGICAL MANAGEMENT OF COLON INJURIES

1. Primary repair is safe.

2. Handsewn and stapled anastomoses have equal complication rates.

3. A preoperative dose of antibiotic therapy, to be continued for 24 hours, is advantageous.

7. **How should the surgical incision and penetrating wound be managed?**
   Wounds should be left open (for delayed primary closure) to decrease the incidence of wound infection and fascial dehiscence.

8. **What complications are associated with colonic injury and its treatment?**
   - Wound infection (≤ 65% if the skin incision is closed primarily; do not be tempted to close a dirty incision)
   - Intraabdominal abscess (20%)
   - Fascial dehiscence (10%)
   - Stomal complications (5%)
   - Anastomotic leak (5%)
   - Mortality (6%)

RECTAL TRAUMA

9. **How do rectal injuries occur?**
   Similar to colon injuries, most rectal injuries result from penetrating trauma. Blunt pelvic fractures should be assessed with a strong suspicion for rectal (and urethral) injury.

10. **How are rectal injuries diagnosed?**
    A thorough examination is crucial, and the diagnosis is suggested by the course of the projectiles and the presence of blood on digital rectal examination. If rectal trauma is suspected, the patient should undergo proctoscopy to look for hematomas, contusions, lacerations, or gross blood. If the diagnosis is in question, radiographs with soluble-contrast enemas should be performed.

11. **How are patients with intraperitoneal rectal injuries treated differently from those with extraperitoneal injuries?**
    The portion of the rectum proximal to the peritoneal reflection is called the intraperitoneal segment. Injuries of this portion are treated similar to colonic injuries.

12. **What are the four basic principles for managing simple extraperitoneal rectal injuries?**
    1. **Diversion:** either a loop or an end-sigmoid colostomy is appropriate.
    2. **Drainage:** a retroanal incision should be used to place Penrose or closed-suction drains near the perforation site.

3. **Repair:** appropriate, when possible
4. **Washout:** irrigation of the distal rectum with isotonic solution until the effluent is clear. The role of washout remains controversial, but it may benefit patients whose rectum is full of feces.

13. **How are complex extraperitoneal rectal injuries managed?**
   In patients with massive pelvic trauma and an associated rectal injury, an abdominoperineal resection may be required for adequate debridement and hemostasis. An abdominoperineal resection is also required in rare instances in which anal sphincters have been destroyed.

14. **What complications are associated with rectal trauma and its treatment?**
   They are similar to those in colonic injuries. In addition, pelvic osteomyelitis may occur. In this case, debridement may be necessary, and culture-specific intravenous antibiotics should be administered for 2–3 months.

15. **What is the role of antibiotics in colorectal trauma?**
   Antibiotics are important. They should be initiated preoperatively (you need a good blood level at the time you make your incision) and ended quickly (12–24 hours postoperatively). Broad-spectrum, combination therapy is superior to single-agent therapy.

BIBLIOGRAPHY

1. Berne J, Velmahos G, Chan LS, et al: The high morbidity of colostomy closure after trauma: Further support for the primary repair of colon injuries. Surgery 123:157–164, 1998.
2. Burch J, Franciose R, Moore E: Trauma. In Schwartz S (ed): Principles of Surgery, 8th ed. New York, McGraw-Hill, 1999, pp 155–221.
3. Demetriades D, Murray J, Chan LS, et al: Handsewn versus stapled anastomosis in penetrating colon injuries requiring resection: A multicenter study. J Trauma 52:117–121, 2002.
4. Demetriades D, Murray J, Chan L, et al: Penetrating colon injuries requiring resection: Diversion or primary anastomosis? An AAST prospective multicenter study. J Trauma 50:765–775, 2001.
5. Velmahos G, Vassiliu P, Demetriades D, et al: Wound management after colon injury: Open or closed? A prospective randomized trial. Am Surg 68:795–801, 2002.

CHAPTER 29

PELVIC FRACTURES

Steven J. Morgan, M.D., and Wade R. Smith, M.D.

1. **What are the first steps in the evaluation and treatment of a patient with pelvic trauma?**
   The ABCs (airway, breathing, and circulatory assessment). The answer to this first trauma question is always the same. Trauma patients with displaced pelvic fractures have a high incidence of associated injuries to the head, chest, and abdomen.

2. **What are the sources and potential volume of bleeding in the displaced pelvic fracture?**
   Pelvic fractures bleed from exposed cancellous bone surfaces, pelvic veins, and pelvic arteries. Cadaveric injection studies have demonstrated that 90% of patients with trauma fatalities with pelvic fractures bleed to death from exposed bone and injured veins. Only 10% bleed from arteries. The total volume the pelvis can hold is 4–6 L before a tamponade effect slows venous and bone bleeding.

3. **Should a Foley catheter be placed in trauma patients with displaced pelvic fractures?**
   Yes. Contraindications include urethral injuries, which should be suspected when blood is observed at the penile meatus or vaginal introitus. A manual rectal examination in men and a bimanual examination in women are mandatory to exclude an open fracture into the vagina or rectum or a high-riding prostate. If a urethral injury is present, a suprapubic catheter can be easily inserted percutaneously, and both a urethrogram and cystogram are performed.

4. **What is the incidence of urologic injury associated with pelvic fractures?**
   The overall incidence is 16%.

5. **What are the commonly used radiographic classification schemes for pelvic fractures?**
   The mechanistic classification describes pelvic fractures as anteroposterior compression (APC), lateral compression (LC), vertical shear (VS), or combined mechanism (CM). The Tile classification categorizes fractures into three groups, A, B, or C, with numbered subgroups based on increasing severity of ligamentous and bony disruption.

6. **What is an open pelvic fracture?**
   An open fracture has been contaminated via a laceration in the skin, vagina, or rectum. When an open pelvic fracture is suspected, patients should receive a rectal examination with an anoscope, as well as a vaginal examination performed bimanually and with a speculum. With open fractures, the morbidity and mortality rates are increased both in the acute period (because of hemorrhage) and in the delayed period (because of infection). Open injuries in the rectal or perirectal region often require a diverting colostomy to prevent deep pelvic infection.

7. **When is acute mechanical stabilization of a pelvic fracture indicated?**
   Open-book and vertical shear fractures with displacement may benefit from acute mechanical stabilization. When hemodynamic instability persists in the face of ongoing aggressive

resuscitation, pelvic stabilization with a beanbag, external wrap, or external fixation device may help to decrease pelvic bleeding by decreasing pelvic volume (tamponade effect), stabilizing fracture surfaces, and promoting clot formation.

8. **What is the role of angiography in an acute pelvic fracture?**
   It is both diagnostic and therapeutic. Angiography can identify and embolize arterial bleeding caused by pelvic fractures. But only a low percentage of pelvic bleeding is from arterial injury. Suspicion should be increased when patients with hypotension fail to respond to pelvic ring stabilization and aggressive fluid resuscitation.

9. **Why do patients die from pelvic fractures?**
   Mortality is usually caused by associated injuries rather than the pelvic fracture. Only 2% of patients with a pelvic fracture experience isolated trauma to the pelvis. For example, patients with LC pelvic fractures are more likely to die secondary to associated head injuries rather than from pelvic hemorrhage. Death related to pelvic hemorrhage is generally seen in patients with massive pelvic displacement associated with APC or VS injury patterns. Early stabilization and mobilization, however, decrease the mortality from 26% to 6%.

KEY POINTS: BLOOD LOSS FROM PELVIC FRACTURES

1. 90% of deaths related to pelvic bleeding result from venous and bony bleeding.

2. The remaining 10% are due to arterial bleeding—most commonly from the superior gluteal artery.

3. Normally the pelvis can hold 4–6 L of blood before a tamponade effect occurs.

4. Pelvic wraps or fixation can limit bleeding, reduce bony shear, and promote clot formation.

5. Angiography is therapeutic and diagnostic, but only 10% of injuries are predominantly arterial.

10. **What is external fixation?**
    External fixation by the use of pins placed into the iliac wings and connected to a frame or by pins placed into the bone just superior to the acetabulum and connected to a C clamp can be used as a temporary method of fracture reduction and stabilization. External fixation does not prevent vertical and posterior displacement of the pelvis in the case of complete posterior disruption. The fixation device must be placed in a manner that permits abdominal access for laparotomy, diagnostic imaging, and the definitive operative approach for open reduction and internal fixation.

11. **Is there a role for pneumatic antishock garments (PASGs) in the treatment of pelvic fractures?**
    PASGs are falling out of favor in the treatment of pelvic fractures. Their potential role is limited to emergency transportation and initial stabilization of patients with a complex pelvic fracture. PASGs can reduce displacement of anteroposterior compression fractures but may increase the displacement of a lateral compression fracture. The garment also restricts access to the patient, compromises pulmonary reserve, and is associated with increased risk of compartment syndrome.

12. **When can patients with a pelvic fracture ambulate?**
    Patients with fractures involving only the anterior pelvic ring, such as unilateral or bilateral pubic rami fractures, may bear weight immediately. If the fracture pattern involves the posterior structures, such as the sacroiliac joint or iliac wing, patients must not bear weight for 10 weeks.

13. **What is the most common source of arterial bleeding associated with a pelvic fracture?**
The superior gluteal artery.

14. **Which gender and what portion of the urethra is most commonly injured in patients with a displaced pelvic fracture?**
The male urethra is more commonly injured. The urethra passes through the urogenital diaphragm or pelvic floor, transitioning in an abrupt fashion from the membranous to the bulbous urethra. The urethra at this point is attenuated and relatively fixed above, accounting for the large number of injuries at the membranous bulbous junction. The female urethra is much shorter and the pelvic floor is less well developed, allowing for greater mobility of the female urethra (or perhaps it is because girls are smarter, more cautious, and do not get injured as often). The most common site of urethral injury in girls and women is at the bladder neck.

15. **Describe the mechanism that results in a bladder rupture.**
The bladder is both an intraperitoneal and extraperitoneal structure. Compression of a distended bladder results in an intraperitoneal rupture along the bladder dome. Extraperitoneal rupture, a more common injury, results from the laceration of the bladder by displaced pubic rami fracture fragments.

16. **What are the three radiographic views required to evaluate patients with pelvic fractures?**
1. Anteroposterior pelvis view
2. Inlet view
3. Outlet view

17. **What is the appropriate insertion location for a diagnostic peritoneal lavage catheter in the presence of a pelvic fracture?**
A supraumbilical location avoids inadvertent decompression of the pelvic hematoma and a false-positive result.

18. **What percent of patients with an unstable pelvic fracture will suffer an associated neurologic injury?**
Associated injuries of the lumbosacral plexus, sacral foramina, and sacral canal are reportedly as high as 50%.

19. **What is a potential pitfall of aggressive blood transfusion of hemodynamically unstable pelvic fracture patients?**
Coagulopathy. Forty percent of patients with unstable pelvic fractures may require $\geq$ 10 units of blood. Fresh frozen plasma and platelets should be transfused early in the resuscitation.

20. **What is the significance of an L5 transverse process (TP) fracture in a patient with a pelvis fracture?**
A TP fracture at the level of L5 may indicate vertical instability of the pelvic fracture. The iliolumbar ligaments attach to the TP and the iliac wing, often resulting in the avulsion of the TP when the pelvis vertically displaces.

WEB SITE

http://www.east.org/tpg/pelvis.pdf

BIBLIOGRAPHY

1. Biffl WL, Smith WR, Moore EE, et al: Evolution of a multidisciplinary key clinical pathway for the management of unstable pelvis fractures. Ann Surg 233:843–850, 2001.

2. Buehle R, Browner B, Morandi M: Emergency reduction for pelvic ring disruptions and control of associated hemorrhage using the pelvic stabilizer. Tech Orthop 9:258–266, 1995.

3. Burgess AR, Eastridge BJ, Young JW, et al: Pelvic ring disruptions: Effective classification system and treatment protocols. J Trauma 30:848–856, 1990.

4. Cook RE, Keating JF, Gillespie I: The role of angiography in the management of haemorrhage from major fractures of the pelvis. J Bone Joint Surg 84B:178–182, 2002.

5. Gruen GS, Leit ME, Gruen RJ, Peitzman AB: The acute management of hemodynamically unstable multiple trauma patients with pelvic ring fractures. J Trauma 36:706–713, 1994.

6. Kellam JF, Browner BD: Fractures of the pelvic ring. In Browner BD, et al (eds): Skeletal Trauma, 2nd ed. Philadelphia, W.B. Saunders, 1997.

7. Perez JV, Hughes TM, Bowers K: Angiographic embolisation in pelvic fracture. Injury 29:187–191, 1998.

8. Poole GV, Ward EF: Causes of mortality in patients with pelvic fractures. Orthopaedics 17:691–696, 1994.

9. Routt ML, Simonian PT, Ballmer E: A rational approach to pelvic trauma: Resuscitation and early definitive stabilization. Clin Orthop 318:61–74, 1995.

10. Starr AJ, Griffin DR, Reinert CM, et al: Pelvic ring disruptions: Prediction of associated injuries, transfusion requirement, pelvic arteriography, complications, and mortality. J Orthop Trauma 16:553–561, 2002.

11. Tile M: Pelvic ring fractures: Should they be fixed? J Bone Joint Surg 70B:1–12, 1988.

12. Velmahos GC, Toutouzas KG, Vassiliu P, et al: A prospective study on the safety and efficacy of angiographic embolization for pelvic and visceral injuries. J Trauma 53:303–308, 2002.

CHAPTER 30

UPPER URINARY TRACT INJURIES

Fernando J. Kim, M.D., and Siam Oottamasathien, M.D.

1. What is the most common type of renal trauma in the United States, blunt or penetrating?

Blunt, by far.

2. Do most kidney injuries require surgery?

No. Fewer than 2% of blunt injuries require surgery, and many penetrating injuries can also be treated nonoperatively.

3. Are pediatric kidneys more susceptible to major injury?

Yes. Because of children's weaker abdominal muscles, less-ossified thoracic cage, decreased perirenal fat, and increased renal size in relation to the rest of the body, the risk for renal injury is greater in the pediatric population.

4. When should potential renal trauma be investigated?

All blunt trauma patients with gross hematuria or with microscopic hematuria and shock (systolic blood pressure < 90 mmHg) should be closely examined. Penetrating injuries with any degree of hematuria should be imaged. For pediatric patients, liberal use of studies is advisable. When children spill < 50 red blood cells (RBCs) per high-powered field (hpf) on microscopic urinalysis, significant renal injury is rare. Furthermore, shock is not a useful guide in children.

5. When does one suspect renal trauma?

The mechanism of injury, physical examination (e.g., flank ecchymosis, location of penetrating wounds), and associated injuries (e.g., rib fractures) should raise suspicion of renal trauma. Although the degree of hematuria does not correlate with the degree of renal injury, when hematuria is out of proportion to the history of trauma, it suggests preexisting renal abnormality (e.g., hydronephrosis, ectopic kidney, tumor, cystic disease, vascular malformation). Conversely, renal pedicle injuries (grade 4) may bleed little because of arterial interruption.

6. What imaging study is best to evaluate renal trauma?

Computed tomography (CT) scan of the abdomen and pelvis with and without intravenous (IV) contrast should be performed, but it is pivotal that the perfusion and excretion phases (10 minutes after IV contrast is administered) are obtained during the study.

7. What is a single-shot IVP, and when do you perform it?

It is an extremely abbreviated form of intravenous pyelogram (IVP) performed in emergent cases when a full evaluation is not permitted. A bolus (2 mL/kg contrast agent) is injected intravenously, and the first film should be obtained at approximately 10 minutes, with additional films at 10-minute intervals as necessary for diagnosis. Intraoperative IVP is recommended when renal damage is first suggested (e.g., retroperitoneal hematoma) during emergency surgery for other injuries.

8. How is renal trauma classified?

Grade 1: contusion

Grade 2: superficial laceration

Grade 3: deep laceration without collecting system damage
Grade 4: contained renal pedicle injury or deep laceration and collecting system damage
Grade 5: shattered kidney or avulsion of renal hilum
Grade 1, 2, and 3 injuries are safe to watch with nonoperative management, whereas grades 4 and 5 typically require operative intervention for repair or removal. Grade 4 injury (pedicle injury) is picked up by ipsilateral urographic nonfunction and nominal bleeding. Grade 5 injury is manifested by urographic nonfunction, parenchymal shattering, and significant gross hematuria.

9. **What are the different kinds of renal pedicle trauma?**
The renal pedicle may be interrupted by thrombosis or complete avulsion; both events are characterized by urographic nonvisualization and minimal hematuria. The most common site of arterial interruption is the junction of the proximal and middle thirds of the main renal artery. Although hematuria is often absent, one may see transitory gross hematuria or microhematuria, emphasizing the requirement for urinalysis in all circumstances.

10. **How long can a nonperfused kidney tolerate warm ischemia?**
Irreversible renal damage may be seen in kidneys after 30 minutes of warm ischemia, and after 8 hours of ischemia, renal salvage is minimal. Recently, single reports of renovascular trauma with intimal tear treated with endovascular stents have been encouraging.

11. **What is the significance of delayed gross hematuria?**
This occurs 3–4 weeks after trauma and may indicate an arteriovenous fistula. Selective embolization is the next step if conservative therapy (bed rest) fails. Rarely, operative intervention, usually for partial nephrectomy, is necessary.

12. **How do you deal with unexpected retroperitoneal bleeding noted at operation?**
A pulsatile hematoma suggests a major vascular injury, and exploration should be preceded by vascular control (both proximal and distal) and preparation for rapid blood replacement. Stable hematomas (above the pelvic brim) may be left undisturbed unless studies (preoperative or intraoperative) disclose severe renal damage. When doubt exists, exploration is justified, with the likelihood of losing a kidney.

13. **How are patients with posttraumatic urine extravasation managed?**
When urine extravasation is caused by a major laceration into the collecting system and coexists with significant persistent bleeding, surgical correction is advised. Otherwise, urine extravasation commonly resolves promptly. Reimaging at 48–72 hours defines cases requiring drainage, stenting, or operative repair.

14. **What is included in conservative management of renal trauma?**
Conservative management includes bed rest until gross hematuria has subsided. Strenuous activity is avoided until microhematuria has subsided (usually within 3 weeks). Patients followed for grade 5 renal trauma should undergo ultrasonography, CT scan of the abdomen and pelvis, or urography at 6 weeks. Hospitalization is not required during these periods.

15. **What is the likelihood of subsequent hypertension?**
Documented posttraumatic hypertension occurs in < 2% of patients and is renin mediated. Onset generally occurs within the first several months of injury. The mechanisms of posttraumatic hypertension are renal artery stenosis or occlusion, renal parenchymal compression (extravasation of blood or urine), and posttrauma arteriovenous fistula.

16. **How are most ureters damaged?**
In the civilian world, excluding iatrogenic injuries, penetrating trauma is responsible for 4% of ureteral injuries, and 1% are caused by blunt trauma.

KEY POINTS: PRINCIPLES OF URETERAL REPAIR

1. Primary tension-free anastomosis is preferred over stent with absorbable suture.

2. For a distal injury in the lower third of the ureter, perform ureteroneocystostomy; suspend the bladder if tension exists.

3. For middle third injuries, perform end-to-side transretroperitoneal ureteroureterostomy.

4. For proximal injury with significant length loss, use nephrostomy tube for drainage.

17. **How do you evaluate and identify ureteral injury?**
    The site and mechanism of trauma should prompt the surgeon to suspect ureteral injury. The clinical manifestations are characteristically subtle and often obscured by coexisting injury and complaints. The majority of gunshot wounds and stabbings that injure the ureter also injure bowel, colon, liver, spleen, blood vessels, or pancreas. Hematuria is often microscopic, but it may be absent. Extravasation of contrast may be detected with noninvasive (IVP and CT scan) and invasive (anterograde and retrograde ureteropyelogram) imaging studies. If ureteral injury is suspected during laparotomy, indigo carmine (1 vial IV bolus) should be given to identify the site of leakage (blue coloration).

18. **What are the potential consequences of missed ureteral injury?**
    Fever, leukocytosis, azotemia, flank pain, ileus, urinoma, or urinary fistula. Presentation is often delayed by several weeks after the injury.

19. **What are the principles of ureteral repair?**
    Devitalized tissue must be debrided, and the two ends of the ureters should be mobilized, spatulated, and anastomosed (tension free) over a ureteral stent using absorbable suture. Placement of a drain should be performed without rubbing on the fresh anastomosis. Distal injuries permit direct implantation of the ureter into the bladder. Midureteral injuries may be repaired by primary anastomosis. Pediatric patients are more susceptible to proximal complete ureteral disruption. Urgent surgical repair is mandatory. Rarely, when nephrectomy is not an option and ureteral damage prevents standard methods of reconstruction, other elective and more complex surgical reconstructive techniques may be applied. These include kidney autotransplantation, ileal interposition, transureteroureterostomy, Boari flap with nephropexis, and ureterocalicostomy.

20. **The distal ureter is injured and ureteral reimplantation with a psoas hitch (tack up the bladder to the psoas muscle) is performed. Postoperatively, the patient complains of anterior thigh numbness. What did you do wrong?**
    The genitofemoral nerve lies on the anterior aspect of the ileopsoas muscle. You caught this nerve when you synched this to the tendon of the psoas muscle.

WEB SITES

1. http://www.east.org/tpg/GUmgmt.pdf

2. http://www.acssurgery.com/abstracts/acs/acs0510.htm

BIBLIOGRAPHY

1. Armstrong PA, Litscher LJ, Key DW, McCarthy MC: Management strategies for genitourinary trauma. Hosp Phys 34:19–25, 1998.

2. Campbell EW Jr, Filderman PS, Jacobs SC: Ureteral injury due to blunt and penetrating trauma. Urology 40:216–220, 1992.

3. Carroll PR, McAninch JW, Klosterman PW, et al: Renovascular trauma: Risk assessment, surgical management, and outcome. J Trauma 30:547–552, 1990.

4. Kim FJ: Urologic trauma. In Feliciano DV, Moore EE, Mattox KL (eds): Trauma Companion Handbook, 4th ed. New York, McGraw-Hill, 2002.

5. McAninch JW: Traumatic and Reconstructive Urology. Philadelphia, W.B. Saunders, 1996.

6. McAninch JW, Santucci R: Genitourinary trauma. In Walsh PC, Retik AB, Vaughan ED, Wein AJ (eds): Campbell's Urology, 8th ed. Philadelphia, W.B. Saunders, 2002, pp 3707–3744.

7. Moore EE, Shackford SR, Pachter HL, et al: Organ injury scaling: Spleen, liver, and kidney. J Trauma 29:1664–1666, 1998.

8. Peterson NE: Genitourinary trauma. In Feliciano DV, Moore EE, Mattox KL (eds): Trauma, 4th edition. Norwalk, CT, Appleton & Lange, 1996, pp 661–694.

9. Skinner EC, Parisky YR, Skinner DG: Management of complex urologic injuries. Surg Clin North Am 76:861–878, 1996.

CHAPTER 31

LOWER URINARY TRACT INJURY AND PELVIC TRAUMA

Fernando J. Kim, M.D., and Siam Oottamasathien, M.D.

1. **What are the causes of bladder injury?**
   Iatrogenic manipulation and penetrating or blunt trauma. Because of the rich detrusor blood supply, bladder injury is usually accompanied by hematuria. Other signs may include suprapubic pain, inability to void, or incomplete recovery of catheter irrigation.

2. **What types of bladder injury may occur with blunt trauma?**
   Laceration or perforation may be either intra- or extraperitoneal. Hematuria with a normal cystogram defines bladder contusion in the absence of upper tract injury. Extraperitoneal injuries constitute the majority of bladder trauma and tend to concentrate at the bladder base or parasymphyseal area. These can be managed conservatively with urinary catheter drainage for at least 10 days. Intraperitoneal (IP) ruptures typically occur when the bladder is distended at the time of trauma, causing a blowout of the dome of a bladder. IP vesical rupture should be surgically repaired using a two-layer closure with absorbable sutures and placement of suprapubic and urethral catheters.

KEY POINTS: MANAGEMENT OF BLADDER INJURY DUE TO BLUNT TRAUMA

1. Diagnose with CT cystography and retrograde cystourethrography.

2. Extraperitoneal injuries are more common and may be managed conservatively with a Foley catheter for 10 days.

3. Intraperitoneal injuries are more likely if the bladder is distended at the time of injury; they require surgical repair with suprapubic and Foley drainage postoperatively.

3. **What is the likelihood of a bladder injury in patients with a fractured pelvis?**
   Extraperitoneal bladder injury occurs in 10% of all pelvic fractures. Conversely, approximately 85% of blunt bladder injury is associated with pelvic fracture. Bladder injuries occur more often with parasymphyseal pubic arch fractures and more often with bilateral than unilateral fractures. Isolated ramus fractures produce bladder laceration in 10% of cases.

4. **How is bladder injury evaluated?**
   Both computed tomography (CT) cystography and retrograde cystourethrography provide great diagnostic accuracy for bladder rupture. The bladder should be filled under gravity with a total of 300–400 mL of a 50% dilution of standard radiocontrast agent using the Foley catheter. Films should include anteroposterior, lateral, and oblique views. Finally, a postvoid film should be obtained. When renal or distal ureteral injury is suspected, upper tract imaging (intravenous pyelogram [IVP] or CT scan) should precede the cystogram.

5. **What are the retrograde cystourethrographic patterns of bladder injury?**
    Extraperitoneal injury allows contrast agent to escape adjacent to the symphysis, but it is confined to the bladder base by the intact peritoneum. Intraperitoneal extravasation produces a "sunburst" appearance from the bladder dome, which may collect in the paracolic gutters, outline loops of bowel, or pool under the liver or spleen. It is pivotal to obtain postvoid films.

6. **How is bladder rupture managed?**
    Extraperitoneal lacerations can be managed with an indwelling catheter for 7–10 days, at which time cystogram usually confirms resolution of extravasation. Intraperitoneal lacerations require operative repair. Bladder contusion requires catheter drainage until gross bleeding has subsided.

7. **When should urethral injury be investigated?**
    The mechanism of injury (e.g., crushing or deceleration/impact, straddle injuries) and associated trauma (e.g., pelvic fracture), blood at the meatus, penile or scrotal swelling and ecchymosis, upward prostatic displacement on digital rectal examination, and inability to void or to pass a urethral catheter (do not try this) should be investigated.

8. **When a patient presents with a pelvic fracture, is concomitant urethral injury a major concern?**
    Yes. Urethral trauma occurs in 10% of pelvic fractures; it is more common with anterior disruption of the pelvic ring, including 20% of unilateral and 50% of bilateral parasymphyseal fractures. Posterior (prostatomembranous) avulsion is associated with potentially disabling sequelae and requirements for complex and challenging operative corrections. In contrast, more distal urethral injuries avoid impotence and incontinence issues and are more surgically accessible.

9. **How is urethral injury best assessed?**
    Retrograde urethrography must always be performed before inserting a Foley catheter. Incomplete urethral transection produces local contrast dye extravasation and bladder opacification. Total avulsion produces extensive local extravasation, and no contrast dye gets into the bladder. Incomplete transection is more common with anterior (50%) than posterior (10%) urethral injuries.

10. **How is urethral injury managed?**
    For incomplete transection regardless of site, either catheter stenting across the defect or diversion by suprapubic cystostomy permits resolution. With complete urethral transection, the bladder should be decompressed initially via suprapubic cystostomy. Early restoration of continuity by placement of a bridging urethral catheter should be performed endoscopically. A bridging catheter reduces complex scarring and avoids subsequent surgery in many patients.

11. **What are the complications of urethral injury?**
    Strictures, incontinence, and impotence (associated with traumatic prostatic displacement). Iatrogenic complications are associated with retropubic dissection.

12. **What is the differential diagnosis in blunt scrotal trauma?**
    Testicular rupture, hematocele, scrotal hematoma, intratesticular hematoma, and testicular torsion. Ultrasonography helps sort this out.

13. **What is the sonographic sign of testicular rupture?**
    The sign is loss of the normal homogenous echo texture of the testicle, with areas of irregular hyper- or hypoechogenicity.

14. **How are patients with acute testicular rupture managed?**
Management includes surgical exploration and debridement of extruded, nonviable tubules and evacuation of the hematoma. After proper hemostasis is achieved, the tunica albuginea should be closed with running absorbable suture.

15. **What is the most common cause of penile fractures?**
Penile fracture is a rupture of the corpus cavernosum, most commonly associated with sexual intercourse, masturbation, or an abnormally forced bending of the erect penis. Characteristically the patient hears a popping sound, followed by pain and detumescence.

16. **What are the physical examinations findings with a penile fracture?**
Injury to the tunica albuginea causes formation of hematoma and deviation of the shaft to the opposite side of injury. If Buck's fascia is intact, the hematoma will be confined to the penis; disruption of Buck's fascia allows spread of the hematoma under Colles' and Scarpa's fascia onto the perineum and abdominal wall.

17. **How are penile fractures managed?**
Surgically. A retrograde urethrogram should be performed when urethral injury is suspected. Closure of the defect (or defects) along the tunica albuginea and evacuation of hematoma are performed after degloving the penis.

18. **In penile amputation injuries, how should the amputated portion of the penis be preserved for transport?**
The amputated portion of the penis should be wrapped in saline-soaked gauze, placed in a plastic bag with ice slush surrounding the bag.

19. **How is major scrotal skin loss managed?**
If primary repair is not possible, meshed split-thickness skin grafts may be used to cover the testis. When delayed repair is necessary, thigh pouches should be created until permanent reconstruction is feasible.

20. **A 50-year-old woman complains of urine leakage from her vagina after a hysterectomy. What is the most likely diagnosis?**
Unrecognized bladder injury during hysterectomy with subsequent urine extravasation into the surgical field and drainage via the vaginal cuff suture line leads to formation of vesicovaginal fistula.

21. **What is the best time to repair a vesicovaginal fistula secondary to an uncomplicated hysterectomy?**
Although 3–6 months after injury has been recommeded in the past, early repair can be successful if there is minimal inflammation and there are no complicating factors.

WEB SITES

1. http://www.east.org/tpg/GUmgmt.pdf

2. http://www.acssurgery.com/abstracts/acs/acs0510.htm

BIBLIOGRAPHY

1. Armstrong PA, Litscher LJ, Key DW, McCarthy MC: Management strategies for genitourinary trauma. Hosp Phys 34:19–25, 1998.

2. Jacob TD, Gruen GS, Udekwu AO, Peitzman AB: Pelvic fracture. Surg Rounds (Aug):583, 1993.

3. Jordan GH: Lower Genitourinary Tract Trauma and Male External Genital Trauma (Nonpenetrating Injuries, Penetrating Injuries, and Avulsion Injuries). In American Urological Association Update Series, Vol. XIX, Lesson 11, part 2. Baltimore, American Urological Association, 2000.

4. Kim FJ: Urologic trauma. In Feliciano DV, Moore EE, Mattox KL (eds): Trauma Companion Handbook, 4th ed. New York, McGraw-Hill, 2002.

5. McAninch JW: Traumatic and Reconstructive Urology. Philadelphia, W.B. Saunders, 1996.

6. Peterson NE: Current management of urethral injuries. In Rous S (ed): 1998 Urology Annual. New York, Appleton-Century-Crofts, 1988, pp 143–179.

7. Peterson NE: Traumatic posterior urethral avulsion. Mongr Urol 7:61, 1986.

8. Spirnak JP: Pelvic fracture and injury to the lower urinary tract. Surg Clin North Am 68:1057, 1988.

CHAPTER 32

EXTREMITY VASCULAR INJURIES

Kyle H. Mueller, M.D., and William H. Pearce, M.D.

1. **What are the "hard signs" of arterial injury?**
   - Distal circulatory deficit: ischemia or diminished or absent pulses
   - Bruit
   - Expanding or pulsatile hematoma
   - Arterial (pulsatile) bleeding

2. **What are the four ways in which an arterial injury may present?**
   1. Hemorrhage
   2. Thrombosis
   3. Arteriovenous fistula
   4. Pseudoaneurysm

3. **What are the "soft" signs of arterial injury?**
   - Small- or moderate-sized stable hematoma
   - Adjacent nerve injury
   - Shock not explained by other injuries
   - Proximity of penetrating wound to a major vascular structure

4. **What are the symptoms of acute arterial occlusion?**
   The six P's: pain, pallor, pulse deficit, paresthesia, paralysis, and poikilothermia (cold).

5. **What initial screening test is used to evaluate an extremity for occult vascular injury?**
   Calculation of arterial pressure indices (APIs).

6. **What are the APIs for the upper extremity and lower extremity called?**
   An API for the upper extremity is the wrist brachial index (WBI).
   An API for the lower extremity is the ankle brachial index (ABI).

7. **How are WBI and ABI measured, and what is considered a normal value?**
   A hand-held Doppler and blood pressure cuff are used to measure systolic blood pressure in the brachial, radial, ulnar, dorsalis pedis (DP), and posterior tibial (PT) arteries bilaterally. The ABI for each leg is the highest DP or PT divided by the highest brachial pressure. The WBI for each arm is the highest radial or ulnar artery pressure divided by the highest brachial pressure. A value of 1.0 is normal.

8. **What API value raises concern for arterial injury, and what is the sensitivity and specificity?**
   - An API value < 0.9 has a sensitivity of 95% and specificity of 97% for major arterial injury.
   - An API > 0.9 has a negative predictive value of 99%.

9. **When the API value is < 0.9 in an injured extremity, what should be the next diagnostic test?**
   Arteriography to establish the diagnosis and plan for operative intervention.

10. **What abnormalities on arteriography determine a positive test result?**
    - Obstruction of flow
    - Extravasation of contrast
    - Early venous filling or arteriovenous fistula
    - Wall irregularity or filling defect
    - False aneurysm (pseudoaneurysm)

11. **What study should be performed for patients with proximity injury or soft signs (API > 0.9)?**
    Duplex ultrasonography to rule out occult vascular injury.

12. **What occult vascular injuries can be detected by duplex ultrasonography?**
    - Intimal flap
    - Pseudoaneurysm
    - Arteriovenous fistula
    - Focal vessel narrowing
    - Nonoperative observation of these injuries is safe and effective: 89% of them do not require surgery

13. **What is a pseudoaneurysm?**
    It is a disruption of the arterial wall leading to a pulsatile hematoma contained by fibrous connective tissue (but not all three arterial wall layers). (See Figures 32-1 and 32-2.)

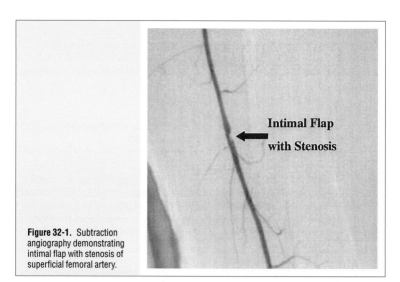

Figure 32-1. Subtraction angiography demonstrating intimal flap with stenosis of superficial femoral artery.

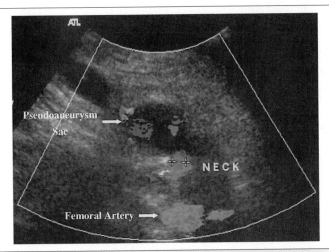

Figure 32-2. Duplex ultrasound of common femoral artery demonstrating pseudoaneurysm sac and associated neck between pseudoaneurysm sac and femoral artery after percutaneous access for angiography.

14. **What is a true aneurysm?**
    Dilatation of all three layers of the vessel wall (i.e., intima, media, and adventitia).

15. **What is the most effective way to control arterial bleeding in an injured extremity?**
    Direct digital pressure.

16. **What means of controlling vascular injury should be avoided? Why?**
    A tourniquet should be avoided because collateral circulation is occluded and leads to increased tissue ischemia.
    Blind clamping should also be avoided because it causes further vessel damage, making reconstruction more difficult.

17. **How should a patient with an extremity vascular injury be prepared and draped in the operating room?**
    The entire involved extremity should be in the sterile field. The major arterial trunk proximal to the site of injury (for proximal control) and a portion of lower extremity permitting access to saphenous vein should be included in the sterile field.

18. **What else should be prepared and draped for proximal extremity injuries?**
    The chest should be prepped for proximal injuries of the upper extremity. The abdomen should be prepped for proximal injuries of the lower extremity. (Access to the chest or abdomen may be necessary to obtain proximal vascular control.)

19. **What are the operative principles relative to repair of vascular injuries?**
    - Perform longitudinal incisions over vessels to be explored.
    - Initial dissection should be away from the site of suspected injury and adjacent hematoma.
    - Obtain proximal and distal control of the injured vessel.
    - Debride the injured vessel.
    - Perform primary repair if tension free (fully extend extremity to ensure tension-free repair).
    - Repair with autogenous interposition vein graft if there is inadequate length (tension).

20. **What is the best conduit to use if primary repair is not possible? Why?**
Saphenous or cephalic vein from the uninjured extremity to preserve venous flow.

21. **Should injuries to major veins of the extremities be repaired?**
Yes. Repair of a major vein enhances the success of a concomitant arterial repair by improving out-flow. Late thrombosis often occurs after venous repair, but initial patency helps by allowing collateral circulation to develop. This may also reduce the incidence of postoperative venous insufficiency.

22. **When should injured major veins be ligated?**
Major veins should be ligated rather than repaired when the patient is hemodynamically unstable or the repair is too complex.

23. **What complications can develop after ligation of major extremity veins?**
Possible complications include rapid increase in muscle compartment pressure, leading to compromised venous or arterial flow and compartment syndrome. Also, postoperative venous stasis may occur, which can be alleviated with intermittent pneumatic calf compression and leg elevation.

24. **What is a compartment syndrome?**
Development of pathologically elevated tissue pressures (preventing perfusion) within nonexpansile envelopes (inside fascial compartments) of the arm or leg.

KEY POINTS: COMPARTMENT SYNDROME

1. Pathologically elevated tissue pressures in nonexpansile fascial compartments prevent tissue perfusion.

2. The most common cause is ischemia-reperfusion injury following traumatic extremity injuries.

3. The earliest clinical sign is numbness in the first dorsal webspace associated with compromise of the deep peroneal nerve. Other signs: pain with passive joint motion, pain out of proportion to injury, tense and tender muscle compartments.

4. Distal pulses are evident until late in the diagnosis and should *not* be used to rule out compartment syndrome.

5. Hand-held manometer is used to measure muscular compartments.
Normal pressure = < 10 mmHg; pathologic pressure = > 30 mmHg.

6. Treatment is emergent fasciotomy.

25. **What is the most common cause of a compartment syndrome?**
Ischemia-reperfusion injury when ischemia depletes intracellular energy stores and then reperfusion leads to toxic oxygen radicals, causing cellular swelling and interstitial fluid accumulation.

26. **What is the earliest sign of compartment syndrome after vascular repair of an extremity?**
Neurologic deficit in the distribution of the peroneal nerve with weak dorsiflexion and numbness in the first dorsal webspace.

27. **Are there any other signs of a developing compartment syndrome of an extremity?**
- Increased pain with passive motion of the ankle
- Pain out of proportion to clinical findings (ischemia hurts)

- Tense muscle compartments that are tender to palpation
Distal pulses can remain intact.

28. **How is the objective diagnosis of a compartment syndrome made?**
By measuring compartment pressures with a percutaneous needle and pressure transducer. Criteria for compartment syndrome are as follows:
- When diastolic pressure-compartment pressure is ≤ 20 mmHg or
- When mean arterial pressure-compartment pressure is ≤ 30 mmHg

29. **What is the treatment for compartment syndrome of an extremity?**
Emergent fasciotomy, with decompression of the four compartments of the lower leg (anterior, lateral, superficial posterior, and deep posterior) or decompression of the forearm compartments.

30. **What is the result of untreated compartment syndrome?**
Loss of perfusion promotes eventual myoneuronecrosis.

31. **Which are the most commonly injured arteries in the upper extremity?**

Brachial artery	30% (most frequently caused by catheterization for arteriography)
Radial or ulnar artery	20%
Axillary artery	10%
Subclavian artery	5%

32. **Which are the most commonly injured arteries in the lower extremity?**

Superficial femoral artery	20%
Popliteal artery	10%
Common femoral artery	< 5%
Anterior, posterior tibial, and peroneal arteries	< 5%
Deep femoral artery	2%

33. **Can a patient with an extremity arterial injury have palpable distal pulses?**
Yes. In $\leq 20\%$ of proven arterial injuries, a distal pulse is palpable (often because of collateral circulation).

34. **What orthopedic injuries commonly have associated vascular injuries?**
- Supracondylar humerus fractures are associated with brachial artery injuries.
- Knee dislocations are associated with popliteal artery injuries.
- Femur fractures can be associated with injury to the superficial femoral artery.

35. **For an injured extremity with concomitant fracture and vascular injury, which repair should be performed first?**
The vascular repair should be performed first to restore flow and reverse tissue ischemia.

36. **After reducing or fixing an extremity fracture, what must you always do?**
Evaluate the distal pulses to ensure adequate vascular inflow (especially if fixation or any manipulation follows a vascular repair).

37. **What is the likely diagnosis in a patient with repetitive palmar trauma and finger ischemia or necrosis?**
Hypothenar hammer syndrome (HHS). The mechanism is thought to be repetitive palmar trauma in patients with preexisting palmar artery fibrodysplasia. (The arteriogram shows digital artery occlusions with segmental ulnar artery occlusion or "corkscrew" elongation.) (See Figure 32-3.)

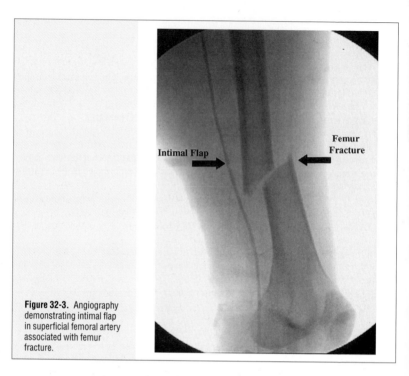

Figure 32-3. Angiography demonstrating intimal flap in superficial femoral artery associated with femur fracture.

38. **What complications can occur after angiography when a percutaneous closure device is used on the femoral artery?**
   - Thrombosis, ischemia, or both when the closure suture involves the posterior wall (back wall) of the artery
   - Infected pseudoaneurysm
   - Distal embolization when a hemostatic plug closure device is used

WEB SITES

1. http://www.east.org/tpg/lepene.pdf

2. http://www.surgery.ucsf.edu/eastbaytrauma/Protocols/ER%20protocol%20pages/extremity.htm

BIBLIOGRAPHY

1. Ferris BL, Taylor LM Jr, Oyama K, et al: Hypothenar hammer syndrome: Proposed etiology. J Vasc Surg 31:104–113, 2000.
2. Rutherford RB (ed): Vascular Surgery, 5th ed. Philadelphia, W.B. Saunders, 2000, pp 862–870.
3. Schwartz SI (ed): Principles of Surgery, 7th ed. New York, McGraw-Hill, 1999, pp 158–177.

CHAPTER 33

FACIAL LACERATIONS

Lawrence L. Ketch, M.D.

1. What distinguishes facial from other lacerations?
Appearance is clearly of primary importance. Quality of the final result depends on strict adherence to basic principles of wound management and painstaking technique. Copious irrigation, judicious debridement, gentle tissue handling, meticulous hemostasis, and minimization of sutures combined with early stitch removal are critical to an optimal result. Fine suture and sharp instruments should be used; eversion of the wound margin with layered closure, obliteration of dead space, and lack of tension are mandatory.

2. What factors influence treatment for the wound?
The mechanism of injury, the clinical assessment of contamination, and the time elapsed since wounding dictate treatment. Clean lacerations, heavily contaminated wounds, crush injuries, and bites are treated very differently.

3. How are clean lacerations repaired?
They should be irrigated with normal saline or Ringer's lactate. Only the surrounding skin should be prepared, and no antiseptic should be introduced into the wound. Regional anesthesia is preferred because of the potential for spread of contamination with direct injection of the wound margin. Epinephrine should be avoided because it devitalizes tissue and potentiates infection. Wounds should be repaired in layers with absorbable suture in deep tissue. The smallest number of sutures necessary to overcome the natural resting wound tension should be used. Sutures should be removed within 3–5 days, and the wound margin should be subsequently supported with Steri-strips.

4. How are dirty lacerations repaired?
Heavily contaminated wounds should remain open after irrigation and debridement to undergo delayed closure. Because of cosmetic considerations, however, this approach is unacceptable in the face. For this reason, meticulous debridement of devitalized tissue and removal of all foreign material is essential. The wound should be cultured before copious irrigation, and a broad-spectrum antibiotic should be instituted prophylactically. The patient must be informed of the potential of a postrepair infection.

KEY POINTS: FACIAL LACERATIONS

1. Appearance is of paramount importance.

2. Clean lacerations are treated with minimal, tension-free, fine monofilament suture placement and early suture removal (3–5 days).

3. Heavily contaminated wounds are irrigated, debrided, and repaired with administration of antibiotics.

4. Human and animal bites are highly prone to infection; therefore, antibiotics and delayed closure are necessary.

5. N-butyl-2-cyanoacrylate (Dermabond) is used to repair pediatric facial lacerations.

5. **What factors influence suture selection?**
Any method of suturing provokes tissue damage, impairs host defense, increases scar prolifera-tion, and invites infection. Presence of a single silk suture in a wound lowers the infective threshold by a factor of 10,000. Therefore, fine, monofilament suture, just strong enough to overcome the resting wound tension, should be used. Use as few sutures as possible. Wounds with little or no retraction may be closed with tape alone.

6. **Which wounds are suitable for closure with tissue adhesives?**
N-butyl-2-cyanoacrylate may suffice for cutaneous closure of low-tension lacerations in children (preferred method) and adults. This adhesive effectively closes low-tension lacerations. This method is fast and relatively painless. It has a low complication rate and produces excellent cos-metic outcomes. In many instances, if initial wound orientation is against Langer's lines, it may, in fact, offer an advantage over conventional manual suturing.

7. **Should eyebrows be shaved when facial lacerations are repaired?**
No. They provide a landmark for realignment of disrupted tissue edges and do not always grow back.

8. **How should crush avulsion injuries with associated skin loss be repaired?**
Nonviable elements must be surgically excised because they predispose to infection and lead to excessive scarring. If viability is in doubt, the wound should be irrigated thoroughly and left open with moist dressings. A delayed closure can be accomplished when the questionable areas have declared themselves. It is often prudent to close facial tissue as it lies; this technique often produces a less obtrusive scar than straight-line debridement and closure.

9. **How should bites be treated?**
Both animal and human bite wounds are big-time contaminated and prone to infection. The wound should be left open and closed in a delayed fashion. Antibiotic prophylaxis is indicated. If the wound becomes infected, the sutures must be removed and the wound allowed to drain and heal. The patient should be informed that a scar revision will be necessary.

10. **Should skin grafts or flaps be used for primary closure of a wound?**
Complicated tissue transfer techniques have no place in the acute treatment of facial wounds. Closure should be achieved in the simplest way possible and complex reconstructive efforts should be deferred until the scar has matured (months). When tissue loss prevents closure, it may be necessary to use a thin split-thickness skin graft for coverage.

11. **When are antibiotics indicated in the treatment of facial lacerations?**
Copious irrigation, debridement, and gentle tissue handling are more pertinent to the prevention of infection than the use of antibiotics in clean and clean-contaminated wounds. Antibiotic cov-erage is indicated, however, in crush avulsion injuries, bites, and heavily contaminated injuries.

12. **What determines the quality of the scar?**
Location of the wound, age of the patient, and type and quality of skin determine it. Lesser deter-minants are the type and quantity of suture material and wound care. Final appearance depends little on the method of suture. Contusion, infection, retained foreign body, improper orientation of laceration, tension, and beveling of edges predict a poor outcome. Differences among suture materials are negligible; however, the technical factors of suture placement to produce wound eversion and time to removal affect the final result.

13. **When should scars be revised?**
A scar usually has its worst appearance at 2 weeks to 2 months after suturing. Scar revision should await complete maturation, which may take 4–24 months. A good rule of thumb is to

undertake no revisions for at least 6–12 months after initial repair. The maturation of the wound may be assessed by its degree of discomfort, erythema, and induration.

CONTROVERSIES

14. **What controversies exist regarding the care and repair of facial lacerations?**
    There is little controversy about the care and repair of facial lacerations. Attention to basic principles of wound care usually produces a satisfactory scar. Because of the cosmetic considerations in facial trauma, primary repair in some instances is undertaken for the sake of appearance despite the risk of infection that would be deemed unacceptable in other areas of the body.

BIBLIOGRAPHY

1. Adame N Jr, Bayless P: Carotid arteriovenous fistula in the neck as a result of a facial laceration. J Emerg Med 16:575–578, 1998.
2. Amiel GE, Sukhotnik I, Kawar B, Siplovich I: Use of N-butyl-2-cyanoacrylate in elective surgical incisions: Long-term outcomes. J Am Coll Surg 189:21–25, 1999.
3. Farion KJ, Osmond MH, Hartling L, et al: Tissue adhesives for traumatic lacerations: A systematic review of randomized controlled trials. Acad Emerg Med 10:110–118, 2003.
4. Hollander JE, Richman PB, WerBlud M, et al: Irrigation in facial and scalp lacerations: Does it alter outcome? Ann Emerg Med 31:73–77, 1998.
5. Keyes PD, Tallon JM, Rizos J: Topical anesthesia. Can Fam Physicians 44:2152–2156, 1998.
6. Mitchell RB, Nanez G, Wagner JD, Kelly J: Dog bites of the scalp, face, and neck in children. Laryngoscope 113:492–495, 2003.
7. Quinn J, Wells G, Sutcliffe T, et al: A randomized trial comparing octylcyanoacrylate tissue adhesive and sutures in the management of lacerations. JAMA 277:1527–1530, 1997.
8. Simon HK, Zempsky WT, Burns TB, Sullivan KM: Lacerations against Langer's lines: To glue or suture? J Emerg Med 16:185–189, 1998.

CHAPTER 34

BASIC CARE OF HAND INJURIES

Michael J.V. Gordon, M.D., and Lawrence L. Ketch, M.D.

1. **What are the goals of hand repair?**

   Functional considerations override cosmesis in the treatment of hand trauma. There are no minor hand injuries. Initial diagnosis and management determine the final result; expert secondary repair cannot overcome primary errors in diagnosis or decision making.

2. **What determines the final outcome of a hand injury?**

   It is determined by minimal sacrifice of tissue and primary healing accomplished by early wound closure. Minimization of scar tissue by control of edema, prevention of infection, early wound closure, and vigorous physical therapy produce the optimal functional outcome.

3. **What factors influence treatment of hand trauma?**

   Mechanism, location, and timing of injury; hand dominance; occupation; age; and general health of the patient.

4. **How common are occupational hand injuries?**

   Hand injuries result in more days lost from work than any other type of occupational injury.

5. **What are the essentials of examination of the hand?**

   Inspection of position, color, and temperature often reveals the injury. Location suggests possible injury to underlying structures. Motor, sensory, and Doppler ultrasonic examination are confirmatory. All injuries must be radiographed, and surgical exploration provides the definitive diagnosis.

6. **How and where should hand injuries be explored?**

   Hand wounds should be explored under tourniquet control with adequate analgesia using delicate instruments in a well-lighted surgery suite. Visual magnification is usually mandatory.

7. **How is emergency hemostasis of injured hands achieved?**

   In the acute setting (outside the operating suite), no tourniquet should be applied, and there should be no blind clamping of any structures. Hemostasis may be achieved by elevation of the extremity and with direct compression of the wound. This approach prevents injury to delicate underlying structures that are tough to see.

8. **How are fingertip injuries treated?**

   If < 1 cm of pulp is disrupted, the wound will heal spontaneously with daily cleansing and dressing with nonadherent, moist gauze. Larger defects may require a skin graft, which can often be provided by defatting the amputated piece. Bone exposure necessitates flap coverage if digital length is to be maintained. Digital nerves cannot be repaired distal to the distal interphalangeal (DIP) joint.

9. **What is the classification system for fingertip amputations?**

   Classification for fingertip amputations is based on the amount of remaining sensate volar skin. Although the favorably angulated amputation commonly removes some nail and bone, the volar skin is available for easy coverage. This amputation type is "favorable" for treatment by dressings only, allowing wound repair by contraction and epithelialization. The volarly angulated amputation angle is "unfavorable" for conservative management and usually requires a reconstructive procedure. (Image from Ditmars DM Jr: Fingertip and nail bed injuries. In Kasdan ML (ed): Occupational Hand and Upper Extremity Injuries and Disease. Philadelphia, Hanley & Belfus, 1991, with permission.) (See Figure 34-1.)

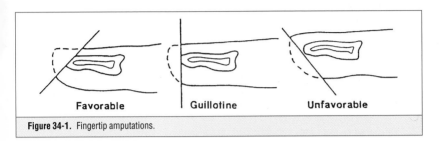

Figure 34-1. Fingertip amputations.

10. **How are nail bed injuries repaired?**
    Repair of the disruption of the germinal matrix must be meticulously approximated under magnification and the nail bed splinted, preferably with the avulsed part. Subungual hematomas should be evacuated by a hot-tipped paperclip or battery-powered electric cautery. Repair of the disruption of the sterile eponychial fold must be maintained for 3 weeks with Xeroform gauze or with the original nail. Often, nail bed disruption cannot be diagnosed without removal of the nail.

11. **What is the initial management of flexor tendon?**
    Flexor tendon laceration is not an emergency, and repair should not be undertaken in the emergency department. If a hand surgeon is unavailable, the wound should be copiously irrigated and sutured and prophylactic antibiotics instituted. This injury can wait for definitive repair.

12. **What is the proper management of an open fracture?**
    Open fractures should be cultured and then undergo copious lavage with normal saline or Ringer's lactate. Broad-spectrum antibiotic coverage should be instituted, and the hand should be splinted in the position of function with a bulky dressing.

13. **What is the proper treatment for hand infection?**
    The extremity should be immobilized and elevated, and parenteral antibiotics should be given. The patient should be immediately referred for possible surgical drainage.

14. **What is the proper management of human bites?**
    After cleansing of the wound, a radiograph should be taken. The wound should be left open—never closed. Antibiotics should be started, and the wound should be rechecked at 24 and 48 hours. If evidence of infection is present, parenteral antibiotics should be instituted and referred for possible surgical drainage. The so-called fight bite occurs over the metacarpophalangeal (MCP) joint or proximal interphalangeal joint when a clenched fist is impaled on the front teeth of an adversary. This often inoculates the MCP joint with anaerobic streptococci. When infection is diagnosed, immediate arthrotomy and lavage should be performed.

15. **How are injection injuries treated?**
    Despite their innocuous appearance, injection injuries may cause profound destruction of hand structures. Any such injury requires immediate hospitalization with prompt and extensive decompression, drainage, and debridement.

KEY POINTS: CARPAL TUNNEL SYNDROME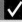

1. Symptoms: numbness, tingling, pruritus of the palm, thumb, middle, and index fingers.

2. Mechanical cause is compression of median nerve and carpal tendons.

3. Women are affected twice as often as men; the syndrome is more common after 40 years of age.

4. Predilection for people who perform repetitive manual labor.

---

16. **What is carpal tunnel syndrome (CTS)?**
    CTS is the most common peripheral compression neuropathy; it is signaled by numbness and tingling of the hand.

17. **Is CTS more common in older or younger people? Men or women?**
    CTS is more common in people older than age 40 years, but an increasing number of young people with CTS have been reported in recent years, usually those whose jobs involve repetitive manual labor. Women are affected approximately twice as often as men.

18. **What are the most preventable causes of deformity in hand injuries?**
    Edema and infection lead to increased scarring and restricted function. Prolonged immobilization in a poor position also impairs function, as does delayed skin closure. Failure to obtain a radiograph leads to a missed diagnosis with delay in recognition of an injury.

19. **What is the proper emergency department treatment of all hand injuries?**
    The patient should be sedated and the wound cultured and irrigated. A thorough examination must be performed and a sterile compression dressing placed. The upper extremity should be splinted, tetanus prophylaxis should be administered, and broad-spectrum antibiotic coverage should be instituted for crush avulsion or heavily contaminated wounds. Radiographs of the hand should always be obtained.

20. **What are the guidelines for replantation of an amputated finger?**
    There are no absolute guidelines. A microsurgeon who is a member of a replantation team should be consulted. If replantation is planned, parts should not be immersed directly in water or put directly on ice or dry ice. The part should be copiously irrigated, wrapped in a moist sponge, and placed in a sterile plastic container; the plastic container should be placed in an ice-water slurry for transport.

WEB SITE

http://www.ninds.nih.gov
  Search: carpal tunnel

BIBLIOGRAPHY

1. Dunn R, Watson S: Suturing versus conservative management of hand lacerations. Hand lacerations should be explored before conservative treatment. Comment on Br Med J 325(7359):299, 2002. Br Med J 325(7372):1113, 2002.

2. Hansen TB, Carstensen O: Hand injuries in agricultural accidents. J Hand Surg 24B:190–192, 1999.

3. Irvine AJ: Suturing versus conservative management of hand lacerations. Incisions are not lacerations. Comment on Br Med J 325(7359):299, 2002. Br Med J 325(7372):1113, 2002; author reply 325(7372):1113, 2002.

4. Lee SJ, Montgomery K: Athletic hand injuries. Orthop Clin North Am 33:547–554, 2002.

5. McAuliffe JA: Hand care in the new millennium: Surgeons' perspective. J Hand Ther 12:178–181, 1999.

6. Riaz M, Hill C, Khan K, Small JO: Long-term outcome of early active mobilization following flexor tendon repair in zone 2. J Hand Surg 24B:157–160, 1999.

7. Taras JS, Lamb MJ: Treatment of flexor tendon injuries: Surgeons' perspective. J Hand Ther 12:141–148, 1999.

8. Van der Molen AB, Matloub HS, Dzwierzynski W, Sanger JR: The hand injury severity scoring system and workers' compensation cases in Wisconsin, USA. J Hand Surg 24B:184–186, 1999.

CHAPTER 35

BURNS

Paulus C. Bauling, MBChB, M.Med., FACS

1. **Why is it essential to have sound clinical knowledge of urgent and emergent burn care?**
   The events of September 11, 2001, have vividly underlined the fact that wars, plane crashes, nuclear and industrial accidents, and many other potential disasters can produce large numbers of burn-injured victims in an instant.

2. **How prevalent are burn injuries and deaths from burns?**
   Roughly, 1.5 million burn injuries occur annually in the United States. Approximately 75,000 of these patients are hospitalized annually. About one half of those hospitalized need the skills of specialized burn centers.

   In 1998, 146,941 trauma-related deaths occurred in the United States (population of 270,248,524). This equates to 54.4 deaths per 100,000 people. Of the quoted trauma deaths recorded in 1998, 3813 were burn deaths, representing 1.4 burn deaths per 100,000 people per year. Thus, based on 1998 data, more than 10 people die per day in the United States because of a burn injury.

3. **Where do burn injuries occur?**
   Eighty percent of burn-related injuries occur in the home, mostly in low-income, multifamily dwellings.

4. **Who is at risk of suffering burns?**
   The male-to-female ratio for burn injuries is roughly 2:1. The combined annualized death rate for children younger than 5 years and adults age 65 or older is five to six times higher than for the rest of the population.

   Work-related burn injuries account for most of the male/female disparity, with accidents in the petrochemical and transportation industries responsible for a significant proportion. Alcohol abuse and illicit drug activity also increase the risk of burn injury and death.

   The incidence of burn injuries and deaths in the United States is substantially higher than that of the rest of the industrialized world. Data published in 1995 reveal that New York City (population, 7 million) had more deaths than all of Japan (population, 120 million). The U.S. city of Baltimore, roughly the same size as Amsterdam in the Netherlands, recorded a 13 times higher fire death rate than Amsterdam's in 1990.

5. **Who should provide care for patients with burn injuries?**
   This is determined by the severity of the injury and the ability of the provider. All level I, II, and III trauma centers should have well-defined protocols and well-established affiliations with specialized burn centers. A list of these burn centers can be found on the Internet at the American Burn Association's Web site (www.ameriburn.org) and the American College of Surgeon's Web site (www.facs.org/dept/trauma).

6. **What are the outcomes of the victims of burn injuries?**
   Of the roughly 75,000 burn victims hospitalized annually in the United States, approximately 3800 died in 1998, equating to a mortality risk of 7.6%. Pediatric burn centers record mortalities

between 2% and 3%. Mortality for those older than 50 years is more than three times higher than the national mean. Above 70 years of age, mortality exceeds one in three victims.

7. **Which factors influence burn outcomes most profoundly?**
Using logistic regression analysis on 1665 burn injuries treated in single specialty burn centers, three risk factors were identified with essentially equal weight in predicting mortality. The three factors were burn size of > 40% total body surface area (TBSA), patient age older than 60 years, and presence of inhalation injury to the lungs. The cumulative probability of death when one or more of these factors is presented in Table 35-1.

TABLE 35-1. MORTALITY RATES ASSOCIATED WITH BURN INJURY	
Number of Risk Factors Present	Mortality
0	0.3%
1	3%
2	33%
3	90%

8. **Do any other variables influence survival?**
Ethanol abuse and illicit drug abuse can be added to the three factors listed above, increasing the risk of death by a factor of two to four times.

9. **As a single mode of injury, why do burns pose such a devastating challenge and threat to victims?**
   - Extensive damage to the skin (considered the largest single organ in the body and consuming almost 20% of the cardiac output) sets the stage for bacterial invasion.
   - Because humans are almost 70% water, enclosed by a complex integumentary system, serious derangements in fluid homeostasis occur when the skin envelope is destroyed.
   - Heat-induced denaturation of integumentary proteins enter the circulation. Systemic infection or sepsis remains the dominant precipitant of organ failure and death; this points to a burn injury–related immune dysfunction or failure.

10. **What happens to the body of a burn victim?**
The pathophysiologic damage is both local and systemic.

11. **What happens locally?**
The injury site may be divided into three zones by standard light microscopy: an inner zone of necrosis, a middle zone of stasis, and an outer zone of hyperemia. In the **zone of necrosis**, all proteins are denatured; all microvascular and macrovascular structure and function are destroyed. Surrounding this central zone is a **zone of stasis**. Here, cellular morphology is intact but cells are swollen with microstructural changes with extravasation of leukocytes and red blood cells into the interstitial space, increased interstitial fluid, and capillary stasis. A third **zone of hyperemia** then gently transitions into the adjacent normal tissues where no abnormalities are seen.

12. **What changes occur systemically?**
Systemic events become clinically significant beyond an injury size of 10% TBSA. Two important abnormalities occur: (1) a trend to fluid retention with generalized edema, caused by an increased systemic microvascular permeability of very rapid onset (minutes to hours) and

(2) a definite and reproducible decrease in cardiac output that gradually resolves over 12–36 hours to evolve into an ensuing cardiovascular *hyperdynamism* at 36 hours postinjury. To summarize, *the pump is failing, and the microvasculature is leaking.*

KEY POINTS: FACTORS STRONGLY ASSOCIATED WITH MORTALITY AFTER BURN INJURY

1. Burn size > 40% TBSA

2. Patient age > 60 years

3. Presence of inhalation injury

4. One risk factor: 3% mortality rate; all three risk factors: 90% mortality rate

13. **How can burn victims be managed in a rational way from the time of injury?**
    Five phases of care can be identified:
    1. Burn first aid
    2. Prehospital care
    3. Emergency department
    4. Transport to burn unit
    5. Stabilization in burn unit or patient room

14. **What can first responders do when witnessing a burn injury?**
    First, do no harm. No ice, butter, dry ice, or any other substance should be applied to the wound after extinguishing the fire. Instead, focus on caring for the patient's needs. If the burn is minor (< 10% TBSA), running tepid tap water over the burn with a hand-held shower for 20 minutes is beneficial. The time and effort required to apply wet soaks with towels appears to provide no benefit and may provoke hypothermia. If stranded in a remote area, encourage oral fluid intake and cover the wound with clean towels. Aspirin or ibuprofen may benefit the patient and the wound. Elevate any burned extremities and encourage full range of motion of all joints.

15. **What actions are needed from prehospital providers (i.e., after the prehospital crew arrives, what are their priorities)?**
    The American College of Surgeons' Committee on Trauma (ACS-COT) advises that all ambulance crews follow "scoop and run" procedure guidelines for all burn victims within 60 minutes of an appropriate hospital (level I or II trauma center or burn facility). Attempt to place an intravenous (IV) line en route, but this is *not* essential if the travel time is < 60 minutes. Lines may be placed through burned skin, preferably in antecubital veins.

16. **How does the hospital-based emergency department contribute to the care of the patients with major burns?**
    Urgency in caring for the victim, not the wound, is pivotal for the ultimate survival of the victim:
    A = Airway—Look for soot in the pharynx and for extensive facial burns.
    B = Breathing—Identify hoarseness, or stridor. Listen for breath sounds on both sides.
    C = Circulation—Place two peripheral IV lines, start fluids as lactated Ringer's solution; calculate the Parkland formula = 4 mL × kg body weight × % body burn [half of volume in first 8 hours; other half over 16 hours].
    D = Neurologic deficit—Examine central nervous system (CNS) and cranial nerves; assess the neurologic status of burned extremities.
    E = Expose and examine the skin, log roll and meticulously determine burn size on the posterior body, and then cover and preserve body heat. The patient's environment should be heated to 90° F.

F = Fluid therapy should be assessed for effect as demonstrated by 1 mL of urine output per kilogram of body weight every hour.

Pain management and psychoemotional support are also vitally important. Avoid overdosing with narcotics.

17. **What initial yardstick determines the severity of a burn injury?**
Burn wound size, which is expressed as a percentage of the total body surface, determines the severity. Remember that the Parkland formula for fluid resuscitation uses the burn wound size to calculate the volume of resuscitation. Therefore, overestimation of burn size leads to overestimation of fluid requirements, which may lead to excessive edema (including such unwanted outcomes as abdominal compartment syndrome). Underestimation of burn size may lead to persistent shock.

Contrary to popular belief, the depth of a burn injury has much less impact on the severity of the injury. The depth of injury also remains an area in which accurate clinical diagnosis, even by experts, is lacking. Burn depth, however, does determine whether a wound will heal on its own or whether skin grafting has to be done.

18. **How are burns sized?**
This determination is done clinically, with the aid of three important clinical tools:
1. The **volar surface of the victim's opened hand** (including fingers) = 0.8–1.0% of TBSA; most useful for the sizing of small, scattered wound areas
2. **Rule of nines:** most commonly used; easy to memorize; not very accurate; usually overestimates
   Adult head = 9%
   Total upper extremity = 9%
   Total lower extremity = 2 × 9%
   Anterior torso = 2 × 9%
   Posterior torso including buttocks = 2 × 9%
   Genitals = 1%
Note that adults and children differ significantly by the difference in the relative size of the head (9% in adults, 15% in infants). By contrast, a thigh in an infant is much smaller than in adults (6% versus 10%).
3. **Lund and Browder chart**: more accurate; time consuming; requires practice; not easy to memorize

19. **Besides the actual skin injury, what other associated injuries may occur?**
Inhalation injury is diagnosed in ± 10% of all hospitalized burn victims. Other physical trauma is frequently associated with explosions or merely the attempts to escape the fire. Awareness of associated trauma justifies the importance of a careful Advanced Trauma Life Support (ATLS)–guided trauma evaluation.

20. **How is inhalation injury defined?**
In contrast to the visible and somewhat quantifiable external burn injury to the skin, the inhalation of heat, carbon monoxide (CO), cyanide, and other toxic or noxious vapors is less visible and less quantifiable, yet very dangerous. Four separate mechanisms of injury to the airways are sometimes incorrectly grouped as inhalation injury:
1. **CO intoxication:** CO is a product of incomplete combustion of organic or synthetic materials. CO has a 250 times greater affinity for hemoglobin than does oxygen, causing a decrease in blood oxygen content with possible hypoxic neurologic, cardiac, and kidney damage. Levels around 5% are routinely found in cigarette smokers, burn victims become symptomatic around 15–20%, and life is threatened around 30%. Management is by administration of 100% oxygen, which reduces the half-life of carboxyhemoglobin from 200 to 40 minutes.

2. **Heat damage to upper airways:** Although building fires can reach temperatures of 1000°F, the countercurrent mechanism of blood flow in upper air passages that normally helps us warm very cold air in the winter is equally capable of cooling down the air to temperatures > 100°F. However, prolonged breathing of superheated air or steam provokes damage to the naso-, oro-, and laryngopharynx and, most critically, the vocal folds. Even minimal vocal-fold edema presents as altered phonation or hoarseness and may rapidly progress to stridor, acute laryngeal edema, asphyxia, and death. Therefore, patients with altered phonation (see question 21) need immediate endotracheal intubation. Intubation is then usually necessary for 2–3 days or until airway edema has subsided.

3. **Inhalation of toxic smoke components** that are produced by the combustion of modern synthetic materials used in the interior decoration of houses, buildings, and cars. Examples include plastics, vinyl, paints, carpets, synthetic fabrics, and floor tiling. The overall mortality from this kind of injury (for which the term *parenchymal inhalation* lung injury could be more descriptive and appropriate) approaches 50%. The ultimate effect of the inhaled toxins is direct damage to airway mucosa, necrosis of mucociliary brush border, and death of surfactant-producing type 2 alveolar pneumocytes, leading to pulmonary failure.

4. **Cyanide poisoning:** The combustion of many synthetic materials also produces cyanide gas, which binds to the cytochrome enzyme system and inhibits mitochondrial function and cellular respiration. Blood cyanide levels should be assessed in all patients with CO levels > 10%. A toxicology center should be contacted. Sodium nitrite is usually administered intravenously, followed by IV sodium thiosulfate.

21. **How is inhalation injury diagnosed and managed?**
It is diagnosed and managed with the following five entities:
1. Obvious hoarseness or stridor
2. Substantial head and neck or facial burns
3. Entrapment in enclosed space or direct proximity to an explosion
4. Extensive total body burns (> 50% in young adults; less in elderly individuals)
5. Event history of superheated steam

In the absence of these findings, immediate airway intervention (intubation) is not warranted, because endotracheal intubation immediately sets the stage for other respiratory complications, including pneumonia. Laryngoscopy or dynamic pulmonary function testing (flow-loop) may be helpful but are not essential or of definitive value. Repeated clinical assessment (e.g., respiratory rate, progressive hoarseness, use of accessory muscles) is more helpful than special tests. Sit the patient up as soon as possible, when stabilized, to help limit edema in head and neck and airway.

The diagnosis and management of **CO poisoning** rests on the blood level of CO, but all victims of dwelling fires should receive 100% oxygen through a non-rebreathing mask until the CO level is documented < 10%. Levels > 15% justify endotracheal intubation with 100% oxygen. The diagnosis of **smoke inhalation** is determined by the event history (e.g., when the victim has been trapped in an enclosed space for a significant period of time). The presence of soot in the mouth or in expectorated sputum is not diagnostic in itself. Significant smoke inhalation mandates endotracheal intubation. CO levels are critical, as well as a cyanide level, *if the CO level is > 10%.*

22. **What treatment has most influenced the outcome of burn victims over the past 100 years?**
Adequate and timely fluid resuscitation.

23. **Why should fluid be resuscitated, and by what route?**
All patients with burns > 10% TBSA should receive fluid. Fluid resuscitation through the gastrointestinal tract with an orogastric tube is used quite often in pediatric burn centers. In adults, the IV route is mandatory.

24. **How is fluid therapy managed?**
The fluid management plan has two components. First, determine the burn wound size and the patient's weight in kilograms, calculate the hourly fluid rate by the Parkland formula, and administer lactated Ringer's solution at the hourly rate calculated.

The second component of the plan is just as important. Monitor the effectiveness of your fluid therapy plan and adjust it promptly when indicated. Our goals are a hemodynamically normalized individual, with a urine output of 0.5–1.0 mL of urine per kilogram body weight per hour. Avoid bolus therapy. Simply adjust your hourly rate. Be aggressive when you have to increase the hourly rate and very cautious when you decrease it in response to excessive urine flow.

25. **What should be done if this treatment algorithm fails to achieve clinical improvement and patient stabilization?**
Failure to respond to the Parkland formula is indicative of a poor prognosis. However, some additional measures may be beneficial but are not currently considered as part of the standard of care. These include the use of hypertonic saline solutions in massive burns, early use of colloids in massive burns, and the early use of inotropes (dopamine is preferred in most burn texts). Finally, at least two prospective studies have failed to show benefit of invasive cardiac monitoring in the absence of preinjury cardiac disease.

26. **How are fluid requirements calculated when there has been a delay in the initiation of therapy?**
Sometimes delay is unavoidable. In an attempt to address a perceived backlog of fluid resuscitation, current teaching is to proportionally increase the fluid volume in an attempt to get the desired total volume for 8 hours into the patient before the 8-hour period elapses. This remedy does require some common sense—one should not apply this guideline if the patient arrives at the resuscitation site later than 3 hours after the injury. Instead, administer fluids based on blood pressure, pulse, and urine output.

27. **What is the best way to care for burn wounds initially?**
Early on, these wounds need simple coverage with a surgically clean or, if available, sterile sheet or surgical drape. The ACS-COT burn and trauma guidelines state that definitive wound care need not occur up to 24 hours postinjury. No ointment or specific antibacterial treatment is initially required. The patient should be kept warm because exposure precipitates systemic hypothermia.

For definitive wound care, the entire patient is washed or showered, and residual debris and damaged epidermis are removed. Then the extent of the injury is mapped, usually on a Lund and Browder chart, along with very preliminary attempts to determine the depth of the injury. A burn wound is usually a mosaic of different areas injured to varying degrees (depths). All burn wounds deepen to some extent over the first 48–96 hours, so a better prediction of which areas require grafting will come with time.

If appropriate wound care is applied, healing should occur within 14–18 days in areas where germinal cells are present in sufficient numbers. Wherever an area of burn injury is identified as a full-thickness injury, healing will never occur; these areas require skin grafting.

28. **Why and how is the depth of a burn injury graded?**
This depends on the presence of skin appendages (hair follicle and sweat gland) that carry the germinal layer deep into the dermis, from which re-epithelialization can occur. On the day of injury, the visual ability to differentiate burn wound that will heal from that which will not is poor (50% accurate). Over time (next 3–7 days), the accuracy of clinical prediction will improve somewhat (≤ 90%). The following table helps to elucidate these aspects. (See Table 35-2.)

Fourth-degree burns involve damage to structures deeper than the dermis (e.g., fat, muscle, bone, tendon, nerve, joint capsule). Burns are designated as fifth degree when tissue is lost, blown off, or vaporized by the burn or blast.

TABLE 35-2. DEPTH OF INJURY WITH CLINICAL SIGNS AND PROBABLE OUTCOME

Depth of Injury	Clinical Signs and Symptoms	Outcome
First degree (superficial injury limited to epidermis)	Erythema of the skin with mild to moderate discomfort.	Wounds heal spontaneously in 5–10 days; damaged epithelium peels off, leaving no residual effects.
Second degree Superficial (involves entirety of epidermis and superficial portion of dermis)	Wounds are blistered or weeping, erythematous, and painful.	Wounds heal spontaneously within 2–3 weeks without residual scarring and with good-quality skin; pigmentation may be altered.
Deep (involves deeper dermis, but viable portions of epidermal appendages remain)	Skin is desiccated, blistered, white eschar often seen. Wounds are occasionally moist and difficult to distinguish from third-degree burn.	Wounds heal spontaneously beyond 3–4 weeks; hypotrophic scarring often occurs and, occasionally, unstable epithelium. For best results, remove eschar by tangential excision and cover with split-thickness skin graft.
Third degree (all epidermal appendages destroyed)	Avascular, waxy, white, leathery brown or black, insensate eschar.	Unless small in size (< 2 cm in diameter), wounds require removal of eschar and coverage with skin graft for healing.

29. **When should surgical excision of the burn wound begin?**

    It should start as soon as possible, but it should be blended with common sense and pragmatism, which implies a hemodynamically "normalized" patient with no signs of sepsis or other contraindication to major surgery. This can be as soon as 24 hours after injury in small to moderate size burns (≤ 30% depending on age) but may take up to 4–10 days in unstable, septic, or frail patients. The overall goal remains to remove the infected or necrotic burned tissue as soon as possible without unduly stressing the patient. It is better for the patient to have a large surgically created wound than a wound containing large amounts of burn-damaged tissue exuding proinflammatory cytokines. Excisional strategies include staged excisions in several sessions, not exceeding 2 hours of operating time. Some authorities stop excising tissue as soon as 75% of the patient's blood volume has been transfused. Burn wound excision can be a huge physiological stress, but is vastly safer than any alternative.

30. **How is the excised area managed?**

    A significant advance in burn management occurred in the early 1970s when Janzekovic demonstrated that excised wounds should be immediately grafted with skin. This remains the goal. If donor sites are insufficient, cadaver skin, pigskin, or biosynthetic products (e.g., Integra, Biobrane, or Transcyte) can be used for wound coverage. These areas require autografting subsequently. Cultured autologous keratinocytes are an attractive theoretical alternative, but they still lack consistent high-percentage engraftment when used on large areas.

31. **What is the impact of a severe burn injury on the body?**
    A big burn is on the top of the list of diseases or injuries that are best avoided. The metabolic response peaks at 2.5 times the basal metabolic rate (BMR) in all burns > 50% TBSA. This maximal acceleration of the body's metabolism by burn injury leads to rapid and severe catabolism, further aggravated by periods of septicemia as well as heat loss through increased evaporation. Recent evidence suggests that growth hormone (HGH) therapy may have benefits in massively burned patients, but problems with glucose control are substantial during HGH-therapy. Several recent studies have also demonstrated the benefit of using beta-adrenergic receptor blockade (metoprolol) early in burns, with substantial benefits toward ameliorating the hypermetabolism.

32. **How can we best supply fuel to the metabolic furnace of the body?**
    Nutritional support of the burn victim is paramount. However, the total reliance on the gut as the primary route of nutritional support (as opposed to IV nutrition) has been slow to achieve acceptance. Total enteral nutrition may have the added benefit of maintaining the intestinal barrier function, which is purported to reduce septic events by preventing bacterial translocation. Currently, the concept of immuno-nutrition is in vogue, but it is fraught with intense controversy surrounding the role of glutamine and, more especially, arginine.

33. **What major life-threatening complications may occur during the healing period?**
    Septicemia, sepsis or septic shock, pneumonia, multiple organ dysfunction, and multiple organ failure.

34. **What is the role of antibiotics in burn care?**
    Antibiotics are never administered prophylactically for burn injuries. Fewer than 10% of all burn injuries require systemic antibiotics during the entire course of treatment. However, early and appropriate antibiotic therapy is a critically important and life-saving tool in the management of *established* infections in burn patients. The key to appropriate antibiotic therapy is the *early* diagnosis of an infective or septic event and wise selection of the appropriate drug or drugs based on the unique infectious profile of the burn victim. The antibiotic selected must be adjusted after culture and sensitivity information becomes available.
    One real dilemma of burn care, however, is that a raised core body temperature does not always indicate infection or sepsis. It is important to view abnormal temperature readings in conjunction with other aberrations in clinical, biochemical (C-reactive protein; procalcitonin), and microbiologic data. Such warning signs include sudden changes in hemodynamic parameters, mental status, general appearance of the patient (he or she suddenly looks ill or is unwilling to cooperate), arterial blood gas changes, sudden intolerance of enteric feeding, thrombocytopenia, glucose intolerance, and oliguria.

35. **How are chemical burn injuries approached?**
    Brush off all chemicals that remain in powdered form on the victim. Thereafter, immediate and prolonged irrigation (30 minutes) of the contaminated skin should be done with running tap water; in the case of alkali burns, irrigate for 60 minutes. Some chemicals may be absorbed; therefore, immediate contact with a toxicology center is indicated.

36. **How are patients with electrical burns managed?**
    An injury caused by electricity may either be an electrical **flash** burn or **contact or conduction** injury. In electrical flash injury, the air or atmosphere is ionized by the electrical discharge, without conduction of current through the body. Thus, the injury is only cutaneous. A true electrical flash burn most frequently heals without much grafting. Airway compromise is rare. In electrical conduction injury, however, tissue is damaged through the actual transfer of electrical energy through the patient from entry point to exit. Thermal energy is generated within the tissues because of the relative resistance to the conduction of current, with resultant protein

denaturation and cell death. Different structures (e.g., bone, skin, muscle, nerve, tendon, lung) exhibit different electrical conductivity, resulting in unpredictable conduction pathways. Thus, the skin is often only minimally involved at the entry and exit sites, with extensive muscle, nerve, tendon, and even bone necrosis in erratic patterns. Neurologic injury, compartment syndrome, and myoglobinuria are frequent complications. Rapid tissue decompression (i.e., fasciotomy) is essential with early and repeated reexploration to remove necrotic tissue. The goal of fluid therapy should be to achieve high urine volumes (> 1.0–1.5 mL/kg/h). Alkalinization of the urine is also beneficial.

37. **After burn injuries have healed, what important issues remain to be addressed in the rehabilitation period?**
The rehabilitation of a burn victim must begin on the day of admission and is a total team effort that involves physiatrists, plastic surgeons, occupational therapists, physical therapists, nutritionists, psychologists, social workers, pulmonologists, microbiologists, pharmacists, speech therapists, and nurses. Rehabilitation of the mind and body must occur in concert.

38. **Are burnt children just small adults with burn injuries?**
No. Children really are different, so a pediatrician should be consulted.

39. **Does this chapter provide a complete review of contemporary burn care?**
No, this is just an overview. Please review the bibliography below. Injury by lightning, ionizing radiation, and cold also warrant special attention.

WEB SITE

http://www.ameriburn.org/

BIBLIOGRAPHY

1. Demling RL: Burn care in the immediate resuscitation period. In American College of Surgeons: Surgery: Principles and Practice. Chicago, American College of Surgeons, 2002.

2. Gibbons J: Prevention. In Gibbons J (ed): Fire! 38 Lifesaving Tips for You and Your Family. Seattle, Ballard Publishing, 1995, pp 15–64.

3. Heyland DK, Novak F, Drover JW, et al: Should immuno nutrition become routine in critically ill patients? JAMA 29:944–953, 2001.

4. McDonald-Smith GP, Saffle JR, Edelman L, et al: National Burn Repository 2002 Report. Chicago, American Burn Association, 2002.

5. McGill V, Kahn S, Gamelli RL, et al: The impact of substance use on mortality and morbidity from thermal injury. J Trauma 38:931–934, 1995.

6. Pruitt BA, Goodwin CW, Mason AD Jr: Epidemiological, demographic and outcome characteristics of burn injury. In Herndon DN (ed): Total Burn Care, 2nd ed. London, W.B. Saunders, 2002, pp 16–33.

7. Ryan CM, Sheridan RL, Tompkins RG, et al: Objective estimates of the probability of death from burn injuries. N Engl J Med 338:362–368, 1998.

CHAPTER 36

PEDIATRIC TRAUMA

David A. Partrick, M.D., and Denis D. Bensard, M.D.

1. **What is the leading cause of death in children in the United States?**
   Injuries cause more death and disability in children from ages 1 to 18 years than all other causes combined. Unintentional injury deaths account for 65% of all injury deaths in children under 19 years of age. Each year, approximately 20,000 children and teenagers die as a result of injury and 50,000 children suffer permanent disabilities. Each year, nearly one child in four receives medical treatment for an injury. The estimated annual cost is $15 billion.

2. **What age groups are at particular risk for traumatic death?**
   Infants younger than age 2 years have a consistently higher mortality rate for the same level of injury. During adolescence, however, injury takes the greatest toll, accounting for nearly 80% of deaths.

3. **What primary mechanisms account for pediatric traumatic injuries?**
   Blunt (90%), penetrating (9%), and crush injuries (< 1%). Motor vehicle accidents are the most common cause of injury (50%) and death in childhood.

4. **What is the incidence of injuries by body region?**
   Multiple (50%), extremities (20%), head and neck (15%), abdomen (3%), face (2%), and thorax (1%).

5. **What is the overall mortality from injury in children?**
   2% of all injured children and 3% of hospitalized injured children.

6. **What is the mortality rate of injuries by mechanism?**
   See Table 36-1.

TABLE 36-1. MORTALITY RATE BY MECHANISM OF INJURY	
Mechanism	**Mortality (%)**
Beating	13
Gunshot wound	8
Motor vehicle accident	5
Pedestrian	5
Motorcycle	3
Bicycle	2
Sport	1
Fall	1
Other	3

7. **Are boys and girls equally susceptible to injury?**
No. Boys are injured twice as often as girls. Boys and men are at a 4 times greater risk for "successful" suicide (although boys try it less often), 3 times greater risk for drowning, 2.5 times greater risk for homicide, and 2 times greater risk for motor vehicle-related trauma. The second X chromosome is clearly protective.

8. **How is a child's airway different from an adult's?**
Children are at increased risk of airway obstruction because of their large tongue; floppy epiglottis; increased lymphoid tissue; and short, small-diameter trachea. Uncuffed endotracheal tubes are appropriate in children younger than age 8 years to minimize vocal cord trauma, subglottic edema, and ulceration. The narrowest part of a child's airway is the cricoid ring, which functions as a seal for the uncuffed endotracheal tube.

9. **What is the appropriate size of endotracheal tube to place in a child?**
The endotracheal tube should be the same size as the child's small finger. For newborns, use a 3-mm tube; children in first year of life, 4-mm tube; children older than 1 year, internal diameter of the endotracheal tube = 18 + patients's age in years ÷ 4 (but, in an urgent situation do not resort to extensive calculations; simply look at the child's pinky).

10. **What if oral endotracheal intubation cannot be accomplished?**
A needle cricothyrotomy is preferable to surgical cricothyrotomy and can be performed with a 14-gauge catheter. Conceptually, this is the same as jet insufflation in adults. Surgical cricothyrotomy is much more difficult in small children and has a high association with secondary subglottic stenosis.

11. **What is a child's total blood volume?**
80 mL/kg (8% of body weight).

12. **What is the first sign of significant blood loss in children?**
Tachycardia. Young children are incredibly tough and have a remarkable tolerance to blood loss. Hemorrhage of 30% of blood volume may result in no blood pressure change, but such blood loss does cause a rapid increase in heart rate. A child's cardiac output depends largely on heart rate; unlike adults, children have a limited capacity to increase stroke volume.

13. **What are signs of hypovolemic shock in children?**
Tachycardia (progressing to bradycardia), altered mental status, respiratory compromise, delayed capillary refill (> 2 sec), and decreased or absent peripheral pulses.

14. **Is hypotension a reliable indicator of blood loss in children?**
No. Fewer than half of injured children with documented hypotension have an identifiable insult resulting in significant volume loss. Hypotension is often associated with an isolated closedhead injury, especially in children younger than age 6 years.

15. **Why are children at increased risk for hypothermia during resuscitation?**
The child's surface area is large relative to internal body mass—an unclothed child can lose heat fast. Cold intravenous fluids and inhaled gases can exacerbate hypothermia, leading to hypoxemia, which causes pulmonary hypertension and progressive metabolic acidosis. Particularly vulnerable are infants < 6 months of age, who lack significant subcutaneous fat and an effective shivering mechanism.

16. **What sites are preferred for venous access in children?**
Two large-bore intravenous (IV) catheters should be inserted percutaneously in the upper extremities. The second choice is percutaneous access to the distal saphenous vein (or a cutdown).

KEY POINTS: PEDIATRIC HEMODYNAMICS

1. Blood volume: 80 mL/kg.

2. The first sign of hypovolemia is tachycardia, which progresses to bradycardia.

3. Hypotension is *not* a reliable indicator of blood loss; children can lose 30% of blood volume without detectable change in blood pressure.

4. Preferred IV access routes in order: (1) two large-bore upper extremity IVs; (2) distal saphenous vein or cutdown; (3) intraosseous access.

5. Resuscitation fluid is lactate Ringer's, 20 mL/kg × 2; then packed red blood cells (10 mL/kg) if instability continues.

17. What if you cannot establish an IV line?
The intraosseous route is safe and actually requires less time than a venous cutdown. The antero-medial surface of the proximal tibia is used most commonly, with the needle placed 3 cm distal to the tibial tuberosity. The proximal femur, distal femur, and distal tibia are other potential sites. Saline, glucose, blood, bicarbonate, atropine, dopamine, epinephrine, diazepam, antibiotics, phenytoin, and succinylcholine have been administered successfully via the intraosseous route. Complications are rare and result primarily from infection or extravasation. Intraosseous volume resuscitation facilitates subsequent cannulation of the venous circulation.

18. What are the appropriate crystalloid and blood resuscitation volumes in children?
Administer 20 mL/kg of Ringer's lactate solution or normal saline by bolus. A response is a decrease in heart rate and an increase in urinary output. The 20-mL/kg bolus should be repeated if assessment reveals inadequate tissue perfusion. If evidence of shock persists after two bolus infusions of crystalloid solution, 10 mL/kg of packed red blood cells (type specific if available or O-negative) should be administered. Unfortunately, a favorable response to resuscitation does not exclude a big abdominal or thoracic injury.

19. Why are head injuries more common in children than adults?
Similar to Olympic ski jumpers, children lead with their heads. Until age 10 years, children's heads are larger in relation to the body than heads of adults. Central nervous system injury is the leading cause of death among injured children and, thus, is the principal determinant of outcome.

20. What types of head injuries are more common in children?
Epidural hemorrhage is the most common; subdural hemorrhage is relatively rare. However, mortality from subdural hemorrhage is 40% versus 4% for an epidural bleed. Pediatric patients also tend to sustain injuries that produce diffuse edema rather than focal, space-occupying lesions.

21. Can children have significant chest trauma without rib fractures?
Absolutely. The chest wall is much more compliant in children than in adults; thus, kinetic energy is transmitted more readily to structures within the thorax. A child with significant blunt chest trauma is at increased risk of life-threatening contusion to the lungs or heart even with no or relatively few rib fractures. Furthermore, pneumothorax may prove rapidly fatal in children because of a more mobile mediastinum. When present, rib fractures in children reflect non accidental trauma. Thoracic injury is the second leading cause of death (after head trauma) in children.

22. **What types of thoracic injuries are common or uncommon in children?**
Pulmonary contusion, traumatic asphyxia, and tracheobronchial injuries are common. Traumatic aortic rupture, flail chest, diaphragmatic rupture, and open pneumothorax are unusual.

23. **What is the frequency of abdominal organ injury in blunt trauma?**
In decreasing order of frequency, they are spleen, liver, kidneys, intestine, pancreas, urinary bladder, and major blood vessels. Approximately one third of children with major trauma have significant intraperitoneal injuries that must be recognized and treated expeditiously.

24. **How accurate is physical examination in the evaluation of pediatric blunt abdominal trauma?**
Poor. Physical examination is misleading in ≤ 50% of injured children.

25. **What are the advantages and disadvantages of diagnostic peritoneal lavage (DPL) in children?**
DPL is 96% accurate in detecting intraabdominal injury. However, it may lead to nontherapeutic laparotomy rates of 15%.

26. **What are the advantages and disadvantages of computed tomography (CT) in children?**
Abdominal CT scan is safe, noninvasive, and can assess retroperitoneal structures as well as identify specific organ injuries. CT is critical in the decision to manage children nonoperatively. Disadvantages include insensitivity for hollow visceral injury and the need for IV and enteral contrast agents. In addition, CT is time consuming (spiral CT may prove better) and requires patient transport and sedation. A trip to the scanner leaves patients vulnerable and unmonitored. Thus, CT is risky in unstable patients.

27. **Is ultrasonography effective in the evaluation of children with abdominal trauma?**
Yes. It is simple, fast, readily available, and can be performed at the bedside. In addition, it is noninvasive and easily repeatable. The sensitivity and specificity of a focused abdominal ultrasonographic examination for traumatic injury exceeds 95%. Abdominal ultrasound is best used as a triage tool to detect significant intraperitoneal fluid, thus identifying hemodynamically unstable patients who might benefit from a laparotomy.

28. **Is there a reliable method to diagnose hollow visceral injury in children?**
No. Serial physical examinations remain the gold standard. Repeat physical examination by the trauma surgical team is mandatory.

29. **What are the "soft signs" of pediatric intraabdominal injury?**
- Lap-belt ecchymosis corresponds to a high incidence of solid organ injury, hollow viscus injury, and lumbar spine injury.
- Gross hematuria has a 30% risk for significant intraabdominal injury not even involving the genitourinary system.
- Elevation of the liver enzymes aspartate aminotransferase (> 250 U/L) or alanine aminotransferase (> 450 U/L) corresponds to a 50% risk for liver injury.
- Children with documented pelvic fracture have at least a 20% risk for associated intraabdominal injury.
- Children with severe neurologic impairment (Glasgow Coma Scale score < 8) frequently suffer concurrent intraabdominal injury.

30. **What should be suspected in children with seat-belt or handlebar injuries?**
The **seat-belt complex** consists of ecchymosis of the abdominal wall, a flexion–distraction injury to the lumbar spine (Chance fracture), and intestinal injury. Approximately 30% of children with the seat-belt sign have an associated intestinal injury.

   A **handlebar injury** classically causes disruption of the pancreas at the junction of the body and tail, where the pancreas crosses the vertebral column and is vulnerable to anterior blunt compression.

31. **Does the presence of hemoperitoneum in children require laparotomy?**
No. Unlike in adults, < 15% of children with hemoperitoneum require laparotomy for control of bleeding or repair of an injury.

32. **Do all children with solid organ injuries require operative repair?**
No. Selective nonoperative management of solid organ injuries has revolutionized the management of pediatric trauma and is even gaining acceptance as safe and effective in the management of solid organ injuries in adults.

33. **When is nonoperative management of solid organ injury in children appropriate?**
When the vital signs remain stable, 50% of the blood volume is replaced, and no other significant intraabdominal injuries are present. The decision for nonoperative management versus laparotomy should be based on the child's physiologic condition and not on the extent of injury as documented radiographically.

34. **What are the indications for operative intervention for solid organ injuries?**
Massive bleeding on presentation and transfusion of > 50% of blood volume (40 mL/kg) within 24 hours of injury.

35. **What is SCIWORA?**
Spinal cord injury without radiologic abnormalities (SCIWORA) is a problem unique to children. A child's spine has increased elasticity, shallow and horizontally oriented facet joints, anterior wedging of the vertebral bodies, and poorly developed uncinate processes. The spinal cord can be completely disrupted in young children without apparent disruption of the vertebral elements. However, most patients have evidence of spinal cord injury on magnetic resonance imaging. Two thirds of SCIWORA cases are seen in children ≤ 8 years of age.

36. **What is the hallmark of SCIWORA?**
A documented neurologic deficit that may have changed or resolved by the time the child arrives in the emergency department. The danger is that immediate reinjury of the same area may produce permanent disability. Many children with SCIWORA tend to develop neurologic deficits hours to days after the reported injury. Therefore, spinal immobilization should continue, and thorough neurosurgical evaluation is essential in any child with reliable evidence of even a transient neurologic deficit.

37. **What percentage of pediatric deaths attributed to injury are caused intentionally?**
Twenty-five percent. More than 80% of deaths from head trauma in children younger than 2 years are caused by intentional abuse.

38. **What signs are suspicious for nonaccidental trauma (NAT)?**
   - History of failure to thrive
   - Delay in obtaining medical care

- Multiple previous injuries
- Absent or uninterested caregiver
- Fluctuating or conflicting histories
- History inconsistent with the injury or developmental level of the victim

Suspicious physical findings include bite, pinch, slap, or cord marks or bruises in various stages of healing; multiple or bilateral skull fractures; a skull fracture in a fall < 4 feet; and retinal hemorrhages (from shaking).

39. **List the characteristics of shaken-baby syndrome.**
    - Retinal hemorrhage
    - Subdural or subarachnoid hemorrhage
    - Little evidence of external trauma
    - Age < 2 years

40. **What fracture patterns are suspicious for NAT?**
    - Multiple rib fractures of different ages
    - Extremity fractures such as metaphyseal "chip" or "bucket-handle" fractures
    - Diaphyseal spiral fracture in children < 9 months of age
    - Transverse midshaft long-bone fracture
    - Femur fracture in infants < 2 years of age
    - Fracture of the acromion process of the scapula
    - Proximal humerus fracture

41. **What percentage of NAT cases involve burn injuries? What are their characteristics?**
    20% of abuse cases involve burns. Scalding by hot water is the most common. Specific patterns of injury may raise suspicion of abuse, including burns involving the buttocks and perineum (bathing trunk distribution), back, dorsum of the hand, and stocking-glove distribution. Cigarette burns look like circular punched-out ulcers of similar size.

42. **What are the necessary steps in evaluation of children with suspected NAT?**
    Any child with suspected NAT should have a detailed physical examination, head CT scan, skeletal survey (babygram), and retinal funduscopic examination. The appropriate child protective services should be contacted immediately.

43. **How common is postinjury multiple organ failure in children?**
    It is rare. With equivalent injury severity, multiple organ failure in children is much lower than in adults and carries a much lower mortality.

WEB SITE

http://www.emedicine.com/med/topic3223.htm

BIBLIOGRAPHY

1. American College of Surgeons Committee on Trauma: Recognition of Physical Child Abuse. Chicago, American College of Surgeons, 1997.
2. Calkins CM, Bensard DD, Moore EE, et al: The injured child is resistant to multiple organ failure: a different inflammatory response? J Trauma 53:1058–1063, 2002.

3. Dare AO, Dias MS, Li V: Magnetic resonance imaging correlation in pediatric spinal cord injury without radiographic abnormality. J Neurosurg 97(1 suppl):33–39, 2002.

4. Mazzola CA, Adelson PD: Critical care management of head trauma in children. Crit Care Med 30(11 suppl): S393-S401, 2002.

5. Mehall JR, Ennis JS, Saltzman DA, et al: Prospective results of a standardized algorithm based on hemodynamic status for managing pediatric solid organ injury. J Am Coll Surg 193:347–353, 2001.

6. Partrick DA, Bensard, DD, Janik JS, et al: Is hypotension a reliable indicator of blood loss from traumatic injury in children? Am J Surg 184:555–560, 2002.

7. Partrick DA, Bensard DD, Moore EE, et al: Ultrasound is an effective triage tool to evaluate blunt abdominal trauma in the pediatric population. J Trauma 45:57–63, 1998.

8. Stafford PW, Blinman TA, Nance ML: Practical points in evaluation and resuscitation of the injured child. Surg Clin North Am 82:273–301, 2002.

APPENDICITIS

Alden H. Harken, M.D.

CHAPTER 37

1. **What is the classic presentation of acute appendicitis?**
   Periumbilical pain that migrates to the right lower quadrant (RLQ) in a patient who is anorexic.

2. **Where is McBurney's point?**
   One third the distance between the anterosuperior iliac spine and the umbilicus.

3. **What is McBurney's point?**
   The point of maximal tenderness in acute appendicitis.

4. **Was McBurney a cop from Boston?**
   Probably. Another McBurney was a surgeon from New York who, in collaboration with a surgeon named Fitz, coined the term *appendicitis* in classic papers published in 1886 and 1889.

5. **What are the typical laboratory findings of a patient with appendicitis?**
   - White blood cell (WBC) count: 12,000–14,000
   - Negative urinalysis results (no WBCs)
   - Negative pregnancy test result

6. **What layers does the surgeon encounter on exposing the appendix through a Rockey-Davis incision?**
   Skin, subcutaneous fat, aponeurosis of the external oblique muscle, internal oblique muscle, transversalis fascia and muscle, and peritoneum.

7. **Who was Rockey-Davis?**
   Rockey-Davis was a pair of surgeons—A.E. Rockey and G.G. Davis—who developed RLQ transverse, muscle-splitting incisions that extend into the rectus sheath.

8. **What is the blood supply to the appendix and right colon?**
   The ileocolic and right colic arteries.

9. **Does surgery for appendicitis involve a risk of mortality?**
   No surgical procedure is devoid of risk.

	Mortality rate
Nonperforated appendix	< 0.1%
Perforated appendix	≤ 5.0%

10. **What patient groups are at higher risk of death from perforated appendicitis?**
    1. Very young patients (younger than 2 years)
    2. Elderly patients (older than 70 years) who exhibit diminished abdominal innervation and present late
    3. Diabetic patients, who present late because of diabetic visceral neuropathy
    4. Patients taking steroids, steroids mask everything

11. **What is the role of ultrasound in the diagnosis of acute appendicitis?**
Ultrasound can be both negatively and positively helpful. It is nice to see a perfectly normal right fallopian tube and ovary (to rule out an ectopic pregnancy and tubo-ovarian abscess [TOA]). It is also reassuring to see an inflamed, edematous appendix.

12. **Is laparoscopic appendectomy replacing the traditional approach?**
Surgeons are now facile with laparoscopic cholecystectomy, colectomy, and hiatus herniorrhaphy. The normal appendix can be removed easily and safely via the laparoscope, but the inflamed or perforated appendix is tougher. Laparoscopic appendectomy probably should be reserved for the normal appendix.

13. **What is a "white worm"?**
A normal appendix.

14. **What is the differential diagnosis of right lower quadrant pain?**

Meckel's diverticulum	TOA
Diverticulitis	Pelvic inflammatory disease
Ectopic pregnancy	Carcinoid tumor
Crohn's disease	Cholecystitis

KEY POINTS: APPENDICEAL CARCINOID

1. 60% of carcinoid tumors occur in the appendix; 0.03% of appendectomies reveal incidental carcinoid.

2. This malignant but slow tumor spreads to lymph nodes, liver, and right heart.

3. If tumor size is < 2 cm and does not involve the base of the appendix, appendectomy alone may suffice; however, bowel should be assessed because of 30% chance of synchronous lesion.

4. If tumor size is > 2 cm or involves the base of the appendix, right hemicolectomy is necessary.

15. **What is a Meckel's diverticulum?**
Meckel's diverticulum is a congenital omphalomesenteric mucosa remnant that may contain ectopic gastric mucosa. It is found in 2% of the population, 2 feet upward from the ileocecal valve. It becomes inflamed in 2% of patients (i.e., the rule of 2's).

16. **Can chronic diverticulitis masquerade as appendicitis?**
Yes. Fifty percent of patients aged 50 years and older have colonic diverticula. The appendix is just a big cecal diverticulum. Thus, it makes sense that appendicitis and diverticulitis should look, act, and smell alike.

17. **Can a woman with a negative pregnancy test present with an ectopic pregnancy?**
Yes. The fallopian tube must be inspected for a walnut-sized lump. Appropriate surgical therapy is a longitudinal incision to "shell out" the fetus with subsequent repair of the tube. This approach (as opposed to salpingectomy) is designed to preserve fertility. Methotrexate also may precipitate spontaneous evacuation.

18. **Can Crohn's disease initially present as appendicitis?**
Yes; this presentation is typical. Crohn's disease is boggy, edematous, granulomatous inflammation of the distal ileum. Traditional surgical dictum suggests that it is appropriate to

remove the appendix in patients with Crohn's disease unless the cecum at the appendiceal base is involved.

19. **Is it possible to confuse appendicitis with a TOA?**
   Of course. An ovarian abscess buried deep in an inflamed, edematous, matted right adnexa can be treated successfully with intravenous antibiotics alone. Do not drain pus into the free peritoneal cavity—this will only make the patient sicker.

20. **Can pelvic inflammatory disease (PID) resemble appendicitis?**
   PID can look exactly like appendicitis except for a positive "chandelier sign." On pelvic examination, manual tug on the cervix moves the inflamed, painful adnexae, and the patient hits the chandelier. Patients with PID should be treated with antibiotics (either orally or intravenously, depending on how sick the patient is).

21. **How does one deal with an appendiceal carcinoid tumor?**
   Carcinoid tumors may present anywhere along the gastrointestinal tract; 60%, however, are in the appendix. An obstructing carcinoid tumor, much like a fecalith, can lead to appendicitis—and in 0.3% of appendectomies, carcinoid tumors are the culprit. Most carcinoid tumors are small (< 1.5 cm) and benign; 70% are located in the distal appendix. They are effectively treated with appendectomy alone. A large carcinoid tumor (> 2.0 cm) at the appendiceal base, especially with invasion into the mesoappendix, must be considered malignant and mandates a right hemicolectomy.

22. **Can appendicitis be mistaken for acute cholecystitis?**
   Occasionally, yes. Both entities reflect acute, localized, intraperitoneal inflammation. Laboratory studies may be identical: WBC count of 12,000–14,000, negative urinalysis result, and negative pregnancy test result. Thus, if one is thinking "appendicitis," the major difference may be only right upper versus right lower quadrant pain. Laparoscopic cholecystectomy is possible for acute cholecystitis, but conversion to an open procedure should be more frequent.

WEB SITES

1. http://www.acssurgery.com/abstracts/acs/acs0324.htm

2. http://www.pmppals.org/appendiceal_carcinoid.htm

BIBLIOGRAPHY

1. Fitz RH: Perforating inflammation of the vermiform appendix with special reference to its early diagnosis and treatment. Trans Assoc Am Physicians 1:107, 1886.
2. Meakins JL: Appendectomy and appendicitis. Can J Surg 42:90, 1999.
3. Rockey AE: Transverse incisions in abdominal operations. Med Rec 68:779, 1905.
4. Samuel M: Pediatric appendicitis score. J Pediatric Surg 37:877–881, 2002.
5. Urbach DR, Cohen MM: Is perforation of the appendix a risk factor for tubal infertility and ectopic pregnancy? An appraisal of the evidence. Can J Surg 42:101–108, 1999.

CHAPTER 38

GALLBLADDER DISEASE

Jeff Cross, M.D.

1. **What is the prevalence of gallstones in Western society for women and men 60 years of age?**
   Women, 50%; men, 15%, although there is formidable ethnic predilection with gallstones endemic in Native Americans.

2. **What percentage of asymptomatic gallstones convert to symptomatic gallstones?**
   10% at 5 years, 15% at 10 years, and 18% by 15 years.

3. **What is the incidence of gallbladder perforation in patients with acute cholecystitis?**
   5%.

4. **What organisms require antibiotic coverage?**
   Escherichia coli, Klebsiella species, *Streptococcus faecalis, Clostridium welchii, Proteus* species, *Enterobacter* species, and anaerobic *Streptococcus* species.

5. **What percent of patients with common duct gallstones have positive bile bacterial culture findings?**
   90%.

6. **Has the frequency of cholecystectomy increased in the laparoscopic era?**
   Yes. It has increased 500,000 operations per year to > 700,000 per year.

KEY POINTS: GALLSTONES

1. Overall incidence in U.S.: women > 60 years old, 50%; men > 60 years old, 15%.

2. Genetic predisposition in Native Americans.

3. 15–20% of patiens with gallstones become symptomatic.

4. If gallstones become symptomatic, cholecystectomy is required.

5. In the U.S., 75% of gallstones are cholesterol stones; in Asia, pigment stones are more common.

7. **What percent of patients undergoing cholecystectomy experience missed common duct gallstones?**
   2%.

8. **After a laparoscopic cholecystectomy, what is the difference between retained common duct gallstones and choledocholithiasis?**
Gallstones found within 2 years of cholecystectomy are considered retained gallstones. Patients who develop choledocholithiasis more than 2 years after cholecystectomy are arbitrarily defined as having recurrent rather than retained common duct gallstones.

9. **What is the incidence of acalculus cholecystitis?**
10% of all cases of cholecystitis.

10. **How does laparoscopic intraoperative ultrasound (LUS) compare with laparoscopic intraoperative cholangiography (LIOC)?**
The sensitivity of LUS is high (90%) and comparable to that of LIOC. Potential advantages of LUS include less time and less dissection than LIOC. Disadvantages include less sensitivity in detecting gallstones in the intrapancreatic portion of the common bile duct.

11. **What is postcholecystectomy syndrome?**
Unexplained pain, similar to that noted preoperatively, occurred in 20% of patients in previous decades. The incidence of this "wastebasket" diagnosis has decreased recently in that more specific causes can now be identified.

12. **What are these more specific causes of postcholecystectomy pain?**

Common duct gallstones	Cystic duct remnant
Retained gallbladder	Stenosing papillitis
Traumatic stricture	Biliary dyskinesia

13. **What is the conversion rate from laparoscopy to the open approach in acute cholecystitis and in symptomatic cholelithiasis?**
10% for acute cholecystitis and 5% for symptomatic cholelithiasis.

14. **When a patient presents with acute cholecystitis, is there a difference in mortality and morbidity for cholecystectomy performed early compared with cholecystectomy performed late after the patient "cools down"?**
No.

15. **What is the incidence of common bile duct injury in the laparoscopic era?**
0.7% for laparoscopic cholecystectomy and 0.5% for open cholecystectomy.

16. **When, if ever, should laparoscopic cholecystectomy be performed during pregnancy?**
Most attacks of acute biliary colic during pregnancy resolve spontaneously. In order to avoid a surgically induced abortion, cholecystectomy should be performed after delivery. If surgery is necessary, however, the second trimester is preferred for any surgical intervention.

17. **What is the prevalence of gallbladder carcinoma found incidentally during cholecystectomy?**
Open, 1%; laparoscopic, 0.1%.

18. **Why is cholecystectomy increasing in the pediatric population?**
Gallstone identification has increased because of the more liberal use of ultrasonography in patients with abdominal pain.

19. **Should patients with asymptomatic gallstones undergo laparoscopic cholecystectomy?**

   No. The risk of observation of patients with asymptomatic gallstones is less than or equal to the risk of operation.

20. **In what groups of patients with asymptomatic gallstones is prophylactic cholecystectomy beneficial?**

   ■ Patients with congenital hemolytic anemia who have gallstones at the time of splenectomy
   ■ Obese patients undergoing bariatric surgery who have already developed gallstones

21. **What is the optimal timing for laparoscopic cholecystectomy in acute cholecystitis?**

   Within 72 hours of the onset of symptoms. Procedures performed within the first 20 hours generally are easier because the area of dissection is not yet maximally inflamed. Fibrosis and increased blood vessel proliferation have not yet occurred.

WEB SITES

1. http://www.acssurgery.com/abstracts/acs/acs0316.htm

2. http://www.acssurgery.com/abstracts/acs/acs0315.htm

BIBLIOGRAPHY

1. Adamsen S, Hansen OH, Funch-Jensen P, et al: Bile duct injury during laparoscopic cholecystectomy: A prospective nationwide series. J Am Coll Surg 184:571–578, 1997.

2. Behari A, Sikora SS, Wagholiker GD, et al: Long-term survival after extended resections in patients with gallbladder cancer. J Am Coll Surg 196:82–88, 2003.

3. Bender JS, Zenilman ME: Immediate laparoscopic cholecystectomy as definitive therapy for acute cholecystitis. Surg Endosc 9:1081–1084, 1995.

4. Ghumman E, Barry M, Grace PA, et al: Management of gallstones in pregnancy. Br J Surg 84:1646–1650, 1997.

5. Kolecki R, Schirmer B: Intraoperative and laparoscopic ultrasound. Surg Clin North Am 78:251–271, 1998.

6. Koo KP, Thirlby RC: Laparoscopic cholecystectomy in acute cholecystitis: What is the optimal timing for operation? Arch Surg 131:540–545, 1996.

7. Machi J, Tateishi T, Oishi A, et al: Laparoscopic ultrasonography versus operative cholangiography during laparoscopic cholecystectomy: Review of the literature and a comparison with open intraoperative ultrasonography. J Am Coll Surg 188:361–367, 1999.

8. Mirza DR, Narsimhan KL, Ferraz Neto BH, et al: Bile duct injury following laparoscopic cholecystectomy. Referral pattern and management. Br J Surg 84:786–790, 1997.

9. Moody F: Post cholecystectomy problems. In Cameron J (ed): Current Surgical Therapy. St. Louis, Mosby, 1998, pp 434–438.

10. Nakano KJ, Waxman K, Rimkus D, et al: Does gallbladder ejection fraction predict pathology after elective cholecystectomy for symptomatic cholelithiasis? Am Surg 68:1052–1056, 2002.

11. Sharp K, Peach S: Common bile duct stones. In Cameron J (ed): Current Surgical Therapy. St. Louis, Mosby, 1998, pp 410–415.

12. Stewart DJ, Lobo DN, Scholefield JH: Colonic gallstone ileus. J Am Coll Surg 196:154, 2003.

CHAPTER 39

PANCREATIC CANCER

Nathan W. Pearlman, M.D.

1. **What are the general features of pancreatic cancer?**
   There are about 30,000 new cases per year in the United States, and more than 29,000 deaths, so it is a highly lethal disease. In most cases, histology is adenocarcinoma. About 80% arise in the head of the gland, and 20% arise in the body and tail. About 20% of patients have localized (potentially curable) disease at diagnosis; the remainder are inoperable either because of regional spread (portal vein, superior mesenteric artery) or widespread metastases (liver, peritoneum).

2. **What are the presenting signs of pancreatic cancer?**
   - Painless jaundice: 40% of patients
   - Pain (epigastric, right upper quadrant, back) with jaundice: 40%
   - Metastatic disease (e.g., hepatomegaly, ascites, lung nodules) with or without jaundice: 20%.

3. **Why is there such a high rate of advanced disease at diagnosis?**
   The pancreas is retroperitoneal and relatively insensate, and symptoms of disease are uncommon unless the pancreatic or biliary duct is obstructed or the process (pancreatitis, cancer) extends outside the gland.

4. **A previously healthy 73-year-old patient presents with pruritus, dark urine, and icteric sclerae after recent overseas travel. What is a reasonable differential diagnosis?**
   1. Gallstones
   2. Cancer of the extrahepatic bile ducts
   3. Cancer of the pancreas
   4. Hepatitis

5. **What is the first step in evaluating the patient?**
   The first step is liver function tests to determine the degree of jaundice and hepatic dysfunction. Then ultrasound is done to determine whether the cause is intrahepatic (normal bile ducts) or extrahepatic (dilated bile ducts). Ultrasound can detect stones in the gallbladder or common duct with about 95% accuracy. Thus, if a jaundiced patient has normal bile ducts on ultrasound, the problem is intrahepatic cholestasis, probably from hepatitis.

6. **What if an ultrasound shows dilated extrahepatic bile ducts?**
   Proceed to endoscopic retrograde cholangiopancreatography (ERCP) or transhepatic cholangiogram to determine whether the obstruction is high or low in the common bile duct and to determine its likely cause (stricture, stone, tumor). The biliary tract can be decompressed with an internal stent at this time, allowing liver function to improve before major surgery. If stones are present, endoscopic sphincterotomy should be performed, allowing the stones to pass and simplifying future surgery.

7. **When should computed tomography (CT) scan be used instead of ERCP?**
ERCP is best for determining intraluminal anatomy. CT scan provides other information, such as size of the tumor (if one is present), degree of regional spread (portal vein, lymph nodes), and presence or absence of liver metastases.

8. **In this case, ultrasound, ERCP, and CT scan show dilated extrahepatic bile ducts, a mass in the head of the pancreas, and no obvious cause other than cancer. The tumor seems separate from the portal vein, and there are no liver metastases. What should be done next?**
If the patient is a poor operative risk, one should consider percutaneous or endoscopic ultrasound-guided fine-needle aspiration (FNA) to document cancer, if possible, and endoscopic stenting of the bile duct; surgery probably is not a good option. If the patient is a good operative risk, the next step is surgery. The clinical picture is accurate in at least 90% of cases, and FNA adds no useful information at this time. If no malignant tissue is obtained, surgery is still indicated because the needle may have missed the lesion, sampling only the pancreatitis that surrounds all such tumors.

KEY POINTS: DIAGNOSTIC WORK-UP OF JAUNDICED PATIENT

1. Liver function tests: determine degree of jaundice (obstructive versus nonobstructive) and hepatic dysfunction.

2. Ultrasound of right upper quadrant: rules out gallstones, evaluates intrahepatic vs. extrahepatic ductal dilatation.

3. If hepatic ducts are dilated: ERCP or PTC to delineate site of mechanical obstruction.

4. CT: evaluates size of tumor if present, degree of regional spread, and/or liver metastases

9. **We are in the operating room, the abdomen is open, and the discussion revolves around taking out the tumor. What is a Whipple procedure?**
This is a removal of the gallbladder, distal common duct, duodenum, and the portion of pancreas to the right of the portal vein—in essence, a proximal pancreatectomy. In some centers, it is also routine to remove the gastric antrum, with or without a vagotomy.

10. **What is distal pancreatectomy? A total pancreatectomy?**
Distal pancreatectomy removes the portion of gland to the left of the portal vein, along with the spleen. Total pancreatectomy combines both procedures—again, with antrectomy in some centers.

11. **Why remove gallbladder, duodenum, and stomach if the problem is in the pancreas?**
After the ampulla of Vater is removed, the gallbladder does not function well and forms gallstones. The second and third portions of the duodenum share a blood supply with the head of the pancreas and are usually devascularized when the head is removed. Historically, the gastric antrum was removed to improve resection margins. Vagotomy was added to reduce the incidence of marginal ulceration at the anastomosis between the gastric remnant and jejunum.

Removing the antrum adds little to the scope of the operation, however, and marginal ulceration can be prevented by placing the gastrojejunostomy downstream from where bile and pancreatic secretions enter the gut. Thus, many surgeons now perform a pylorus-preserving Whipple procedure whenever possible, preserving the vagus nerve as well. Survival is the same as with more radical procedures, and the long-term function is somewhat better.

12. **How does one determine whether to perform a Whipple procedure, distal pancreatectomy, or total pancreatectomy? What is the cure rate?**
Whipple procedures are used for mobile tumors in the head without signs of lymph node metastases at the celiac axis or root of mesentery. Distal pancreatectomy is used for lesions of the body and tail unaccompanied by signs of spread. Total pancreatectomy is generally reserved for a few select situations in which cancer involves most of the gland but nowhere else; this is a rare event. Median survival with each procedure is about 20 months, and 5-year survival is about 15%. This procedure has about 3% operative mortality and 25% morbidity in centers with extensive experience; in other settings, the operative risk and complication rate can be much higher.

13. **What should be done if there are nodal metastases at the celiac axis or root of mesentery?**
The patient cannot be cured with surgery, so the goal is palliation. If obstructive jaundice is present, a biliary-enteric bypass should be performed. If a tumor obstructs the duodenum, a gastroenterostomy should also be carried out. Some surgeons believe gastroenterostomy should be done routinely for cancers of the pancreatic head, regardless of whether duodenal compromise is present, because ≤ 30% of patients without this problem at the time of surgery may require gastroenterostomy for problems of gastric emptying in the future.

14. **Do any other signs of inoperability exist?**
Most pancreatic tumors lie near the portal vein and adhere to or invade the vein as they expand. Most surgeons consider attachment to the portal vein a sign of incurability. Some surgeons, however, remove the affected portion of vein, if this is the only sign of inoperability, and bridge the gap with a graft. Survival in such patients is actually about the same as in similar patients undergoing resection but without vein involvement.

15. **A patient is found to have unsuspected spread to the celiac axis. You carry out a biliary and gastric bypass. Is there anything else you can offer the patient, either surgically or nonsurgically?**
Some of these patients, if suffering from preoperative back pain, can be relieved of this by intraoperative alcohol celiac ganglion block. Alternatively, such treatment can be carried out postoperatively by an interventional radiologist. Most patients with locally advanced disease (i.e., no liver or peritoneal metastases) benefit from postoperative radiotherapy combined with chemotherapy, either 5-fluorouracil or gemcitabine. Many of them will achieve pain relief with this regimen, and median survival is now about 10–15 months (almost as good as with resection).

16. **What about patients with liver or peritoneal metastases? What happens to them?**
Unfortunately, the best that we have to offer this group is palliative chemotherapy. They have a median survival of about 6 months.

17. **With cure rates so low, why are surgeons so eager to do Whipple procedures?**
Unfortunately, this represents the only chance for cure. In addition, pancreatic resection—when carried out safely—probably offers the best long-term palliation in those destined to die of their disease. Finally, the outlook after pancreatic resection may improve in the future with preoperative chemoradiotherapy or newer forms of postoperative adjuvant therapy, so the future does have at least some hope.

WEB SITE

http://www.ascsurgery.com/abstracts/acs/acs0304/htm

BIBLIOGRAPHY

1. Bluemke DA, Fishman EK: CT and MR evaluation of pancreatic cancer. Surg Oncol Clin North Am 7:103–124, 1998.

2. Fuhrman GM, Leach SD, Staley CA, et al: Rationale for en bloc resection in the treatment of pancreatic adenocarcinoma adherent to the superior mesenteric-portal vein. Ann Surg 223:154–162, 1996.

3. Harrison LE, Klinstra D, Brennan MF: Portal vein resection for adenocarcinoma of the pancreas: A contraindication for resection? Ann Surg 224:342–349, 1996.

4. Jemal A, Thomas A, Taylor M, Thun M: Cancer statistics, 2002. Ca Cancer J Clin 52:23–47, 2002.

5. Kozuch P, Petryk M, Bruckner H: A comprehensive update on the use of chemotherapy for metastatic pancreatic adenocarcinoma. Hematol Oncol Clin North Am 16:123–128, 2002.

6. Neuberger TJ, Wade UP, Swope TJ, et al: Palliative operations for pancreatic cancer in the hospitals of the U.S. Department of Veterans Affairs from 1987–1991. Am J Surg 166:632–637, 1993.

7. Ryan DP, Willett CG: Management of locally advanced adenocarcinoma of the pancreas. Hematol Oncol Clin North Am 16:95–103, 2002.

8. Schafer M, Mulhaupt B, Clavien P-A: Evidence-based pancreatic head resection for pancreatic cancer and pancreatitis. Ann Surg 236:137–148, 2002.

CHAPTER 40

ACUTE PANCREATITIS

Clay Cothren, M.D., and Jon M. Burch, M.D.

1. **What are the common causes of acute pancreatitis?**
   Gallstones (45%), alcohol (35%), and other (20%).

2. **What are the uncommon causes?**
   Hyperlipidemia, hypercalcemia (hyperparathyroidism, multiple myeloma), iatrogenic factors
   (endoscopic retrograde cholangiopancreatography), drugs (didanosine, thiazide diuretics,
   H_2 blockers, tetracycline, azathioprine), infections (mumps, coxsackievirus), pancreas divisum,
   and scorpion bites (favorite pimp question on rounds). Approximately 10% of cases are considered truly idiopathic.

3. **What are the characteristic symptoms?**
   Acute onset of severe epigastric pain that is boring in nature and often radiates to the back.
   Pain frequently is accompanied by nausea and vomiting.

4. **What may be found on physical examination?**
   Diffuse abdominal tenderness, abdominal distention, a "board-like" abdominal guarding,
   and hypoactive bowel sounds. Patients may be febrile, tachycardic, and dehydrated. Evidence
   of jaundice or identification of gallstones on right upper quadrant ultrasound is associated with
   a biliary cause of pancreatitis.

5. **What is the appropriate therapy for mild to moderate pancreatitis?**
   The critical component of supportive therapy is fluid resuscitation to maintain urine output
   (place a Foley catheter). Nasogastric decompression in the presence of vomiting, pain medications, alcohol withdrawal prophylaxis, and avoidance of oral feeding until the patient clinically
   improves should also be done.

6. **Which is the better laboratory test, amylase or lipase?**
   Serum lipase has somewhat greater sensitivity and specificity; however, an isolated elevation of lipase with a normal amylase is unlikely to be caused by pancreatitis. Serum
   amylase levels tend to peak sooner than lipase levels, which may remain elevated for
   4–5 days. Up to 30% of patients with pancreatitis have normal amylase levels, most notably
   alcoholics with chronic "burned-out" pancreatitis. The absolute levels do not correlate
   with severity of disease, although an amylase level > 500 most likely derives from the
   pancreas.

7. **What other disease states cause hyperamylasemia?**
   Perforated peptic ulcers, small bowel obstruction, parotid inflammation or tumor, and ovarian
   tumors are associated with elevated amylase levels.

8. **What are Ranson's indices (criteria)?**
   Ranson's indices are 11 measurements that are useful in predicting the occurrence (and severity) of pancreatitis.

On admission	After the initial 48 hours
Age > 55 years	Rise in blood urea nitrogen > 5 mg/dL
White blood cell count > 16,000 K	Decrease in hematocrit level > 10%
Glucose > 350 mg/dL	Calcium < 8 mg/dL
Lactate dehydrogenase > 350 U/L	PaO_2 < 60 mmHg
Aspartate aminotransferase (AST) > 250 µ/L	Base deficit > 4 mmol/L
	Fluid sequestration > 6 L

9. How do Ranson's indices relate to mortality?

Number of criteria	Mortality rate (%)
0–2	5
3–4	15
5–6	50
7–8	100

KEY POINTS: ACUTE PANCREATITIS

1. Causes: gallstones (45%), alcohol (35%), other (10%), idiopathic (10%).

2. Symptoms: acute onset of epigastric pain that radiates to back with associated nausea and/or emesis.

3. Lab tests: elevated amylase and/or lipase (more sensitive).

4. CT can be diagnostic, especially in severe cases.

5. Management is supportive; 10% of cases progress to hemorrhagic or necrotizing pancreatitis.

10. **What is necrotizing pancreatitis?**
The inflammation and edema of acute pancreatitis may progress with subsequent devitalization of pancreatic and peripancreatic tissue. Pancreatic necrosis occurs in approximately 20% of acute episodes.

11. **Why is it important to differentiate acute pancreatitis from necrotizing pancreatitis?**
The presence and extent of necrosis are key determinants of the clinical course. Approximately 70% of patients with pancreatic necrosis develop infected pancreatic necrosis; infection accounts for 80% of all deaths from pancreatitis and is an absolute indication for surgery.

12. **What is the optimal method for diagnosing pancreatic necrosis with or without associated infection?**
Dynamic computed tomography (CT) scans with contrast allow visualization and differentiation of healthy perfused parenchyma from patchy, poorly perfused necrotic tissue. CT-guided aspirate of the necrotic tissue should be sent for Gram stain and culture to determine the presence of infection.

13. **When is surgery indicated in patients with pancreatitis?**
Infected pancreatic necrosis is the only absolute indication for surgery. Open drainage is best accomplished via a bilateral subcostal incision, placement of the greater omentum over the transverse colon to prevent enteric fistulas, and removal of necrotic material from the lesser sac. The patient may require multiple trips to the operating room for repeated debridement; the abdomen is not formally closed until only viable tissue remains.

14. **When should antibiotic therapy be added?**
Patients with mild cases of pancreatitis should be treated with supportive measures because antibiotics do not alter the course or septic complications of the disease. In cases of necrotizing pancreatitis, randomized trials have shown a decreased incidence of sepsis in patients treated with the broad-spectrum antibiotic imipinem. Patients who have more than three Ranson's criteria or are at high risk should be considered for early antibiotic treatment.

15. **What is the most common complication of acute pancreatitis?**
Patients who develop pancreatic pseudocysts typically present with persistent abdominal pain, nausea and vomiting, and an abdominal mass. One should wait 6–12 weeks for the pseudocyst to "mature" before undertaking operative or endoscopic drainage.

16. **What is the significance of hypoxemia early in the course of pancreatitis?**
Patients with necrotizing pancreatitis may develop respiratory failure requiring mechanical ventilation. In addition, they may become hemodynamically unstable and progress to multiple organ failure. Hypoxemia is an ominous sign.

17. **What is the natural history of gallstone pancreatitis?**
Attacks recur. Cholecystectomy is curative and is performed before patient discharge.

18. **What is the natural history of alcoholic pancreatitis?**
Attacks recur. Abstinence from alcohol should be encouraged because many patients develop chronic pancreatitis.

WEB SITE

http://www.emedicinehealth.com/articles/10597–1.asp

BIBLIOGRAPHY

1. Baron TH, Morgan DE: Acute necrotizing pancreatitis. N Engl J Med 340:1412–1417, 1999.
2. Bosscha K, Hulstaert PF, Hennipman A, et al: Fulminant acute pancreatitis and infected necrosis: Results of open management of the abdomen and "planned" reoperations. J Am Coll Surg 187:255–262, 1998.
3. Bradley EL: A clinically based classification system for acute pancreatitis. Arch Surg 128:586–590, 1993.
4. Branum G, Galloway J, Hirchowitz W, et al: Pancreatic necrosis: Results of necrosectomy, packing, and ultimate closure over drains. Ann Surg 227:870–877, 1998.
5. Folsch UR, Nitsche R, Ludtke R, et al: Early ERCP and papillotomy compared with conservative treatment for acute biliary pancreatitis. N Engl J Med 336:237–242, 1997.
6. Gotzinger P, Sautner T, Kriwanek S, et al: Surgical treatment for severe acute pancreatitis: Extent and surgical control of necrosis determine outcome. World J Surg 26:474–478, 2002.
7. Hwang T, Chang K, Ho Y: Contrast-enhanced dynamic computed tomography does not aggravate the clinical severity of patients with acute pancreatitis. Arch Surg 135:287–290, 2000.
8. LeMee J, Paye F, Sauvanet A, et al: Incidence and reversibility of organ failure in the course of sterile or infected necrotizing pancreatitis. Arch Surg 136:1386–1390, 2001.
9. Pederzoli P, Bassi C, Vesentini S, Campedelli A: A randomized multicenter clinical trial of antibiotic prophylaxis of septic complications in acute necrotizing pancreatitis with imipinem. Surg Gynecol Obstet 176:480–483, 1993.
10. Powell JJ, Miles R, Siriwardena AK: Antibiotic prophylaxis in the initial management of severe acute pancreatitis. Br J Surg 85:582–597, 1998.

11. Rau B, Pralle U, Uhl W, et al: Management of sterile necrosis in instances of severe acute pancreatitis. J Am Coll Surg 181:279–288, 1995.

12. Schoenberg MH, Rau B, Beger HG: New approaches in surgical management of severe acute pancreatitis. Digestion 60(suppl S1):22–26, 1999.

13. Uhl W, Roggo A, Kirschstein T, et al: Influence of contrast-enhanced computed tomography on course and outcome in patients with acute pancreatitis. Pancreas 24:191–197, 2002.

14. Windsor JA, Hammodat H: Metabolic management of severe acute pancreatitis. World J Surg 24:664–672, 2000.

DIAGNOSIS AND THERAPY OF CHRONIC PANCREATITIS

Clay Cothren, M.D., and Jon M. Burch, M.D.

CHAPTER 41

1. **What is chronic pancreatitis?**
   The classic syndrome consists of smoldering abdominal pain and evidence of pancreatic insufficiency. Histologically, chronic inflammation results in destruction of the functioning endocrine and exocrine pancreatic cells.

2. **What is the most common cause?**
   Alcohol abuse accounts for 75% of cases.

3. **Is chronic pancreatitis the result of acute pancreatitis?**
   Patients may not have had acute pancreatitis, although alcoholism is common to both. One hypothesis is the inflammation from recurrent bouts of acute pancreatitis causes interstitial acinar fibrosis with secondary dilatation of the main pancreatic duct. The average age for chronic pancreatitis is paradoxically 13 years less than for acute disease.

KEY POINTS: CHRONIC PANCREATITIS

1. 75% of cases are due to alcohol abuse.

2. Symptoms include smoldering abdominal pain and evidence of pancreatic insufficiency (diabetes, steatorrhea).

3. 30% of patients may not mount hyperamylasemia due to "burned-out" pancreas.

4. Common complications include pseudocyst, abscess, fistula, obstructive jaundice, malnutrition.

---

4. **What are the signs of pancreatic insufficiency?**
   Insulin-dependent diabetes mellitus (found in up to 30% of patients) and steatorrhea (in 25%).

5. **How much of the pancreas must be destroyed before diabetes develops?**
   Approximately 90%.

6. **What is steatorrhea? How does one confirm the diagnosis?**
   Steatorrhea is soft, greasy, foul-smelling stools. A 72-hour fecal fat analysis may be done to confirm the diagnosis. The D-xylose test shows normal results, and the Schilling test is not sensitive for pancreatic insufficiency. Patients with steatorrhea are treated with a variable combination of low-fat diets, pancreatic enzymes, antacids, and cimetidine.

7. **Is serum amylase elevated in patients with chronic pancreatitis?**
   No. The serum amylase level is usually normal in cases of "burned-out" pancreatitis.

8. **What are the complications of chronic pancreatitis?**
    Pancreatic pseudocyst, abscess, or fistula may occur. Obstruction of the biliary tree with result-ant jaundice may be caused by areas of fibrosis. Malnutrition and narcotic addiction are more likely to coexist than actual complications of pancreatic insufficiency.

9. **What is a possible source of upper gastrointestinal bleeding (UGIB) in a patient with chronic pancreatitis?**
    Although gastritis and peptic ulcer disease are more common causes of UGIB, splenic vein thrombosis with associated gastric varices and hypersplenism also should be considered. (Your attending will love this answer!)

10. **What is the "chain of lakes"?**
    In performing endoscopic retrograde cholangiopancreatography (ERCP), contrast dye is intro-duced directly into the pancreatic duct; sequential areas of narrowing followed by dilatation of the duct cause the appearance of a "string of beads" or "chain of lakes."

11. **What are the indications for surgery?**
    There are no steadfast rules. Relative indications include unabating pain refractory to medical management, a dilated main pancreatic duct, biliary or gastric outlet obstruction, pancreas divi-sum, and suspicion of malignancy.

12. **Which operative procedures are commonly performed?**
    The Peustow procedure (a lateral Roux-en-Y pancreaticojejunostomy) lays the Roux limb of bowel directly upon the "chain of lakes" duct to provide longitudinal head-to-tail drainage. Distal pancreatectomy may be used for isolated distal disease or retrograde drainage into a pancreati-cojejunostomy. A modified Whipple operation (i.e., pancreaticoduodenectomy) can also remove a nonfunctioning but painful pancreas.

13. **What is the result of such operations?**
    Pain relief occurs in 70% of patients at the end of 1 year and in 50% of patients at the end of 5 years.

WEB SITES

1. http://www.emedicinehealth.com/articles/10597-1.asp

2. http://www.ascsurgery.com/abstracts/acs/acs0304.htm

BIBLIOGRAPHY

1. American Gastroenterological Association: AGA technical review: Treatment of pain in chronic pancreatitis. Gastroenterology 115:765–776, 1998.

2. Beger HG, Schlosser W, et al: The surgical management of chronic pancreatitis: Duodenum-preserving pancrea-tectomy. Adv Surg 32:87–104, 1999.

3. Fernandez-del Castillo C, Rattner DW, Warshaw AL: Standards for pancreatic resection in the 1990s. Arch Surg 130:295–300, 1995.

4. Mergener K, Baillie J: Chronic pancreatitis. N Engl J Med 332:1379–1385, 1995.

5. Steer ML, Waxman I, Freedman S: Chronic pancreatitis. N Engl J Med 332:1482–1490, 1995.

6. Wiersema M: Diagnosing chronic pancreatitis: Shades of gray. Gastrointest Endosc 48:102–106, 1998.

CHAPTER 42

PORTAL HYPERTENSION AND ESOPHAGEAL VARICES

Ramin Jamshidi, B.S., B.S., and Gregory V. Stiegmann, M.D.

1. **Describe the blood supply to the liver.**
   Total hepatic blood flow is roughly 1500 mL/min, or 25% of cardiac output. The hepatic artery normally supplies about 30% of blood flow, and the portal vein contributes 70%. The hepatic artery and portal vein each supply 50% of the liver's oxygen, however. With portal hypertension, portal flow decreases and the relative contribution of the hepatic artery necessarily increases.

2. **How is portal hypertension defined?**
   The portal venous pressure is normally 5–10 mmHg; > 20 mmHg is defined as portal hypertension. Direct measurement is risky, so the hepatic venous pressure gradient (HVPG) is used instead. This is the change in hepatic vein pressure when flow is occluded by wedging a balloon catheter into it (analogous to the estimation of left atrial pressure by wedging a pulmonary artery). A normal HVPG is 2–6 mmHg; > 12 mmHg is considered portal hypertension.

3. **What is hepatopetal flow?**
   Appropriate portal blood flow into the liver is termed *hepatopetal flow*. Reversal of flow in the portal vein can occur with greatly increased hepatic vascular resistance and is called *hepatofugal flow*. In this case, the hepatic artery must provide the dominant blood flow to the liver.

4. **What are the most common causes of portal hypertension?**
   - In the world: schistosomiasis
   - In the United States: chronic hepatitis C virus infection or alcoholic cirrhosis (Laennec's disease)
   - In children: extrahepatic portal venous occlusion (as in portal vein thrombosis) or biliary atresia

5. **What are schistosomiasis and Katayama fever?**
   Infection by a freshwater blood fluke that causes an initial dermatitis ("swimmer's itch") and rash followed after 1–2 months by fever, myalgias, abdominal pain, and bloody diarrhea (Katayama fever). As these parasites mate and lay eggs in the venous system, the resulting inflammation causes chronic obstructing fibrosis of the organs and vessels, which is manifested by portal hypertension. Katayama fever lasts a few weeks and is second only to malaria as a cause of chronic tropical illness. Treat with praziquantel.

KEY POINTS: CHRONIC PANCREATITIS

1. Portal venous pressure > 20 mmHg (normal = 5–10 mmHg).

2. Most common cause in the United States is alcoholic cirrhosis.

3. Anatomic causes characterized as presinusoidal, sinusoidal, or postsinusoidal.

4. Complications include ascites, esophageal varices, encephalopathy, hypersplenism, hemorrhoids.

5. Initial management is medical; surgery is reserved for refractory cases.

6. **How can the causes of portal hypertension be classified anatomically?**
   Presinusoidal:
   - Extrahepatic: portal or splenic vein thrombosis, congenital biliary atresia, extrinsic compression (e.g., tumor)
   - Intrahepatic: primary biliary cirrhosis, schistosomiasis, hepatic metastases, polycystic disease, sarcoidosis

   Sinusoidal: hepatic cirrhosis (e.g., viral infection, alcohol, hemochromatosis)
   Postsinusoidal: Budd-Chiari syndrome, inferior vena cava obstruction, right heart failure

7. **List the four major anatomic connections between the portal and systemic venous systems.**
   1. Left gastric (coronary) vein to the esophageal vein (potential esophageal varices)
   2. Inferior mesenteric vein through the superior hemorrhoidal veins to the hypogastric vein (potential rectal varices)
   3. Portal vein to umbilical vein to superficial veins of the abdominal wall (potential caput medusae)
   4. Mesenteric veins to perilumbar veins of Retzius into the inferior vena cava (potential retroperitoneal hemorrhage)

   Note that the reason these anastomoses can shunt blood (around the liver) is that the splanchnic veins lack one-way valves.

8. **Define sinistral portal hypertension.**
   Derived from *sinister*, the Latin word for "left," this is "left-sided" portal hypertension specifically caused by splenic vein thrombosis or obstruction. This causes shunting from the short gastric branches of the splenic vein to the left gastric vein, resulting in gastric varices. Splenectomy is the definitive treatment.

9. **What are the common complications of portal venous hypertension?**
   - Ascites and spontaneous bacterial peritonitis
   - Hemorrhage from esophageal varices (the major cause of mortality)
   - Hypersplenism
   - Rectal varices (hemorrhoids)
   - Portosystemic encephalopathy
   - Portal hypertensive gastropathy and colopathy

10. **What impact can portal hypertension have on other organ systems?**
    - Hyperdynamic circulation (decreased systemic vascular resistance with increased cardiac output and low blood pressure)
    - Hepatorenal syndrome
    - Hepatopulmonary syndrome or portopulmonary hypertension

11. **Liver function is classified according to what system?**
    The modified Child-Turcott-Pugh system defines three classes of liver disease based on mortality; the points should be totalled from Table 42-1.
    Class A (5–6 points): 85% 2-year survival
    Class B (7–9 points): 60% 2-year survival
    Class C (≥ 10 points): 35% 2-year survival

12. **What is MELD?**
    The **M**ayo **e**nd-stage **l**iver **d**isease score is a completely objective measure of disease calculated with international normalized ratio (INR), bilirubin, and creatinine. In 2002, MELD was adopted by the United Network for Organ Sharing (UNOS) for determining liver transplantation priority.

TABLE 42-1. CHILD–TURCOTT–PUGH SYSTEM OF SCORING LIVER DISEASE			
Parameter	1 Point	2 Points	3 Points
Albumin (g/dL)	> 3.5	2.8–3.5	< 2.8
Bilirubin (mg/dL)	> 2	2–3	> 3
International normalized ratio	< 1.7	1.7–2.2	> 2.2
Ascites	None	Moderate	Severe
Encephalopathy	None	Moderate	Severe

13. **How is MELD calculated?**

$$\text{MELD} = 10 \times [0.957 \times \ln (\text{creatinine mg/dL}) + 0.378 \times \ln (\text{bilirubin mg/dL}) + 1.120 \times \ln (\text{INR}) + 0.643 \text{ (0 if cholestatic/alcoholic)}]$$

Result is rounded to the nearest integer.

14. **How common are esophageal varices?**
At time of diagnosis of cirrhosis, approximately 30% of patients have esophageal varices, and the incidence of new varix formation in patients with known cirrhosis is roughly 6% per year. There is a 50% point prevalence of varices in cirrhotic patients. However, bleeding occurs in only about one third of patients with varices.

15. **Is upper gastrointestinal bleeding in cirrhotic patients with documented varices always variceal?**
Good test-taking skills tell you the answer must be no. Twenty percent of these patients bleed from another source (e.g., alcoholic gastric ulcerations, peptic ulcer disease). This also includes patients with ascites, spider angiomata, and asterixis.

16. **Are gastric varices a common bleeding source in patients with portal hypertension?**
No. Only about 5% of variceal bleeds in cirrhotic patients are caused by gastric varices. Portal hypertension with gastric varices and no esophageal varices is usually associated with splenic vein thrombosis. Gastric varices bleed much less frequently—but more severely—than their esophageal counterparts.

17. **What factors are predictive of variceal bleeding?**
- Size of varices (the most important factor), which increases vessel wall tension
- Red wale markings on the varices (longitudinal "whip marks") from decreased wall thickness
- Severity of liver disease
- Active alcohol abuse

All told, variceal hemorrhage occurs in 30% of patients within 2 years of varix documentation.

18. **Does the degree of portal hypertension predict bleeding?**
Surprisingly, no. Bleeding risk correlates poorly with the magnitude of portal pressure. However, bleeding rarely occurs with HVPG <12 mmHg; this threshold pressure is considered necessary but not sufficient for bleeding.

19. **An initial variceal bleed is associated with what mortality and rebleeding risk?**
Thirty percent of these patients die within 6 weeks, with one third to one half of rebleeds occurring in the first 10 days. If untreated, up to 75% of patients rebleed within the first year.

20. **Should selective or nonselective beta blockers be used in the treatment of esophageal varices?**

*Non*selective beta blockade best minimizes bleeding by lowering blood pressure and reducing splanchnic flow. Beta$_1$-adrenergic antagonism causes splanchnic vasoconstriction by reflex activation of alpha receptors and decreases myocardial contractility. Beta$_2$ blockade prevents splanchnic and peripheral vasodilation. Nadolol is the drug of choice.

21. **What are the major components of acute variceal bleed management?**
    - Fluid or blood product resuscitation (be careful not to worsen ascites with excess crystalloid)
    - Pharmacologic agents to lower portal pressure and flow to limit bleeding)
    - Endoscopy to confirm diagnosis and treat by banding or sclerotherapy
    - Antibiotic prophylaxis
    - Lactulose catharsis (GI bleeding increases protein load—blood is protein—and may worsen encephalopathy)
    - Tamponade, surgery, or transjugular intrahepatic portosystemic shunting (TIPS) if refractory or an early recurrent bleed

22. **What pharmacologic treatments are used in acute variceal bleeding?**

Vasopressin (start at 0.2 U/min intravenously [IV] and increase the level while watching the electrocardiogram) decreases splanchnic perfusion and thus portal pressure. Be careful; systemic vasoconstriction can cause myocardial or mesenteric ischemia and infarction.

Terlipressin (2 mg IV every 4 hours) is a synthetic vasopressin analog with fewer side effects and simpler dosing. This has shown clear promise in randomized controlled trials but is not yet available in the United States.

Octreotide (50 µg IV bolus, then 25 µg/h IV) is a synthetic somatostatin analog that decreases portal blood flow by selective splanchnic vasoconstriction, so side effects are limited. Octreotide acts through vasoactive peptides substance P and glucagon.

23. **What endoscopic treatments are used in acute variceal bleeding?**
    - **Sclerotherapy:** intravariceal injection of a sclerosing chemical
    - **Endoscopic band ligation (EBL):** direct strangulation of varices with rubber bands, similar to hemorrhoid banding

    Either technique typically controls acute bleeding in ≤ 90% of variceal bleeding, but although sclerotherapy can be easier in the face of a large bleed, band ligation is safer (less chance of perforation) and tends to require fewer retreatments. (See Figure 42-1.)

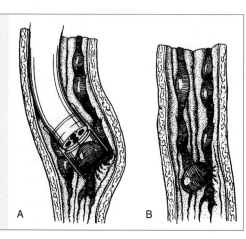

Figure 42-1. Endoscopic band ligation. *A,* The endoscope is positioned over a varix and suction is applied to draw it into the ligator. A rubber band is then ejected over the base of the lesion. *B,* The band strangulates the varix, which sloughs off and passes through the body in about 5–7 days.

24. **Why should antibiotics be given to cirrhotic patients admitted for GI bleeding?**
    These patients have almost twice the risk of developing bacterial infections while hospitalized than do cirrhotic patients admitted for other reasons (nosocomial infection rates approach 50%). Spontaneous bacterial peritonitis, bacteremia, and pneumonia are the most common infections. Short-term antibiotic prophylaxis decreases infection incidence and early rehemorrhage with a resultant increase in survival. Norfloxacin, 400 mg given orally every day for 7 days, is a proven regimen.

25. **What is a Sengstaken-Blakemore tube?**
    A large nasogastric tube with two inflatable balloons that can be used to tamponade both the esophagus and the gastric cardia. The gastric balloon is inflated in the stomach (insert 150 mL of saline plus 25 mL of Gastrografin so that you can confirm appropriate positioning by radiograph) and pull this inflated balloon gently up against the gastroesophageal junction. Most bleeds occur in the distal 5 cm of esophagus, so if bleeding continues, the esophageal balloon should be inflated as well. In order to prevent balloon-induced esophageal ischemia or rupture, do not inflate this balloon to > 30 mmHg (portal venous pressure) and limit use to 24 hours. Half of patients rebleed after balloon deflation, and 10–25% suffer aspiration pneumonia. (See Figure 42-2.)

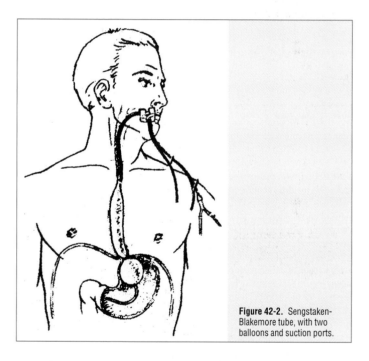

Figure 42-2. Sengstaken-Blakemore tube, with two balloons and suction ports.

26. **What are the options for preventing recurrent variceal bleeds?**
    Without treatment, 75% of patients rebleed within 1 year. Beta-blockers reduce this to 40%; when combined with sclerotherapy, the rate is 35%, and when combined with EBL, the rate is reduced to 25%. The lowest rebleeding rates are thus accomplished with EBL and chronic nadolol. Interestingly, EBL with beta blockade has demonstrated no difference in 2-year survival when compared with beta-blocker and nitrate treatment alone. Shunt surgery and TIPS are slightly better than all these options at 15% rebleeding per year, but these invasive interventions also increase morbidity.

27. **How should a patient with recurrent variceal bleeds be treated?**
Primary treatment should be EBL combined with beta blockade. Failing this treatment, the second-line option is to decompress the portal venous system by shunting blood away with a portosystemic anastomosis. The decision of open versus radiologic shunting is based on the urgency and the patient's fitness for surgery.

28. **What is TIPS?**
TIPS is a percutaneous radiologic technique for diverting portal vein blood directly into the inferior vena cava. Under fluoroscopy, a stent is placed through the hepatic parenchyma to link the hepatic and portal veins. Although TIPS relieves ascites and is superior to EBL in lowering variceal bleed risk, it also exacerbates encephalopathy without any decrease in mortality. New or worsened encephalopathy occurs in at least 25% of patients after TIPS. Stent stenosis and dysfunction occurs in 30% by 1 year and 50% by 2 years. (See Figure 42-3.)

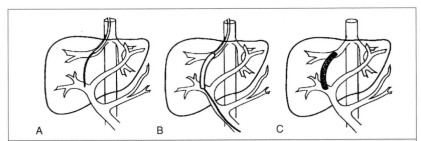

Figure 42-3. TIPS placement. *A,* From a hepatic vein, a needle punctures through the liver to reach a portal vein. *B,* The tunnel is widened with a balloon catheter. *C,* A permanent stent is placed. (From McNally PR (ed): GI/Liver Secrets, 2nd ed. Philadelphia, Hanley & Belfus, 2001.)

29. **Describe the basic options for surgical shunting.**
Nonselective (central) shunt: portovacal and mesocaval shunts nonselectively decompress the portal venous system, thus risking hepatofugal flow and worsening hepatic failure. Large amounts of portal blood (not detoxified in the liver) in the systemic circulation worsen encephalopathy. Creating a smaller diameter conduit (partial shunt) helps preserve some anterograde portal flow and limits this effect.
Selective splenorenal (Warren) shunt: anastomosis of the distal splenic vein to the left renal vein with ligation of the left gastric. This does not decompress as thoroughly and, therefore, this technique enjoys a lower risk of encephalopathy.
As a rule, the more central the shunt site, the more extensive the portal decompression, but the tradeoff is the increased risk of encephalopathy (as demonstrated by TIPS).

30. **How can you estimate operative mortality for elective portosystemic shunting?**
Perioperative mortality correlates well with Child-Pugh class (this was the original purpose of the classification). Classes A, B, and C demonstrate 5%, 10%, and 40% mortality, respectively, at 30 days.

31. **Is there a definitive treatment for recurrent variceal bleeding?**
Liver transplantation provides portal decompression and restores hepatic function. Listing criteria are strict, and the psychological assessment of the "reformed alcoholic" is particularly arduous. Prior TIPS or shunting operations are not contraindications to transplant.

CONTROVERSY

32. **How should a patient with known esophageal varices be treated to prevent an initial variceal bleed?**
The combination of beta blocker and nitrate is used for primary prophylaxis, but endoscopic band ligation is at least equivalent to pharmacotherapy without the side effects (one third of patients cannot tolerate beta-blockers because of fatigue or bronchospasm, and 20% cannot tolerate nitrates secondary to pounding headaches). These treatments reduce the incidence of an initial bleed from 30% to < 10% and the mortality from 30% to 20%. Endoscopic band ligation was previously suggested for prophylaxis only in class C disease, but mounting evidence suggests that EBL is more effective than pharmacotherapy in all patients. The effect of combined EBL and beta blockade in primary prophylaxis remains to be established but makes great intuitive sense.

WEB SITE

http://www.emedicine.com/med/topic1889.htm

BIBLIOGRAPHY

1. Hayes PC: Primary prophylaxis of variceal hemorrhage: A randomized controlled trial comparing band ligation, propranolol, and isosorbide mononitrate. Gastroenterology 123:735–744, 2002.

2. Hegab AM, Luketic VA: Bleeding esophageal varices: How to treat this dreaded complication of portal hypertension. Postgrad Med 109:75–86, 2001.

3. Jensen DM: Endoscopic screening for varices in cirrhosis: Findings, implications, and outcomes; Gastroenterology 122:1620–1630, 2002.

4. Lo GH, Chen WC, Chen MH, et al: Banding ligation versus nadolol and isosorbide mononitrate for the prevention of esophageal variceal rebleeding. Gastroenterology 123:728–734, 2002.

5. Lui HF, Stanley AJ, Forrest EH, et al: Gastroesophageal variceal hemorrhage. N Engl J Med 345:669–681, 2001.

6. Tait KS, Krige J, Terblanche J: Endoscopic band ligation of oesophageal varices. Br J Surg 86:437–446, 1999.

7. Tierney LM, McPhee SJ, Papadakis MA (eds): Current Medical Diagnosis and Treatment, 41st ed. New York, McGraw-Hill, 2002, pp 606–609.

CHAPTER 43

GASTROESOPHAGEAL REFLUX DISEASE

Michael E. Fenoglio, M.D., and Lawrence W. Norton, M.D.

1. **What symptoms suggest gastroesophageal reflux disease (GERD)?**
   Substernal burning after meals or at night, associated occasionally with regurgitation of gastric juices, is one symptom. Discomfort is relieved by standing or sitting. Dysphagia, a late complication of GERD, is caused by mucosal edema or stricture of the distal esophagus. However, no symptom is specific for GERD, and therapeutic decisions should not be made on symptoms alone.

2. **What is the difference between heartburn and GERD?**
   Heartburn is a lay term for mild, intermittent reflux of gastric content into the esophagus without tissue injury. It is relatively common among adults. GERD implies esophagitis with varying degrees of erythema, edema, and friability of the distal esophageal mucosa. It occurs in 10% of the population.

3. **What causes GERD?**
   The underlying abnormality of GERD is functional incompetence of the lower esophageal sphincter (LES), which allows gastric acid, bile, and digestive enzymes to damage the unprotected esophageal mucosa. Achalasia, scleroderma, and other esophageal motility disorders are sometimes associated with GERD.

4. **Is hiatal hernia an essential defect in patients with GERD?**
   No. Not all patients with GERD have a hiatal hernia, and not all patients with a hiatal hernia have GERD. A total of 50% of patients with GERD have an associated hiatal hernia.

5. **What studies are useful to diagnose GERD?**
   Endoscopy with biopsy is essential in diagnosing GERD. Barium swallow with or without fluoroscopy can diagnose reflux but cannot identify esophagitis. Twenty-four-hour esophageal pH testing associates reflux with symptoms and is useful in some patients. Gastric secretory or gastric emptying tests are occasionally helpful. Manometry of the esophagus and LES is required whenever an esophageal motility disorder is suspected and before any surgical intervention.

6. **What is the initial management of a patient suspected of having GERD?**
   - Change diet to avoid foods known to induce reflux (e.g., chocolate, alcohol, and coffee).
   - Avoid large meals before bedtime.
   - Stop smoking.
   - Do not wear tight, binding clothes.
   - Elevate the head of the bed 4–5 inches.
   - Take antacids when symptomatic.
   - Weight loss can be very effective in reducing GERD symptoms.

7. **If initial treatment fails, what should be recommended?**
   About 50% of patients show significant healing with H2 blockers, but only 10% of these patients remain healed 1 year later. Metoclopramide promotes gastric emptying but rarely relieves symptoms consistently in the absence of acid reduction.

KEY POINTS: DIAGNOSTIC WORK-UP OF GERD

1. Underlying anatomic abnormality may cause functional incompetence of the lower esophageal sphincter (LES).

2. Endoscopy and biopsy are paramount in diagnosis.

3. Swallow studies delineate possible anatomic causes.

4. 24-hour pH monitoring can link reflux to patient's symptoms.

5. Manometry of the LES is required if esophageal motility disorder is suspected.

8. **What is the role of proton pump inhibitor (PPI) in GERD?**
   PPIs (omeprazole and others) irreversibly inhibit the parietal cell hydrogen ion pump and are > 80% successful in healing severe erosive esophagitis. Two thirds of patients who continue the medication remain healed. A concern in prolonged PPI therapy is hypergastrinemia secondary to alkalinization of the antrum. Gastrin is trophic to gastrointestinal mucosa, but the initial fear of induced neoplasia has not been borne out by follow-up studies.

9. **When should operation for GERD be recommended?**
   Failure of nonoperative (medical) therapy is the primary indication for surgery. Noncompliance with prescribed treatment is a frequent cause of failure and even stricture unresponsive to dilation. With PPIs, most patients' symptoms can be controlled for long periods of time. Current recommendations for surgical intervention include: (1) failed medical therapy (e.g., intractable disease, intolerance or allergy to medications, noncompliance, and recurrence of symptoms while on medical therapy), (2) complications (e.g., stricture, respiratory symptoms, medicosocial changes, and premalignant mucosal changes), (3) patient preference (e.g., cost—long-term medical prescriptions can be expensive—or lifestyle issues).

10. **What is the goal of surgical treatment?**
    Operations for GERD attempt to prevent reflux by mechanically increasing LES pressure and, in most procedures, to restore a sufficient length of distal esophagus to the high-pressure zone of the abdomen. Hiatal hernia, when present, is reduced simultaneously.

11. **What procedures can accomplish this goal and how do they do it?**
    1. In the **Nissen fundoplication**, which is used in > 95% of patients, the fundus of the stomach is mobilized, wrapped around the distal esophagus posteriorly, and secured to itself anteriorly (i.e., 360-degree wrap). The procedure alters the angle of the gastro-esophageal junction and maintains the distal esophagus within the abdomen to prevent reflux. The operation is performed transabdominally by either laparotomy or laparoscopy. (See Figure 43-1.)
    2. The **Belsey Mark IV operation** accomplishes the same anatomic changes but is done via a thoracotomy. (See Figure 43-2.)
    3. The **Hill gastropexy** restores the esophagus to the abdominal cavity by securing the gastric cardia to the preaortic fascia. (See Figure 43-3.)
    4. The **Toupet (partial) fundoplication** is used in patients who have associated motility disorders. Because the wrap is not circumferential, the incidence of postoperative dysphagia is significantly reduced with this partial wrap compared with a full 360-degree wrap (Nissen fundoplication). However, long-term durability may not be as good as with a Nissen fundoplication. This operation can be done transabdominally by either laparotomy or laparoscopy. (See Figure 43-4.)

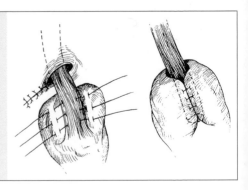

Figure 43-1. In the **Nissen fundoplication,** which is used in > 95% of patients, the fundus of the stomach is mobilized, wrapped around the distal esophagus posteriorly, and secured to itself anteriorly (i.e., 360° wrap). The procedure alters the angle of the GE junction and maintains the distal esophagus within the abdomen to prevent reflux. The operation is performed transabdominally by either laparotomy or laparoscopy.

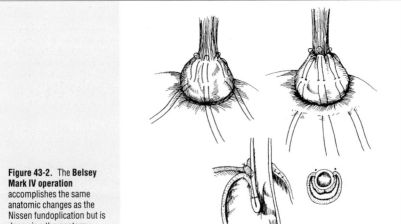

Figure 43-2. The **Belsey Mark IV operation** accomplishes the same anatomic changes as the Nissen fundoplication but is done via a thoracotomy.

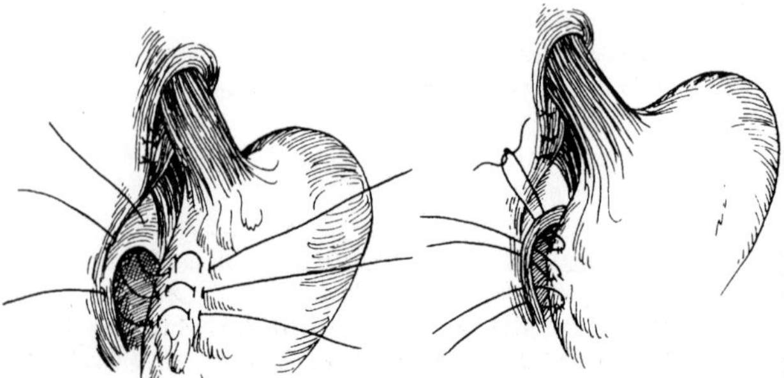

Figure 43-3. The **Hill gastropexy** restores the esophagus to the abdominal cavity by securing the gastric cardia to the preaortic fascia.

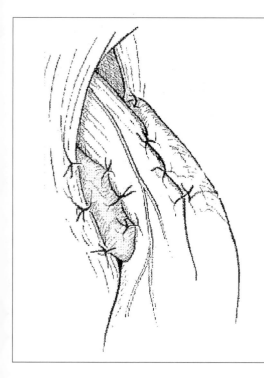

Figure 43-4. The **Toupet (partial) fundoplication** is used in patients who have associated motility disorders. Because the wrap is not circumferential, the incidence of postoperative dysphagia is significantly reduced with this partial wrap compared with a full 360° wrap (Nissen fundoplication). However, long-term durability may not be as good as with a Nissen fundoplication. This operation can be done transabdominally by either laparotomy or laparoscopy.

12. **What are the success rates for such procedures?**

All of the procedures described in question 11 eliminate GERD in almost 90% of patients who are followed for 10 years. But the Nissen fundoplication wins in comparison studies. Recurrent symptoms should be thoroughly worked up because they are frequently associated with other disorders and not recurrent GERD.

13. **What are the long-term complications of such procedures?**

The repair may fail, with recurrence of reflux, after any of these operations. Incorrect placement or slippage of the stomach wrap can complicate Nissen fundoplication and the Belsey Mark IV procedure. Dysphagia and the inability to belch (i.e., gas-bloat syndrome) result from too tight a wrap.

14. **How can stricture from GERD be managed?**

Pliable (unfixed) strictures can be dilated. Fixed strictures require surgical repair. A Thal patch expands the stricture by interposing a piece of stomach.

CONTROVERSIES

15. **Is GERD better treated in the long term by PPI therapy or Nissen fundoplication?**

PPIs really work in resolving esophagitis and eliminating symptoms of GERD, but the long-term side effects are not fully known. Fundoplication potentially frees the patient from daily medicine (this has been challenged recently) and may cause morbidity in ≤ 10% of patients.

16. **Should a Nissen fundoplication be performed by laparoscopy or laparotomy?**
The same procedure can be accomplished by either approach. Postoperative morbidity and mortality is comparable. The distinct advantages of laparoscopy are less postoperative pain, shorter hospitalization, and earlier return to work.

17. **Can this disease be treated by other minimally invasive means?**
Yes. Other endoscopic methods include:
- Endoluminal suturing
- Radiofrequency treatment of the LES
- Injection of bulk-forming agents around the LES

WEB SITE

http://www.emedicine.com/med/topic857.htm

BIBLIOGRAPHY

1. Bremner RM, DeMeester TR, Crookes F, et al: The effect of symptoms and nonspecific motility abnormalities on outcomes of surgical therapy for gastroesophageal reflux. J Thorac Cardiovasc Surg 107:1244–1250, 1994.

2. DeMeester TR, Peters JH, Bremner CG, Chandrasoma P: Biology of gastroesophageal reflux disease: Pathophysiology relating to medical and surgical treatment. Annu Rev Med 50:469–506, 1999.

3. Hinder RA, Filipi CJ, Wetscher G, et al: Laparoscopic Nissen fundoplication is an effective treatment for gastroesophageal reflux disease. Ann Surg 220:472–481, 1994.

4. Lagergren J, Bergstrom R, Lindgren A, Nyren O: Symptomatic gastroesophageal reflux as a risk factor for esophageal adenocarcinoma. N Engl J Med 340:825–831, 1999.

5. Lord RV, Kaminski A, Oberg S, et al: Absence of gastroesophageal reflux disease in a majority of patients taking acid suppression medications after Nissen fundoplication. J Gastrointest Surg 6:3–9, 2002.

6. Peters JH, DeMeester TR (eds): Minimally Invasive Surgery of the Foregut. St. Louis, Quality Medical Publishing, 1994.

7. Roy-Shapira A, Stein HJ, Scwartz D, et al: Endoluminal methods of treating gastroesophageal reflux disease. Dis Esophagus 15:132–136, 2002.

8. Spechler SJ: Comparison of medical and surgical therapy for complicated gastroesophageal reflux disease in veterans. N Engl J Med 326:786–792, 1992.

9. Spechler SJ, Lee E, Ahnen D, et al: Long-term outcome of medical and surgical therapies for gastro-esophageal reflux disease: follow-up of a randomized controlled trial. JAMA 285:2331–2338, 2001.

10. Spivak H, Lulcuk S, Hunter JG: Laparoscopic surgery of the gastroesophageal junction. World J Surg 23:356–367, 1999.

11. Triadafilopoulos G, DiBaise JK, Nostrant TT, et al: The Stretta procedure for the treatment of GERD: 6 and 12 month follow-up of the U.S. open label trial. Gastrointest Endosc 55:149–156, 2002.

12. Trus TL, Laycock WS, Waring JP, et al: Improvement in quality of life measures after laparoscopic antireflux surgery. Ann Surg 229:331–336, 1999.

13. Watson DI, Jamieson JG, Pike GK, Davies N, et al: Prospective randomized double-blind trial between laparoscopic Nissen fundoplication and anterior partial fundoplication. Br J Surg 86:120–130, 1999.

CHAPTER 44

ESOPHAGEAL CANCER

Casey M. Calkins, M.D.

1. **What are the risk factors for developing esophageal cancer?**
   Both alcohol and tobacco increase the risk of carcinoma of the esophagus by a factor of 10.
   Additional risk factors include Barrett's esophagus with dysplasia, carcinogen exposures
   (e.g., nitrosamines in the Eastern world), vitamin and trace element deficiencies, and Plummer-
   Vinson syndrome.

2. **What is the epidemiology of carcinoma of the esophagus?**
   Esophageal cancer accounts for 1% of all cancers and 2% of cancer-related deaths.
   Generally, it is three times more common in men and occurs most commonly in the seventh
   decade of life. Worldwide, 95% of all esophageal cancers are of squamous cell origin;
   however, in the Western world, the relative incidence of adenocarcinoma has increased
   dramatically over the past 20 years because of the comparable increase in the incidence of
   Barrett's esophagus.

3. **What is Barrett's esophagus, and how does it relate to esophageal cancer?**
   Chronic reflux of gastric contents into the esophagus may lead to Barrett's esophagus,
   which is characterized by replacement of the normal squamous esophageal mucosa with
   a glandular columnar mucosa resembling the stomach. This is also called *intestinal metapla-
   sia*. If Barrett's esophagus progresses to high-grade dysplasia, patients have a fortyfold
   increased risk of esophageal adenocarcinoma. Patients with high-grade dysplasia are traditionally treated by esophagectomy; however, photodynamic therapy (PDT) may eliminate
   dysplastic Barrett's mucosa, obviating surgical resection. PDT remains unapproved
   and experimental.

4. **What are the most common presenting symptoms of esophageal cancer?**
   Dysphagia occurs in 85% of patients. Others symptoms include weight loss (60%), chest or epigastric pain (25%), regurgitation of undigested food (25%), hoarseness caused by recurrent
   laryngeal nerve involvement (5%), cough or dyspnea (3%), and hematemesis (2%).

5. **What is the diagnostic work-up for patients presenting with these symptoms?**
   1. History and physical examination
   2. Upper gastrointestinal series (contrast study of the upper GI tract)
   3. Upper endoscopy with biopsies of all concerning luminal structures
   4. Computed tomography (CT) scan of chest and abdomen to define nodal and potential
      metastatic disease
   5. Endoscopic ultrasound (EUS) to define the T stage (i.e., size) of the primary mass and
      regional lymph node involvement with possible fine-needle aspiration (FNA) biopsy
   6. Positron emission tomography (PET) scan to define distant metastatic spread

6. **What is the anatomic distribution of esophageal cancer?**
   The esophagus is divided into three anatomic segments: upper, middle, and lower thirds. Fifteen
   percent of esophageal cancers arise in the upper third, 50% in the middle third, and 35% in the
   lower third.

KEY POINTS: ESOPHAGEAL CARCINOMA

1. Most common in older patients with dysphagia (85% of cases) and weight loss (60% of cases).

2. Major causative factors are alcohol and tobacco (10-fold increase in risk).

3. Diagnosis is made by upper GI endoscopy and biopsy.

4. Most common variant is adenocarcinoma; second most common is squamous cell cancer.

5. Radiographic work-up is necessary to stage disease.

7. **What is neoadjuvant chemotherapy? What are its advantages and disadvantages?**
   This is chemotherapy, radiation therapy, or both to the primary lesion before surgical resection. The advantages include:
   - Potential downstaging (to shrink the tumor or treat locoregional lymph node involvement)
   - Early treatment of micrometastatic disease
   - Treatment is better tolerated before surgical stress
   - Calibrates the patient's ability to tolerate major surgery
   - Verification of primary tumor's sensitivity to the chemotherapy or radiation therapy
   The disadvantages include:
   - Delay in treatment of the primary lesion, particularly when the primary tumor progresses despite neoadjuvant therapy
   - Selection for chemoresistant cell lines

8. **What are the surgical options for treatment of carcinoma of the esophagus?**
   Surgery alone or combined with chemoradiotherapy offers the only hope for cure. The surgical approaches include: (1) transabdominal resection of lesions located at the gastroesophageal junction; (2) resection with intrathoracic anastomosis by left thoracoabdominal (Sweet procedure) or combined midline laparotomy and right thoracotomy (Ivor-Lewis procedure); and (3) transhiatal esophagectomy with cervical anastomosis. Laser therapy, esophageal stenting procedures, and dilatation are reserved for palliation.

9. **What are the risks of surgery?**

Death	Anastomotic stricture
Hemorrhage	Local recurrence of cancer
Anastomotic leak	Dysphagia
Empyema and sepsis	

10. **What is the natural history of esophageal cancer?**
    In a collected series of almost 1000 untreated patients, the 1- and 2-year survival rates were 6.0% and 0.3%, respectively. Untreated patients typically succumb to progressive malnutrition complicated by aspiration pneumonia, sepsis, and death. Formation of a fistula between the aorta or pulmonary artery and the esophagus or pulmonary tree is a somewhat more dramatic (or perhaps merciful) mode of exit. Treated or untreated, esophageal cancer is a bad disease.

11. **Describe the stages of esophageal cancer and the respective 5-year survival rate after esophagectomy.**
    Stage I is cancer confined to the inner layer (muscularis mucosae or submucosa), and 5-year survival is as high as 80%. **Stage II** describes tumors that are confined to the layers outside the submucosa with local lymph node involvement, and 5-year survival can be as high as

35%. **Stage III** tumors have either invaded surrounding structures (lung, aorta, or trachea) irrespective of regional lymph node involvement or go through the wall of the esophagus with nodal involvement. The 5-year survival is typically < 10%. **Stage IV** esophageal cancer has spread to nonregional lymph nodes (supraclavicular or celiac nodes) or distant organs (lung, liver, bone). Essentially, all patients with stage IV disease die within 2 years of diagnosis.

12. **What is an "R0" (or "R zero") resection, and how does it impact survival?**
All gross disease is removed, and microscopically, the margins of resection are negative for tumor. Achieving an R0 resection is the surgeon's goal and is the most robust predictor of a favorable outcome after surgery for esophageal cancer. An R1 resection represents removal of all gross disease, yet resection margins are microscopically positive for tumor. The overall 5-year survival (any stage) for patients with microscopically positive margins decreases by an order of magnitude (e.g., 30% down to 3%).

WEB SITES

1. http://www.emedicine.com/med/topic741.htm

2. http://www.acssurgery.com/abstracts/acs/acs0309.htm

BIBLIOGRAPHY

1. Cordero JA: Self-expanding esophageal metallic stents in the treatment of esophageal obstruction. Am Surg: 66:958–959, 2000.

2. Hofstetter W: Treatment outcomes of resected esophageal cancer. Ann Surg 236:376–384, 2002.

3. Kato H: Comparison of PET and computerized tomography in the use of the assessment of esophageal carcinoma. Cancer 15:921–928, 2002.

4. Kelsen DP: Chemotherapy followed by surgery compared with surgery alone for localized esophageal cancer. N Engl J Med 339:1979–1984, 1998.

5. Oesophageal Cancer Group: Surgical resection with or without preoperative chemotheraphy in oesophageal cancer. Lancet 359:1727–1733, 2002.

6. Overholt BF: Photodynamic therapy in the management of Barrett's esophagus with dysplasia. J Gastrointest Surg 4: 129–130, 2002.

7. Reed C: Techniques of esophageal surgery. Chest Surg Clin North Am 5:379–574, 1995.

8. Salazar JD: Does cell-type influence post-esophagectomy survival in patients with esophageal cancer? Dis Esophagus 11:168–171, 1998.

9. Shumaker DA: Potential impact of preoperative EUS on esophageal cancer management and cost. Gastrointest Endosc 56:391–396, 2002.

10. Swaroop VS: Re: Practice guidelines for esophageal cancer. Am J Gastroenterol 94:2319–2320, 1999.

11. Urba S: Combined modality therapy for esophageal cancer—standard of care? Surg Oncol Clin North Am 11:377–386, 2002.

12. Walsh T: A comparison of multimodal therapy and surgery for esophageal adenocarcinoma. N Engl J Med 335:462–467, 1996.

CHAPTER 45

ACID-PEPTIC ULCER DISEASE

Frank H. Chae, M.D.

DUODENAL ULCER DISEASE

1. **What is the risk of duodenal ulcer disease?**
   The lifetime risk for duodenal ulcer is about 1 in 14. It usually occurs between ages 20 and 60 years, with peak incidence in the fourth decade of life. It is more common in males. Hemorrhage is the most common cause of hospital admission. The annual number of deaths in the United States is about 10,000 deaths caused by duodenal ulcers.

2. **What is the role of *Helicobacter pylori* in duodenal ulcer?**
   Helicobacter pylori, a gram-negative bacillus, is strongly associated with peptic ulcer disease. It is isolated from antral mucosa in 80% of patients with peptic ulcer disease. Ulcers may occur in the absence of *H. pylori*. These ulcers occur in the setting of hyperacid secretion, normal acid secretion, or after acid reduction operations such as vagotomy. Recurrent or multiple ulcerations may indicate an underlying endocrine disease. The breakdown of the duodenal mucosal barrier probably also contributes to ulcerogenesis.

3. **Is acid hypersecretion necessary for peptic ulcer disease?**
   No. Gastric hypersecretion of acid and pepsin plays an important role in ulcer formation; however, only 40% of ulcer sufferers manifest acid hypersecretion.

4. **What are the clinically important complications of *H. pylori* infection?**
   Peptic ulcer disease: As noted, *H. pylori* is present in 80% of peptic ulcers. Conversely, 50% of the general population harbors this organism, but only a small percentage of people develop ulcers. *H. pylori* may be part of the indigenous human gastric flora; antigens were detected in pre-Columbian Central American mummies whose last meal was 1700 years ago.
   Gastric carcinoma: *H. pylori* is strongly linked to gastric cancer and is now classified as a group I carcinogen. It may also cause mucosa-associated lymphoid tissue lymphoma.
   Barrett's esophagus is a possible *H. pylori*–associated disease, although it is more commonly associated with chronic gastroesophageal reflux.
   H. pylori probably synergizes with nonsteroidal anti-inflammatory drug (NSAID) use.

5. **What is the most commonly used test for *H. pylori*?**
   The **CLO test** detects the presence of *H. pylori*. *H. pylori* releases urease, which breaks down urea to ammonia and bicarbonate, thus increasing the pH. The CLO test can be performed at the time of endoscopy by obtaining scrapings from the antral mucosa.
   If endoscopy is not available, the **enzyme-linked immunosorbent assay** (ELISA) may be used to detect anti–*H. pylori* IgA and IgG antibody titers.
   Direct culture of the organism should be reserved for cases in which antibiotic resistance becomes the issue.

6. **What other risk factors are associated with duodenal ulcer disease?**
   - Cigarette smoking is a major risk factor; its cessation is a key component of ulcer therapy.

- Blood group O is associated with higher incidence of duodenal ulcer, as are leukocyte antigens HLA-B5, B12, and BW35.
- NSAIDs promote ulcer formation by suppressing systemic prostaglandin production.
- Chronic pancreatitis, cirrhosis, emphysema, and alpha-1 antitrypsin deficiency are also associated with the condition.

7. **Which endocrine disorder is associated with severe ulcer disease?**
   Patients with multiple endocrine neoplasia (MEN) type I have a 75% incidence of gastrinoma with severe ulcer diathesis.

8. **What other endocrine disorders should be screened?**
   Pituitary tumor and hyperparathyroidism should be suspected when MEN type I is considered.

9. **What are the clinical presentations of peptic ulcer disease?**
   - Pain is usually epigastric in origin, although radiation to the back may indicate pancreatic involvement. It is often relieved by food or antacid ingestion. Nausea and vomiting may occur.
   - Upper gastrointestinal (GI) bleeding.
   - Gastric outlet obstruction (GOO) may result from pyloric spasm, inflammatory mass constriction, duodenal scarring, or fibrosis.
   - Perforation is a surgical emergency with a mortality rate as high as 10%. Perforation may occur without a history of peptic ulcer disease, especially if the ulcer is situated on the anterior surface of the duodenum.

10. **How does the location of the ulcer affect its clinical presentation?**
    Anterior wall ulcers (usually first portion of duodenum) may perforate and cause peritonitis with free air in the abdomen. Posterior ulcers may erode into the gastroduodenal artery or pancreas.

11. **What are the differential diagnoses of epigastric pain?**
    In addition to peptic ulcer disease, gastroesophageal reflux disease, gastritis, gastric carcinoma, biliary tract disease, pancreatitis or pancreatic carcinoma, aortic aneurysm, intestinal angina (ischemia), and myocardial ischemia should be considered.

12. **What initial test should be performed when evaluating epigastric pain of presumed GI origin?**
    Flexible esophagogastroduodenoscopy (EGD) is preferred, although the upper GI contrast study with barium may be acceptable. The CLO test can be performed at the time of the EGD if indicated. Ultrasound should be performed if gallbladder or vascular diseases are suspected. A lateral-view angiogram for intestinal angina, computed tomography (CT) scan for aneurysm, and a baseline electrocardiogram should be obtained because ischemic heart disease is always possible.

13. **How are patients with duodenal ulcer treated?**
    - **Diet:** Aspirin and NSAIDs must be discontinued. Alcohol and nicotine should be avoided.
    - **Antacids:** Neutralizing gastric pH may alleviate symptoms, but its impact on ulcer healing is not well defined.
    - **H_2 receptor antagonists:** The use of cimetidine or ranitidine prevents gastric acid secretions by blocking the H_2 histamine receptor.
    - **Sucralfate:** A protective-barrier medicine adheres to the ulcer base, providing a protective coating. Medications that decrease acid secretion should not be used at the same time because sucralfate requires an acidic environment to be activated.
    - **Proton pump inhibitors:** Omeprazole blocks the hydrogen-potassium adenosine triphosphatase pump in the gastric parietal cells and inhibits hydrogen ion release. It usually is reserved for failures of first-line therapy (i.e., H_2 receptor antagonists).

- ■ **H. pylori eradication:** If *H. pylori* infection is diagnosed, the combination of triple therapy (bismuth, tetracycline, and metronidazole) with an H$_2$ receptor antagonist regimen appears to provide a 90% cure rate. Erythromycin, amoxicillin-omeprazole, or erythromycin-omeprazole may be added for initial failures.

14. **What are the recurrence rates after medical therapy?**
Approximately 80% of duodenal ulcers heal in 6 weeks. The recurrence rate within 1 year of treatment is 70%; thus, repeated treatment may be necessary.

15. **What complications are associated with medical therapy?**
H$_2$ receptor antagonists may induce mental status changes and gynecomastia. Cimetidine, in particular, may affect hepatic metabolism of warfarin, phenytoin, theophylline, propranolol, and digoxin, leading to abnormal serum levels. Omeprazole may cause hypergastrinemia by blocking gastric acid secretion. *H. pylori* resistance to antibiotics may develop, especially to metronidazole; therefore, a triple combination of at least two antimicrobials with an acid inhibitory drug is recommended as initial therapy.

16. **How should recurrent or multiple ulcers be evaluated?**
In addition to the previously mentioned workup, serum gastrin levels should be obtained to evaluate for possible endocrine disorder. Patients should not be taking omeprazole when gastrin levels are measured. In Zollinger-Ellison syndrome, gastrin hypersecretion from the pancreatic islet tumor results in multiple or intractable ulcers (normal serum gastrin, < 200 pg/mL; Zollinger-Ellison syndrome, usually > 500 pg/mL).

17. **How do you evaluate a borderline serum gastrin value (200–500 pg/mL)?**
The secretin stimulation test may be used to diagnose Zollinger-Ellison syndrome. An intravenous bolus of secretin (2 U/kg) should result in an increase of gastrin of 150 pg/mL within 15 minutes if the patient has this syndrome.

KEY POINTS: *HELICOBACTER PYLORI*

1. *H. pylori* is a gram-negative urease-producing bacillus.

2. It has a strong association with peptic ulcer disease (80% of ulcer patients).

3. It is linked to development of mucosa-associated lymphoid tissue lymphoma (MALT).

4. Is is associated with development of gastric carcinoma.

5. *H. pylori* infection is diagnosed by EGD biopsy and CLO test.

6. Treatment includes triple antibiotic therapy supplemented with acid-reduction medication (90% cure rate).

18. **What are the indications for operative treatment of duodenal ulcers?**
Failure of medical management to control pain, bleeding (< 6 units of packed red blood cell transfusions in 24 hours or, better yet, two thirds of the patients calculated blood volume loss in 24 hours), and obstruction are the usual indications. Perforation of the ulcer is usually treated surgically unless the patient presents 24 hours after the event without peritonitis and the Gastrografin upper GI series confirms that the perforation has been well sealed (usually with omentum).

19. **What operations are used to treat duodenal ulcers?**
    - Truncal vagotomy and pyloroplasty (V and P) or gastrojejunostomy
    - Truncal vagotomy and antrectomy with Billroth I or II anastomosis
    - Subtotal gastrectomy with Billroth I or II anastomosis
    - Selective vagotomy (just the vagal branches to the parietal cells in the stomach)
    - Total gastrectomy

20. **What are Billroth I and Billroth II anastomoses?**
    The **Billroth I** operation is an anastomosis between the duodenum and the gastric remnant (gastroduodenostomy). The **Billroth II** operation is constructed by sewing a loop of jejunum to the gastric remnant (gastrojejunostomy). Either method is acceptable.

21. **Which procedure is preferred, Billroth I or Billroth II?**
    Billroth I has the advantages of eliminating the duodenal stump and requiring only one suture line instead of two (as in Billroth II). Duodenal stump blowout is a critical surgical emergency that requires immediate laparotomy. Afferent loop syndrome (i.e., sludging of stuff in the loop that is not in the enteric stream) is also a complication of Billroth II. Bile reflux gastritis may occur in both procedures. Billroth I is more physiologic; thus, it results in better protein and fat digestion. Billroth I is more susceptible to gastric outlet obstruction with ulcer or tumor recurrence; therefore, a Billroth I hook-up is not recommended for patients with gastric carcinoma.

22. **What is afferent loop syndrome?**
    Postprandial abdominal pain often is relieved by bilious vomiting. A narrowing at the junction of the stomach and duodenal side of a Billroth II anastomosis leads to biliary and pancreatic fluid build-up within the afferent limb of the intestine. Pain is relieved when the fluid content is emptied into the stomach, which may result in bilious vomiting and severe reflux gastritis.

23. **How is afferent loop syndrome prevented?**
    Prevention requires avoidance of a long or twisted afferent limb with too narrow an anastomosis during Billroth II construction. A Billroth I procedure eliminates this possible problem.

24. **Who was Billroth?**
    Christian Albert Theodor Billroth (1829–1894) was an Austrian surgeon credited with performing the first successful gastric resection in 1881 and introducing innovations to intestinal bypass surgery. The father of modern American surgery, William Halsted, was once an apprentice to Billroth in Vienna.

25. **How does alkaline or bile reflux gastritis occur?**
    Reflux of bile and pancreatic secretions into the stomach after a Billroth II (sometimes Billroth I) anastomosis may cause marked gastric irritation, leading to chronic postprandial pain. Persistent pain should be evaluated with endoscopy, and surgical reconstruction should be considered, usually with a Roux-en-Y gastrojejunostomy from a 40-cm efferent jejunal limb.

26. **What is selective vagotomy?**
    In this limited proximal vagotomy, the gastric parietal cells are selectively denervated. Fibers to antrum, pylorus, liver, biliary tract, and the rest of the intestinal tract are left **intact**, thereby precluding the need for a gastric emptying procedure. Recurrence of ulcer disease may be 10% or greater, but its side effects, namely dumping (caused by resection of the pylorus) or diarrhea (caused by the vagotomy), are minimized to 2%.

27. **What is dumping syndrome?**
    Resection of the pylorus can lead to uncontrolled, rapid emptying of hyperosmolar gastric contents into the proximal small bowel. The osmotic and glucose load in the intestine sucks

intravascular volume into the gut, making the patient transiently hypovolemic. The physiologically appropriate adrenergic response to this volume shift produces tachycardia, sweating, flushing, weakness, nausea, abdominal cramps, and even syncope. Ingesting a small, dry, low-carbohydrate meal (to limit the available osmols) may prevent this syndrome. Anticholinergic drugs also may help. As many as 20% of patients experience the dumping syndrome in the early postoperative period, but only 2% develop chronic problems.

28. **What must accompany truncal vagotomy?**
Truncal vagotomy denervates the stomach, resulting in gastric hypomotility. Some gastric emptying procedure such as a pyloroplasty or a side-to-side gastroduodenostomy should be performed.

29. **What is a Heinecke-Mikulicz pyloroplasty?**
A pyloduodenal incision along the longitudinal axis followed by a transverse closure flops the pylorus open and promotes gastric emptying.

30. **What is a Finney pyloroplasty?**
A side-to-side gastroduodenal anastomosis that transects and defunctionalizes the pylorus and promotes gastric emptying

31. **What is a Jaboulay pyloroplasty?**
This gastric emptying procedure comprises a side-to-side gastroduodenal anastomosis that does not transect the pylorus. It is ideal if severe pyloric scarring is present.

32. **What are the rates of ulcer recurrence after surgical treatment?**

Vagotomy and pyloroplasty:	10%
Vagotomy and antrectomy:	2%
Highly selective vagotomy:	10%
Subtotal gastrectomy:	1%
Total gastrectomy:	< 1%

33. **What is the mortality rate of these operations?**

Vagotomy and pyloroplasty:	1%
Vagotomy and antrectomy:	2%
Highly selective vagotomy:	0.1%
Subtotal gastrectomy:	2%
Total gastrectomy:	5%

34. **How are patients with perforated duodenal ulcers treated?**
The patient must be resuscitated first, following the ABCs of airway, breathing, and circulation. The stomach contents are emptied via nasogastric tube. Surgical closure by omental patch (Graham closure) is widely practiced. For hemodynamically stable patients, oversewing of the ulcer followed by a selective vagotomy is appropriate. Antrectomy with vagotomy to remove the ulcer is appropriate if the patient has an intractable peptic ulcer.

35. **What (ulcer-specific question) should you always ask before you proceed to the operating room?**
Past history of ulcer disease. Choice of operation will depend on acute versus chronic ulcer disease.

36. **What is the long-term result after Graham closure of a perforated ulcer?**
One third of patients remain asymptomatic, one third have symptoms controlled by medical treatment, and one third require an additional ulcer operation.

37. **What are the complications of surgery for duodenal ulcers?**
Duodenal stump leakage may occur within the first week after antral resection and Billroth anastomosis. Treatment consists of prompt reoperation to drain and control the leak. Total parenteral nutrition may be required as a "bowel rest" adjunct.
Gastric retention may occur because of edema at the anastomosis or atony of the stomach after vagotomy. It usually resolves spontaneously in 3–4 weeks.
Bleeding may occur from a suture line, a missed ulcer, or other gastric mucosal lesions. Most postgastrectomy bleeding ceases spontaneously, but endoscopy may be necessary in some cases.

38. **Where do ulcers recur after operation?**
Ulcers usually recur adjacent to the gastric anastomosis on the intestinal side (i.e., jejunum, duodenum).

39. **Why do they recur?**
The responsible factors are inadequate gastric resection, incomplete vagotomy, inadequate drainage of the gastric remnant (stasis of gastric contents proximal to the anastomosis), or retained gastric antrum (gastrin-producing cells) after a Billroth II procedure.

40. **How do you treat pyloric stenosis?**
Fluid resuscitation and nasogastric tube decompression should be initiated. Metabolic alkalosis may result from prolonged vomiting (loss of hydrogen ions) and should be corrected with normal saline infusion. Either vagotomy with gastrojejunostomy or resection of the stenosis with a Billroth II bypass is acceptable. Partial gastrectomy is required less often.

GASTRIC ULCER DISEASE

41. **What is the most important factor in managing gastric ulcers?**
All gastric ulcers must be evaluated for malignancy. The incidence of malignancy is about 10%.

42. **How is gastric ulcer evaluated?**
Biopsy is mandatory. Esophagogastroduodenoscopy (EGD) with multiple biopsies (typically, six) of the ulcer crater is the best method. Upper GI series may be helpful, but biopsy is not possible. The CLO test can be performed at the time of the EGD to detect *H. pylori*. Benign ulcers usually heal by 12 weeks. Intractability should arouse suspicion for malignancy.

43. **How are gastric ulcers classified?**

Type I	At the incisura or most inferior portion of the lesser curvature
Type II	Gastric ulcer + duodenal ulcer
Type III	Prepylorus
Type IV	Gastroesophageal junction or proximal cardia
Type V	Any ulcer from NSAID or aspirin use

44. **Which is the most common type of gastric ulcer?**
Type I.

45. **How do benign gastric ulcers differ from duodenal ulcers?**
Benign gastric ulcers are difficult to treat and have a higher rate of recurrence and complications. Gastric ulcer disease and gastric carcinoma have a probable common etiologic factor, which is atrophic gastritis induced by *H. pylori*. By contrast, factors associated with duodenal ulcer may protect against gastric cancer.

46. **How is *H. pylori* related to gastric ulcer disease?**
H. pylori colonization induces chronic active gastritis, which is associated with ulcer formation, although a direct cause-and-effect link has not been clearly established. Other factors such as focal defect in acid neutralization that allows acid diffusion into the stomach mucosa or hyper-secretion of acid (in cases of type II and III ulcers) may play important roles.

47. **What is a "trial of healing"?**
A combination of H2 receptor antagonists or hydrogen pump inhibitors with anti–*H. pylori* medications, if indicated, may be tried for 6–12 weeks. A second EGD should be performed to evaluate the ulcer. An additional trial of 12 weeks is acceptable provided that the biopsy results for malignancy are negative.

48. **What is the aim of *H. pylori* eradication in the setting of gastric ulcer?**
Therapy aimed at *H. pylori* eradication is associated with increased ulcer healing and decreased ulcer relapse. Several series have shown decreases in recurrences from 50% to < 10% with *H. pylori* eradication. *H. pylori* is strongly linked to gastric cancer and is now classified as a group I carcinogen. It also may cause mucosa-associated lymphoid tissue lymphoma.

49. **How are patients with *H. pylori* infection treated?**
They should be given a triple therapy of bismuth, metronidazole, and tetracycline, usually supplemented with acid-reducing medications.

50. **Does gastric ulcer healing guarantee a benign ulcer?**
No. Gastric ulcers with foci of malignancy may heal completely on medical therapy.

51. **What are the indications for operative therapy of benign gastric ulcers?**
Hemorrhage, perforation, obstruction, and intractability (the same as duodenal ulcers).

52. **What is the definitive procedure used for benign gastric ulcers?**
Hemigastrectomy or antrectomy (including the ulcer) without vagotomy for types I and IV ulcers is the standard procedure. Type I and IV ulcers have low or normal acid levels. For types II and III, vagotomy should be added.

53. **What are the options under emergent (i.e., hemorrhage or perforation) conditions?**
Hemodynamically stable: truncal vagotomy and distal gastrectomy
Unstable: truncal vagotomy and drainage procedure with biopsy followed by excision and over-sewing of ulcer

54. **What is the rebleeding rate if the ulcer is left in situ?**
33%.

55. **What is giant gastric ulcer?**
An ulcer > 3 cm in diameter, usually located along the lesser curvature. The malignancy risk is about 30% and increases with the diameter. Early surgical resection is indicated because of the risk of malignancy. Vagotomy may be added.

56. **What is Cushing's ulcer?**
A stress ulcer found in critically ill patients with central nervous system injury. Typically, single, deep, and with tendency to perforate.

57. **What is Curling's ulcer?**
A stress ulcer found in critically ill patients with burn injuries.

58. **What is Dieulafoy ulcer?**
Erosion of the gastric mucosa overlying a vascular malformation, which often leads to hemorrhage. Chronic inflammation is not associated with this lesion.

59. **What is a marginal ulcer?**
An ulcer found near the margin of the gastroenteric anastomosis, usually on the small bowel side.

60. **When does stress gastritis occur? Why?**
Sixty percent of them occur within 24–48 hours after trauma, shock, or sepsis. Usually, mucosal erosions begin proximally in the stomach and travel distally. These are eventually seen in nearly all critically ill patients. The integrity of cellular barrier in the lamina propria is compromised, probably from decreased blood supply, leading to back diffusion of acid; erosion of submucosa; and, finally, bleeding.

61. **How are patients with bleeding stress gastritis treated?**
Blood clots should be removed from the stomach lumen by nasogastric tube suction and lavage. Fibrinolysins from clots increase bleeding. Stomach pH should be kept above 4.0 with acid-reducing medications.

WEB SITE

http://www.emedicine.com/med/topic1776.htm

BIBLIOGRAPHY

1. Calam J, Baron JH: ABC of the upper gastrointestinal tract: Pathophysiology of duodenal and gastric ulcer and gastric cancer. Br Med J 323:980–982, 2001.

2. Correa P, Willis D, Allison MJ, et al: *Helicobacter pylori* in pre-Columbian mummies. Gastroenterology 114(suppl 4):A956, 1998.

3. Hansson LE, Nyren O, Hsing AW, et al: The risk of stomach cancer in patients with gastric or duodenal ulcer disease. N Engl J Med 335:242–249, 1996.

4. Kokoska ER, Kauffman GL: *Helicobacter pylori* and the gastroduodenal mucosa. Surgery 130:13–16, 2001.

5. Leung WK, Graham DY: Ulcer and gastritis. Endoscopy 33:8–15, 2001.

6. Rollhauser C, Fleischer DE: Nonvariceal upper gastrointestinal bleeding. Endoscopy 34:111–118, 2002.

7. Rosin D, Rosenthal RJ, Bonner G, et al: Gastric MALT lymphoma in a *Helicobacter pylori*-negative patient: A case report and review of literature. J Am Coll Surg 192:652–657, 2001.

8. Schwesinger WH, Page CP, Sirinek KR, et al: Operations for peptic ulcer disease: Paradigm lost. J Gastrointest Surg 5:438–443, 2001.

9. van Lanschot JJ, van Leerdam M, van Delden OM, Fockens P: Management of bleeding gastroduodenal ulcers. Dig Surg 19:99–104, 2002.

CHAPTER 46

SMALL BOWEL OBSTRUCTION

Joyce A. Majure, M.D.

1. **Name three mechanisms of bowel obstruction, and give examples and incidence of each type.**
   1. **Extrinsic compression:** adhesions (60%), malignancy (20%), hernias (10%), volvulus, and others (5%)
   2. **Internal blockage** of the lumen by abnormal materials (obturation): bezoars, gallstone, worms, or foreign body (usually obstructs at the ileocecal valve)
   3. **Mural disease** encroaching on the lumen (inflammatory bowel disease [5%]), fibrous stricture secondary to trauma, ischemia, or radiation, intussusception)

2. **What are the most common symptoms of small bowel obstruction (SBO)?**
   1. **Abdominal pain**—initially nonspecific, often colicky, coinciding with waves of peristalsis trying to pass the point of obstruction
   2. **Bloating**—the more distal the obstruction, the more severe the abdominal distention caused by proximal bowel dilatation
   3. **Vomiting**—bilious, frequent, and profuse with proximal obstruction, less frequent but larger volume and often feculent with distal obstruction
   4. **Obstipation**—failure to pass gas or stool; occasionally, the patient has a few loose stools early on, as the bowel distal to the obstruction empties

3. **What are the pertinent questions in the patient's history?**
   - Any previous abdominal or pelvic surgery?
   - Any previous SBO?
   - Any history of cancer? What type, and how treated? Any radiation?
   - Any previous abdominal infections or inflammation (include pelvic inflammatory disease, appendicitis, diverticulitis, inflammatory bowel disease, perforation, and trauma)?
   - Any history of gallstones?
   - Current medications, particularly anticoagulants, anticholinergics, chemotherapy, or diuretics?

4. **What are the findings on physical examination?**
   The patient is often dehydrated and may have a low-grade fever, postural hypotension, and abdominal distention. Bowel sounds may be hyperactive with "tinkles and rushes" or may be totally silent if the patient has delayed seeking treatment. Percussion usually reveals diffuse tympani, and thin, elderly patients may even have visible loops of distended small bowel. Palpation may increase the abdominal pain, but localized tenderness or peritoneal signs indicate likely strangulation or another diagnosis.

5. **Is a rectal examination necessary?**
   Absolutely. The rectal examination may reveal signs of cancer, such as a rigid rectal shelf from carcinomatosis, and blood on hemoccult examination may herald ischemia or strangulation or may indicate inflammatory bowel disease. An obturator hernia can best be palpated transrectally or transvaginally.

6. **Where should the examiner look for obstructing hernias?**
   Examine the groins near the pubic tubercle and along the inguinal floor, check the femoral triangles for bulging or tenderness, do a rectal examination to look for obturator hernia (see question 5), and palpate all existing incisions. Check all trocar sites from previous laparoscopic surgeries.

7. **What is the most inexpensive way to confirm the diagnosis?**
   The "four-way abdominal series" (flat and upright abdominal films, plus posterolateral [PA] and lateral chest radiographs) is diagnostic about 75% of the time. Look for:
   - Air-fluid levels in dilated small intestine (also known as "stair steps" or "string of pearls" sign)
   - Absent or minimal air in the distal colon and rectum
   - "Ground glass" appearance and obscuring of the psoas shadows by extraperitoneal fluid
   - Sometimes a single distended loop of small bowel with a "beak" at each end, indicating a closed loop obstruction in an otherwise gasless abdomen or a single fixed loop that remains in the same location on both supine and upright films
   - Chest radiographs may demonstrate an infiltrate, with accompanying ileus, rather than SBO. The lateral chest radiograph is the most sensitive for identifying free air in the abdomen; this necessitates an urgent laparotomy for perforated viscus

8. **What other imaging studies can be used?**
   Oral contrast studies with water-soluble contrast (Gastrografin) help to distinguish partial from complete obstruction, intraluminal tumor or foreign body, and inflammatory bowel disease; they may also define the point of obstruction. Recent studies indicate that Gastrografin may actually help resolve partial obstructions by its osmotic effect.
   Computed tomography (CT) and **magnetic resonance imaging (MRI)** can both help delineate bowel obstructions. MRI has the advantage of speed (6–10 minutes using the HASTE [half Fourier single shot turbo spin echo] technique), no need for contrast agent, and a higher accuracy rate. A recent Mayo Clinic series also claims superior accuracy (95% versus 71%). Ultrasound has not proven useful.

9. **Which laboratory studies are indicated?**
   1. **Complete blood cell count (CBC)** to check for leukocytosis or unexpected anemia
   2. **Urinalysis** to look for urinary tract infection (which may also cause an ileus and present with a similar picture to SBO) and to assess hydration (urine-specific gravity)
   3. **Chemistry panel** to check for electrolyte abnormalities such as hypokalemic or hypochloremic metabolic alkalosis (associated with vomiting of acid gastric contents), hyponatremia, and prerenal azotemia (elevated blood urea nitrogen [BUN] and creatinine levels)
   4. **Amylase** to rule out pancreatitis; this can also be elevated, although not as high, with ischemic bowel

10. **What are the initial steps in treatment?**
    Nasogastric suction and intravenous fluids should be instituted to restore electrolyte and fluid balance, and a Foley catheter should be placed to monitor urine output. As soon as resuscitation is complete, prompt surgical intervention is mandatory for complete obstructions and for anyone with signs and symptoms of strangulation.

11. **How can I distinguish between a complete and partial obstruction?**
    - **Clinically:** If partial, the patient may continue to pass small amounts of gas or stool. Pain and distention decreases rapidly with nasogastric suction.
    - **Radiographically:** Radiographs show gas moving into the colon (partial obstruction)
    - **With oral contrast studies:** Barium or water-soluble contrast agent given via the nasogastric tube passes into the colon in partial obstructions

12. **What conditions should be included in the differential diagnosis?**
    Ileus from other causes (e.g., as urinary tract infection, pneumonia, hypokalemia), viral gastroenteritis, appendicitis (usually with perforation), ureteral stone, diverticulitis, mesenteric thrombosis, and obstructing colon cancer should be included.

KEY POINTS: SMALL BOWEL OBSTRUCTION

1. Most common cause is adhesive disease, followed by hernias.

2. Malignancy must be considered as a possible cause.

3. Treatment involves NG decompression, fluid and electrolyte repletion, and expectant management.

4. Surgical intervention is required if strangulation or closed loop obstrution is suspected.

13. **What are the three types of SBO, based on bowel viability?**
    1. **Simple obstruction:** Nothing passes the point of obstruction, but the vascular supply is not compromised. It may be partial and resolve with nonoperative management.
    2. **Strangulated obstruction:** The mesentery is twisted or there is so much dilation of the bowel that arterial or venous flow is cut off and the bowel becomes ischemic. Urgent surgery is mandatory.
    3. **Closed loop obstruction:** The bowel is obstructed proximally and distally, usually for a short segment, and that segment becomes massively dilated and susceptible to strangulation as well as perforation. Urgent surgery is mandatory.

14. **What are the "five classic signs" of strangulation? How accurate are they?**
    1. Continuous pain (not colicky)
    2. Fever
    3. Tachycardia
    4. Peritoneal signs (localized guarding or tenderness, rebound tenderness)
    5. Leukocytosis
    These signs usually indicate irreversible ischemia. Persistent pain, progressive fever, and leukocytosis are indications for surgery.

15. **What is the mortality rate of SBO?**
    - **Simple obstruction:** Mortality ~ 5% if operated within 24 hours
    - **Strangulated obstruction:** Mortality rate ~ 25%. The mortality depends on the patient's resiliency (comorbid disease); but strangulation escalates the mortality by fivefold.

16. **What operative interventions may be needed for treatment of SBO?**
    - Open or laparoscopic lysis of adhesions at the point of obstruction
    - Reduction and repair of hernia
    - Resection of obstructing lesions with primary anastomosis
    - Resection of strangulated segment with primary anastomosis
    - Bypass of obstructing lesions (used mostly for carcinomatosis)
    - Placement of long tube down through the duodenum and into the small bowel (a Baker tube is the most commonly used)

17. **Describe criteria for distinguishing viable from dead bowel at the time of operation.**
Pink color, peristalsis, and arterial pulsations are the most obvious way to identify viable intestine. In questionable cases, Doppler ultrasound can detect arterial pulsations, but the most reliable is the intravenous injection of fluorescein dye with use of a Wood's lamp. Viable bowel fluoresces purple.

18. **What is the risk of development of SBO after initial laparotomy? After previous laparotomy for SBO? Which operations are associated with high rates of SBO?**
Approximately 15% of all patients undergoing laparotomy eventually develop an SBO. About 12% of patients with a prior SBO develop another. The more recurrences, the higher the recurrence rate. Total or subtotal colectomy has a 1-year rate of 11% and a 30% rate at 10 years. Hysterectomy also carries a high rate of SBO: about 5% for routine procedures and up to 15% after radical hysterectomy.

19. **What can surgeons do to decrease the risk of SBO?**
- Use powderless gloves or wash off glove powder from gloves.
- Avoid suturing through the peritoneum at closure.
- Use barrier film between the incision and small intestine.

20. **What is the role of laparoscopy in SBO?**
Laparoscopic lysis of adhesions is usually reserved for patients who have not had multiple previous laparotomies. Approximately one third of them can be treated successfully by laparoscopy alone, one third require a minimal laparotomy ("lap-assisted"), and about one third require a full open laparotomy. Recent series claim more than 80% success.

21. **What can be done for patients with multiply recurrent bowel obstructions for adhesions?**
Long tube placement, either via nasogastric, gastrostomy, or jejunostomy with the tube advanced through to the ileocecal valve, can be done. The long tube is left in position for approximately 7 days and reportedly allows the bowel to reform adhesions in more gentle curves. Many other techniques have been tried and abandoned, including Noble plication (i.e., suturing the bowel in orderly loops) and adding various irrigants (e.g., heparin, Dextran, saline) to the peritoneal cavity before closure.

22. **Name five complications associated with surgery for SBO.**
1. Enterotomy
2. Prolonged ileus
3. Wound infection
4. Abscess
5. Recurrent obstruction

23. **Name products purported to decrease adhesion formation.**
- Oxidized cellulose (Interceed)
- Sodium hyaluronate and carboxymethylcellulose (Seprafilm)
- Icodextrin (Adept; investigational)
- 0.5% Ferric hyaluronate gel (Intergel; investigational)

WEB SITES

1. http://www.acssurgery.com/abstracts/acs/acs0305.htm
2. http://www.emedicine.com/EMERG/topic66.htm

BIBLIOGRAPHY

1. Bass BN, Jones B, Bulkley GB: Current management of small-bowel obstruction. Adv Surg 31:1, 1997.

2. Beall DP, Fortman BJ, Lawler BC, Regan F: Imaging bowel obstruction: A comparison between fast magnetic resonance imaging and helical computed tomography. Clin Radiol 57:719–724, 2002.

3. Beck DE, Opelka FG, Bailey HR, et al: Incidence of small-bowel obstruction and adhesiolysis after open colorectal and general surgery. Dis Colon Rectum 42:241–248, 1999.

4. Choi HK, Chu KW, Law WL: Therapeutic value of Gastrografin in adhesive small bowel obstruction after unsuccessful conservative treatment: a prospective randomized trial. Ann Surg 236:1–6, 2002.

5. DeCherney AH, diZerega GS: Clinical problem of intraperitoneal postsurgical adhesion formation following general surgery and the use of adhesion prevention barriers. Surg Clin North Am 77:671–688, 1997.

6. Helton WS: Intestinal obstruction. In ACS Surgery: Principles and Practice. New York, WebMD Professional Publishing, 2003, pp 263–280.

7. Leon EL, Metzger A, Tsiotos GG, et al: Laparoscopic management of small bowel obstruction: Indications and outcome. J Gastrointest Surg 2:132–140, 1998.

CHAPTER 47

INTESTINAL ISCHEMIA

Thomas F. Rehring, M.D.

1. **What is the arterial supply to the gut?**

   The foregut (stomach and duodenum) receives its blood supply from the celiac artery, the midgut (jejunum to the proximal descending colon) from the superior mesenteric artery (SMA), and the hindgut (the remainder of the intraperitoneal gut) from the inferior mesenteric artery (IMA).

2. **Name the potential collateral pathways between the celiac axis and SMA. SMA and IMA? Iliac and IMA?**

   The pancreaticoduodenal arteries form the major collaterals between the celiac artery and the SMA. The gastroduodenal artery gives off the superior pancreaticoduodenal artery that encircles the head of the pancreas and anastomoses with the inferior pancreaticoduodental artery, the first branch of the SMA.

   The SMA and IMA have two main connections. The marginal artery of Drummond lies within the mesentery of the colon and is made up of branches of the ileocolic, right, middle, and left colic arteries. The arc of Riolan (meandering mesenteric artery) is more central and connects the middle colic branch of the SMA and the left colic branch of the IMA.

   The internal iliac artery gives rise to the middle rectal artery, which can provide flow to the superior rectal and thus the IMA.

3. **For extra credit, for whom is the marginal artery of Drummond named? What about the arc of Riolan?**

   Hamilton **Drummond**, a British surgeon, proved the anastomotic connection that bears his name by ligating the origins of the right, middle, and left colic arteries and demonstrating flow to the sigmoidal arteries in 1913 and 1914.

   Jean **Riolan** (1577–1657) was a well-known French anatomist who (ironically) opposed Harvey's theory of circulation but is acknowledged to be the first person to point out the communication between the SMA and IMA.

4. **Name the common causes of acute intestinal ischemia.**

   Acute SMA embolism (50% of all cases), acute SMA thrombosis, nonocclusive mesenteric ischemia (NOMI), mesenteric venous thrombosis, vasculitis, and iatrogenic causes (e.g., inotropic agents, aortic surgery).

5. **What is the mortality rate of patients with acute mesenteric ischemia?**

   Although the prognosis of embolic occlusion is somewhat better because of the dramatic presentation, the diagnosis of acute mesenteric ischemia is often made after infarction. The result is a high mortality rate (75%), regardless of cause. Despite advances in diagnosis, intervention, and critical care, this figure has gone unchanged for more than 30 years.

6. **What is a "paradoxical embolus"?**

   A paradoxical embolus occurs in the setting of a venous thrombus embolizing to the arterial circulation via a cardiac defect (typically an atrial septal defect allowing right-to-left shunting).

7. **What is the diagnostic triad of acute *embolic* intestinal ischemia?**
Sudden onset of (1) severe abdominal pain, (2) bowel evacuation (vomiting or diarrhea), and (3) a history of cardiac disease (arterial emboli). An additional hallmark is pain out of proportion to physical findings.

8. **How does the presentation of patients with acute *thrombotic* occlusion differ?**
Thrombotic occlusion typically presents in elderly patients with diffuse atherosclerotic occlusive disease or in patients with a history consistent with chronic mesenteric ischemia (see question 25). Particularly in the former group of patients, acute embolic occlusion may be indistinguishable from thrombotic occlusion.

9. **Which laboratory value is diagnostic of acute intestinal ischemia? Is acidosis?**
No laboratory values are diagnostic for acute intestinal ischemia. Metabolic acidosis is a late finding and implies advanced ischemia or infarction. Similarly, elevated lactate and elevated phosphate levels are nonspecific and frequently late findings. Although leukocytosis is found in the majority of patients, no laboratory studies are specific. The diagnosis is pursued on clinical suspicion alone.

KEY POINTS: DIAGNOSTIC TRIAD OF ACUTE EMBOLIC INTESTINAL ISCHEMIA

1. Sudden onset of severe abdominal pain out of proportion to physical exam.

2. Sudden bowel evacuation (vomiting or diarrhea).

3. History of cardiac disease (e.g., atrial fibrillation that accounts for embolic source).

4. *No* laboratory findings (e.g., lactate level) are diagnostic; metabolic acidosis is a *late* finding.

5. Emergent arteriography is indicated.

10. **When acute intestinal ischemia is suspected, what study is diagnostic?**
Emergent arteriography is diagnostic. It is important to include lateral views of the aorta to visualize the visceral vessels.

11. **How do the operative findings differ in patients with atherosclerotic occlusion and patients with SMA embolism?**
An SMA embolus usually lodges 3–4 cm distal to its origin, and thus beyond the proximal jejunal and middle colic arteries. Therefore, the proximal 6–10 inches of jejunum are usually spared. Thrombotic occlusion occurs directly at the ostia, where the atherosclerotic narrowing is most severe, causing ischemia of the entire midgut.

12. **What is the appropriate management of an SMA embolus? Is there a role for thrombolysis?**
Immediate heparinization, urgent exploration, embolectomy, assessment of bowel viability, and resection of any infarcted bowel. Postoperative anticoagulation is essential to avoid further embolization.
Thrombolysis currently has little or no role in the treatment of acute mesenteric ischemia. Revascularization of bowel must be pursued rapidly, and bowel viability must be ascertained directly.

13. **How is visceral ischemia of thrombotic origin managed?**
    The general management follows that of an embolism; however, mesenteric ischemia from thrombotic occlusion is the end stage of progressive atherosclerotic occlusion. Therefore, thrombectomy alone is not sufficient; bypass or endarterectomy of the proximal diseased vessel or vessels is necessary. Again, bowel viability is assessed after reperfusion.

14. **Which intraoperative tests help surgeons determine bowel viability?**
    Both systemic intravenous infusion of fluorescein, which is evaluated using a Wood's lamp, and intraoperative Doppler examination of the bowel are helpful, but ultimately the decision is based on clinical judgment.

15. **When the extent of bowel viability is in question, what should be done?**
    All nonviable and necrotic bowel should be resected. The surgeon should schedule a second-look operation 12–24 hours later to evaluate the bowel of marginal viability. Some segments that were initially questionable may become clearly viable or necrotic during this period.

16. **How much small intestine is required to maintain adequate nutrition?**
    About 100 cm of small intestine is required to maintain adequate nutrition. The distal ileum and ileocecal valve are the most important segments to retain for vital bowel absorption and function.

17. **Should a second-look operation be canceled because a patient improves?**
    Never. The decision is made in the operating room based on findings at the time of surgery. No clinical parameters within the ensuing 12–24 hours accurately indicate the status of the bowel in question.

18. **What is NOMI?**
    NOMI accounts for approximately 25% of acute ischemic cases; arterial spasm is the most common cause. This typically occurs in critically ill patients with systemic hypoperfusion. In such low-flow states, splanchnic blood flow is reduced in attempts to preserve perfusion to cardiac and cerebral beds. Pharmacologic agents such as ergot alkaloids, digitalis, and vaso-constrictors are the "usual suspects." Cocaine-induced mesenteric ischemia has also been reported.

19. **How is NOMI diagnosed and managed?**
    Angiography documents vasospasm in the absence of an anatomic occlusion. The right colon is most commonly affected because of its less consistent collateral blood flow. It is associated with (and may be exacerbated by) the concomitant use of digitalis in patients with systemic hypoperfusion. In severe cases associated with multisystem organ failure, the mortality rate approaches 75%. Treatment consists of hemodynamic optimization, weaning of inotropes, and selective arterial infusion of vasodilators (papaverine) through the angiogram catheter. Surgical intervention is reserved for intestinal infarction or perforation.

20. **If mesenteric vein thrombosis (MVT) is suspected, which test is best?**
    The signs and symptoms of MVT are similar to those of acute intestinal ischemia, but they are often subtler. Delay in diagnosis is thought to contribute to the reported high mortality rate of 50%. Contrast-enhanced computed tomography (CT) scan remains the gold standard for diagnosis.

21. **What are the risk factors for MVT? How is it treated?**
    Approximately half of patients with MVT have an underlying hypercoagulable state. Other causes include splenectomy, portal hypertension, visceral infections, pancreatitis, malignancy, and blunt abdominal trauma.

Treatment of MVT includes anticoagulation, broad-spectrum antibiotics, treatment of the underlying cause, and supportive measures. Surgery is reserved for resection of nonviable bowel. Venous thrombectomy has not proven to be of effective long-term benefit. The use of thrombolytic agents has been explored but only in anecdotal reports. Furthermore, access to the splanchnic venous circulation for directed lysis is difficult.

22. **What is the primary cause of *chronic* mesenteric ischemia?**
Atherosclerosis. In general, symptoms do not occur unless two of the three major arteries are narrowed or occluded. Bowel infarction may be forestalled by development of collaterals.

23. **What is the one unique risk factor for chronic mesenteric ischemia that differs from other atherosclerotic phenomena?**
It occurs more frequently in women.

24. **What are the clinical features of patients with chronic mesenteric ischemia?**
Weight loss is the most consistent sign of chronic mesenteric ischemia. Patients gradually and sometimes unknowingly become afraid to eat (food fear) because of postprandial pain (intestinal angina). In the absence of weight loss, the diagnosis of chronic intestinal ischemia is unlikely. Conversely, in patients with severe atherosclerosis and weight loss of unknown cause, mesenteric ischemia should be strongly considered. An epigastric bruit is an important sign suggestive of mesenteric occlusive disease.

25. **How should patients with chronic mesenteric ischemia be evaluated?**
Noninvasive ultrasound duplex scanning may provide important physiologic information about the celiac axis and SMA. However, this procedure is technician dependent and not widely available. If unavailable or equivocal, mesenteric angiography should be performed. If surgical intervention is considered, arteriography is essential.

26. **What are the goals of arterial bypass in chronic mesenteric ischemia?**
Resolution of symptoms, improved nutrition, and prevention of visceral infarction.

27. **If mesenteric revascularization is entertained, what five essential decisions must be considered?**
- Surgical approach (transabdominal, retroperitoneal, thoracoabdominal)
- Which and how many vessels to revascularize
- Endarterectomy or bypass
- If bypass, antegrade or retrograde
- If bypass, what type of conduit (vein versus prosthetic)

See also question 32.

28. **What is ischemic colitis?**
Ischemic colitis is circulatory insufficiency of the colon that may result from occlusive, nonocclusive, and pharmacologic (e.g., cocaine, nonsteroidal anti-inflammatory drugs) causes. Seven percent of all patients having nonemergent abdominal aortic aneurysm surgery and as many as 60% of patients who survive a ruptured abdominal aortic aneurysm suffer from ischemic colitis. Most cases are mild, typically involving only the mucosa and resulting in abdominal pain and bloody diarrhea. Severe disease (15% of cases) is characterized by transmural gangrenous infarction that presents with clear signs of peritonitis and bloody diarrhea.

29. **How is ischemic colitis diagnosed and treated? What are its prognostic implications?**
The diagnosis is made by endoscopy. In idiopathic cases, angiography demonstrates patent large vessels because the responsible emboli or lesions are believed to involve peripheral,

end-arterial vessels. Mild disease is typically treated conservatively with bowel rest, vigorous hydration, and broad-spectrum antibiotics. Severe disease requires surgical resection. Overall mortality rates are about 50%, but in patients requiring colon resection, the mortality rate may exceed 85%. The high mortality in the latter group is attributed to endotoxemic shock and multisystem organ failure.

CONTROVERSIES

30. **What is celiac compression syndrome (Dunbar's syndrome)?**
    Celiac compression is a rare and controversial disorder most commonly described in women (female-to-male ratio = 4:1) between the ages of 20 and 50 years. Patients appear to suffer from chronic mesenteric ischemia without angiographic evidence of atherosclerotic disease. The mechanical compression is believed to be caused by the left crus of the diaphragm (i.e., marginal arcuate ligament), and diagnosis occasionally is confirmed by demonstrating transient celiac compression during expiration. The associated pain is the result of a complicated and still heavily debated redirection of flow (foregut steal) away from the SMA. Effective treatment has required not only release of the compression but also bypass to improve the likelihood of pain resolution.

31. **Which is the preferred treatment for chronic mesenteric ischemia, antegrade or retrograde visceral artery bypass? Is it necessary to reconstruct more than one mesenteric vessel?**
    As they apply to intestinal bypass, the terms *antegrade* and *retrograde* refer to the origin of the graft from the aorta as either proximal to the celiac axis or distal to the SMA, respectively. The stated advantages of antegrade bypass are less kinking of the graft and possibly better blood flow characteristics. The disadvantages are that supraceliac exposure is technically more difficult and clamping may result in renal or spinal cord ischemia. Retrograde bypass grafts are more difficult to position to avoid kinking.

    Recent series suggest that the results for single- or multiple-vessel reconstruction in either antegrade or retrograde fashion are excellent, with symptom-free survival rates > 90% at 5 years.

32. **What is the role of percutaneous transluminal angioplasty (PTA) in chronic mesenteric ischemia?**
    The endovascular treatment of chronic mesenteric ischemia is a relatively new technique. The obvious avoidance of surgery is an important advantage, but the rare complications of dissection and embolus can be devastating in arterial beds without adequate collaterals. Success rates approximate 70%; restenosis and recurrent symptoms are reported in 50% of patients. No prospective trials have compared PTA with arterial bypass; however, retrospective reviews suggest that initial results with either technique are similar with regard to morbidity, death, and recurrent stenosis. However, symptom recurrence rates are higher with PTA.

WEB SITE

http://www.emedicine.com/emerg/topic311.htm

BIBLIOGRAPHY

1. Fisher DF Jr, Fry WJ: Collateral mesenteric circulation. Surg Gynecol Obstet 164:487–492, 1987.

2. Gewertz BL, Schwartz LB: Mesenteric ischemia. Surg Clin North Am 77:275–502, 1997.

3. Hallisey MJ, Deschaine J, Illescas FF, et al: Angioplasty for the treatment of visceral ischemia. J Vasc Interv Radiol 6:785–791, 1995.

4. Kasirajan K, O'Hara PJ, Gray BH, et al: Chronic mesenteric ischemia: Open surgery versus percutaneous angioplasty and stenting. J Vasc Surg 33:63–71, 2001.

5. Kazmers A: Operative management of acute mesenteric ischemia. Ann Vasc Surg 12:187–197, 1998.

6. Kazmers A: Operative management of chronic mesenteric ischemia. Ann Vasc Surg 12:299–308, 1998.

7. Park WM, Cherry KJ Jr, Chua HK, et al: Current results of open revascularization for chronic mesenteric ischemia: a standard for comparison. J Vasc Surg 35:853–859, 2002.

8. Taylor LM: Management of visceral ischemic syndromes. In Rutherford RB (ed): Vascular Surgery, 5th ed. Philadelphia, W.B. Saunders, 2000.

CHAPTER 48

DIVERTICULAR DISEASE OF THE COLON

Gregory P. Victorino, M.D., Jyoti Arya, M.D., and Lawrence W. Norton, M.D.

1. **What is a colonic diverticulum?**

   A protrusion of mucosa and submucosa through the muscular layers of the bowel wall. It has no muscular covering. Because diverticula do not involve all layers of the bowel wall, they are really "false" diverticula. Diverticulum formation may be related either to weakness of the bowel wall at the sites of vessel perforation or to increased intraluminal pressure caused by low dietary fiber and constipation.

2. **What is the difference between diverticulosis and diverticulitis?**

   Diverticulosis is colonic diverticula without associated inflammation. Diverticulitis is inflammation and infection. Only 15% of patients with diverticulosis develop diverticulitis.

3. **How does a diverticulum cause pain?**

   Pain apparently results from perforation of the diverticulum The resulting leakage may be scant and contained within pericolic fat or extensive, involving the mesentery, other organs, or the peritoneal cavity. Sigmoid diverticulitis typically causes pain in the left lower quadrant.

4. **Where in the colon are diverticula usually located?**

   In the United States, 95% of all diverticula occur in the left colon, primarily in the sigmoid colon. Diverticula, however, may occur anywhere in the colon. In Asia, right colonic diverticula are more common.

5. **At what age is diverticulitis most common?**

   The sixth or seventh decade of life. Patients younger than 50 with diverticulitis tend to have more complications. Younger patients are more likely than older patients to have right colonic diverticulitis.

6. **What strategy may decrease diverticulitis in patients with diverticula?**

   A diet high in fiber. Large bulk in the colon decreases segmentation and intraluminal pressure.

7. **What is the best imaging test for diagnosing acute diverticulitis?**

   Computed tomography (CT) scan, which can also diagnose local complications of diverticulitis.

8. **What complications can result from perforation of a colonic diverticulum?**
   - Inflammatory phlegmon or abscess in the bowel mesentery
   - Peritonitis
   - Intra-abdominal abscess
   - Internal fistula
   - Bowel obstruction

9. **Can diverticular disease cause bleeding?**

   Yes. Diverticulosis (not -*itis*) is a common cause of lower gastrointestinal bleeding. Bleeding from diverticulitis is uncommon.

10. **How can the site of diverticular bleeding be localized?**

It is localized with angiography performed via the inferior mesenteric artery and, if necessary, the superior mesenteric artery. Tagged red blood cell studies are less useful. Colonoscopy is rarely helpful.

KEY POINTS: LOCALIZATION OF LOWER GI BLEEDING

1. Common causes: diverticulosis, cancer, angiodysplasia.

2. Proctosigmoidoscopy without prep is helpful in ruling out rectal source of bleeding (more proximal bleeding lmiits the utility of endoscopy).

3. Tagged red blood cell nuclear scans are useful for slower GI bleeding (detects bleeding at 0.2–0.5 mL/min).

4. Arteriography is the preferred imaging modality because it can be therapeutic and detects bleeding at 0.5–2 mL/min.

5. Start arteriography with the IMA, then the SMA, then the celiac axis if necessary; administer vasopressin or embolize (85% success rate).

11. **When should an operation be performed for a bleeding colonic diverticulum?**

Replacement of 5–6 units of blood (two thirds of a patient's blood volume) within 24 hours and rebleeding during hospitalization are standard indications for resection of the segment of colon containing a bleeding diverticulum.

12. **If bleeding is life threatening but cannot be localized within the colon, what treatment is required?**

Subtotal colectomy with ileostomy and closure of the distal sigmoid colon at the peritoneal reflection (Hartmann's operation) or total abdominal colectomy with ileorectal anastomosis is required.

13. **Which three procedures may be used when perforation of the diverticulum results in an abscess? Which has the lowest operative mortality rate?**

1. Diverting colostomy and abscess drainage (first of three stages)
2. Resection of involved colon with proximal colostomy and distal mucous fistula or closure by Hartmann's operation (first of two stages)
3. Resection with primary anastomosis (one stage)

Operative mortality is lowest after resection and proximal colostomy for fecal diversion. Despite reports of success with the one-stage procedure, most surgeons favor a safer two-stage approach for perforated diverticulitis (this strategy requires a second operation after 3 months for colostomy takedown and colonic re-anastomosis).

14. **What is the clinical evidence of a vesicocolic or ureterocolic fistula after diverticular perforation?**

Pneumaturia, fecaluria, and chronic urinary tract infections (polymicrobial).

15. **What procedure is required to repair a vesicocolic fistula?**

A staged procedure was the standard until recently. Now most patients can be treated with a single procedure that includes sigmoid resection, colonic anastomosis, and primary repair of bladder defect with absorbable suture. A Foley catheter is usually left in place for 10 days after surgery. Some viable tissue should be placed between the colonic and bladder repairs to prevent a recurrent fistula.

WEB SITE

http://www.acssurgery.com/abstracts/acs/acs0327.htm

BIBLIOGRAPHY

1. Bouillot JL, Berthou JC, Champault G, et al: Elective laparoscopic colonic resection for diverticular disease: Results of a multicenter study in 179 patients. Surg Endosc 16:1320–1323, 2002.

2. Eijbouts QA, de Haan J, Berends F, et al: Laparoscopic elective treatment of diverticular disease. A comparison between laparoscopic-assisted and resection-facilitated techniques. Surg Endosc 14:726–730, 2000.

3. Faynsod M, Stamos MJ, Arnell T, et al: A case-control study of laparoscopic versus open sigmoid colectomy for diverticulitis. Am Surg 66:841–843, 2000.

4. Gooszen AW, Tollenaar RA, Geelkerken RH, et al: Prospective study of primary anastomosis following sigmoid resection for suspected acute complicated diverticular disease. Br J Surg 88:693–697, 2001.

5. Schwesinger WH, Page CP, Gaskill HV 3d, et al: Operative management of diverticular emergencies: Strategies and outcomes. Arch Surg 135:558–562, 2000.

6. Simpson J, Scholefield JH, Spiller RC: Pathogenesis of colonic diverticula. Br J Surg 89:546–554, 2002.

7. Wolff BG, Devine RM: Surgical management of diverticulitis. Am Surg 66:153–156, 2000.

8. Young-Fadok TM, Roberts PL, Spencer MP, et al: Colonic diverticular disease. Curr Probl Surg 37:457–514, 2000.

CHAPTER 49

ACUTE LARGE BOWEL OBSTRUCTION

Elizabeth C. Brew, M.D.

1. **What are the mechanical causes of large bowel obstruction?**
   The three most common mechanical causes are carcinoma (50%), volvulus (15%), and diverticular disease (10%). Extrinsic compression from metastatic carcinoma is another cause of obstruction. Less frequent causes include stricture, hernia, intussusception, benign tumor, and fecal impaction.

2. **How is the diagnosis made?**
   1. The patient complains of crampy abdominal pain and bloating. Nausea and vomiting occur later in large bowel obstruction and may be feculent. An acute onset of symptoms is more consistent with volvulus compared with the gradual development of obstructive complaints from patients with colon carcinoma.
   2. Physical examination reveals abdominal distention and high-pitched bowel sounds. Rectal examination may reveal an obstructing rectal cancer or evidence of fecal impaction. Absence of bowel sounds and localized tenderness may be signs of peritonitis. Progression of symptoms accompanied by a high fever or tachycardia requires immediate operative attention.
   3. Flat and upright abdominal radiographs reveal dilated colon proximal to the obstruction. An upright chest radiograph may show free air under the diaphragm if a perforation has occurred.

3. **How is the diagnosis confirmed?**
   A contrast enema (barium or water-soluble contrast) is necessary to delineate the level and nature of an obstruction. A volvulus can be identified by a "bird's beak" narrowing at the neck of the volvulus. Sigmoidoscopy or colonoscopy is an essential part of the evaluation; it allows visualization of the colon and may be therapeutic in the case of a sigmoid volvulus.

4. **What is the role of computed tomography (CT) scanning in the diagnosis of large bowel obstruction?**
   CT scans may be valuable in distinguishing between mechanical obstruction or pseudo-obstruction. It can help with the diagnosis of diverticulitis or colon carcinoma. However, plain radiographs, colonoscopy, and physical examination exceed the benefits of CT scanning in the evaluation of large bowel obstruction.

5. **Why is tenderness in the right lower quadrant (RLQ) important?**
   The cecum is the area that is most likely to perforate. When the cecum reaches 15 cm at its widest diameter, the tension on the wall is so great that decompression is essential to prevent perforation. The larger diameter of the cecum causes more tension of the cecal wall at the same intraluminal pressure (law of Laplace). The other area at risk for perforation is the site of a primary colon cancer.

6. **Where is the obstructing cancer usually located?**
   Most obstructing colorectal carcinomas occur in the splenic flexure, descending colon, or hepatic flexure. In contrast, lesions of the right colon usually present with occult bleeding. Cecal and rectal cancers are uncommon causes of obstruction.

KEY POINTS: CAUSES OF LARGE BOWEL OBSTRUCTION

1. Carcinoma: most common cause: 50%

2. Volvulus: 15%

3. Diverticular disease: 10%

4. Stricture, hernia, intussusception, fecal impaction: 25%

7. **What is a volvulus? Where is it located?**
A volvulus is an abnormal rotation of the colon on an axis formed by its mesentery and occurs either in the sigmoid colon (75%) or cecum (25%). **Sigmoid volvulus** occurs in an older population when chronic constipation causes the sigmoid colon to elongate and become redundant. **Cecal volvulus** requires a hypermobile cecum as a result of incomplete embryologic fixation of the ascending colon.

8. **When is surgery indicated?**
Surgery is performed early in colon obstruction. Urgent laparotomy is necessary in patients with suspected perforation or ischemia. Danger signs are quiet abdomen, RLQ tenderness, and increasing pain. The patient's cardiopulmonary status should be assessed and optimized preoperatively. It is essential to correct dehydration and administer perioperative antibiotics. Marking of possible stoma sites and deep venous thrombosis prophylaxis are other important preoperative considerations.

9. **Which operation should be performed for a large bowel obstruction?**
The traditional procedure for a large bowel obstruction has been a decompressing colostomy. However, careful assessment of the patient's condition, viability of the bowel, location of the obstruction, and absence of intra-abdominal contamination often allow resection with or without a primary anastomosis. In fact, an initial diverting colostomy has not been shown to have any survival advantage and incurs the risk of further surgeries.
An **obstructing carcinoma** may be resected satisfactorily under emergency conditions in 90% of patients. Carcinomas of the right and transverse colon (proximal to the splenic flexure) are routinely treated with resection and primary anastomosis. Recently, obstructing cancers of the descending colon have been treated either with resection and colostomy or intraoperative lavage followed by resection and primary anastomosis. Techniques for nonoperative decompression of the colon, such as balloon dilation, laser therapy, and stent placement, are under investigation. Theoretically, these techniques will allow palliation, bowel preparation, and elective colon resection.
A **volvulus** should be reduced and resected. Reduction of a sigmoid volvulus can be achieved nonoperatively by sigmoidoscopy or hydrostatic decompression with a contrast enema. The recurrence rate of volvulus after simple nonoperative reduction is 75%. Surgical therapy includes detorsion with colopexy or sigmoid colectomy. Cecal volvulus can be treated similarly with nonoperative decompression, cecopexy, or surgical resection.
The optimal treatment of **diverticular disease** is initial bowel rest; intravenous antibiotics; and percutaneous abscess drainage, if necessary. Colon resection and primary anastomosis can be performed after adequate bowel preparation.

0. **What are the nonmechanical causes of large bowel obstruction?**
Paralytic ileus (i.e., colonic pseudoobstruction) or toxic megacolon.

11. **What is Ogilvie's syndrome?**

Ogilvie's syndrome is an acute paralytic (adynamic) ileus or pseudoobstruction (i.e., enormous dilation of the colon without a mechanical distal obstructing lesion). Patients present with a massively dilated abdomen and a small amount of pain. Nonoperative management, including bowel rest, intravenous fluids, and gentle enemas, is the therapy of choice. Gastrografin enema or colonoscopy is diagnostic and therapeutic. Neostigmine is another treatment modality in patients with colons > 10 cm in diameter.

12. **What is toxic megacolon?**

Toxic megacolon is dilatation of the entire colon secondary to acute inflammatory bowel disease. The disease is manifested by acute onset of abdominal pain, distention, and sepsis. Initial therapy includes intravenous fluid resuscitation, nasogastric decompression, and broad-spectrum antibiotics. If symptoms do not resolve within a few hours, the patient requires an operation to avoid perforation. Surgical therapy most often consists of an emergency abdominal colectomy with formation of an ileostomy.

WEB SITE

http://www.emedicine.com/emerg/topic65.htm

BIBLIOGRAPHY

1. Adler DG, Baron TH: Endoscopic palliation of colorectal cancer. Hematol Oncol Clin North Am 16:1015–1029, 2002.
2. Dauphine CE, Tan P, Beart RW Jr, et al: Placement of self-expanding metal stents for acute malignant large-bowel obstruction: A collective review. Ann Surg Oncol 9:574–579, 2002.
3. Frager D: Intestinal obstruction: Role of CT. Gastroenterol Clin North Am 31:777–799, 2002.
4. Lopez-Kostner F, Hool GR, Lavery IC: Management and causes of acute large-bowel obstruction. Surg Clin North Am 77:1265–1290, 1997.
5. Murray JJ, Schoetz DJ, Coller JA, et al: Intraoperative colonic lavage and primary anastomosis in nonelective colon resection. Dis Colon Rectum 34:527–531, 1991.
6. Paran H, Silverberg D, Mayo A: Treatment of acute colonic pseudo-obstruction with neostigmine. J Am Coll Surg 190(3):315–318, 2000.
7. Tan SG, Nambiar R, Rauff A, et al: Primary resection and anastomosis in obstructed descending colon due to cancer. Arch Surg 126:748–751, 1991.

CHAPTER 50

INFLAMMATORY BOWEL DISEASE

Anthony J. LaPorta, M.D., and Gilbert Hermann, M.D.

1. **What two clinical entities encompass the diagnosis of inflammatory bowel disease?**
Crohn's disease and ulcerative colitis (acute or chronic).

2. **Although the two diseases often overlap, they usually can be distinguished by clinical criteria. What are the major clinical differences?**
Rectal bleeding is unusual in Crohn's disease but common in chronic ulcerative colitis. An abdominal mass and anal complications (fissure, fistula) are more common in Crohn's disease.

3. **What are the major radiologic differences between the two diseases?**
Terminal ileal involvement, skip areas, internal fistulas, and "thumb printing" are rare or absent in chronic ulcerative colitis but common in Crohn's disease.

4. **What are the major histologic differences?**
Granulomas in the intestinal wall and adjacent lymph nodes are absent in ulcerative colitis but occur in 60% of patients with Crohn's disease. The inflammatory process in Crohn's disease involves the entire bowel wall. In ulcerative colitis, the inflammation usually is limited to the mucosa and submucosa.

5. **Although Crohn's disease may affect the gastrointestinal (GI) tract from the pharynx to the anus, what are the most common clinical patterns of GI involvement?**
Small bowel only: 28%; both ileum and colon (ileocolitis): 41%; and colon only: 27%. Crohn's involvement of the colon is also called *Crohn's colitis* or *granulomatous colitis*.

6. **Crohn's colitis and ulcerative colitis are often difficult to distinguish clinically. What are the major differences at colonoscopy?**
Crohn's disease is focal and predominantly right sided. The mucosa has a cobblestone appearance with transverse ulcerations in affected areas. Biopsies reveal transmural disease with possible focal granulomas. On colonoscopy, chronic ulcerative colitis may appear as a diffuse disease. However, if only a portion of the colon is involved, it is on the left side and almost always involves the rectum. Pathologic changes involve the mucosa and submucosa.

7. **What are the major indications for surgery in Crohn's disease?**
It depends on the site of involvement. Enterocutaneous or enteroenteral fistulas (controversial), abscess, and intestinal obstruction are the most common surgical indications for small intestinal and ileocolic types. Perianal disease, medical failure, ileocolic fistulas, and abscess formation are the most common indicators for surgery in Crohn's colitis.

8. **What are the major indications for surgery in ulcerative colitis?**
Medical intractability (including failure to thrive in children, diarrhea, weight loss, and abdominal pain), toxic megacolon with or without perforation, and concern about the development of colonic cancer (controversial, but real).

KEY POINTS: DIFFERENCES BETWEEN CROHN'S DISEASE AND ULCERATIVE COLITIS

1. Rectal bleeding is uncommon in Crohn's disease but common in chronic ulcerative colitis.

2. Terminal ileal involvement, skip areas, internal fistulas, and "thumb printing" are common in Crohn's disease but rare or absent in chronic ulcerative colitis.

3. In ulcerative colitis, the inflammation is usually limited to the mucosa and submucosa, whereas in Crohn's disease it involves the entire bowel wall.

9. **What is the surgical treatment of ulcerative colitis?**
Total colectomy with ileoanal pouch anastomosis is the standard. A total colectomy with a Brooke ileostomy was the classic surgical approach and is still applicable in some situations. A Kock (continent) pouch can be used for younger (age < 55 years) patients who do not wish to wear an ileostomy bag or who have lost their ileoanal pouch. Ileorectal anastomosis has been advocated by some (controversial), but this leaves disease behind.

10. **What are the surgical procedures for the complications of Crohn's disease?**
Complications requiring surgery are usually corrected by removing all areas of bowel involved in the complication. Strictureplasty as opposed to resection is now preferred in selected cases of small bowel obstruction. When resection is necessary, grossly clear margins are satisfactory. Skip areas should be preserved unless they are directly adjacent to resected intestine.

11. **What should the patient be told about the possibility of recurrence after surgery?**
With chronic ulcerative colitis, surgery is definitive and curative. With Crohn's disease, however, the aim of surgery is to treat the complications (i.e., obstruction and sepsis). Recurrence of Crohn's disease can be expected in a high percentage of cases if the patient is followed long enough. Small bowel recurrence after total colectomy for Crohn's colitis does occur.

12. **How do you evaluate the placement of a stoma?**
The location of a stoma is a major factor in patient morbidity. Placement is optimal at the summit of the infraumbilical bulge within the rectus muscle. This is usually within a triangle formed by lines between the umbilicus to the anterior superior iliac spine, umbilicus to the pubis, and the inguinal ligament. All scars and creases should be avoided.

13. **Does Crohn's disease have a genetic basis?**
The patients described by Crohn et al. in the original article were a 14-year-old boy and his 32-year-old sister. Genetic studies have identified two loci, IBD1 and IBD2 on chromosomes 16 and 12, respectively, that are linked to inflammatory bowel disease. New data suggest that these mutations affect the innate bacterial reaction to lipopolysaccharides, leading to an exaggerated immune response, causing the tissue damage in Crohn's disease. Similar studies also have links to chromosomes 14q and 6p.

14. **What is the difference between an enteroclysis and a small bowel follow-through?**
Enteroclysis is a procedure performed by a radiologist with a catheter placed at the duodenal-jejunal junction. Because the rate of barium entering the intestine and thus distention of the intestine can be controlled, this study provides a superior demonstration of the luminal contour,

valvulae conniventes, and mucosal surface. Thus, it is superior to the small bowel follow-through for the evaluation of short obstructing lesions but is a technically more demanding procedure for the radiologist and the patient.

15. **What is a Brooke ileostomy?**
    The Brooke ileostomy is the "rosebud" or full-thickness ileostomy folded over on itself for approximately 1 cm above the skin. This prevents the erosion of the skin and high-output serositis that is common with an ostomy that is flush with the skin.

16. **What is pouchitis, and which patients are likely to have it?**
    Pouchitis is an inflammation of indeterminate origin, possibly related to bacterial overgrowth, that occurs in the ileal pouch after ileal-pouch anal anastomosis. This complication is common (25%) when this procedure is performed for ulcerative colitis, but it is rare when this same procedure is performed for familial polyposis. Patients with pouchitis are effectively treated with metronidazole, ciprofloxacin, or 5-amino salicylic acid. They rarely require ileal diversion or pouch excision.

CONTROVERSIES

17. **Should all patients with enteroenteral fistulas secondary to Crohn's disease have surgery when the fistula is discovered?**
    For: Such patients ultimately do poorly, develop further intraperitoneal septic complications, and almost always require surgery.
    Against: Many of these patients do well without operative treatment until they develop symptoms. It is fine to wait for symptoms.

18. **Should all patients with ulcerative colitis that is documented for 10 years, whether the disease is active or not, undergo a colectomy to avoid the risk of carcinoma of the colon?**
    For: The risk of colon cancer in ulcerative colitis increases by approximately 1% per year 10 years after the diagnosis.
    Against: Using surveillance colonoscopy and biopsy, only patients whose colons show dysplastic changes need a colectomy.

19. **Is ileorectal anastomosis an acceptable operation after colectomy for ulcerative colitis?**
    For: The patients have reasonably normal bowel habits and avoid the complications associated with anal reconstructive procedures.
    Against: At least 50% of patients eventually require reoperation for recurrence of disease. The remaining rectum also may be a site for the development of cancer.

20. **Is standard (Brooke) ileostomy a good way to handle the terminal ileum after total colectomy for chronic ulcerative colitis?**
    For: The complication rate is very low. More than 90% of patients lead satisfactory lives.
    Against: Psychosocial and sexual problems are associated with the use of external appliances, particularly in the teenage group, among whom chronic ulcerative colitis is quite common.

21. **Is the continent Kock pouch a good procedure after colectomy for chronic ulcerative colitis?**
    For: It avoids use of an external appliance and is quite easy to manage.
    Against: Approximately 25% of all patients who have a Kock pouch require a revision due to slippage of the valve mechanism, thus rendering the pouch incontinent.

22. **Is an ileoanal anastomosis with a surgically constructed ileoanal reservoir a good operation after colectomy for chronic ulcerative colitis?**
For: It avoids external appliances or ostomies, so it is well accepted by patients. Currently, this is the most commonly performed operation after colectomy.
Against: It is more difficult technically to construct; thus, the complication rate is higher. The average number of bowel movements is five per day, and there may be soilage at night. Pouchitis remains a problem.

23. **Do all ileal pouch anal anastomoses require a temporary diverting ileostomy?**
For: The diverting ileostomy protects the reservoir and its suture lines by diverting the fecal stream until it is healed, thus lowering the complication rate.
Against: The triple-stapled ileal pouch anal anastomosis has a low complication rate and low rate of small bowel obstruction. Thus, avoidance of the diverting ileostomy returns the patient to a functional life sooner.

BIBLIOGRAPHY

1. Duerr RH: The genetics of inflammatory bowel disease. Gastroenterol Clin North Am 31:63–76, 2002.
2. Farouk R: Functional outcomes after ileal pouch-anal anastomosis for chronic ulcerative colitis. Ann Surg 231:919–926, 2000.
3. Fazio V: Current status of surgery for inflammatory bowel disease. Digestion 59:470–480, 1998.
4. Heuschen UA, Hinz U, Allemeyer EH, et al: One- or two-state procedure for restorative protocolectomy: Rationale for a surgical strategy in ulcerative colitis. Ann Surg 234:788–794, 2001.
5. Hurst RD, Michelassi F: Strictureplasty for Crohn's disease: Techniques and long term results. World J Surg 22:359–363, 1998.
6. Present DH, Rutgeerts P Targan S, et al: Infliximab for the treatment of fistulas in patients with Crohn's disease. N Engl J Med 340:1398–1405, 1999.
7. Solomon MJ, Schmitz M: Cancer and inflammatory bowel disease: Bias, epidemiology, surveillance, and treatment. World Surg 22:352–358, 1998.
8. Stocchi L, Pemberton JH: Pouch and pouchitis. Gastroenterol Clin North Am 30:223–241, 2001.
9. Sugerman HJ: Ileal pouch anal anastomosis without ileal diverson. Ann Surg 232:530–541, 2000.
10. Wolff BG: Factors determining recurrence following surgery for Crohn's disease. World J Surg 22:364–369, 1998.

CHAPTER 51

UPPER GASTROINTESTINAL BLEEDING

G. Edward Kimm, Jr., M.D., and Allen T. Belshaw, M.D.

1. **What is upper gastrointestinal (GI) bleeding?**
   Bleeding from proximal to the ligament of Treitz (the transition point between duodenum and jejunum).

2. **What are the most common causes of upper GI bleeding?**
   In descending order of frequency, they are gastritis, duodenal ulcer, esophageal varices, benign gastric ulcer, esophagitis, and Mallory-Weiss tear. All other causes account for < 5% of cases.

3. **What is the overall mortality rate of upper GI bleeding?**
   Approximately 10%. Mortality is usually associated with comorbid factors such as cardiac, pulmonary, hepatic, and renal disease as well as age (> 60 years) and large transfusion requirements (> 5 units of blood). Patients who rebleed during the same hospitalization have a mortality rate of 30%.

4. **What is the most common presentation of upper GI bleeding?**
   Eighty percent of patients present with **melena** (blood is a cathartic, and patients pass black, tarry, or maroon-colored stools) or **hematochezia** (bright red blood in the rectum). **Hematemesis** (bright red or coffee-ground emesis) is diagnostic of an upper source of GI bleeding. **Occult bleeding** may present only with guaiac-positive stool.

5. **How much GI blood loss is necessary to cause melena?**
   As little as 50 mL. Occult bleeding (guaiac- or Hematest-positive) can be detected with as little as 10 mL of blood loss.

6. **A 45-year-old man presents to the emergency department with massive hematemesis, tachycardia, and hypotension. What should the initial approach be?**
   Acute GI hemorrhage requires a prompt and systematic approach. As in all critically ill patients, initially assess the ABCs (airway, breathing, circulation). Start two large-bore intravenous (IV) lines, and give 1 L of Ringer's lactate while monitoring the patient. Place a nasogastric tube (NGT) and Foley catheter and irrigate the NGT with saline. Send blood for type and crossmatch and coagulation and liver function tests.

7. **This patient stabilizes after your interventions. Is a medical history of any value in determining a cause of the bleeding?**
   Yes. The following are pertinent:
   - Previous symptoms of peptic ulcer disease or nonsteroidal anti-inflammatory drug use: bleeding duodenal or gastric ulcer
   - History of gastroesophageal reflux disease: esophagitis
   - Heavy alcohol use: gastritis or bleeding varices
   - Recent retching or vomiting: Mallory-Weiss tear
   - Weight loss: upper GI malignancy

8. **What physical finding may be helpful in establishing the source of bleeding?**
    Physical examination is generally not helpful. The stigmata of liver disease (jaundice, caput medusa, ascites, muscle wasting) raise the suspicion of variceal bleeding or multiple superficial gastric erosions.

9. **What percentage of patients with known esophageal varices are bleeding from the varices on presentation?**
    Only 50%.

10. **Does bilious or clear NGT aspirate rule out an upper GI source of hemorrhage?**
    No. Although NGT aspiration can be useful in directing the search for a bleeding site, one should keep in mind that the false-negative rate may be as high as 20%.

11. **What studies can be used to determine the source of bleeding?**
    Esophagogastroduodenoscopy (EGD) is the first and best test. Barium studies may miss a significant source of upper GI bleeding, such as erosive gastritis, and interfere with other more definitive tests, especially arteriography. Nuclear scans are of limited value in acute upper GI hemorrhage.

12. **What is the sensitivity of EGD?**
    EGD identifies the source of bleeding in up to 95% of cases. EGD has the advantage of directly visualizing the source of blood loss and provides the opportunity to biopsy a lesion and perform therapeutic maneuvers such as cauterizing a bleeder in a duodenal ulcer.

KEY POINTS: UPPER GI BLEEDING

1. Upper GI bleeding is defined as bleeding proximal to the ligament of Treitz.

2. The most common causes are gastritis, duodenal ulcer, esophageal varices, benign gastric ulcer, esophagitis, and Mallory-Weiss tear.

3. Eight percent of patients present with melena or hematochezia.

4. EGD identifies the source of bleeding in 95% of cases.

13. **How can EGD be used to control nonvariceal bleeding?**
    Electrocautery and injection of vasoconstrictors are well-established techniques. Other modalities such as argon beam coagulation, hemoclips, and cyanoacrylates (super glue) are promising.

14. **What amount of bleeding is required to see a "blush" on arteriography?**
    Less than 5 mL per minute. Although angiography is the most invasive of these tests, the catheter can be left in place and used for delivery of therapeutic vasopressin or embolization.

15. **What treatment options are available to control variceal bleeding?**
    Upper endoscopy with sclerotherapy or band ligation. In experienced hands, placement of a Sengstaken-Blakemore tube (a double balloon tube that permits direct tamponade of both gastric and esophageal varices) temporarily controls bleeding in 90% of cases. IV infusion of vasopressin or octreotide should decrease blood flow to the varices but is less successful in patients with more severe liver disease.

16. **What are the indications for surgery in patients with upper GI hemorrhage?**
About 10% of patients eventually require surgery. Indications include:
- Persistent hypotension or shock (failure of resuscitative therapy)
- Recurrent bleeding while on maximal medical therapy
- High-risk patients with significant comorbid disease
- Large transfusion requirements (transfusion of more than two thirds of the patient's blood volume in 24 hours)

17. **What is the surgical approach to an unstable patient with a nonlocalized upper GI bleed who does not respond to initial resuscitation?**
At laporotomy start with a generous gastroduodenotomy centered over the pylorus. If this does not reveal a source of bleeding, proceed with a proximal gastrotomy.

18. **A patient presents with hematemesis and has a remote history of an abdominal aortic aneurysm repair. What uncommon cause of upper GI bleeding needs to be considered?**
Aortoduodenal fistula. Any patient with a history of aortic surgery and evidence of GI bleeding should be aggressively worked up for aortoenteric fistula. The study of choice is endoscopy.

19. **What is a Dieulafoy's ulcer?**
A gastric vascular malformation with an exposed submucosal artery, usually within 2–5 cm of the gastroesophageal junction. It presents with painless hematemesis, often massive (fortunately, this is uncommon).

20. **A patient recently admitted with a traumatic liver laceration is treated nonoperatively and later develops painless hematemesis. What do you suspect? How should you treat this patient?**
Hemobilia, another rare cause of upper GI bleeding, usually occurs after liver trauma or hepatic resection. Treatment consists of angiographic embolization.

21. **What are other rare causes of upper GI bleeding?**
Watermelon stomach, portal hypertensive gastropathy, arteriovenous malformations, upper GI neoplasm, duodenal diverticulum, and pancreatitis (resulting in erosion into the splenic artery or splenic vein thrombosis with portal hypertension).

BIBLIOGRAPHY

1. Cameron JL: Current Surgical Therapy, 7th ed. St. Louis, Mosby, 2001.

2. Conrad SA: Acute upper gastrointestinal bleeding in critically ill patients: Causes and treatment modalities. Crit Care Med 30:365–368, 2002.

3. Fallah MA, Prakash C, Edmundowitz S: Acute gastrointestinal bleeding. Med Clin North Am 84:1183–1208, 2000.

4. Jamieson GG: Current status of indications for surgery in peptic ulcer disease. World J Surg 24:256, 2000.

5. Savides TJ, Jensen DM: Therapeutic endoscopy for nonvariceal gastrointestinal bleeding. Gastroenterol Clin North Am 29:465–487, 2000.

CHAPTER 52

LOWER GASTROINTESTINAL BLEEDING

Kathleen Liscum, M.D.

1. **Describe the treatment of a patient who presents with lower gastrointestinal (GI) bleeding.**
   Treatment begins with the ABCs (airway, breathing, circulation). Place two large-bore intravenous (IV) catheters in the upper extremities. Obtain hemoglobin and hematocrit levels, blood type, and cross-match. A Foley catheter should be placed to help monitor volume status.

2. **What is the next step in evaluating the patient?**
   A nasogastric tube should be placed to rule out an upper GI source. If the aspirate is bilious, the examiner can be fairly certain that the source is distal to the ligament of Treitz. However, if the aspirate reveals no bile, the patient may still be bleeding in the duodenum with a competent pylorus.

3. **What are the two most common causes of massive lower GI bleeding?**
   Diverticular hemorrhage (diverticulosis) and bleeding vascular ectasias. Diverticular disease was previously thought to be the most common cause of lower GI bleeding, but vascular ectasias are now quite frequent.

4. **What are the other causes of blood per rectum?**

Colon cancer	Inflammatory bowel disease
Polyps	Anorectal disorders (e.g., hemorrhoids, fissure)
Ischemic colitis	Meckel's diverticulum
Infectious colitis	

5. **After a thorough history and physical examination, what is the first step toward identifying the specific site of bleeding?**
   Anoscopy and rigid proctosigmoidoscopy to rule out anorectal fissures and an extraperitoneal source.

6. **Name four options for localizing lower GI bleeding.**
   1. Tagged red blood cell scan
   2. Sulfur colloid scan
   3. Angiography
   4. Colonoscopy

7. **Discuss the differences between sulfur colloid scan and tagged red blood cell (RBC) scan.**
   The **sulfur colloid scan** can be accomplished quickly and detects bleeding as minimal as 0.1 mL/min. The radiolabeled sulfur colloid is cleared quickly by the liver and spleen, which may obscure the bleeding site if it is located in the hepatic or splenic flexure. The test is complete within 20 minutes of administration of the radionuclide.

   The **tagged red blood cell scan** requires a 60-minute delay while the autologous RBCs are labeled with isotope. The test detects bleeding as slow as 0.5 mL/min. Because the tagged cells stay in the patient's system, it is also helpful in identifying the source when the patient is bleeding intermittently. The study takes at least 2 hours.

8. **What is the role of angiography?**
Angiography detects bleeding rates of 0.5–1.0 mL/min but only if the patient is actively bleeding. When a bleeding site is identified, the angiographic appearance may provide further insight into the cause of the bleeding. Whereas diverticular bleeding is often seen as extravasation of contrast, vascular ectasias may be identified by a vascular tuft or early filling vein.

9. **What therapeutic options are available with angiography?**
(1) Infusion of vasopressin (Pitressin) into a selected vessel and (2) embolization of the bleeding vessel.

KEY POINTS: LOWER GI BLEEDING

1. The most common causes of massive lower GI bleeding are diverticular hemorrhage and bleeding vascular ectasias.

2. The most common cause of lower GI bleeding in children is Meckel's diverticulum.

3. After a thorough history and physical exam, the first steps in identifying the specific site of bleeding are anoscopy and rigid proctosigmoidoscopy.

4. Tagged red blood cell scan, sulfur colloid scan, colonoscopy, and angiography are four options for localizing lower GI bleeding.

5. Indications for surgery include patients who have received 6 U of blood without resolution of bleeding and patients who continue to bleed after vasopressin or embolization.

10. **Which patients should have angiographic embolization of the bleeding site?**
Most surgeons believe that embolization should be reserved for patients who are poor operative risks in that a 15% complication rate is associated with the procedure. Patients may perforate or develop a stricture as a result of bowel wall ischemia.

11. **What is the role of vasopressin infusion?**
Vasopressin is only a temporizing measure. Control of the bleeding with vasopressin allows time for resuscitation and essentially converts an emergent case into an urgent one. Vasopressin occasionally may be used as the only treatment for diverticular bleeding. If the patient has a repeated episode of bleeding after weaning from vasopressin, the surgeon must decide between embolization and surgery.

12. **Do lower GI hemorrhages ever spontaneously resolve?**
Spontaneous resolution occurs in 75% of patients with vascular ectasias and 90% of patients with diverticular bleeding.

13. **What are the indications for operative intervention?**
When the patient has received 6 units of blood (two thirds of the patient's blood volume in 24 hours) without resolution of bleeding. Any patient who continues to bleed or has recurrent bleeding after vasopressin or embolization should undergo resection.

14. **What is the role of blind subtotal colectomy in the management of patients with massive lower GI bleeding?**

Blind subtotal colectomy is limited to the small group of patients in whom a specific bleeding source cannot be identified. The procedure is associated with a 16% mortality rate. Younger patients tend to tolerate the procedure better than elderly patients. Older patients often suffer with severe diarrhea, urgency, and incontinence. However, blind segmental colectomy is associated with an even higher mortality rate (40%) and a 50% rebleeding rate.

15. **What is the most common cause of lower GI hemorrhage in the pediatric population?**

Meckel's diverticulum.

BIBLIOGRAPHY

1. American Society for Gastrointestinal Endoscopy: The role of endoscopy in the patient with lower gastrointestinal bleeding. Gastrointest Endosc 48:685–688, 1998.

2. Belaiche J, Louis E, D'Haens G, et al: Acute lower gastrointestinal bleeding in Crohn's disease: Characteristics of a unique series of 34 patients. Belgian IBD Research Group. Am J Gastroenterol 94:2177–2181, 1999.

3. Cynamon J, Atar E, Steiner A, et al: Catheter-induced vasospasm in the treatment of acute lower gastrointestinal bleeding. J Vasc Interv Radiol 14:211–216, 2003.

4. Gunderman R, Leef JA, Lipton MJ, Reba RC: Diagnostic imaging and the outcome of acute lower gastrointestinal bleeding. Acad Radiol Suppl 2:S303–S305, 1998.

5. Mallant-Hent RC, Van Bodegraven AA, Meuwissen SG, Manoliu RA: Alternative approach to massive gastrointestinal bleeding in ulcerative colitis: Highly selective transcatheter embolization. Eur J Gastroenterol Hepatol 15:189–193, 2003.

6. So JB, Kok K, Hgoi SS: Right-diverticular disease as a source of lower gastrointestinal bleeding. Am Surg 65:299–302, 1999.

7. Wilcox CM, Clark WS: Causes and outcome of upper and lower gastrointestinal bleeding: The Grady Hospital experience. South Med J 92:44–50, 1999.

CHAPTER 53

COLORECTAL POLYPS

Carlton C. Barnett, Jr., M.D., and Michael B. Wallace, M.D., M.P.H.

1. **What are polyps?**
   A polyp is an elevation of the mucosal surface that can occur anywhere in the gastrointestinal (GI) tract. Two thirds of polyps occur in the rectosigmoid and descending colon.

2. **What are the major types of polyps?**
   1. **Pedunculated polyps** have a head attached by a stalk to the mucosa of the colon or rectum. The stalk usually is covered with normal mucosa.
   2. **Sessile polyps** rest on a broad base.
   In both types, the muscularis mucosa is an important landmark for differentiating invasive from noninvasive lesions. Lymphatics and veins do not extend across the muscularis mucosa. Submucosal lesions such as carcinoids and lipomas may resemble colorectal polyps.

3. **At what age do polyps occur?**
   Adenomatous colorectal polyps occur infrequently under the age of 30 years. The incidence increases with age. However, autopsy series report a microscopic frequency as high as 70% in patients older than age 45 years. The clinical incidence is 25% for persons older than age 60 years.

4. **Which polyps have no malignant potential?**
   Hyperplastic (metaplastic) polyps are small (1–5 mm) and constitute > 90% of the polyps in the colon and rectum. Unlike adenomatous polyps, hyperplastic polyps are caused by failure of mucosal cells to spread over the mucosal lumen. These cells then accumulate on the luminal surface, forming a polyp.
   Hamartomas are collections of normal tissue in abnormal places (within the colonic mucosa).
   Inflammatory polyps are common in diseases such as ulcerative colitis, Crohn's disease, and schistosomiasis. They represent islands of healed or healing mucosal epithelium that are not permanent. The appearance of inflammatory polyps actually reflects the severity of the underlying disease. Lipomas may occur in polypoid form with head and stalk.

5. **Which polyps have malignant potential?**
   Adenomatous polyps may be precursors for cancer. There are three histologic types of adenomatous polyps. Polyps containing > 75% glandular elements are called tubular, those containing > 75% villous elements are termed villous, and those containing > 25% of both glandular and villous elements are tubulovillous.

6. **Are some types of polyps more frequently associated with adenocarcinoma?**
   Yes. Villous polyps are "bad actors." Coutsoftides et al. reported 5.6%, 16%, and 41% incidences of adenocarcinoma in tubular, villotubular, and villous adenomas, respectively.

7. **What is the relationship between polyp size and risk of adenocarcinoma?**
   Polyps < 2 cm have a 2% risk of containing cancer, 2-cm polyps have a 10% risk, and polyps > 2 cm have a cancer risk of 40%. Sixty percent of villous polyps are > 2 cm, and 77% of tubular polyps are < 1 cm at the time of discovery.

8. **What are juvenile polyps?**

Polyps that occur in the colon and rectum of infants, children, and adolescents. Histologically, they consist of large mucus-filled glands with lots of connective tissue. The cause of these polyps is unclear. They may represent a response to inflammation, or they may be hamartomas. Juvenile polyps may present as rectal bleeding or as lead points for intussusception. They should be left alone unless they cause trouble, at which point endoscopic polypectomy is sufficient treatment.

9. **How are colorectal polyps diagnosed?**

Fecal occult blood test (FOBT) is the most common test in the United States that leads to the discovery of polyps. Sigmoidoscopy and colonoscopy confirm the diagnosis. Colonoscopy has the advantage of being both diagnostic and potentially therapeutic.

KEY POINTS: COLORECTAL POLYPS

1. A polyp is an elevation of the mucosal surface that can occur anywhere in the GI tract.

2. Hyperplastic polyps are small and constitute > 90% of polyps in the colon and rectum.

3. Polyps containing > 75% glandular elements are called *tubular,* those with > 75% villous elements are termed *villous,* and those containing > 25% of both glandular and villous elements are called *tubulovillous.*

4. Fecal occult blood test is the most common test in the United States that leads to the discovery of polyps.

10. **What are the risks of colonoscopy?**

Bleeding and perforation. For diagnostic colonoscopy, these risks are extremely low—1.0% and 0.2%, respectively. Both risks are still < 1% for therapeutic colonoscopy. Bleeding usually stops on its own and rarely necessitates laparotomy.

11. **How can one determine whether endoscopic polypectomy is adequate treatment?**

In general, if a margin > 1 mm can be obtained, there is no invasion of the muscularis mucosa, and the histologic grade of the lesion is I or II (well to moderately differentiated), the patient should be offered endoscopic polypectomy. Patients with margins < 1 mm, invasion into vessels or lymphatics, and histologic grade III (poorly differentiated) lesions should undergo colon resection, unless comorbid medical conditions contraindicate surgery.

12. **What are the screening recommendations to detect polyps?**

There is broad consensus that persons in otherwise good health should undergo periodic screening for colorectal cancer and polyps beginning at age 50 years in average-risk individuals and age 40 years (or 10 years before the index person's age) in patients with a family history of cancer (excluding genetic colon cancer syndromes discussed below). Colonoscopy every 10 years is the most commonly used strategy, but FOBT with flexible sigmoidoscopy every 5 years for FOBT-negative patients is permissible. All patients who are FOBT positive and those with adenomatous polyps > 5 mm found on sigmoidoscopy should undergo full colonoscopy. To date, FOBT is the only screening test demonstrated in high-quality randomized clinical trials to reduce the risk of death from colorectal cancer. The risk reduction for death is similar to that of mammography (15–33%), depending how the testing is done. The sensitivity and specificity of FOBT is 40% and 96%, respectively, for colorectal polyps. Sigmoidoscopy and colonoscopy are 90% sensitive and 99% specific for polyps. Sigmoidoscopy, however, does not allow for evaluation of the proximal colon, thus lowering the overall effectiveness of this screening technique. Although colonoscopy is highly effective, it must be performed by trained individuals and carries the risk of anesthesia, thus, compromising its value as a screening tool.

13. **What are the screening recommendations for patients with known polyps?**
Patients with low risk (one to three tubular adenomas) should have repeat colonoscopy at 5 years. If patients are found to have multiple polyps or high-grade lesions, they should undergo colonoscopy at more frequent intervals (every 2 years). If patients are found to have no new lesions after one screening cycle, screening can be extended to every 5 years.
Malignant polyps should be removed based on the criteria discussed in question 12. Follow-up endoscopy should be performed at 3 months to ensure that no residual tumor is present at the polypectomy site. After this, follow-up should be the same as for multiple adenomatous lesions.

14. **Which clinical syndromes are associated with colorectal polyps?**
Familial adenomatous polyposis (FAP) or **adenomatous polyposis coli** (APC) is inherited as an autosomal dominant trait characterized by multiple adenomatous polyps throughout the GI tract. Diagnosis is made clinically by observing at least 100 adenomatous polyps in the colon; more than 1000 are found in many cases. FAP is caused by the loss of the APC tumor suppressor gene(s) on the long arm of chromosome 5. Multiple family members often are diagnosed with colorectal cancer, generally at a young age. Bleeding, diarrhea, and abdominal pain are common presenting symptoms. FAP is associated with nearly a 100% risk of cancer. FAP is also associated with small bowel, especially periampullary polyps, cancer, and mandibular osteoma.
Gardner syndrome is also associated with loss of the APC gene. Patients have polyposis, as do patients with FAP, but they also have osteomas of the skull, epidermoid cysts, retinal pigmentation abnormalities, and multiple soft tissue tumors.
Turcot syndrome is also associated with APC mutations and is characterized clinically with central nervous system tumors and multiple adenomatous polyps.
Peutz-Jeghers syndrome consists of multiple hamartomatous polyps throughout the alimentary tract. These polyps are associated with cutaneous melanotic spots on the lips, within the oropharynx, and on the dorsum of the fingers and toes. The malignant potential is very low.

15. **What is the natural history of APC?**
In a review of more than 1000 cases of adenomatous polyposis coli, the mean age at diagnosis of polyps was 34 years, and the mean age at diagnosis of colorectal cancers was 40 years. The mean age of death was 43 years. It is now recommended that patients with APC undergo colectomy at age 25 years. Patients are also at risk for the late development of foregut adenocarcinoma. Despite prophylactic total colectomy, this group of patients will not have a normal life expectancy.

16. **What are the surgical treatment options for APC?**
Treatment options include total proctocolectomy with permanent ileostomy, abdominal colectomy with rectal preservation, abdominal colectomy with ileorectal anastomosis, and ileal pouch-anal anastomosis. In patients in whom the rectum is preserved, yearly endoscopic surveillance is necessary.

17. **What role do genetic defects play in the progression of colorectal polyps to adenocarcinoma?**
The progression of adenomatous polyps to colorectal cancer is believed to involve an accumulation of genetic defects via the activation of protooncogenes or the inactivation of tumor suppressor genes. Colon polyps have provided the best available model of genetic mutations in the progression of normal tissue to cancer. Vogelstein and others have provided an elegant

description of genetic events demonstrating that polyps accumulate mutations first in the APC and *ras* oncogenes. Larger, more advanced polyps carry alterations of a tumor suppressor gene on chromosome 18, and carcinomas are associated with inactivation of the tumor suppressor gene *TP53* with coincident loss of function of p53 protein.

18. **What role do oncogenes play in the development of adenocarcinoma from adenomatous polyps?**
Oncogenes are copies of normal cellular genes that have been activated by mutation. Activating mutations of one allele of an oncogene can disrupt normal cell growth and differentiation and increase the likelihood of neoplastic transformation. The Ki-*ras* gene is the most commonly mutated oncogene in sporadic colonic neoplasia. Point mutations in the K-*ras* gene have been observed in approximately 40% of sporadic colorectal adenomas and carcinomas. Analysis of mutations in DNA from cells shed into the stool has been proposed as a potentially useful way to screen for colorectal cancer. In addition, activation of the tyrosine kinase of the *c-src* gene product pp60^{s-src} is frequent in polyps of high malignant potential; the activity of tyrosine kinase is significantly elevated above the level of primary tumors in liver metastases.

WEB SITE

http://www.asge.org

BIBLIOGRAPHY

1. Ahnen DJ, Feigl P, Quan G, et al: Ki-ras mutation and p53 overexpression predict the clinical behavior of colorectal cancer: A Southwest Oncology Group study. Cancer Res 58:1149–1158, 1998.

2. Bond JH: Polyp guideline: Diagnosis, treatment and surveillance for patients with nonfamilial colorectal polyps. Ann Intern Med 119:836–843, 1993.

3. Cooper HS, Deppisch LM, Gourley WK, et al: Endoscopically removed malignant colorectal polyps: Clinicopathologic correlations. Gastroenterology 198:1657–1665, 1995.

4. Darmon E, Cleary KR, Wargovich MJ: Immunohistochemical analysis of p53 overexpression in human colonic tumors. Cancer Detect Prevent 18:187–195, 1994.

5. Hahn WC, Weinberg RA: Rules for making human tumor cells. N Engl J Med 347:1593–1602, 2002.

6. Iwama T: The impact of familial adenomatous polyposis coli (FAP) on the tumorigenesis and mortality: Its rational treatment. Ann Surg 217:101, 1993.

7. Nivatvongs S, Rojanasakul A, Reimann HM, et al: The risk of lymph node metastasis in colorectal polyps with invasive adenocarcinoma. Dis Colon Rectum 34:323–328, 1991.

8. Ransahoff DF, Sandler RS: Screening for colorectal cancer. N Engl J Med 346:40–44, 2002.

9. Shih IM, Wang TL, Traverso G, et al: Top-down morphogenesis of colorectal tumors. Proc Natl Acad Sci USA 27:2640–2645, 2001.

10. Stein BL, Coller JA: Management of malignant colorectal polyps. Surg Clin North Am 73:47–66, 1993.

11. Talamonti MS, Roh MS, Curley SA, Gallick GE: Increase in activity and level of pp60c-src in progressive stages of human colorectal cancer. J Clin Invest 91:53–60, 1993.

CHAPTER 54

COLORECTAL CARCINOMA

Kathleen Liscum, M.D.

1. **What are the top three causes of cancer deaths in the United States?**
   Lung, breast or prostate, and colon cancer.

2. **List a few of the presenting symptoms of patients with colorectal cancer.**
   Intermittent rectal bleeding, vague abdominal pain, fatigue secondary to anemia, change in bowel habits, constipation, tenesmus, and perineal pain.

3. **What options are available to evaluate a patient who has guaiac-positive stools?**
   To evaluate the entire colon and rectum, one may perform a barium enema and proctoscopy or a colonoscopy. Colonoscopy is 10 times more expensive but is more sensitive for lesions < 1 cm.

4. **List at least five risk factors for colorectal cancer.**
   Prior adenomatous polyps, family history of colorectal cancer, age older than 40 years, chronic ulcerative colitis, Crohn's colitis, history of colon cancer, exposure to pelvic radiation for prostate or cervical cancer, and familial polyposis. Hamartomatous polyps (Peutz-Jeghers syndrome), inflammatory polyps, and hyperplastic polyps are not considered premalignant.

5. **What are the current screening recommendations of the American Cancer Society for colorectal cancers?**
   A yearly digital rectal examination with testing for occult blood for patients age 40 years and older. Additionally, for patients older than age 50 years, a flexible sigmoidoscopy is recommended every 3–5 years.

6. **In what part of the colon or rectum are most cancers found?**
   Historically, there has been a higher incidence of cancers in the rectum and left colon. However, over the past 50 years, there has been a gradual shift toward an increased incidence of right colon cancers. This change in pattern may reflect improvement in early detection.

7. **Surgical options for colorectal cancer are dependent on the tumor location. What operation should be performed for a patient with a lesion at 25 cm from the anal verge?**
   A sigmoid colectomy.

8. **What about a lesion at 9 cm from the anal verge?**
   A low anterior resection (LAR).

9. **What about a lesion at 4 cm from the anal verge?**
   An abdominoperineal resection (APR). This requires a permanent colostomy.

10. **What is the significance of finding adenomatous polyps in a patient's colon?**
    This patient is six times more likely to develop colorectal cancer than a patient without polyps. Evidence suggests that all colon cancers arise from adenomatous polyps. The "adenoma-carcinoma

KEY POINTS: COLORECTAL CARCINOMA

1. Presenting symptoms may include intermittent rectal bleeding, vague abdominal pain, fatigue secondary to anemia, change in bowel habits, constipation, tenesmus, and perineal pain.

2. The current recommendations of the American Cancer Society for screening are a yearly digital rectal exam with testing for occult blood at age 40 years and for patients over 50 a flexible sigmoidoscopy every 3–5 years.

3. Patients with lymph node involvement should receive chemotherapy postoperatively to treat micrometastases.

sequence" describes this transformational process. Patients with familial adenomatous polyposis (FAP) typically harbor more than 100 polyps, which cover the colonic mucosa. If these patients go untreated, they will, without exception, develop adenocarcinoma of the colon by age 40 years.

11. **How does the surgeon prepare the patient's colon for an operation?**
Bowel preparation includes both a mechanical cleansing and appropriate antimicrobial prophylaxis. This combination has resulted in significant decrease in morbidity and mortality from colon surgery. Mechanical cleansing can be accomplished by lavage with polyethylene glycol (Go-Lytely) or a combination of cathartics and enemas (Fleet's Prep).
   Antimicrobial prophylaxis should cover the expected aerobic and anaerobic flora of the gut. Significant controversy exits over whether the antibiotics should be given enterally (e.g., neomycin, 1 g, and metronidazole [Flagyl], 1 g, three times orally at 4-hour intervals the evening before surgery) or parenterally (e.g., cefotetan, 2 g intravenously within 1 hour before surgery). Many clinicians give both to obtain both intraluminal and systemic protection.

12. **What is Dukes' staging system?**
In 1932, Dr. Dukes described a staging system for rectal cancer. He originally described the following:
Dukes A   Tumor confined to bowel wall
Dukes B   Tumor invading through the bowel wall
Dukes C   Tumor cells found in the regional lymph nodes
Since his original article was published, this classification has been modified several times. One of the most commonly used modifications is the inclusion of Dukes' D stage, which indicates distant metastases.

13. **Which patients with colorectal cancer require adjuvant (postoperative) therapy?**
Patients with lymph node involvement (Dukes' C) should receive chemotherapy postoperatively to treat micrometastases. Two large studies have documented a survival advantage for these patients. However, no studies have documented a survival advantage for patients with Dukes' B disease treated with chemotherapy.
   Patients with rectal cancer with a significant chance of local recurrence (Dukes' B and C) should be treated with radiation therapy. This may be given preoperatively, postoperatively, or with a combined "sandwich" technique.

WEB SITE

http://www.nejm.org

BIBLIOGRAPHY

1. Colorectal Cancer Collaborative Group: Adjuvant radiotherapy for rectal cancer: A systematic overview of 22 randomised trials involving 8507 patients. Lancet 358:1291–1304, 2001.

2. Jass JR: Pathogenesis of colorectal cancer. Surg Clin North Am 82:891–904, 2002.

3. Levin B, Brooks D, Smith RA, Stone A: Emerging technologies in screening for colorectal cancer: CT colonography, immunochemical fecal occult blood tests, and stool screening using molecular markers. CA Cancer J Clin 53:44–55, 2003.

4. Lynch HT, de la Chapelle A: Hereditary colorectal cancer. N Engl J Med 348:919–932, 2003.

5. National Institutes of Health Consensus Conference: Adjuvant therapy for patients with colon and rectal cancer. JAMA 264:1444–1450, 1990.

6. Ransohoff DF: Screening colonoscopy in balance issues of implementation. Gastroenterol Clin North Am 31:1031–1044, 2002.

7. Salz LB, Minsky B: Adjuvant therapy of cancers of the colon and rectum. Surg Clin North Am 82:1035–1058, 2002.

8. US Multisociety Task Force on Colorectal Cancer: Colorectal cancer screening and surveillance: Clinical guidelines and rationale—update based on new evidence. Gastroenterology 124:544–560, 2003.

CHAPTER 55

ANORECTAL DISEASE

Eric L. Sarin, M.D., and John B. Moore, M.D.

1. **What aspect of the initial patient encounter is most important in the diagnosis of anorectal disease?**
Clinical history, including duration of complaints, exacerbating or alleviating issues, precipitating events, dietary and bowel habits, and current or previous treatments. This may not sound glamorous, but you will never encounter a more grateful patient than one whose rectal problem you have solved.

2. **What is the most common cause of painless, bright red blood per rectum?**
Internal hemorrhoids.

3. **What are the proximal and distal anatomic landmarks of the anal canal? What is its average length?**
The anal canal starts at the anorectal junction (which is the upper border of the internal sphincter muscle or puborectalis muscle) and ends at the anal verge. The average length is only 3–4 cm. The midpoint of the anal canal is called the dentate line.

4. **What is the anatomic and surgical significance of the dentate line?**
The dentate line is the location of the anal crypts that drain the intramuscular and intersphincteric anal glands, which are the site of anorectal abscesses and fistulas in ano. Above the dentate line, the anal canal receives visceral innervation (involuntary control), is covered by columnar epithelium, and is the origin of internal hemorrhoids. Below the dentate line, the anal canal receives somatic innervation (voluntary control), is lined with squamous epithelium, and is the location of external hemorrhoids.

ANORECTAL ABSCESS AND FISTULA IN ANO

5. **What is the most common cause of anorectal abscess?**
Ninety percent result from cryptoglandular infection.

6. **What are the four potential anorectal spaces used to classify anorectal abscesses?**
   1. Perianal (area of the anal verge)
   2. Ischiorectal (area lateral to the external sphincter muscles, extending from the levator ani muscles to the perineum)
   3. Intersphincteric (area between the internal and external sphincter muscles, continuous inferiorly with the perianal space and superiorly with the rectal wall)
   4. Supralevator (area superior to the levator ani muscles, inferior to the peritoneum, and lateral to the rectal wall)

7. **Define fistula in ano.**
A fistula is an abnormal communication between any two epithelial-lined surfaces. The internal opening of the fistula in ano involves the anoderm at the dentate line, whereas the external orifice is located at the anal margin.

8. **What is the incidence of fistula in ano after appropriate surgical incision and drainage of acute anorectal abscesses?**
50%.

9. **What is the most important factor leading to the successful surgical eradication of anorectal abscesses or fistulas?**
You must know anorectal anatomy, including the potential spaces (just memorize the answers to questions 4 and 6).

10. **What is Goodsall's rule?**
The location of the internal opening of an anorectal fistula is based on the position of the external opening. An external opening posterior to a line drawn transversely across the perineum origi-nates from an internal opening in the posterior midline. An external opening, anterior to this line, originates from the nearest anal crypt in a radial direction.

11. **What is the most important determinant of successful surgical treatment of fistula in ano?**
Identification of the internal openings.

12. **What is a seton?**
A seton is a heavy suture placed through the fistulous tract that is then serially tightened, allow-ing slow, controlled transection of the sphincter. The associated fibrous reaction maintains sphincter integrity. Although associated pain is a limiting factor in its use, the technique can effectively change a high fistula into a low fistula with minimal risk of incontinence.

13. **What is the role of fibrin glue in the management of anal fistula?**
Theoretically, the use of fibrin sealant represents an attractive alternative to the morbidity of operative treatment. However, although preliminary results support a marked decrease in post-operative pain and discomfort, 1-year recurrence rates are often > 50%.

ANAL FISSURE

14. **What is the most common location for idiopathic anal fissure?**
90% are posterior, and 10% are anterior.

15. **What are the most common symptoms of anal fissure?**
Tearing anal pain and bleeding with bowel movements.

16. **What is the underlying pathophysiology of fissure in ano?**
Local trauma to the anal canal, internal anal sphincter dysfunction, and ischemia.

17. **What is the differential diagnosis for anal fissure, especially if atypical in location?**
Anorectal abscess, thrombosed hemorrhoid, inflammatory bowel disease, or malignancy.

18. **How do you best diagnose anal fissure?**
By clinical history and visual inspection—*not* by digital examination or anoscopy (which serves only to turn a friendly patient into an irate one).

19. **What are the nonoperative treatment options?**
High-fiber diet; stool-bulking agents; increased hydration; frequent, warm sitz baths; and topical agents containing anti-inflammatory agents, local anesthetics, and vasodilators (nitroglycerin).

20. **What is the most common operation performed to treat intractable fissure in ano?**
Fissurotomy with lateral internal anal sphincterotomy.

KEY POINTS: ANAL FISSURE

1. Ninety percent of idiopathic anal fissures are posterior and 10% are anterior.

2. The most common symptoms are tearing anal pain and bleeding with bowel movements.

3. The diagnosis involves visual inspection—not by digital exam or anoscopy.

4. Nonoperative treatment includes high-fiber diet, warm sitz baths, and topical agents containing anti-inflammatory agents, local anesthetics, and vasodilators.

5. The most common operation is a fissurotomy with lateral internal anal sphincterotomy.

HEMORRHOIDS

21. **What are hemorrhoidal tissues, and what are their normal functions?**
Hemorrhoids are cushions of vascular tissue that contribute to anal continence and protect the sphincter mechanism during defecation. Hemorrhoids are not veins, but sinusoids. Bleeding originates from presinusoidal arterioles, thus explaining the bright red arterial color.

22. **What are the most common causes of pathologic hemorrhoids?**
Constipation, prolonged straining, pregnancy, and internal sphincter dysfunction.

23. **What is the most important difference between internal and external hemorrhoids?**
Whereas internal hemorrhoids are located above the dentate line with visceral innervation, external hemorrhoids are located below the dentate line with somatic innervation. Ablation of internal hemorrhoids causes a pressure sensation with an urge to defecate, but a similar approach to external hemorrhoids causes excruciating pain.

24. **What are the most common complaints associated with pathologic internal hemorrhoids?**
Bleeding, mucus discharge, and prolapsing tissue.

25. **What are the most common complaints associated with external hemorrhoids?**
Pain, inflammation, thrombosis, and difficulty with anal hygiene.

26. **Are there any treatment options for symptomatic internal hemorrhoids based on identifiable physical characteristics?**
Yes. Treatment is based on the degree of prolapse:
Grade 1:　　None
Grade 2:　　Spontaneous reduction
Grade 3:　　Manual reduction
Grade 4:　　Unreducible

27. **How are patients with symptomatic grades 2 and 3 and occasionally grade 4 internal hemorrhoids treated?**
Diet and stool bulking, rubber band ligation, injection sclerotherapy, cryotherapy, infrared photocoagulation, anal dilatation, or electrocautery.

28. **What is the last-resort treatment for recalcitrant symptomatic internal hemorrhoids or combined internal and external hemorrhoids?**
Operative hemorrhoidectomy.

PILONIDAL SINUS DISEASE

29. **What is the most common clinical presentation of a pilonidal sinus?**
Pain and swelling in the sacrococcygeal region, which typically are associated with a (sometimes several) chronic draining sinus tract.

30. **Is pilonidal disease acquired or congenital?**
Acquired. Hair follicles in the midline sacrococcygeal area enlarge and become infected, resulting in an abscess.

31. **How is acute pilonidal abscess treated?**
Incision and drainage (like a fistula in ano, it is necessary to excise the whole tract).

32. **What is the definitive therapy for pilonidal disease?**
Excision of the entire pilonidal cavity and associated sinus tracts down to the fascia with primary or delayed closure.

33. **What theory explains the rarity of pilonidal disease after age 40 years?**
Changes in body habitus.

BIBLIOGRAPHY

1. Beck DE, Wexner SD (eds): Fundamentals of Anorectal Surgery. Philadelphia, W.B. Saunders, 1998.
2. Cho DV: Endosonographic criteria for an internal opening of fistula-in-ano. Dis Colon Rectum 42:515–518, 1999.
3. Cintron JR, Park JJ, Orsay CP, et al: Repair of fistulas-in ano using fibrin adhesive: Long-term follow-up. Dis Colon Rectum 43:944–949, 2000.
4. Corman ML: Anal fistula. In Corman ML: Colon and Rectal Surgery, 4th ed. Philadelphia, Lippincott-Raven, 1998, pp 238–271.
5. Hodgkin W: Pilonidal sinus disease. J Wound Care 7:481–483, 1998.
6. Law WL, Chu KW: Triple rubber band ligation for hemorrhoids: Prospective randomized trial of local anesthetic injection. Dis Colon Rectum 42:363–366, 1999.
7. Park JJ, Cintron JR, Orsay CP, et al: Repair of chronic anorectal fistulae using commercial fibrin sealant. Arch Surg 135:166–169, 2000.
8. Sentovich SM: Fibrin glue for all anal fistulas. J Gastrointest Surg 5:158–161, 2001.

INGUINAL HERNIA

Gregory P. Victorino, M.D., Jyoti Arya, M.D., and James Bascom, M.D.

1. **"Groin" hernia refers to which three hernias?**
   Direct and indirect inguinal hernias and femoral hernias.

2. **Francois Poupart, a French surgeon and anatomist (1616–1708), described a ligament that bears his name. What is the anatomic name of the Poupart ligament?**
   Inguinal ligament, which is a key element in most groin hernia repair.

3. **Franz K. Hesselbach, a German surgeon and anatomist (1759–1816), described a triangle that is the common site of direct hernias. What are the anatomic margins of Hesselbach's triangle?**
   The triangle is defined inferiorly by the inguinal ligament, superiorly by the inferior epigastric vessels, and medially by the rectus fascia. The transversalis fascia forms the floor of the triangle. The original description used Cooper's ligament as the inferior limit but because of the common use of the anterior approach to hernias, the more apparent inguinal ligament was substituted as the inferior limit of the triangle. With the increasing use of preperitoneal approaches to hernia repair, Cooper's ligament is again much more apparent and useful as an anatomic touchstone.

4. **Sir Astley Paston Cooper, an English surgeon and anatomist (1768–1841), described a ligament bearing his name. What is the anatomic name for the ligament and the proper name of Cooper's ligament repair?**
   The anatomic name of Cooper's ligament is iliopectineal ligament. The Cooper's ligament repair or McVay repair was popularized by Chester McVay (1911–1987). With Barry Aston, professor of anatomy at Northwestern University, McVay provided the modern description of the groin anatomy.

5. **Antonio de Gimbernat, a Spanish surgeon and anatomist (1734–1816), had his interesting name attached to the lacunar ligament, which marks the medial margin of a groin area opening. What is the opening? What hernia protrudes into this opening?**
   The opening is the femoral canal, which is defined medially by the lacunar ligament, anteriorly by the inguinal ligament, posteriorly by the pectineal fascia, and laterally by the femoral vein. A femoral hernia protrudes into the femoral canal.

6. **Indirect inguinal hernia (particularly in children) and hydrocele are associated with which congenital abnormality?**
   Persistence of an open processus vaginalis, in the case of a hernia, allows descent of bowel into the inguinal canal. With fluid accumulation, partial obstruction presents as a hydrocele of the spermatic cord.

7. **What are the diagnostic criteria for hernia in an infant or child?**
   - Inguinal, scrotal, or labial lump that may or may not be reducible
   - History of a lump seen by a health care provider

- History of a lump seen by the mother
- The "silk sign" (the feeling of rubbing together two surfaces of silk cloth when gently rubbing together the two surfaces of a hernia sac)
- An incarceration sometimes felt on rectal examination

8. **What can be done to reduce an incarcerated hernia in an infant or child?**
   The four-point program is easier said than done, but it is worth the effort:
   1. Sedate the patient.
   2. Place the patient in the Trendelenburg position.
   3. Apply a cold pack (over petroleum gauze to avoid skin injury) in inguinal area.
   4. In the absence of spontaneous reduction—and if the patient is quiet—use gentle manipulation.

9. **How often can incarceration be successfully reduced? What should be done next?**
   About 80% of incarcerated hernias can be reduced in children; in adults, the percentage is lower. Despite the fact that 80–90% of inguinal hernias occur in boys, most incarcerations occur in girls. The hernia should be repaired electively within a few days after incarceration. The 20% of hernias that are still incarcerated are operated immediately.

10. **What is a Bassini repair?**
    The Bassini repair sutures together the conjoined tendon and the shelving edge of the inguinal ligament up to the internal ring (Figure 56-1). This classic procedure, introduced in 1887 at the Italian Society of Surgery in Genoa, revolutionized hernia repair. Until recently, it has been the standard of repair. After graduation from medical school and while fighting for Italian independence, Eduardo Bassini (1844–1924) was bayoneted in the groin and, as a prisoner, was hospitalized for months with a fecal fistula.

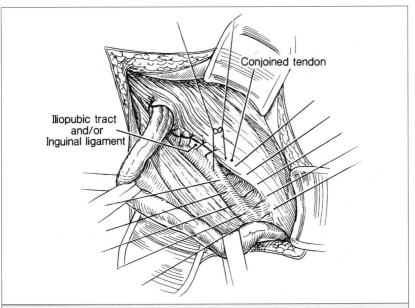

Figure 56-1. The standard right inguinal hernia repair using the conjoined tendon and inguinal ligament.

11. **What is the recurrence rate with indirect and direct hernias that have been repaired with classic Bassini repair technique?**
Over a follow-up period of 50 years, the recurrence rate of adult indirect hernias is 5–10%; of direct hernias, 15–30%.

12. **Describe a McVay hernia repair.**
The line of interrupted sutures starts at a the pubic tubercle and joins the tendinous arch of the transversus abdominis muscle to Cooper's ligament up to the femoral canal. At this point, two or three transitional sutures are placed from Cooper's ligament to the anterior femoral fascia, effectively closing the medial extreme of the femoral canal. The final set of sutures joins the transversus abdominis arch and the anterior femoral fascia. The stitches usually incorporate the inguinal ligament at the upper limit of the repair, the site of the new internal inguinal ring and cord structures. About 15 years ago, McVay described laying in a mesh patch and stitching it, at its periphery, to the same anatomic structures. This application of mesh closely resembles the Lichtenstein repair (see question 17), except that it uses Cooper's ligament.

13. **For what type of hernias is the McVay Cooper's ligament repair most useful?**
Femoral and direct hernias.

14. **What is the Shouldice repair?**
The Shouldice repair, popularized at the Shouldice Clinic near Toronto, imbricates or overlays the transversalis fascia and conjoined tendon with four continuous lines, using two fine-wire sutures. The suture tract runs from the pubic tubercle to a new internal ring. Care is taken with the inferior epigastric vessels. The result is layered approximation of the conjoined tendon to the inguinal ligament tract.

15. **What is the reported recurrence rate for the Shouldice repair?**
The recurrence rate is 1%, the lowest reported rate for nonmesh repairs of inguinal hernias in adults.

16. **For what type of groin hernia is the Shouldice repair not appropriate?**
Femoral hernia.

17. **Describe the Lichtenstein repair.**
The Lichtenstein repair consists of a sutured patch of polypropylene mesh (Marlex, C.R. Bard, Inc., Covington, GA) that covers Hesselbach's triangle and the indirect hernia area. It is considered a tension-free repair because the mesh is sutured in place without pulling ligaments or tissues together as in all other repairs. The mesh is divided at its upper end to wrap closely around the spermatic cord and its associated structures in the normal position of the internal inguinal canal. The Lichtenstein procedure is rapidly becoming the most widely used repair of adult inguinal hernia. The reported recurrence rate is < 1%.

18. **What are the advantages of using the Marlex mesh?**
Central to acceptance and success of the Lichtenstein hernia repair has been the development of and experience with the Marlex mesh. The monofilament mesh is strong, inert, and resistant to infection. The interstices are rapidly and completely infiltrated with fibroblasts, and the mesh is not subject to deterioration, rejection, or fragmentation. (See Figure 56-2.)

19. **For what groin area is the Lichtenstein repair not appropriate?**
Femoral hernia.

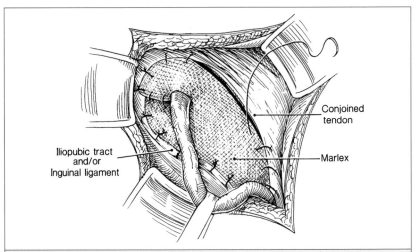

Figure 56-2. The Marlex mesh repair of a right inguinal hernia. Note that the same structures are used but not brought together; thus, the name of the "tension-free" repair.

20. **Which type of repair is acceptable for the femoral hernia?**
Several different repairs can be used. Mesh in the form of a plug can be inserted into the femoral canal and fixed in place. A McVay Cooper's ligament repair can be done. A preperitoneal approach to the hernia can be used to suture or plug the defect. A suture repair or a sartorius facial flap applied from below the inguinal ligament in a femoral approach also may be used. The preperitoneal approach is increasingly used for complicated inguinal and femoral hernias.

21. **What is the preperitoneal or Stoppa procedure?**
The preperitoneal or Stoppa procedure is a groin hernia repair on the internal side of the abdominal wall between the peritoneum and fascial surfaces that do not open into the peritoneal cavity. The anatomic landmarks are very different and initially quite challenging to surgeons accustomed to the external abdominal wall approach. The technique is suited for recurrent hernias in which scarring and obliterated anatomy increase the risk of cord injury and recurrence. Other problems such as large hernias and femoral hernias are corrected with this approach. Conceptually, the laparoscopic hernia repair uses the same approach. (See Figure 56-3.)

22. **Where are the spaces of Retzius and Bogros? Why are they increasingly important?**
Retzius' space is between the pubis and the urinary bladder. Bogros' space is between the peritoneum and the fascia and muscle planes on the posterior aspect of the abdominal wall below the umbilicus and down to Cooper's ligament. Laterally, the space goes to the iliac spines. In either the open Stoppa procedure or the laparoscopic preperitoneal repair, the spaces of Retzius and Bogros are developed for mesh placement and surgical exposure.

23. **How tight around the spermatic cord should a surgically fashioned, internal inguinal ring be?**
About 5 mm, which is less than a fingertip and more than a forceps tip.

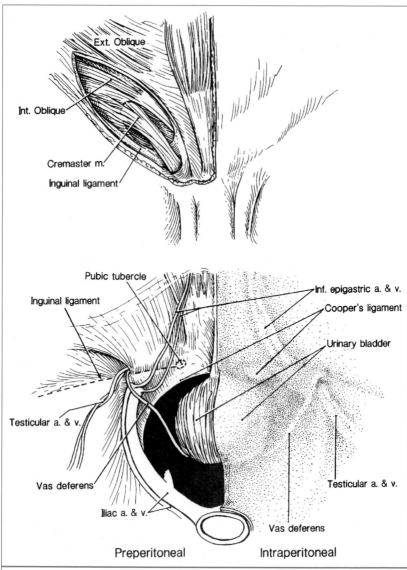

Figure 56-3. The different appearance and landmarks are seen in the anterior view (above) and the posterior view (below) of the inguinal–femoral area. In the posterior view the importance of the inferior epigastric vessels, bladder, and Cooper's ligament as anatomic landmarks is apparent.

24. **What is the common fascial defect of larger indirect and all direct inguinal hernias?**
    Weakness or attenuation of the transversalis fascia.

25. **On examination, the femoral hernia may be confused with what other inguinal hernia?**
    The femoral hernia may be confused with a direct inguinal hernia because of the tendency of the femoral hernia to present at the lateral edge of the inguinal ligament.

KEY POINTS: TYPES OF INGUINAL HERNIA REPAIR

1. The Bassini repair sutures together the conjoined tendon and the shelving edge of the inguinal ligament up to the internal ring.

2. The McVay repair is most useful for femoral and direct hernias.

3. The Shouldice repair imbricates the transversalis fascia and conjoined tendon with four continuous lines, using two fine-wire sutures (not appropriate for femoral hernias).

4. The Lichtenstein repair consists of a sutured patch of polyprolene mesh that covers Hesselbach's triangle and the indirect hernia sac.

26. **What is the difference between an incarcerated and a strangulated hernia?**
Incarcerated: structures in the hernia sac still have a good blood supply but are stuck in the sac because of adhesions or a narrow neck of the hernia sac.
Strangulated: herniated structures, such as bowel or omentum, have lost their blood supply because of anatomic constriction at the neck of the hernia. The herniated, ischemic tissue is, therefore, in various stages of gangrenous changes. Strangulated hernias are surgical emergencies.

27. **What operation is done for an uncomplicated indirect infant hernia?**
High ligation of the hernia sac.

28. **What operation is done for an uncomplicated indirect hernia in young adults?**
The appropriate operation consists of high ligation and possibly one or two stitches in the transversalis fascia to tighten the internal ring. This is the basic Marcy technique, developed by Henry Orlando Marcy (1837–1924); it is smaller and more anatomically focused than the Bassini repair.

29. **What operation is done for an uncomplicated but sizable direct hernia in elderly adults?**
Traditionally, the Bassini or McVay repair was chosen. More recently, because of the low recurrence rate, the Shouldice or Lichtenstein repair is favored.

30. **What organ systems should be reviewed with particular care in the work-up of patients with hernia (especially elderly patients with recent onset of hernia)?**
The gastrointestinal, urinary, and pulmonary systems should be reviewed with particular care. One is looking for causes of chronic strain or sudden forces that may have induced the hernia. Straining during defecation or urination, unusual coughing, or difficulty with breathing, if corrected, may be of great value to the patient and reduce the chance of recurrent hernia.

31. **What is a sliding hernia?**
A sliding hernia is formed when a retroperitoneal organ protrudes (herniates) outside the abdominal cavity in such a manner that the organ itself and the overlying peritoneal surface constitute a side of the hernia sac.

32. **What organs can be found in sliding hernias?**

Colon	Bladder
Cecum	Fallopian tubes
Appendix	Uterus (rare)
Ovary	

33. **What are common operative and postoperative complications of hernia repairs?**

Intraoperative complications

- Injury to the spermatic cord, especially in children
- Injury to the spermatic vessels, resulting in atrophy or acute necrosis of testes
- Injury to the ilioinguinal nerve, genitofemoral nerve, and lateral femoral cutaneous nerve (the lateral femoral cutaneous nerve is uniquely vulnerable in laparoscopic and properitoneal procedures)
- Injury to the femoral vessels

Postoperative complications

- Infection—high risk in children with diaper rash and patients with bowel injury or necrosis
- Hematoma—should resolve in time
- Nerve injury—the nerve is not always divided and, with time, may improve. If pain persists, try lidocaine block for both diagnosis and treatment. If a nerve block is not successful, one may consider reexploration to free the nerve from scar or to excise a postsurgical neuroma.

34. **What are the common sites of hernia recurrence?**

Direct hernias often recur at the pubic tubercle. Indirect hernias recur at the internal ring. The cause is usually related to poorly placed or insufficient stitches. Other possible causes include infection, poor tissue, poor collagen formation, or too much tension at the surgical suture line. A single line of repair under moderate tension fails in a significant number of patients, regardless of adequacy of repair or healing process. Tension is almost always bad in surgery.

35. **How long should the patient avoid heavy lifting after a hernia repair?**

The standard advice for decades has been 6 weeks. The current advice varies from no limitation with the Lichtenstein or preperitoneal repairs to 6 weeks for a Bassini repair. The self-limitation of pain is an excellent guide.

CONTROVERSIES

36. **What are some of the anatomic issues related to inguinal hernias?**

At issue is the **iliopubic tract**, which is central to the Anson/McVay anatomic description of the inguinal area and featured in the McVay Cooper's ligament repair. Although the McVay repair is used in England, the iliopubic tract is not referred to or described in English anatomic texts.

The term **conjoined tendon**, although commonly used, is considered by many to be anatomically inaccurate and misleading. The internal oblique and transversus abdominis muscles that make up the conjoined tendon are obvious and can be used surgically either alone or together. The tendinous edge of the transversus abdominis muscle and the tendinous edge of the internal oblique muscle start at their insertion on the pubic tubercle and course laterally and superiorly to the medial edge of the internal ring. At this point, the tendinous elements diminish, leaving only muscle tissues, and continue laterally and superiorly to their origins.

Whether the lacunar ligament or the iliopubic tract defines the medial border of the femoral canal is controversial. The compromise position is that the iliopubic tract is the border whereas in the normal unstretched state, the lacunar ligament (Gimbernat's ligament) is the border in the presence of hernia (stretched state). At surgery it is enough to say that a palpable, visible curved ligament is present and used in some femoral repairs.

37. **What are some surgical issues in the repair of inguinal hernias?**

The controversy over implanting mesh, as in the Lichtenstein repair, has been resolved in favor of mesh. Another controversy concerns the use of the laparoscope for hernia repair. A further issue is intra-abdominal or preperitoneal placement of mesh. At present, most surgeons accept laparoscopic repair as an alternative for preperitoneal hernia repair. The indications for a preperitoneal approach to hernia repair are still being defined, although the preperitoneal approach is acceptable for repair of recurrent hernia and unusually large or difficult hernias. The preperitoneal approach is used with increasing frequency for repair of femoral hernias. The repair should be appropriate to the circumstance of the hernia. Thus, hernia location and size as well as the patient's age, general condition, and recurrence status should be factored into the strategy of repair.

BIBLIOGRAPHY

1. Avisse C, Delattre JF, Flament JB: The inguinal rings. Surg Clin North Am 80:49–69, 2000.
2. Avisse C, Delattre JF, Flament JB: The inguinofemoral area from a laparoscopic standpoint. History, anatomy, and surgical applications. Surg Clin North Am 80:35–48, 2000.
3. Bendavid R, Howarth D: Transversalis fascia rediscovered. Surg Clin North Am 80:25–33, 2000.
4. Collaboration EH: Laparoscopic compared with open methods of groin hernia repair: Systematic review of randomized controlled trials. Br J Surg 87:860–867, 2000.
5. Collaboration EH: Mesh compared with non-mesh methods of open groin hernia repair. Systematic review of randomized controlled trials. Br J Surg 87:854–859, 2000.

HYPERPARATHYROIDISM

Robert C. McIntyre, Jr., M.D.

CHAPTER 57

1. **What is the prevalence of hyperparathyroidism (HPT)?**
   There are approximately 100,000 new cases of HPT annually in the United States. Primary HPT occurs in 1 in 500 women and in 1 in 2000 men older than 40 years. Approximately 10% of patients with primary HPT are referred for surgery.

2. **What are the symptoms of hyperparathyroidism?**
   "Painful bones, renal stones, abdominal groans, and psychic moans." The three most common symptoms are fatigue, depression, and constipation. The classic symptoms and signs are:
   Bones: arthralgia, osteoporosis, pathologic fractures
   Stones: renal stones, renal insufficiency, polyuria, polydipsia
   Abdominal groans: pancreatitis, peptic ulcer disease, constipation
   Psychic moans: fatigue, weakness, depression

3. **What are the leading causes of hypercalcemia?**
   HPT is the most common cause of hypercalcemia among outpatients and the second most common cause in the hospital setting. The most common cause of hypercalcemia in hospitalized patients is malignancy. Primary HPT and malignancy account for 90% of cases of hypercalcemia.

4. **What is the differential diagnosis of hypercalcemia?**
   Endocrine
   > HPT
   > Hyperthyroidism
   > Addison's disease

   Malignancy
   > Bone metastasis
   > Paraneoplastic syndromes
   > Solid tumors (squamous or small cell lung carcinoma)
   > Hematologic malignancy (myeloma, leukemia, lymphoma)

   Increased intake
   > Milk alkali syndrome
   > Vitamin D intoxication
   > Granulomatous disease
   > Sarcoidosis
   > Tuberculosis

   Miscellaneous
   > Familial hypocalciuric hypercalcemia (FHH)
   > Thiazide use
   > Lithium use

5. **What is the essential laboratory evaluation for HPT?**
   Elevated serum calcium (> 10.3 mg/dL) should be assessed at least twice. Hypercalcemia must be associated with elevation of parathyroid hormone (intact). Serum phosphate levels

are low in nearly 80% of patients. Serum chloride is increased in 40% of patients. A chloride-to-phosphate ratio greater than 33 suggests primary HPT. Increased alkaline phosphatase levels occur only in the setting of advanced bone disease. A 24-hour urine collection for calcium excretion excludes benign FHH. In patients with primary HPT, the 24-hour urine calcium is > 150 mg/day versus < 100 mg/day in those with FHH.

6. **Describe the anatomy of the parathyroid glands.**

The upper parathyroid glands arise from the dorsal part of the fourth brachial pouch along with the lateral lobes of the thyroid. The lower parathyroid glands arise from the dorsal part of the third brachial pouch along with the thymus.

The average weight of a normal parathyroid gland is 35–50 mg. The upper parathyroid gland lies on the posterior portion of the upper half of the thyroid, cephalad to the inferior thyroid artery, and posterior to the recurrent laryngeal nerve. The normal lower parathyroid gland is found on the lateral or posterior surface of the lower pole of the thyroid gland.

Four glands are present in 89% of patients, five in 8%, six in 3%, and < four in 0%.

The upper parathyroid glands' location is more constant. The most common ectopic sites of the upper glands are posterior to the esophagus or in the tracheoesophageal groove down into the posterior superior mediastinum. The lower parathyroid glands are more commonly ectopic and may be in the thyrothymic ligament, thymus, mediastinum (but outside the thymus), or carotid sheath or within the thyroid.

7. **What are the indications for parathyroidectomy?**

All patients with symptomatic HPT or with serum calcium 1 mg/dL above normal should benefit from a parathyroidectomy. Careful history indicates the majority of patients (> 90%) have symptoms. The treatment of asymptomatic patients with minimal elevation (10.3–11.0 mg/dL) of serum calcium is controversial. However, at least four factors favor operation:

1. Patients with untreated primary HPT have an increased death rate caused by cardiovascular disease.
2. Patients with HPT have abnormal quality-of-life scores, and these scores improve to normal after operative success.
3. The cost of parathyroidectomy is equivalent to medical follow-up at 5 years.
4. Experienced endocrine surgeons have a high success rate (≥ 95%) with very low morbidity and mortality rates.

8. **What localization studies are available, and when are they indicated?**

The single best localization study is the sestamibi scan. Other noninvasive localization studies include ultrasound, computed tomography, and magnetic resonance imaging. Invasive localization procedures include arteriography and venous sampling. The tests are most accurate with a single abnormal parathyroid gland. Localization procedures in cases of hyperplasia may be misleading.

Localization studies are not routinely indicated before an initial operation, but they are mandatory before all reoperative parathyroidectomies for persistent or recurrent HPT and in patients with previous thyroid surgery.

Preoperative sestamibi scintigraphy is used by some surgeons for the initial operation to allow a focused parathyroidectomy or minimally invasive radio-guided parathyroidectomy.

9. **What is the pathology of primary HPT?**

Primary HPT is caused by a single adenoma in 87% of cases, hyperplasia in 9%, double adenoma in 3%, and carcinoma in < 1%. In familial HPT, multiple endocrine neoplasia syndromes (MEN I and MEN II), and HPT due to end-stage renal disease, hyperplasia is the rule.

10. **Outline the standard surgical strategy of an initial exploration for primary HPT.**

A meticulously dry, blood-free operative field must be maintained. Tissue in the region of the recurrent laryngeal nerve should not be clamped or divided until the nerve is definitively identified. The standard operation is a bilateral neck exploration. If a solitary adenoma and three normal glands are found, the adenoma is removed and one of the normal glands biopsied. Frozen-section examination confirms that the tissue is parathyroid but is unreliable to differentiate adenoma versus hyperplasia. Four-gland enlargement (hyperplasia) indicates either subtotal parathyroidectomy (leaving approximately 50 mg of well-vascularized parathyroid tissue in the neck) or total parathyroidectomy with autotransplantation of 50 mg of parathyroid tissue. If a remnant is left in the neck, it should be marked with a nonabsorbable suture or staple. In the setting of hyperplasia, a thymectomy eliminates the possibility of thymic supernumerary glands. If more than one enlarged gland is found in association with normal-appearing glands (double adenoma), all abnormal glands should be removed.

KEY POINTS: HYPERPARATHYROIDISM

1. It is the most common cause of hypercalcemia among outpatients and the second most common cause in the hospital setting.

2. The three most common symptoms are fatigue, constipation, and depression.

3. The single best localization study is the sestamibi scan.

11. **Are there any newer alternatives to the standard operative approach?**
Focused parathyroidectomy, minimally invasive radio-guided parathyroidectomy (MIRP), and endoscopic neck exploration are new techniques. A focused parathyroidectomy uses the preoperative localization to guide a parathyroidectomy, avoiding a bilateral exploration. This approach is combined with intraoperative "rapid" parathyroid hormone assay. The parathyroid hormone is measured by a modified assay before operation and 10 minutes after adequate resection. A postresection level < 50% of the preoperative level and within the normal range predicts success. The MIRP uses a sestamibi scan the morning of surgery and an intraoperative gamma probe to guide parathyroidectomy. The ratio of ex vivo radioactivity to background is measured to determine success and, thus, the end of the operation.

12. **What should one do if an adenoma is not found in the usual locations?**
Each normal gland should be biopsied for confirmation and marked. Normal parathyroid glands should not be removed. If three normal glands are identified, the surgeon should assess whether the missing gland is an upper or lower one. A missing upper gland often lies in the tracheoesophageal groove, posterior to the esophagus or in the posterior superior mediastinum. The common mistake is that the upper thyroid is not satisfactorily mobilized and dissection is not carried posterior enough. The location of a missing lower gland is more varied. First, the thyrothymic ligament should be inspected. The thymus then can be resected through the neck incision. If the adenoma is still not found, the surgeon should search for an undescended parathyroid gland. Next, the carotid sheath should be opened. Finally, the thyroid lobe on the side of the missing parathyroid should be palpated or examined by intraoperative ultrasound for nodules. If a nodule is found, a lobectomy is done and the tissue examined by frozen section; it may be an intrathyroidal parathyroid gland. A blind thyroid lobectomy is rarely helpful.

A sternotomy should not be done as part of an initial exploration. If the above maneuvers are unsuccessful in revealing a parathyroid adenoma, the surgeon should stop. A diagram of the location of the identified glands should be made for future reference. Persistent hypercalcemia indicates the need for localization procedures.

13. **What is the outcome of surgery for primary HPT?**

The expected cure rate should be ≥ 95% for patients undergoing an initial exploration for primary HPT. Symptomatic improvement exceeds 95%. Quality-of-life scores return to normal at 6 months. After parathyroidectomy, 80% of symptomatic patients have improvement in bone density and renal function. Even in asymptomatic patients, urinary calcium and deoxypyridinoline levels decrease. Patients have fewer episodes of nephrolithiasis, gout, and peptic ulcer disease. Parathyroidectomy also appears to improve longevity in patients with primary HPT.

14. **What are the complications of parathyroidectomy?**

Permanent recurrent laryngeal nerve injury occurs in < 1% of patients; however, a temporary nerve paresis occurs in 3%. Temporary hypocalcemia occurs in 10% of patients, but permanent HPT occurs in only 2% of cases. An elevated preoperative alkaline phosphatase level and abnormal renal function may predict which patients are likely to have "hungry bone" syndrome.

15. **What are the physical signs of hypocalcemia after surgery?**

Chvostek's sign is spasm of the facial muscles caused by tapping the facial nerve trunk. Trousseau's sign is carpal spasm elicited by occlusion of the brachial artery for 3 minutes with a blood pressure cuff.

16. **How should patients with hypocalcemia be treated?**

Patients with tetany caused by hypoparathyroidism require emergency treatment with intravenous calcium to prevent laryngeal stridor and convulsions. One ampule of 10% calcium gluconate (90 mg elemental calcium per 10 mL) should be given in 100-mL saline over 20 minutes followed by an infusion of calcium (5 ampules of calcium gluconate in 500 cc of saline) at 50 mL/h. Maintaining calcium levels of 7.5–9.0 mg/dL is adequate. Oral calcium should be started as soon as possible in the form of calcium carbonate (Tums or Oscal) at 2–3 g/day in divided doses (3–4 times/day). Calcium citrate is preferred for patients with renal lithiasis because the citrate may be prophylactic against renal lithiasis. In most patients, vitamin D preparations increase intestinal absorption and can be given as calcitriol (Rocaltrol), 0.25–0.75 mg per day.

17. **Define persistent and recurrent HPT.**

Operative success is defined by long-term normocalcemia. Persistent HPT is defined as hypercalcemia within 6 months of surgery; recurrent HPT is defined as hypercalcemia after 6 months.

18. **What is the strategy for managing patients with persistent or recurrent HPT?**

First, the patient should be reevaluated to ensure that the hypercalcemia is caused by primary HPT and not some other cause. Patients should be evaluated for familial hypocalciuric hypercalcemia, which does not warrant reoperation. The severity of disease is evaluated to ensure that repeat operation is justified. Previous operative notes and pathology reports should be reviewed to assist in planning repeat therapy. Localization studies should be used extensively. Before reexploration, vocal cord function should be assessed in all patients.

Repeat cervical exploration is done through the previous incision. Because the strap muscles are usually adherent to the thyroid, a lateral approach through the plane between the sternocleidomastoid and strap muscles may be used instead of the usual medial approach. With positive localization studies or retrospective determination of the side of the missing adenoma, the dissection may be limited if an adenoma is found.

An alternative to repeat exploration is angiographic ablation of parathyroid tissue, which is especially useful for mediastinal adenomas because it avoids a median sternotomy. It is performed by delivering ionic contrast through an arterial catheter wedged into the feeding vessel.

19. **Who performed the first parathyroidectomy?**
In 1925, Felix Mendl performed the first successful parathyroidectomy at the Hochenegg Clinic in Vienna. His patient was Albert, a 34-year-old tram car conductor who could not work because of severe osteitis fibrosa cystica.

20. **Who was Captain Martell?**
An officer in the U.S. Merchant Marine, Captain Martell was the first patient in the United States to undergo surgery for primary HPT. Captain Martell had progressive HPT that reduced his height from 6 feet to a kyphotic 5 feet, 6 inches. After seven operations, the adenoma was finally removed from the mediastinum; however, the captain died in chronic renal failure.

BIBLIOGRAPHY

1. Arici C, Cheah WK, Ituarte PH, et al: Can localization studies be used to direct focused parathyroid operations? Surgery 129:720–729, 2001.

2. Boggs JE, Irvin GL 3d, Molinari AS, Deriso GT: Intraoperative parathyroid hormone monitoring as an adjunct to parathyroidectomy. Surgery 120:954–958, 1996.

3. Burney RE, Jones KR, Coon JW, et al: Assessment of patient outcomes after operation for primary hyper-parathyroidism. Surgery 120:1013–1018, 1996.

4. Chan AK, Duh QY, Katz MH, et al: Clinical manifestations of primary hyperparathyroidism before and after parathyroidectomy: A case-control study. Ann Surg 222:402–412, 1995.

5. Denham DW, Norman J: Cost-effectiveness of preoperative sestamibi scan for primary hyperparathyroidism is dependent solely upon the surgeon's choice of operative procedure. J Am Coll Surg 186:293–305, 1998.

6. Hedback G, Oden A, Tisell LE: The influence of surgery on the risk of death in patients with primary hyper-parathyroidism. World J Surg 15:399–405, 1991.

7. Marx SJ: Hyperparathyroid and hypoparathyroid disorders. N Engl J Med 343:1863–1875, 2000.

8. McIntyre RC Jr, Eisenach JH, Pearlman NW, et al: Intrathyroidal parathyroid glands can be a cause of failed cervical exploration for hyperparathyroidism. Am J Surg 174:750–753; 753–754, 1997.

9. McIntyre RC Jr, Kumpe DA, Liechty RD: Reexploration and angiographic ablation for hyperparathyroidism. Arch Surg 129:499–503, 1994.

10. Molinari AS, Irvin GL 3d, Deriso GT, Bott L: Incidence of multiglandular disease in primary hyperparathyroidism determined by parathyroid hormone secretion. Surgery 120:934–936, 1996.

11. Norman J, Chheda H: Minimally invasive parathyroidectomy facilitated by intraoperative nuclear mapping. Surgery 122:998–1003, 1997.

12. Palmer M, Adami HO, Bergstrom R, et al: Mortality after surgery for primary hyperparathyroidism: A follow-up of 441 patients operated on from 1956 to 1979. Surgery 102:1–7, 1987.

13. Saaristo RA, Salmi JJ, Koobi T, et al: Intraoperative localization of parathyroid glands with gamma counter probe in primary hyperparathyroidism: A prospective study. J Am Coll Surg 195:19–22, 2002.

14. Silverberg SJ, Shane E, Jacobs TP, et al: A 10-year prospective study of primary hyperparathyroidism with or without parathyroid surgery. N Engl J Med 341:1249–1255, 1999.

15. Sivula A, Pelkonen R: Long-term health risk of primary hyperparathyroidism: The effect of surgery. Ann Med 28:95–100, 1996.

16. Sywak MS, Knowlton ST, Pasieka JL, et al: Do the National Institutes of Health consensus guidelines for parathyroidectomy predict symptom severity and surgical outcome in patients with primary hyperparathyroidism? Surgery 132:1013–1019, 2002.

17. Udelsman R: Six hundred fifty-six consecutive explorations for primary hyperparathyroidism. Ann Surg 235:665–670; 670–662, 2002.

CHAPTER 58

HYPERTHYROIDISM

Robert C. McIntyre, Jr., M.D.

1. **What are the symptoms and signs of hyperthyroidism?**

General:	Heat intolerance, perspiration, flushing, tremor, sleep disturbance
Psychological:	Nervousness, emotional lability, anxiety, aggressiveness, delusions
Cardiovascular:	Palpitations, tachycardia, supraventricular dysrhythmias
Respiratory:	Breathlessness, hoarseness
Gastrointestinal:	Increased appetite, weight loss, increased frequency of bowel movements
Reproductive:	Gynecomastia, irregular menses
Bone:	Osteoporosis
Other:	Ophthalmopathy, dermopathy

2. **What causes hyperthyroidism?**

Graves' disease	Factitious thyrotoxicosis
Plummer's disease (toxic nodular goiter)	Iatrogenic hyperthyroidism
	Struma ovarii
Toxic multinodular goiter	Jodbasedow
Thyroiditis (subacute, postpartum)	Pituitary thyrotropin-secreting tumor

3. **How should hyperthyroidism be investigated?**

   A thyroid stimulating hormone (TSH) level is the best intial test. A low TSH with a high serum level of thyroxine (T_4) or triiodothyronine (T_3) is diagnostic. A high TSH with an increase in free T_4 indicates the rare patient with a thyrotropin-producing pituitary tumor.

   After the diagnosis of hyperthyroidism is made, the radioactive iodine uptake (RAIU) can differentiate the many causes.

4. **What are the three treatment options?**

   Antithyroid drugs (ATD), radioiodine, and surgery.

5. **Which drugs are useful for the treatment of hyperthyroidism? What are their mechanisms of action?**

   Methimazole and propylthiouracil (PTU) are the mainstays of treatment. The goal of treatment is remission of Graves' disease during therapy or euthyroidism before treatment with radioiodine or surgery. Both drugs inhibit organification of iodine and coupling of iodothyronines. PTU also inhibits the peripheral monodeiodination of T_4 to T_3. Treatment is started with 20 mg/day of methimazole or 100 mg of PTU 3 times/day. The dose may be reduced after 6 weeks of treatment as the patient shows clinical and biochemical improvement. Therapy is usually maintained for 2 years. Patients must be monitored for side effects, which include rash, pruritus, agranulocytosis, hepatitis, cholestatic jaundice, and lupus-like syndrome.

Beta-adrenergic antagonists ameliorate the signs and symptoms of disease. They should not be used alone except for short periods before radioiodine or surgical therapy. Nadolol (80 mg/day) and atenolol (100 mg/day) are the most common agents.

Iodine given as Lugol's solution (5% iodine and 10% potassium iodide in water, 0.3 mL/day) or potassium iodide (60 mg 3 times/day) inhibits the release of thyroid hormone. It is useful for short-term therapy in preparation for surgery, after radioiodine therapy to hasten the decrease in hormone levels, and for treatment of thyroid storm.

6. **What are the indications for and outcome of drug treatment?**
   ATD therapy is reserved for mild hyperthyroidism and a small gland. Long-term remission of Graves' hyperthyroidism during antithyroid drug therapy occurs in 50% of patients. Relapse is most common in the first 6 months after cessation of treatment.

7. **What is the regimen of radioiodine treatment?**
   Radioiodine is the most common therapy. The usual dose of radioiodine is 10 mCi. If hyperthyroidism is not cured, the dose should be repeated in 6 months. Pretreatment with antithyroid drug therapy should achieve a euthyroid state. Steroids prevent progression of ophthalmopathy. Prednisone is used at a dose of 0.5 mg/kg body weight, starting 3 days after radioiodine therapy and continuing for 1 month. The dose is tapered over 2 months.

   Pregnancy is an absolute contraindication. Women of childbearing age should be evaluated with a pregnancy test before treatment and should avoid pregnancy for 6 months after treatment. Evidence indicates that radioiodine may exacerbate ophthalmopathy.

8. **What is the outcome of radioiodine treatment?**
   Euthyroidism is not achieved for months after treatment. After euthyroidism is achieved, recurrence of hyperthyroidism is rare. Hypothyroidism, the only serious side effect, is dose dependent. It occurs at a rate of 3% per year, affecting 50% of patients at 10 years, and nearly 100% at 25 years.

9. **What are the indications for thyroidectomy for hyperthyroidism?**
   - Pregnant patients who are difficult to treat medically
   - Patients with large goiters and low radioiodine uptake
   - Children
   - Noncompliant patients
   - Patients with nodules suspected to be cancerous
   - Patients with compression of the trachea or esophagus
   - Patients with cosmetic concerns
   - Patients with ophthalmopathy

10. **How should patients be prepared for surgery?**
    Any patient with hyperthyroidism should be rendered euthyroid before surgery. Patients may be treated with antithyroid medication and potassium iodine. Beta-adrenergic antagonists should also be used alone or in combination with the above regimen.

11. **What is the extent of thyroidectomy?**
    The two surgical options for Graves' disease are subtotal thyroidectomy or near-total thyroidectomy. The goal of subtotal thyroidectomy is to preserve 8 g of well-vascularized thyroid tissue to avoid hypothyroidism. Because of the small risk of recurrence (10%), however, some surgeons prefer near-total thyroidectomy. In Plummer's disease, lobectomy or partial thyroidectomy for unilateral lesions and contralateral subtotal thyroidectomy for multiple lesions render the patient euthyroid.

12. **What is the incidence of hypothyroidism after surgery?**
    All patients having a near-total thyroidectomy become hypothyroid and need thyroxine replacement. Hypothyroidism occurs in 50% of patients with subtotal thyroidectomy.

KEY POINTS: HYPERTHYROIDISM

1. A thyroid-stimulating hormone (TSH) level is the best initial test.

2. Methimazole and propylthiouracil are the mainstays of medical treatment.

3. The two surgical options for Graves' disease are subtotal thyroidectomy and near-total thyroidectomy.

13. **What is the appropriate treatment for toxic nodular goiter?**
Hyperthyroidism caused by toxic nodular goiter is permanent and without spontaneous remission; antithyroid drugs are not appropriate long-term therapy. Radioiodine is the most common form of therapy. Larger doses (50 mCi) minimize the risk of persistent hyperthyroidism in such patients, who tend to be older and to have prominent cardiovascular symptoms of hyperthyroidism.

14. **What is the appropriate treatment for hyperthyroidism caused by thyroiditis?**
Subacute thyroiditis should be suspected if the patient has pain and tenderness in the thyroid region. The hyperthyroidism is usually mild and of short duration (i.e., weeks). Patients are treated with a beta-adrenergic antagonist and salicylate or glucocorticoid. Hypothyroidism may occur but is usually not permanent.

15. **What is the appropriate treatment for thyroid storm?**
Thyrotoxic crisis should be treated in the intensive care unit. General measures include hydration, antipyresis (acetaminophen), and nutrition. Specific measures include inhibition of T_4 synthesis and conversion to T_3 with PTU at a dose of 100 mg orally, via nasogastric tube, or rectally every 6 hours. Iodides inhibit T_4 release (saturated solution of potassium iodide, 5 drops by mouth or nasogastric tube every 6 hours). Steroids (dexamethasone, 2 mg every 6 hours) also inhibit T_4 release and conversion to T_3. Beta-adrenergic antagonists (propranolol or esmolol) may control cardiovascular manifestations. The last-resort management option is T_4 removal by plasmapheresis, hemoperfusion, or dialysis.

16. **Who performed the first thyroidectomy?**
Johann von Mikulicz-Radecki performed the first thyroidectomy in 1885.

17. **Which surgeon won the Nobel Prize for his work with thyroid disease?**
Theodor Kocher won the Nobel Prize in medicine in 1909. He was successful in reducing the high mortality rate of thyroidectomy to less than 1%. His most significant achievement was in describing postoperative hypothyroidism as *cachexia strumipriva.*

BIBLIOGRAPHY

1. Bartalena L, Marcocci C, Bogazzi F, et al: Relation between therapy for hyperthyroidism and the course of Graves' ophthalmopathy. N Engl J Med 338:73–78, 1998.

2. David E, Rosen IB, Bain J, et al: Management of the hot thyroid nodule. Am J Surg 170:481–483, 1995.

3. Franklyn JA: The management of hyperthyroidism. N Engl J Med 330:1731–1738, 1994.

4. Franklyn JA, Daykin J, Drolc Z, et al: Long-term follow-up of treatment of thyrotoxicosis by three different methods. Clin Endocrinol (Oxf) 34:71–76, 1991.

5. Kang AS, Grant CS, Thompson GB, van Heerden JA: Current treatment of nodular goiter with hyperthyroidism (Plummer's disease): Surgery versus radioiodine. Surgery 132:916–923, 2002.

6. Miccoli P, Vitti P, Rago T, et al: Surgical treatment of Graves' disease: Subtotal or total thyroidectomy? Surgery 120:1020–1024, 1996.

7. Singer PA, Cooper DS, Levy EG, et al: Treatment guidelines for patients with hyperthyroidism and hypothyroidism. Standards of Care Committee, American Thyroid Association. JAMA 273:808–812, 1995.

8. Torring O, Tallstedt L, Wallin G, et al: Graves' hyperthyroidism: Treatment with antithyroid drugs, surgery, or radioiodine: A prospective, randomized study. Thyroid Study Group. J Clin Endocrinol Metab 81:2986–2993, 1996.

9. Weetman AP: Graves' disease. N Engl J Med 343:1236–1248, 2000.

10. Witte J, Goretzki PE, Dotzenrath C, et al: Surgery for Graves' disease: Total versus subtotal thyroidectomy: Results of a prospective randomized trial. World J Surg 24:1303–1311, 2000.

CHAPTER 59

THYROID NODULES AND CANCER

Robert C. McIntyre, Jr., M.D.

1. **What is the prevalence of thyroid nodules and cancer?**

   Thyroid nodules increase throughout life. Nodules are four times more common in females than in males, and 50% of 50-year-old women have a palpable nodule. After exposure to radiation, nodules develop at approximately 2% annually, reaching a peak at 25 years. Nodules are 10 times more frequent in glands examined by ultrasound, at surgery, or at autopsy. Fewer than 50% of thyroid nodules that appear solitary on physical examination are truly solitary.

   Each year in the United States, there are approximately 15,000 new cases and 1000 deaths due to thyroid cancer. Up to 35% of thyroid glands examined at autopsy contain occult papillary cancer (< 1.0 cm).

2. **What is the importance of the distinction between solitary and multiple thyroid nodules?**

   Traditionally, multiple thyroid nodules were considered benign and solitary thyroid nodules malignant. However, multiple series suggest that a dominant nodule in a multinodular gland carries the same risk of cancer as a solitary nodule (5%).

3. **What is the differential diagnosis of thyroid nodules?**

   Adenoma
   > Macrofollicular (colloid)
   > Microfollicular
   > Embryonal
   > Hurthle cell

   Carcinoma
   > Papillary
   > Follicular
   > Medullary
   > Anaplastic
   > Lymphoma
   > Metastatic

   Cyst
   Nodular goiter with a dominant nodule
   Other
   > Inflammatory diseases (e.g., Hashimoto's thyroiditis)
   > Developmental abnormalities

4. **What features of the history and physical examination indicate a higher risk of cancer?**

   Nodules occurring at the extremes of age are more likely to be cancerous, particularly in males. Rapid growth and local invasion raise the possibility of malignancy, but associated symptoms (e.g., hoarseness, dysphagia) are uncommon. A history of radiation exposure increases the frequency of both benign and malignant nodules. A family history of medullary or papillary thyroid cancer or Gardner's syndrome (i.e., familial polyposis) increases the risk of cancer.

Cancer is more often found in patients with firm, solitary nodules. Fixation to adjacent structures, vocal cord paralysis, and enlarged lymph nodes also are associated with an increased risk of malignancy.

5. **What is the proper laboratory evaluation of a patient with a thyroid nodule?**
   The only biochemical test that is routinely needed is a serum thyroid-stimulating hormone (TSH) concentration to identify patients with unsuspected hyperthyroidism. In patients with suspected medullary thyroid carcinoma (MTC), serum calcitonin should be measured. In patients with known medullary carcinoma, serum calcium levels and 24-hour urine collection for assessment of catecholamines and their metabolic products should be done to exclude multiple endocrine neoplasia (MEN II) before thyroidectomy. Patients with MTC should have lymphocyte-derived DNA analysis for *ret* proto-oncogene mutations.

6. **Which single test best predicts the need for surgical intervention?**
   The single best test to predict the need for surgery is fine-needle aspiration (FNA). If an adequate specimen is obtained, the three possible results are benign (70%), suspicious (15%), and malignant (5%). FNA is most reliable for the diagnosis of papillary carcinoma and in patients with medullary and anaplastic cancer. It is least reliable in distinguishing benign from malignant follicular and Hurthle cell neoplasms. The overall accuracy exceeds 95% in experienced hands. When FNA reveals cancer, it is 97% correct (3% false-positive rate); when it indicates a benign nodule, cancer is present in 4% of cases (4% false-negative rate). When the FNA is suspicious, 30% of nodules are malignant.

7. **What other tests may be useful in the evaluation of a thyroid nodule?**
   Thyroid radionuclide studies with isotopes of either iodine (most common) or technetium often are performed but cannot reliably differentiate malignant from benign nodules. Scans may be useful in patients with indeterminate FNA results and TSH < 1.5 μIU/mL because hyperfunctioning nodules are almost always benign.

   Ultrasound categorizes nodules as cystic, solid, or mixed and is the best measure of the size of a nodule. Ultrasound can be used to determine the presence of other nodules in a patient with a solitary nodule on physical examination. It is particularly useful to follow the size of a nodule. Similar to radionuclide scans, ultrasound cannot distinguish malignant from benign nodules; thus, it is not routinely used in the evaluation of a nodule.

8. **Should a solitary thyroid nodule be suppressed with thyroxine for 3–6 months to determine whether it is benign or malignant?**
   Most nodules change very little over the short term. In one series, 13% of nodules decreased in size, 22% disappeared, 46% did not change, and 19% enlarged. Studies of thyroxine therapy suggest that drug treatment is not superior to placebo in patients with solitary nodules. Most nodules do not change in size, 30% decrease in size, and a few increase in size. Thus, the response to thyroxine is not a reliable indicator of malignancy.

9. **What are the types and distribution of thyroid cancer?**

Papillary	70%
Follicular	20%
Medullary	5%
Anaplastic and lymphoma	5%

10. **What are the axioms of thyroid surgery?**
    - A meticulously dry operative field must be maintained.
    - Tissue in the region of the recurrent laryngeal nerve should not be cut or clamped until the nerve is definitively identified.
    - Every parathyroid gland should be treated as if it were the last functioning gland.
    - If malignancy is suspected, the entire operation should be done as if the lesion were cancer.

11. **What is the minimal extent of thyroidectomy for a solitary thyroid nodule?**
The goal of surgery is to remove all foci of neoplastic tissue and any palpable cervical adenopathy. With the exception of small lesions in the thyroid isthmus, the minimal procedure for suspected malignancy should be lobectomy, including the isthmus (as a diagnostic biopsy). Enucleation is to be avoided. Frozen section is accurate for papillary, medullary, and anaplastic carcinoma. Frozen section is no more accurate than FNA for follicular and Hurthle cell carcinoma. Functioning "toxic" nodules may be resected by a partial lobectomy because they are usually benign. If the lesion is large, a lobectomy is preferred.

12. **What is the most common form of thyroiditis in nodules?**
Hashimoto's thyroiditis, subacute thyroiditis, and Reidel struma (rare). These conditions usually do not require surgery. Thyroidectomy is indicated for compressive symptoms or when cancer cannot be excluded.

13. **What is the surgical therapy for thyroid carcinoma?**
Thyroid carcinoma should be treated by near-total or total thyroidectomy except in young patients with small, well-differentiated tumors (≤ 1 cm) and no evidence of lymph node or extrathyroidal disease. In such cases, lobectomy with resection of the isthmus is adequate therapy. Near-total thyroidectomy eliminates multifocal cancer in the thyroid, allows postoperative radioiodine for the diagnosis and therapy of metastatic disease, decreases the risk of local-regional recurrence, and improves the accuracy of serum thyroglobulin as a marker for persistent or recurrent disease. Enlarged cervical lymph nodes should be removed and examined by frozen section. If metastatic cancer is identified, a neck dissection is performed. "Berry picking" results in an increased rate of regional recurrence and should be avoided in favor of anatomic dissections.
Because medullary thyroid cancer is not responsive to radioiodine or levothyroxine, a total thyroidectomy should be performed. A central neck dissection is mandatory to evaluate metastatic disease. If the central nodes are positive for cancer on frozen section, an ipsilateral modified neck dissection is performed. The contralateral neck may be observed.
Surgery for anaplastic carcinoma is palliative and usually is limited to debulking and tracheostomy for relief of compressive symptoms.

14. **Describe the arterial supply and venous drainage of the thyroid.**
The blood supply to the thyroid gland comes from the superior and inferior thyroid arteries. Occasionally, a midline thyroid imma artery arises from the aortic arch. The superior thyroid artery is the first branch of the external carotid artery. The inferior thyroid artery arises from the thyrocervical trunk.

The three major veins are the superior, middle, and inferior thyroid veins. The superior and middle thyroid veins drain into the internal jugular vein, and the inferior vein drains into the innominate vein.

15. **Describe the anatomy of the recurrent laryngeal nerves.**
The right recurrent laryngeal nerve (RLN) arises from the vagus and loops around the right subclavian artery. The left vagus nerve gives off the left RLN and loops around the aorta. The RLNs run obliquely through the neck, usually in the tracheoesophageal groove. Low in the neck, the nerves are more lateral and course medially as they ascend. The right nerve runs more obliquely than the left. Occasionally, the RLN may branch before entering the larynx, usually on the left side. The motor fibers are usually in the most medial branch. In 1% of cases, the right RLN is not recurrent and enters the neck from a lateral and superior direction.

16. **What defect results from injury to the RLN?**
Injury to a single RLN results in a paralyzed vocal cord, which causes a weak, hoarse voice. Patients also have abnormal swallowing and problems with aspiration. Injury to both nerves causes paralysis of both cords and obstruction of airflow. This situation necessitates a tracheostomy. RLN injury occurs in 1% of thyroidectomies.

17. **Describe the anatomy of the superior laryngeal nerve and the defect that occurs with its injury.**
The superior laryngeal nerve gives off the external laryngeal nerve, which runs medial to the superior pole vessels to enter the cricothyroid muscle. This motor nerve (i.e., Amelita Galli-Curci nerve) increases tension of the vocal cords, allowing for high notes. The internal laryngeal nerve provides the sensory innervation to the posterior pharynx. It lies superior to the thyroid cartilage. Injury to the nerve leads to a weak, low voice that lacks resonance. Patients may also have problems with aspiration.

18. **What is the other major complication of thyroidectomy?**
Permanent hypoparathyroidism occurs in 1% of patients who have had thyroidectomies.

19. **What is the postoperative therapy for well-differentiated thyroid carcinoma?**
Patients with risk factors should be treated with postoperative radioiodine (I-131). Risk factors include older age (> 45 years old), male gender, tumor size, direct local invasion, nodal spread, and distant disease. All patients with well-differentiated thyroid cancer should be treated with levothyroxine (Synthroid) to suppress serum levels of TSH (0.2–0.5 μU/mL). This three-component therapy (i.e., surgery, I-131, levothyroxine) results in the lowest recurrence rate.

20. **How should a patient be followed after therapy for well-differentiated thyroid carcinoma?**
In young, low-risk patients, physical examination of the neck is done every 6 months for 2 years and then yearly thereafter. In high-risk patients, close follow-up includes repeat neck examination in addition to assessment of serum thyroglobulin (Tg) levels, diagnostic radioiodine scans, and cervical ultrasound. Assessment of the serum Tg and scanning depends on the state of the serum TSH. In order to fully evaluate for recurrent disease, the patient should be taken off thyroxine or given recombinent TSH (Thyrogen).
Patients with recurrent cervical disease by palpation or ultrasound should have repeat surgery if the procedure can be performed with low morbidity. After removal of gross disease, patients should be treated with radioiodine. Distant disease should be treated with radioiodine if the metastases take up iodine.

WEB SITE

http://www.acssurgery.com

BIBLIOGRAPHY

1. Cady B: Presidential address: Beyond risk groups—a new look at differentiated thyroid cancer. Surgery 124:947–957, 1998.

2. Duren M, Siperstein AE, Shen W, et al: Value of stimulated serum thyroglobulin levels for detecting persistent or recurrent differentiated thyroid cancer in high- and low-risk patients. Surgery 126:13–19, 1999.

3. Frilling A, Tecklenborg K, Gorges R, et al: Preoperative diagnostic value of [(18)F] fluorodeoxyglucose positron emission tomography in patients with radioiodine-negative recurrent well-differentiated thyroid carcinoma. Ann Surg 234:804–811, 2001.

4. Haugen BR, Ridgway EC, McLaughlin BA, McDermott MT: Clinical comparison of whole-body radioiodine scan and serum thyroglobulin after stimulation with recombinant human thyrotropin. Thyroid 12:37–43, 2002.

5. Hay ID, Grant CS, Bergstralh EJ, et al: Unilateral total lobectomy: is it sufficient surgical treatment for patients with AMES low-risk papillary thyroid carcinoma? Surgery 124:958–964, 1998.

6. Moley JF, DeBenedetti MK: Patterns of nodal metastases in palpable medullary thyroid carcinoma: Recommendations for extent of node dissection. Ann Surg 229:880–887, 1999.

7. Rodriguez GJ, Balsalobre MD, Pomares F, et al: Prophylactic thyroidectomy in MEN 2A syndrome: Experience in a single center. J Am Coll Surg 195:159–166, 2002.

8. Singer PA, Cooper DS, Daniels GH, et al: Treatment guidelines for patients with thyroid nodules and well-differentiated thyroid cancer. American Thyroid Association. Arch Intern Med 156:2165–2172, 1996.

9. Sivanandan R, Soo KC: Pattern of cervical lymph node metastases from papillary carcinoma of the thyroid. Br J Surg 88:1241–1244, 2001.

10. Stojadinovic A, Hoos A, Ghossein RA, et al: Hurthle cell carcinoma: A 60-year experience. Ann Surg Oncol 9:197–203, 2002.

11. Stojadinovic A, Shaha AR, Orlikoff RF, et al: Prospective functional voice assessment in patients undergoing thyroid surgery. Ann Surg 236:823–832, 2002.

12. Udelsman R, Westra WH, Donovan PI, et al: Randomized prospective evaluation of frozen-section analysis for follicular neoplasms of the thyroid. Ann Surg 233:716–722, 2001.

CHAPTER 60

SURGICAL HYPERTENSION

Thomas A. Whitehill, M.D.

1. **What are the surgically correctable causes of hypertension?**
   Renovascular hypertension, pheochromocytoma, Cushing's syndrome, primary hyperaldosteronism (Conn's syndrome), coarctation of the aorta, and unilateral renal parenchymal disease. Surgical hypertension accounts for 5% of all hypertensive patients.

2. **Which form of surgical hypertension is most common?**
   Renovascular hypertension is most common. Although the overall frequency of renovascular hypertension among patients with elevated diastolic blood pressure is about 3%, moderate or severe diastolic hypertension may be caused by renal artery occlusive disease in as many as 25% of cases. Pheochromocytoma, hyperaldosteronism, Cushing's disease, and coarctation of the aorta each are found in only 0.1% of all hypertensive patients.

3. **What are the most common causes of renovascular hypertension?**
   Atherosclerosis causes 70% of cases; it affects men twice as often as women. The second most common cause is fibromuscular dysplasia (25%). Of the many pathologic subtypes, the most common is medial fibrodysplasia (85%); it invariably affects women. Last is developmental renal artery stenosis (10%), which is often associated with neurofibromatosis and abdominal aortic coarctation.

4. **What clinical criteria support the pursuit of investigative studies for suspected renovascular hypertension?**
   Although no clinical characteristics are pathognomonic of renovascular hypertension, the following findings strongly suggest the presence of an underlying renal artery stenotic lesion:
   - Hypertension in very young individuals or in women younger than 50 years of age
   - Rapid onset of severe hypertension after age 50 years
   - Hypertension refractory to three-drug regimens
   - Initial presentation with diastolic blood pressure > 115 mmHg or sudden worsening of presumed preexisting hypertension
   - Accelerated or malignant hypertension
   - Deterioration of renal function after the initiation of antihypertensive agents, especially angiotensin-converting enzyme (ACE) inhibitors
   - Systolic or diastolic upper abdominal or flank bruits

5. **What is the renin-angiotensin-aldosterone system (RAAS)?**
   Renin is released from the juxtaglomerular apparatus of the kidney in response to changes in renal cortical afferent arteriolar perfusion pressure. Renin acts locally and in the systemic circulation on renin substrate (angiotensinogen), a nonvasoactive alpha$_2$ globulin is produced in the liver to form angiotensin I. Angiotensin I undergoes enzymatic cleavage by ACE in the pulmonary circulation to produce angiotensin II, a potent vasopressor responsible for the vasoconstrictive element of renovascular hypertension. Angiotensin II increases adrenal gland production of aldosterone with subsequent retention of sodium and water; this process establishes the volume element of renovascular hypertension.

6. **How do ACE inhibitors work?**

Direct inhibition of ACE decreases concentrations of angiotensin II, which leads to decreased vasopressor activity and decreased aldosterone secretion. Removal of angiotensin II negative feedback on renin secretion leads to increased plasma renin activity.

7. **Should patients with renovascular hypertension be treated medically or surgically?**

Although prospective randomized studies comparing drug and interventional therapy have not been published, surgical treatment and percutaneous transluminal renal angioplasty (PTRA) have been favored over drug therapy by most clinicians. The key is early recognition of the problem.

8. **When should patients with renovascular hypertension be treated with PTRA?**

Clear indications for PTRA include nonorificial atherosclerotic lesions and medial fibrodysplastic lesions limited to the main renal artery.

9. **What findings on history and physical examination should lead to a suspicion of pheochromocytoma?**

Pheochromocytomas are tumors primarily of the adrenal medulla and extraadrenal paraganglia cells. Approximately 90% of them are found within the adrenal gland, and the remaining 10% are scattered along the abdominal paravertebral sympathetic chain or in ganglia located remotely (e.g., urinary bladder, pelvic nerves). Tumors are classified as functioning when they produce catecholamines, always autonomously and usually in great excess. The predictable clinical effects of increased endogenous catecholamine outpouring is sustained hypertension with episodes of increased blood pressure, tachycardia, headache, palpitations, or flushing. Rarely, patients maintain periods of normotension with infrequent and unpredictable paroxysmal episodes of hypertension.

10. **How is pheochromocytoma diagnosed?**

Diagnosis is best confirmed by 24-hour urine collection for excreted catecholamines, metanephrines, and vanillylmandelic acid. The best single test to confirm the diagnosis of pheochromocytoma is still debated; some believe that the metanephrine level is the most precise (85%). Plasma catecholamines are also a specific test, but given the variability of results in individual patients and in many assays, the current approach should continue to emphasize the use of urinary catecholamines. Eighty percent of patients with pheochromocytoma have at least one urinary metabolite greater than twice the normal value. The diagnosis of pheochromocytoma should be followed by studies to localize the tumor.

KEY POINTS: SURGICAL HYPERTENSION

1. The causes of surgically correctable hypertension include renovascular hypertension, pheochromocytoma, Cushing's syndrome, Conn's syndrome, coarctation of the aorta, and unilateral renal parenchymal disease.

2. The most common cause of renovascular hypertension is atherosclerosis.

3. The diagnosis of pheochromocytoma is confirmed by 24-hour urine collection for excreted catecholamines, metanephrines, and vanillylmandelic acid.

4. Conn's syndrome is characterized by hypertension, hypokalemia, hypernatremia, metabolic alkalosis, and periodic muscle weakness and paralysis.

11. **What is the best test to localize a pheochromocytoma?**
    Computed tomography (CT) scanning, magnetic resonance imaging (MRI), and ^{131}I-metaiodoben-zylguanidine (MIBG) scanning are three available imaging modalitites. Because 97% of pheochro-mocytomas are intraabdominal and almost always > 2 cm, an abdominal CT scan (thin cuts through the adrenal bed from the diaphragm to the aortic bifurcation) rarely misses a lesion and provides good anatomic detail. MRI has been increasingly used because 90% of pheochromocy-tomas are characteristically bright on T_2 weighted images. MIBG is best used in patients who are suspected to have extraadrenal, multifocal, or recurrent pheochromocytoma. It is less sensitive than CT and MRI. MIBG is best reserved for patients at higher risk for multiple or extra-adrenal tumors and malignant pheochromocytoma.

12. **Describe the immediate antihypertensive treatment in patients with pheochromocytoma.**
    Hypertension from pheochromocytoma is caused by activation of vascular smooth muscle alpha$_1$-receptors, which results in vasoconstriction. Thus, the best acute treatment is intra-venous administration of an alpha$_1$-antagonist or -blocker; options include phenoxybenzamine, prazosin, or terazosin. Second-line agents include calcium channel blockers and ACE inhibitors. Antiarrhythmic beta-blockade should be avoided initially because these agents cause both unop-posed peripheral alpha$_1$-receptor stimulation and decreased cardiac output (secondary to high vascular resistance). Congestive heart failure may be precipitated by beta-blocking the heart before lowering the blood pressure.

13. **How is primary hyperaldosteronism (Conn's syndrome) diagnosed?**
    Conn's syndrome, which results from autonomous mineralocorticoid hypersecretion, is characterized by hypertension, hypokalemia, hypernatremia, metabolic alkalosis, and periodic muscle weakness and paralysis, often caused by an aldosterone-secreting adenoma. The syndrome is now identified by the combined findings of hypokalemia, suppressed plasma renin activity despite sodium restriction, and high urinary and plasma aldosterone levels after sodium repletion in hypertensive patients.

14. **Why does Cushing's syndrome or Cushing's disease cause hypertension?**
    Both cause hypercortisolism or excessive amounts of glucocorticoids. In the cardio-vascular system, glucocorticoids produce increased cardiac chronotropic and inotropic effects, along with an increased peripheral vascular resistance. Receptors in the distal renal tubules respond to glucocorticoids by increasing tubular resorption of sodium. These receptors belong to a different class from receptors that mediate the more potent actions of aldosterone.

15. **What findings suggest aortic coarctation?**
    Lower blood pressure in the legs than in the arms and diminished or absent femoral pulses. Rib notching may be evident on chest radiograph in patients with long-standing, hemodynami-cally significant coarctation. Bruits may be heard over the chest or abdominal wall. Adults may even develop congestive heart failure and renal failure.

16. **How does aortic coarctation cause hypertension?**
    No single cause has been identified. Mechanical obstruction to ventricular ejection is one com-ponent that leads to upper extremity hytertension. Hypoperfusion of the kidneys with resulting activation of the RAAS probably contributes. Abnormal aortic compliance, variable capacity of collateral vessels, and abnormal setting of baroreceptors also have been implicated.

BIBLIOGRAPHY

1. Blumenfeld JD, Sealey JE, Schlussel Y, et al: Diagnosis and therapy of primary hyperaldosteronism. Ann Intern Med 121:877–885, 1994.

2. Coen G, Calabria S, Lai S, et al: Atherosclerotic ischemic renal disease: Diagnosis and prevalence in an hypertensive and/or uremic elderly population. BMC Nephrol 4:2, 2003.

3. Hansen KJ, Deitch JS, Oskin TC, et al: Renal artery repair: Consequences of operative failures. Ann Surg 277:678–690, 1998.

4. Kebebew E, Duh Q-Y: Benign and malignant pheochromocytoma: Diagnosis, treatment and follow-up. Surg Oncol Clin North Am 7:765–789, 1998.

5. Lairmore TC, Ball DW, Baylin SB, et al: Management of pheochromocytomas in patients with multiple endocrine neoplasia type 2 syndromes. Ann Surg 217:595–603, 1993.

6. Nicholson T: Magnetic resonance angiography for the diagnosis of renal artery stenosis. Clin Radiol 58:257, 2003.

7. Oskin TC, Hansen KJ, Deitch JS, et al: Chronic renal artery occlusion: Nephrectomy versus revascularization. J Vasc Surg 29:140–149, 1999.

8. Palmaz JC: The current status of vascular intervention in ischemic nephropathy. J Vasc Interv Radiol 9:439–543, 1998.

9. Stanley JC: Surgical treatment of renovascular hypertension. Am J Surg 174:102–110, 1997.

10. Wong JM, Hansen KJ, Oskin TC, et al: Surgery after failed percutaneous renal artery angioplasty. J Vasc Surg 30:468–483, 1999.

BREAST MASSES

Christina A. Finlayson, M.D.

CHAPTER 61

1. **What are the three parts of breast screening that assist in the early diagnosis of breast cancer?**
   Breast self-examination (BSE) should begin at age 20 years and should be performed monthly. The breast is usually easiest to examine on the days immediately after the menstrual cycle. BSE can be frustrating to patients, particularly when they have fibrocystic changes, because they are not certain what they are feeling or supposed to feel. The BSE technique should be taught early and reinforced regularly. Women who regularly perform BSE present with tumors 1 cm or smaller more frequently than women who do not perform BSE. BSE has yet to translate into a survival benefit, however. Some women are spooked by repetitive false-positive findings. These women need to rely on their physicians to perform a breast examination once a year.

   Clinical or physician breast examination (CBE) should also begin at age 20 years and should be performed annually for women at average risk for breast cancer. Although tumors between 0.5 and 1.0 cm occasionally can be detected by experienced clinicians, tumors between 1.0 and 1.5 cm are detected 60% of the time. Ninety-six percent of tumors larger than 2.0 cm are identified. CBE should be part of every primary care physician's health maintenance and screening program.

   Screening mammography has had the most substantial impact on the early diagnosis of and subsequent decrease in mortality from breast cancer.

2. **When should routine mammography begin?**
   When mammography screening begins at age 40 years, a 30% or greater decrease in death from breast cancer can be realized. Mammography should be performed annually thereafter.

3. **Does a normal or negative mammogram result guarantee that no cancer is present?**
   No. Mammography has a false-negative rate of at least 15%. For a breast cancer to be detected on mammography, it must have radiographic characteristics that differ from the surrounding tissue. Some tumors, particularly lobular carcinoma, invade breast tissue in a way that does not alter the radiograph.

4. **What is the difference between a screening and a diagnostic mammogram?**
   Screening mammography is done in asymptomatic women to look for clinically occult breast cancer. Two views of each breast are obtained. When a woman has a breast complaint such as a mass or an abnormal screening mammogram, diagnostic mammography is performed. A diagnostic mammogram focuses on the area of clinical concern. Additional views taken at multiple angles or compression views taken with increased magnification help to distinguish between benign and malignant changes.

5. **How are mammographic abnormalities characterized?**
   The American College of Radiology has developed a standard interpretation score to decrease ambiguity in mammographic reporting:
   Bi-Rads   0   Requires further evaluation
             1   Negative (normal examination results without any findings)

     2   Benign (normal examination results with a definitely benign finding)

     3   Probably benign (< 3% chance of malignancy)

     4   Suspicious (30% chance of malignancy)

     5   Highly suspicious or malignant

- **Category 0** is a temporary designation that requires further diagnostic imaging by either ultrasound or compression (magnification) views of the abnormality. After further evaluation, such mammograms are reclassified into one of the other categories.
- **Categories 1 and 2** require no further evaluation; the usual mammographic schedule is not altered.
- For **category 3**, a short-interval (6-month) diagnostic mammogram of the affected breast is recommended. Alternatively, a biopsy may be performed.
- **Categories 4 and 5** require a biopsy.

6. **Which biopsy techniques aid in the diagnosis of mammographic abnormalities?**
   Several image-guided biopsy techniques maximize diagnostic yield while minimizing patient discomfort and loss of normal tissue:

   Tru-cut core biopsy is performed with a 14–18-gauge coring needle. Multiple tissue samples (at least seven) are obtained.

   Stereotactic biopsy is performed with an 11-gauge, vacuum-assisted biopsy needle. Large-core biopsy can remove an entire lesion or area of calcification. A marking clip can be left in the breast at the site of the biopsy. Core biopsy and vacuum-assisted biopsy can be performed with local anesthesia alone.

   The **advanced breast biopsy instrument** (ABBI) removes up to a 2-cm core of breast tissue. It requires local anesthesia and intravenous (IV) sedation and usually is performed in the operating room.

   Needle localization breast biopsy is a surgical procedure that requires the radiologist to place a thin wire into the breast abnormality. In the operating room, the wire and the breast tissue surrounding the wire are removed. This procedure can be done with local anesthesia with or without sedation.

   Although **fine-needle aspiration** (FNA) is excellent for evaluation of palpable abnormalities, its sensitivity and specificity for image-guided biopsy are not acceptable.

   With the exception of FNA (which evaluates cells not intact tissue), each of these techniques is comparable in identifying the pathology associated with the mammographic abnormality. Unfortunately, a 5% false-negative rate is associated with each of these techniques.

7. **What are the characteristics of a dominant breast mass?**
   Identification of a dominant mass, especially in premenopausal women, can be challenging. Typically, a dominant mass can be palpated in three dimensions, and its density is palpably distinct from surrounding breast tissue. Of equal importance are nodule, lump, thickening, and asymmetry. Breast cancer cannot be excluded by physical examination alone. "Failure to be impressed by the physical examination findings" is the most common reason cited for a delay in the diagnosis of breast cancer.

8. **What are the most frequently encountered palpable breast masses?**
   Most dominant masses are benign. Examples include cysts, fibroadenomas, and fibrocystic masses. Carcinoma, although not the most common breast mass, is the reason that all persistent, dominant masses require a diagnosis. Other less common palpable breast masses are lipomas, granulomas, fat necrosis, epidermal inclusion cysts, and lactational adenomas.

9. **What are the distinguishing characteristics of the most common palpable masses?**
   A cyst is a regular, firm or fluctuant, mobile mass that may be tender. A fibroadenoma is smooth, firm, elongated (longer than it is wide), and mobile with discrete borders. Fibrocystic changes are "lumpy-bumpy" breast tissue. There may be a discrete focal area of fibrosis that is more dominant than the

background irregular tissue. Carcinoma is an irregular, hard, painless mass. In advanced stages, it may become fixed to the chest wall or be associated with overlying skin changes. Lobular carcinoma often appears as a soft mass or area of thickening. Because physical examination alone is unreliable in excluding breast cancer, a biopsy must be obtained for all persistent, dominant solid masses.

KEY POINTS: BREAST MASSES

1. A cyst is a regular, firm or fluctuant, mobile mass that may be tender.

2. A fibroadenoma is smooth, firm, elongated, and mobile with discrete borders.

3. Fibrocystic changes are "lumpy-bumpy" breast tissue.

4. Carcinoma is an irregular, hard, painless mass.

10. **A 32-year-old woman presents with the complaint of a breast lump. Which questions about the patient's history are important in the evaluation of the mass?**
The size of the mass, whether it has changed in size, how long it has been present, whether it is painful, skin changes, nipple discharge, and changes in relation to the menstrual cycle are all important. Assessment of risk factors, including personal or family history of breast, ovarian, or other cancers; age at menarche; age at first full-term pregnancy; age at menopause; birth control or hormone replacement use; and history of previous breast biopsy are also important.

11. **The mass identified in question 10 is discrete, not tender, easily palpable, and has gradually increased in size. What is the next step?**
Ultrasound of a discrete mass can determine if it is cystic or solid. Specific ultrasound criteria are used to define a simple cyst. A simple cyst can be aspirated or observed. A complex cyst must be further evaluated by aspiration (to see if it completely resolves) or by excisional biopsy (if it does not). A solid mass requires a tissue diagnosis.

12. **How is a cyst aspiration performed?**
A 22-gauge needle is inserted into the cyst, and fluid is withdrawn. Generally, a 10-mL syringe is adequate. If the cyst is quite deep and difficult to fix between the clinician's fingers, the aspiration can be performed under ultrasound guidance. Aspiration of a cyst is both diagnostic and therapeutic. After aspiration, the mass should resolve completely. If a mass persists or recurs after two aspirations, it should be excised. Cyst fluid may be clear or cloudy yellow, green, gray, or brown. A bloody aspirate obligates excision of the lesion.

13. **What techniques are available for diagnosis of a palpable, solid breast mass?**
FNA, core biopsy, incisional biopsy, and excisional biopsy each have a role:
FNA recovers cells from the mass and requires a dedicated cytopathologist for accurate interpretation. Some (but, not all) benign and malignant lesions can be characterized accurately by FNA, but FNA cannot discriminate between invasive and in situ carcinoma. To be used effectively, it must be correlated with physical examination and breast imaging.
Core biopsy is also a sampling technique that removes 14–18-gauge pieces of tissue for histologic evaluation. Because it is a sampling, there is a risk of missing the lesion and obtaining a false-negative result. Again, correlation with physical examination and imaging is important to avoid missing a cancer.
Incisional biopsy is rarely used today. Its primary role is for a highly suspicious lesion that is a candidate for neoadjuvant treatment and that is not definitively diagnosed on core biopsy.
Excisional biopsy completely removes the target lesion. It provides the most tissue for pathologic evaluation and, in benign disease, is both diagnostic and psychologically therapeutic.

14 . **What is the role for breast imaging in the evaluation of a palpable breast mass?**
Breast imaging helps to define the lesion and screen the remainder of the breast for secondary lesions. In general, breast imaging is performed before biopsy because the artifact from the biopsy can interfere with the interpretation of the study.

In women younger than age 30 years, in whom the risk of malignancy is low, mammography should be reserved for the most suspicious lesions. For women older than age 30 years, evaluation of a mass suspicious for malignancy includes mammography to characterize the mass and to evaluate the remainder of the breast. Ultrasound can reliably differentiate between cystic and solid masses. It is very unusual (< 2%) that ultrasound will fail to identify a clinically significant breast mass.

15 . **What is the "triple negative test" or "diagnostic triad"?**
There are three components to diagnosing a palpable breast abnormality: physical examination, breast imaging, and biopsy. Benign lesions do not have to be removed, but the difficulty is in differentiating between a benign and a malignant lesion. When the characteristics of a mass on physical examination indicate low suspicion for malignancy, the mammogram is benign, and FNA recovers benign cells, the likelihood that the lesion is benign is 98%. Treatment options include excision for definitive diagnosis or observation. If observation is elected, the abnormality should be reexamined within 3 months to confirm that it is stable. If any component of the diagnostic triad is worrisome, definitive diagnosis, usually with excisional biopsy, is necessary.

WEB SITE

http://www.acssurgery.com

BIBLIOGRAPHY

1. Cady B, Steele GD, Morrow M, et al: Evaluation of common breast problems: Guidance for primary care providers. Cancer 48:49–63, 1998.
2. Geller BM, Barlow WE, Ballard-Barbash R, et al: Use of the American College of Radiology BI-RADS to report on the mammographic evaluation of women with signs and symptoms of breast disease. Radiology 222:536–542, 2002.
3. Harris JR, Lippmann ME, Morrow M, et al (eds): Diseases of the Breast, 2nd ed. Philadelphia, Lippincott Williams & Wilkins, 2000.
4. Hendrick RE: Mortality reduction from screening mammography. Breast Diseases 13:303–307, 2003.
5. Morris KT, Vetto JT, Petty JK, et al: A new score for the evaluation of palpable breast masses in women under age 40. Am J Surg 184:346–347, 2002.
6. Singletary SE, Bevers T, Dempsey P, et al: Screening for and evaluation of suspicious breast lesions: NCCN practice guidelines. Oncology 12:89–138, 1998.
7. Thomas DB, Gao DL, Ray RM, Wang, et al: Randomized trial of breast self-examination in Shanghai: Final results. J Natl Cancer Inst 94:1445–1457, 2002.

PRIMARY THERAPY FOR BREAST CANCER

Benjamin O. Anderson, M.D.

CHAPTER 62

1. How is breast cancer diagnosed?

A diagnosis requires tissue confirmation by needle sampling or surgical biopsy. **Excisional biopsy** is the gold standard: the preferred initial diagnostic method has become **core-needle biopsy** or **fine-needle aspiration** (FNA). Needle sampling (1) allows complete operative planning, including decisions about lumpectomy margins or the use of sentinel node mapping and (2) does not distort the breast shape or architecture for future clinical breast examination (CBE) and breast imaging.

2. What are the limitations of needle sampling?

Both FNA and core-needle biopsy can have false-negative results caused by sampling error. If the needle sampling diagnosis is negative for cancer and these findings correlate with the clinical presentation and breast imaging findings (mammogram and ultrasound), all of which suggest a common benign breast process (**concordance**), then the patient may have clinical follow-up examination without further intervention. However, if the needle sampling results do not match the findings from clinical examination or breast imaging (**discordance**), then additional tissue sampling, such as by excisional biopsy, needs to be performed.

3. How do FNA and core-needle biopsy differ?

Whereas core-needle biopsy obtains *histologic* specimens, similar to miniature surgical biopsy, FNA obtains *cytologic* specimens, similar to a Pap smear. As a result, core-needle biopsy can distinguish invasive from noninvasive *(in situ)* cancers, but FNA cannot (also see question 9). Cytologic interpretation requires special training and expertise. A pathologist who is comfortable reading standard surgical breast slides will also be comfortable reading breast core-needle slides, but may not be comfortable reading breast FNA.

4. Why should the breast be imaged before performing a surgical breast biopsy?

Even with good imaging, surgeons can be surprised by histologic findings that reveal more disease in the breast than anticipated. Preoperative imaging helps surgeons optimize surgical outcomes by avoiding these surprises.

The **mammogram**, the road map for breast surgeons, illustrates the distribution of fatty and dense tissues within the breast. Mammography can simultaneously identify additional lesions in the same or opposite breast. Breast **ultrasound** is good for visualizing a specific lesion or mass within the breast. New tests such as breast MRI are currently being evaluated for their ability to assess extent of disease beyond what is seen on standard imaging once cancer is already diagnosed.

5. Does a delay between biopsy and definitive treatment adversely affect cure?

Almost certainly not, if the delay is only for days or weeks. In general, breast cancers evolve slowly. Treatment should be initiated within 3–4 weeks of initial diagnosis. Delays of longer than 3–6 months should be avoided. There is more urgency with pregnancy-associated breast cancer, where tumor growth can be more rapid. It is not appropriate to delay the treatment of a breast cancer until the end of pregnancy, particularly when some chemotherapeutic agents (e.g., doxorubicin [Adriamycin]) can be safely given during pregnancy.

6. **How is breast cancer staged?**
   See Table 62-1.

TABLE 62-1. STAGING OF BREAST CANCER

TNM Stage	Histology	Tumor Size	Nodal Metastases	Distant Metastases
0	Noninvasive	Any	—	—
I	Invasive	≤ 2 cm	No	No
II	Invasive	2–5 cm	No	No
		≤ 5 cm	Yes	
		> 5 cm	No	
III	Invasive	> 5 cm	Yes	No
		Any size	Fixed nodes	
		Skin or chest wall invasion	Yes or no	
IV	Invasive	Any size	Yes or no	Yes

7. **Why is staging of breast cancer important?**
   The stages correlate with likelihood of relapse and fatality. The TNM (tumor, node, metastasis) staging summarizes data about tumor size, axillary node metastases, and distant metastases. Stage 0 cancers are noninvasive cancers (e.g., ductal carcinoma *in situ* [DCIS]); stage I breast cancers are small node-negative invasive cancers; stage II cancers are intermediate-sized cancers with or without axillary nodal metastases; stage III cancers are locally advanced cancers, usually with axillary nodal metastases; and stage IV cancers already have metastasized to distant sites.

8. **What is the overall survival rate after definitive treatment?**
   Stage 0 (DCIS): Nearly 100% 10-year overall survival rate
   Stage I: 90% 10-year overall survival rate
   Stage II: 75% 10-year overall survival rate
   Stage III: 40% 10-year overall survival rate
   A gradual incremental improvement in breast cancer survival over recent years has been attributed to earlier detection and improved systemic therapy. Cytotoxic chemotherapy (e.g., CMF, Adriamycin, paclitaxel [Taxol]), hormonal therapy (e.g., tamoxifen, aromatase inhibitors), and biologic therapy (e.g., herceptin) have progressively improved disease-free and overall survival in breast cancer patients, even those with advanced disease.

9. **What is the difference between noninvasive *(in situ)* and invasive breast cancers?**
   Noninvasive *(in situ)* cancers are malignant cells that remain confined to the duct or lobule in which they originate. *In situ* cancers have minimal chance of spreading to nodes or distant sites. Invasive cancers have traversed the basement membrane of their originating duct or lobule and have metastatic potential. *In situ* cancers do not warrant complete lymph node dissection as part of definitive surgery. Sentinel node mapping is sometimes used in conjunction with surgical treatment of DCIS, particularly if the patient is going to undergo mastectomy or if invasive cancer is also suspected in the breast, but this has not yet been definitively proven.

10. **Where does invasive breast cancer spread (other than to lymph nodes)? Which diagnostic tests are useful for identifying such metastases?**
    Breast cancer can spread to the bones, lung, liver, and brain. **Bone scans** are quite sensitive but less specific for bone metastases. Standard radiographs help distinguish metastases from benign inflammatory conditions. Lung metastases are identified by **chest radiographs** or **computed tomography (CT) scan**. Liver metastases can be identified using **liver function tests** (LFTs), which, unfortunately, are neither specific nor sensitive. Twenty-five percent of breast cancer patients with documented liver metastases have normal LFT results. Liver imaging tests (abdominal ultrasound or CT) are more expensive but are more reliable. Brain metastases are imaged by **head CT or magnetic resonance imaging (MRI) scanning**.

11. **Which tests should be obtained before surgery to screen for metastases?**
    All patients with symptoms suggesting metastatic disease (bone pain, pulmonary symptoms, jaundice, seizures) should be fully evaluated after invasive breast cancer has been diagnosed.
    A standard minimal preoperative workup for invasive disease consists of a **chest radiograph** and **LFTs**. In reality, the utility of these tests among early-stage cancers is quite low. Routine chest radiography identifies unsuspected lung metastases in < 1% of patients. Chest radiography often is justified for other reasons and is useful as a baseline test for future comparison.

12. **What are the alternatives for primary surgical treatment of invasive breast cancer?**
    1. **Modified radical mastectomy:** The combined removal of the breast and axillary lymph nodes has survival benefit equivalent to radical mastectomy, which additionally removes the pectoralis muscles. True radical mastectomy is rarely performed today. The pectoralis *minor* muscle may be removed, with minimal morbidity, in a modified radical mastectomy to facilitate dissection of the highest (level III) lymph nodes.
    2. **Partial mastectomy (lumpectomy or quadrantectomy):** Breast conservation therapy requires the removal of the breast tumor with a margin of normal breast tissue (negative margins), axillary dissection, and postoperative adjuvant breast irradiation. Trials with 20-year follow-up have shown equivalent survival for lumpectomy and radiation, total mastectomy, and radical mastectomy. Mastectomy is preferred when negative margins cannot be achieved.
    3. **Primary irradiation to the breast:** This is largely investigational and cannot currently be considered a standard of care.

13. **What is the National Surgical Adjuvant Breast and Bowel Program (NSABP)?**
    The NSABP is a U.S.-based trialist group that performed many of the crucial randomized trials that have shaped our modern approach to breast cancer therapy. The NSABP proved that breast cancer is largely a systemic problem at the time of diagnosis and that smaller operations can be equivalent to larger ones for curative potential. Most recently, the NSABP has reported that tamoxifen can decrease the chances of high-risk women's developing breast cancer.

14. **What is the significance of the NSABP B-06 trial?**
    NSABP B-06 is a multicenter study that randomized nearly 2000 women with stage I and II tumors (<4 cm) to three treatments: segmental mastectomy (SM; aka, lumpectomy) alone, SM with radiation, and total mastectomy (TM). All patients underwent axillary dissection, and patients with positive nodes received adjuvant chemotherapy. There was **no difference in overall survival rates** between the groups, but radiation therapy decreased local recurrence in the lumpectomized breast. In patients who underwent SM (with or without radiation), there was **no difference in disease-free survival or overall survival rates**, indicating that breast conservation therapy is effective for achieving both local and distant disease control.

KEY POINTS: DIAGNOSIS AND PRIMARY THERAPY FOR BREAST CANCER

1. The excisional biopsy is the gold standard for the diagnosis of breast cancer.

2. The preferred initial diagnostic method has become core-needle biopsy or fine-needle aspiration.

3. The surgical alternatives for treatment of primary invasive breast cancer are modified radical mastectomy, partial mastectomy, and primary irradiation to the breast.

4. NSABP B-06 trial found no difference in overall survival in women with stage I and II breast cancer who underwent either segmental mastectomy, segmental mastectomy with radiation, and total mastectomy, but radiation decreased local recurrence in the lumpectomized breast.

15. **What is the difference among quadrantectomy, lumpectomy, and partial mastectomy?**
There really is no difference because they all refer to removing part of the breast, just in varying amounts. The original quadrantectomy promoted by the Italians in the 1980s included excision of an entire breast quadrant, along with the overlying skin. Standard lumpectomies remove less tissue and do not involve skin removal, but they still demand negative surgical margins for both invasive cancer and DCIS.

16. **Are some patients poor candidates for breast conservation therapy?**
Contraindications (relative or absolute) to breast conservation include (1) cancers that cannot be excised with negative margins without mastectomy, (2) cancers that are too large relative to the breast to obtain acceptable cosmetic results, (3) multicentric cancers, and (4) patients who do not desire or who have a specific contraindication to adjuvant radiation therapy (e.g., during pregnancy).

17. **What is oncoplastic surgery?**
This is a collection of procedures that use combined oncologic and reconstructive principles in performing a partial mastectomy. Large, full-thickness segments of breast are excised, often together with some overlying skin. Using mastopexy techniques, the gland is remodeled on the chest wall in order to preserve the breast's natural shape and appearance without creating an unsightly tissue divot under the skin.

18. **After mastectomy, which patients may undergo immediate breast reconstruction (i.e., during the same operation)?**
Patient selection for immediate reconstruction is controversial. Most agree that patients with noninvasive *(in situ)* or early invasive (stage I and selected stage II) breast cancers may be offered immediate reconstruction using a myocutaneous flap, a breast implant, or a combination of the two. It is disadvantageous to perform immediate reconstruction in patients with locally advanced (stage III) breast cancers because the patients may require postmastectomy chest wall irradiation. Radiation adversely affects the cosmetic outcome in reconstructed tissue flaps and promotes capsular contracture around implants.

19. **When is chest wall radiation therapy indicated after mastectomy?**
In general, mastectomy patients do not require radiation therapy. Exceptions are those with large (>5 cm) primary cancers, positive mastectomy margins, or more than four positive axillary nodes, all of which are associated with heightened locoregional recurrence rates. The possible benefit of radiation with one to three positive axillary nodes is currently being studied.

20. **What is sentinel lymph node mapping for breast cancer?**

Removing normal lymph nodes in a complete axillary lymph node dissection provides important staging information, but with some morbidity, the most notable of which is lymphedema of the arm. Alternatively, with sentinel lymph node mapping, a radioactive tracer (technetium labeled sulfur colloid), a blue dye (lymphazurin), or both are injected into the breast nodule to find the first upstream node(s) to which a primary breast cancer would spread. If the sentinel lymph nodes are negative for cancer, it is not necessary to complete the node dissection.

21. **Are there risks of axillary staging by sentinel lymph node mapping?**

Sentinel node mapping appears most appropriate for smaller breast cancers with clinically normal axillae. The technique may be less reliable with large (T3) cancers and nodes extensively replaced with cancer. Thus, the primary risk of sentinel node mapping is that it may understage a patient by suggesting that the cancer is node negative when, in fact, nodal metastases are present in other "nonsentinel" lymph nodes (i.e., a false-negative result). As a result, the patient may be treated with less aggressive chemotherapy than is appropriate to minimize cancer mortality.

22. **Which tests should be obtained after surgery to screen for metastases or as baseline studies for future comparison?**

The utility of metastatic screening tests correlates with the locoregional tumor and nodal (TN) staging determined at surgery. Patients with locally advanced (stage III and some stage II) cancers are at high risk for developing cancer recurrence with metastases, making additional diagnostic studies valuable. **Bone scan** and **liver imaging (CT or ultrasound)** are helpful baseline studies that occasionally reveal previously unappreciated metastatic disease. Some clinicians use **circulating tumor markers** such as CEA CA-27, 29 to follow treatment results and monitor for evidence of cancer recurrence, although the value of these studies is debatable.

Conversely, baseline studies are best avoided in asymptomatic patients with early cancers because the chance of a false-positive test is vastly higher than the chances of finding clinically occult distant metastases. For example, with stage I breast cancer, the likelihood of a false-positive result on bone scans vastly exceeds the likelihood of a true-positive result. Similarly, **brain imaging (CT or MRI)** generally should be reserved for patients with neurologic symptoms because of low yield in asymptomatic patients.

23. **What is "neoadjuvant" therapy for breast cancer?**

Locally advanced but operable (stage IIIA and some stage II) cancers have a high likelihood of recurrence after surgery. Neoadjuvant therapy (before surgery) is used to decrease the local tumor burden and to begin treatment of micrometastatic disease at the earliest possible time. It is not yet known whether the timing of chemotherapy relative to surgery influences survival time from diagnosis. Neoadjuvant chemotherapy may convert some cancers that otherwise might require mastectomy into potential candidates for breast conservation surgery.

24. **What is "inoperable" breast cancer?**

Inoperable breast cancer has advanced beyond the boundaries of surgical resection. The spread may be regional (internal mammary lymph nodes, stage IIIB) or distant (distant metastases, stage IV). Supraclavicular lymph node metastases, which are beyond the margins of surgical resection, confer the same unfortunate prognosis as metastasis to distant solid organs and currently are staged as such. Primary therapy for advanced cancer is systemic treatment (chemotherapy or hormonal therapy) rather than surgery. Surgery combined with radiation therapy becomes an adjuvant therapy for local control of disease after a good response to systemic treatment.

25. **How is DCIS treated?**

As the earliest form of breast cancer requiring treatment, DCIS has the widest range of treatment choices. Because it lacks metastatic potential, DCIS does not require systemic drug treatment.

Also called intraductal carcinoma, DCIS can be safely treated by breast conservation therapy (lumpectomy plus adjuvant radiation), provided that the disease is excised with negative margins. If negative margins cannot be achieved, then mastectomy is recommended. Axillary dissection for staging is not indicated. Tamoxifen may play a role in breast cancer prevention, and it lowered local recurrence after lumpectomy and radiation in the NSABP B-24 trial.

26. **Can some cases of DCIS be treated by lumpectomy without radiotherapy?**
Using carefully collected retrospective data, Silverstein et al. developed a prognostic index (scoring system) for DCIS based on histologic grade, tumor size, and margin width. Their data suggest that small (< 1 cm), non–high-grade DCIS lesions excised with wide surgical margins do not require radiation therapy in addition to lumpectomy. However, forgoing radiation treatment after lumpectomy for DCIS remains controversial. Recent reports suggest that late local recurrence rates (≤ 25 years) for non–high-grade DCIS may exceed 25%.

27. **How does DCIS management differ from that for lobular carcinoma in situ (LCIS)?**
DCIS is considered a preinvasive malignancy. It is treated surgically with lumpectomy or mastectomy, with or without radiation therapy, similar to how invasive breast cancer is treated. By contrast, LCIS is viewed as a risk factor for the development of subsequent breast cancer and is generally not thought to be "cancer" per se. LCIS does not require surgery.

28. **Why are patients with LCIS not treated surgically?**
LCIS does not invariably degenerate into invasive cancer, but women with proven LCIS have a 25% chance of developing breast cancer during their lifetimes. Unfortunately, the cancer may be ductal or lobular and may develop with equal likelihood in either breast. LCIS is a marker for high breast cancer risk, warranting careful surveillance with serial mammography and physical examination. Because risk is the same in both breasts, bilateral mastectomy is the only logical surgical procedure for this condition, and aggressive therapy simply is not warranted.

29. **Can drugs be used to prevent breast cancer among high-risk women?**
In the NSABP P-01 Tamoxifen Prevention Trial, women at heightened risk for the development of breast cancer (> 1.66% 5-year risk) developed fewer breast cancers when given tamoxifen rather than placebo. For women with LCIS, the 5-year breast cancer incidence was 6.8% in the placebo group and 2.5% in the tamoxifen group, representing a 56% reduction in breast cancers. However, the number of breast cancers that were prevented rivaled the number of tamoxifen-associated complications, including endometrial cancers and thrombotic events. No survival benefit to tamoxifen prophylaxis has yet been observed. At this time, women with LCIS should be offered tamoxifen as an option for treatment and cancer prevention, although they may reasonably decline when presented with the complete data.

WEB SITE

http://www.acssurgery.com

BIBLIOGRAPHY

1. Anderson BO: Prophylactic surgery to reduce breast cancer risk: A brief literature review. Breast J 7:321–330, 2001.

2. Anderson BO, Lawton TJ, Rinn K, et al: Lobular carcinoma in situ. In Silverstein MJ (ed): Ductal Carcinoma in Situ of the Breast, 2nd ed. Philadelphia, Lippincott Williams & Wilkins, 2002, pp 615–634.

3. Fisher B, Anderson S, Bryant J, et al: Twenty-year follow-up of a randomized trial comparing total mastectomy, lumpectomy, and lumpectomy plus irradiation for the treatment of invasive breast cancer. N Engl J Med 347:1233–1241, 2002.

4. Fisher B, Costantino JP, Wickerham DL, et al: Tamoxifen for prevention of breast cancer: Report of the National Surgical Adjuvant Breast and Bowel Project P-1 Study. J Natl Cancer Inst 90:1371–1388, 1998.

5. Fisher B, Bryant J, Wolmark N, et al: Effect of preoperative chemotherapy on the outcome of women with operable breast cancer. J Clin Oncol 16:2672–2685, 1998.

6. Fisher B, Dignam J, Wolmark N, et al: Tamoxifen in treatment of intraductal breast cancer: National Surgical Adjuvant Breast and Bowel Project B-24 randomised controlled trial. Lancet 353:1993–2000, 1999.

7. Heimann R, Karrison T, Hellman S: Treatment of ductal carcinoma in situ. N Engl J Med 341:999–1000, 1999.

8. Morrow M, Strom EA, Bassett LW, et al: Standard for breast conservation therapy in the management of invasive breast carcinoma. Ca Cancer J Clin 52:277–300, 2002.

9. Silverstein MJ, Lagios MD, Craig PH, et al: A prognostic index for ductal carcinoma in situ of the breast. Cancer 77:2267–2274, 1996.

10. Veronesi U, Cascinelli N, Mariani L, et al: Twenty-year follow-up of a randomized study comparing breast-conserving surgery with radical mastectomy for early breast cancer. N Engl J Med 34:1232, 2002.

WHAT IS CANCER?

John A. Ridge, M.D., Ph.D.

CHAPTER 63

1. **What is a neoplasm?**
   A neoplasm is a new growth of tissue (tumor) in which cells grow progressively under conditions that do not prompt the growth of normal cells. A malignant neoplasm (cancer) is composed of cells that invade other tissues and spread.

2. **What kinds of cancers are there?**
   Malignant tumors of epithelial (surface tissue) cells are **carcinomas**. Malignant tumors of mesenchymal (connective tissue) cells are **sarcomas**. Carcinomas and sarcomas are **solid** tumors. Hematologic malignancies, such as leukemia, are **liquid** tumors of mesenchymal origin.

3. **What about skin cancers?**
   Most basal cell and squamous skin cancers are life-threatening only if neglected. They occur in tremendous numbers and are seldom fatal with proper treatment. Although the general principles of cancer management apply to skin cancers, they usually are not considered in the same class with other solid tumors.

4. **Why is cancer bad for you?**
   There is no simple answer. The replacement of normal tissue by tumor eventually causes organ dysfunction. If a tumor outgrows its blood supply and becomes necrotic, local inflammation ensues. Often obstruction (with compromise of the lumen) of the gastrointestinal tract, bile ducts, or airway develops as the tumor grows. Occasionally the cancer bleeds (but life-threatening bleeding is rare). Nerve invasion or inflammation typically cause pain, which may be excruciating. Cancers also may elaborate humoral factors (e.g., gastrin) that cause symptoms.

5. **Are all cancers life-threatening?**
   Cancer is a fatal disease. It is uncommon for a patient with an untreated cancer to die of something else. Currently more than 50% of patients with cancer in the United States are cured.

6. **How do cancers start?**
   No one knows, but cells begin to grow under circumstances when they should not. They stop responding to antigrowth signals, promote their own blood supplies, are seemingly able to replicate endlessly, and do not undergo programmed cell death (apoptosis).

7. **Is this process the same for all cancers?**
   No, the order in which these changes take place seems to vary among types of cancer and even between individual tumors with the same histologic type. Occasionally, a single mutation alone causes cancer, but many genetic alterations are usually involved.

8. **Do all cancers spread?**
   About 25% of patients with solid tumors have detectable metastases at the time of diagnosis. Fewer than 50% of the remainder develop metastases during the course of treatment. At diagnosis, a cancer is usually at least 1 cm in diameter (and often much larger), containing millions of cells. It is surprising that metastases have not occurred in all patients at the time of diagnosis.

9. **How does cancer spread?**
   Most cancer cells that enter the bloodstream or lymphatics do not cause metastases. Only rare malignant cells actually survive to cause distant tumor implants by recruiting new blood vessels. Many cells do not seem to come to rest in tissues conducive to their growth. Perhaps others are extirpated by the immune system.

10. **Does this process have an effect on how surgeons treat patients with cancer?**
    Operations to treat benign conditions are designed to remove as little tissue as possible while creating a new and desirable physiologic or anatomic state. Cancer operations, on the other hand, are designed to remove as much tissue as possible while leaving the patient with acceptable function. Cancer operations typically remove the primary tumor as well as the lymph nodes draining the primary site. Surgical resection is the single most effective treatment for solid tumors.

11. **Why are lymph nodes removed during cancer operations?**
    More than 100 years ago, William S. Halsted (if you don't know the answer to any historical question posed on rounds, you should always guess "Halsted") appreciated that tumor recurrence on the chest wall after mastectomy was related to tumor in remaining lymph nodes. Halsted believed that cancer of the breast spread in an orderly fashion (or perhaps even contiguously) from the primary tumor to regional lymph nodes and eventually to distant sites. He popularized en bloc dissection of the breast with axillary lymph nodes for treatment of breast cancer. Conceptually, this approach was adopted for surgical treatment of most solid tumors.

12. **What is a sentinel lymph node?**
    Sentinel lymph nodes are the first stop for tumor cells metastasizing through lymphatics from the primary tumor. Often there is more than one sentinel node, even for a small tumor. If no tumor is present in a sentinel lymph node, it is unlikely that tumor is present in any of the other nodes. Sentinel lymph node mapping has been used for cancers of many organs (including the skin, breast, colon, thyroid, and head and neck neoplasms). Careful evaluation of sentinel lymph nodes has proven reliable in the staging of melanoma. It will probably prove equally successful in managing breast cancer and head and neck tumors, sparing many patients far more morbid lymphadenectomies (lymph node dissections).

13. **Do solid tumors spread in an orderly way?**
    Not necessarily. Another view of breast cancer behavior became popular by the 1970s. Bernard Fisher postulated that cancer is widespread at its inception. He stated that "breast cancer is a systemic disease . . . and that variations in effective local regional treatment are unlikely to effect survival substantially."

14. **How do these different models of cancer affect treatment?**
    Surgeons who believe that tumors spread in an orderly way tend to perform complete lymph node dissections in concert with resection of the primary tumor. They generally believe that lymphadenectomy will cure some patients who have lymph node involvement without distant metastases and that local recurrence is a preventable cause of death. Surgeons who believe that lymph node metastases are simply markers for systemic disease are usually far less aggressive in performing lymph node dissections because (in their view) removal of lymph nodes that contain tumor will not cure patients who probably already have metastatic disease.

15. **Do we know which model is correct?**
    Both are probably inadequate. Some solid tumors (e.g., squamous cancer of the head and neck, colon cancer) often have no distant disease, even when they have lymph node metastases. Their spread seems to be an orderly process. Other solid tumors (e.g., oat cell lung cancer and prostate cancer) often metastasize widely even when they are small. For such cancers, lymph node involvement is a reliable sign of metastases. Sarcomas seldom metastasize to the

lymph nodes, but patients may develop distant metastases limited to the lungs alone. Remarkably, such patients sometimes are cured by resection of the distant lung lesions.

16. **How else can solid tumors be treated with curative intent?**
Instead of surgical removal of the primary tumor and appropriate lymph nodes, the entire area may be treated with curative radiation. Some types of cancer are more responsive to radiation than others. The side effects of curative radiation treatment are formidable. Similar to those of surgery, they must be explained to the patient. When radiation kills cancer, it injures adjacent normal tissues. The damage to normal tissues continues over the course of the patient's life. Although radiotherapists are getting better at directing their beams, the tolerance of nearby tissues to radiation remains the limiting factor in treatment of cancers with radiation alone.

KEY POINTS: WHAT IS CANCER?

1. A neoplasm is a new growth of tissue in which cells grow progressively under conditions that do not prompt the growth of normal cells.

2. Malignant tumors of epithelial cells are carcinomas.

3. Malignant tumors of mesenchymal cells are sarcomas.

4. About 25% of patients with solid tumors have detectable metastases at the time of diagnosis.

5. Tumor-infiltrating lymphocytes are lymphoid cells that infiltrate solid tumors and appear reactive to autologous tumor antigens.

17. **What is adjuvant therapy?**
Adjuvant means "assisting or aiding," but we use this term to mean assisting after surgical or radiotherapeutic control of the primary tumor. Adjuvant chemotherapy is of documented benefit in the treatment of breast cancer, colorectal cancer, stomach cancer, pancreatic cancer, and ovarian and testicular tumors. Adjuvant radiation therapy is effective in reducing the risk of tumor recurrence around the surgical site. It is often used in treating patients with rectal, breast, head and neck, and stomach cancers as well as sarcomas. Conceptually, both surgery and radiation are local/regional therapies. Although chemotherapy is obviously a systemic treatment, it may help sensitize tumors to radiation. The term "neoadjuvant" doesn't really mean anything, but it is often used to describe preoperative chemotherapy or radiotherapy (which might more accurately be described as "induction" treatment).

18. **What cancer treatments are available in addition to surgery, radiation therapy, and cytotoxic chemotherapy?**
Hormonal manipulation has been used for decades to slow the growth of some tumors. Stimulation of the patient's immune system to combat cancer is potentially promising. This approach may involve vaccines, training of T cells, or enhancement of the immune response. New types of anticancer agents include drugs that interfere with tumor angiogenesis, antibodies and other drugs that interfere with growth factor receptors, other sorts of drugs that alter intracellular signaling, and drugs that restore cell cycle control. The limitation of all of these approaches resides in our inability to specify a target unique to cancer cells. Hence, treatments damage the rest of the patient, with potentially fatal toxicity.

19. **Does the body fight cancer on its own?**
Certainly. Some scientists believe that early cancers are regularly extirpated by the immune system (as we "catch" cancer every day) and that clinical cancers reflect a breakdown in immune surveillance. Immunocompromised patients with transplants or AIDS develop cancers with

frightening frequency. Thus, rejection and sepsis are no longer the most common causes of death among kidney transplant patients—it's cancer. "Spontaneous remissions" of melanoma and renal cell carcinoma do occur and must be immunologically mediated. Indeed, these are the tumors that initially seemed to respond well to "adoptive immunotherapy" and interleukin-2.

20. What is a tumor-infiltrating lymphocyte (TIL)?
TILs are lymphoid cells that infiltrate solid tumors and appear reactive to autologous tumor antigens. Compared with circulating lymphocytes, TILs more aggressively target cancer.

21. What are palliative treatments?
Palliative means "affording relief but not curing."

22 . Give some examples of palliative procedures.
Resection of the primary tumor in the face of distant metastases may be performed to treat bleeding or obstruction. Procedures to bypass intestinal or biliary obstruction in patients with unresectable cancer are common. Tracheotomies are created for patients who are unable to breathe because of upper airway obstruction, and feeding tubes may permit enteral nutrition in patients who cannot eat. Removal of isolated brain metastases often improves the patient's quality of life. Many patients with functioning endocrine tumors benefit from reduction in tumor mass.

23. What is cytoreductive surgery?
Cytoreductive ("debulking") procedures are designed to decrease tumor burden. Simply reducing tumor bulk is seldom sufficient to prolong survival. For cytoreductive surgery to be beneficial, the nonsurgical (adjunctive) therapy must be highly effective—such as radiation for glioblastoma or chemotherapy for ovarian cancer.

CONTROVERSY

24. Is axillary lymph node treatment for breast cancer of therapeutic value, or does it merely help select patients who should receive chemotherapy?
Those who believe that axillary lymph node dissection confers only information about tumor behavior rather than a therapeutic benefit usually cite the National Surgical Adjuvant Breast and Bowel Program (NSABP) B-04 trial. There was no statistically significant difference in survival curves between patients whose axilla was treated initially and patients who received delayed treatment to the axilla. In addition to other problems, however, the study lacked the power to prove the point. To have a 90% chance of detecting a 7% survival difference between the treatment groups, the National Surgical Adjuvant Breast and Bowel Program (NSABP) should have enrolled 2000 patients (not just 550) in each arm. Hence, a substantial survival advantage caused by axillary dissection might not have been recognized. The study was not designed to prove that the two approaches were equivalent, and it has been "overinterpreted." It takes a much larger trial to prove equivalence than to show a difference. Indeed, subsequent randomized trials in the management of breast cancer, as well as evaluation of patterns of care, demonstrate an independent survival advantage conferred by treatment of the axilla. This experience with breast cancer reinforces the importance of actually understanding clinical trials.

WEB SITE

http://www.acssurgery.com

BIBLIOGRAPHY

1. Bland KI, Scott-Conner CEH, Menck H, et al: Axillary dissection in breast-conserving surgery for stage I and II breast cancer: A National Cancer Data Base study of patterns of omission and implications for survival. J Am Coll Surg 188:586–596, 1999.

2. Cabanes PA, Salmon RJ, Vilcoq JR, et al: Value of axillary dissection in addition to lumpectomy and radiotherapy in early breast cancer. Lancet 339:1245–1248, 1992.

3. Fisher B, Jeong J-H, Anderson S, et al: Twenty-five-year follow-up of a randomized clinical trial comparing radical mastectomy, total mastectomy, and total mastectomy followed by irradiation. N Engl J Med 312:674–681, 1985.

4. Hanahan D, Weinberg RA: The hallmarks of cancer. Cell 100:57–70, 2000.

5. Harris JR, Osteen RT: Patients with early breast cancer benefit from effective axillary treatment. Breast Cancer Res Treat 5:17–21, 1985.

6. Hellman S: Natural history of small breast cancers. J Clin Oncol 12:2229–2234, 1994.

7. Krag DN, Weaver DL: Pathological and molecular assessment of sentinel lymph nodes in solid tumors. Semin Oncol 29:274–279, 2002.

8. Rosenberg SA: Progress in human tumor immunology and immunotherapy. Nature 411:380–384, 2001.

9. Whelan TJ, Julian J, Wright J: Does locoregional radiation therapy improve survival in breast cancer? A meta-analysis. J Clin Oncol 18:1220–1229, 2000.

CHAPTER 64

MELANOMA

Mark D. Walsh, Jr., M.D., William R. Nelson, M.D., and Joyesh K. Raj, M.D.

1. **What is melanoma?**
   The term *melanoma* implies a malignant tumor; *malignant melanoma* is redundant. The most malignant of all skin cancers, melanoma usually forms from a preexisting nevus or mole but may develop de novo.

2. **What is the incidence of melanoma?**
   It is the sixth most common cancer in the United States and the fastest rising cancer in men. The lifetime risk in the year 2000 was 1 in 75 versus 1 in 150 in 1985. Over 51,000 new cases of melanoma are reported each year.

3. **What are the types of moles? Which are most prone to malignant change?**
   Intradermal: the most benign form
   Junctional: the junctional component may be the site of melanoma formation
   Compound: intradermal and junctional together; intermediate activity
   Spitz: once called juvenile melanoma, it is actually a spindle cell epithelioid nevus that is quite benign
   Dysplastic: the most likely to turn malignant (especially in dysplastic nevus syndrome)

4. **What are the risk factors in melanoma formation?**
   - Large number of moles (> 50 moles > 2 mm in diameter)
   - Changing nevi
   - Family history of melanoma
   - Light, poorly tanning skin; blonde or reddish-brown hair
   - History of episodic, acute, severe sunburns
   - Dysplastic nevus syndrome, or familial atypical multiple mole melanoma syndrome (FAMMM)
   - History of melanoma

5. **Which skin lesions often mimic a primary melanoma?**
   - Spitz nevus (spindle cell epithelioid nevus)
   - Atypical benign nevus
   - Halo nevus
   - Recurrent benign nevus after inadequate excision
   - Metastatic melanoma to skin
   - Mycosis fungoides
   - Extramammary Paget's disease
   - Bowen's disease
   - Dark sebaceous keratoses
   - Kaposi's sarcoma
   - Pigmented basal cell carcinoma

6. **What is the familial melanoma syndrome?**
   The inherited FAMMM syndrome has been defined as the occurrence of melanoma in one or more first- or second-degree relatives and the presence of > 50 moles of variable size, some of which are atypical histologically. The risk of melanoma in this syndrome runs as high as 100% in the person's lifetime.

7. **Is a specific gene involved in melanoma development in the FAMMM syndrome?**
   Genetic studies have revealed a specific gene (i.e., p16 mapped to chromosome 9) in many people with the FAMMM syndrome.

8. **Are any groups at low risk for melanoma formation?**
   Children younger than 10 years, African Americans, Asians, Native Americans, and dark-complected whites are at low risk.

9. **What are common sites of melanoma development?**
   The most common sites are the posterior trunk in men and lower extremities in women. All sun-exposed areas are possible sites. Uncommon sites for melanoma formation are the soles of the feet, palms, and genitalia. Unusual noncutaneous sites for melanoma formation are the eye, anus, and gastrointestinal tract.

10. **Where is melanoma most common?**
    Melanoma is most common in Australia, especially the northern part of the continent, where light-skinned descendants of the original settlers are exposed to tropical sun.

11. **What are the warning signs of melanoma?**
    Skin lesions that display:
    A = **A**symmetry
    B = Irregular **b**order
    C = **C**olor: variable; spotted; often very black with irregular tan areas; red or pink spots; ulcerated when advanced (bleeds easily)
    D = **D**iameter (> 5–6 mm)
    E = **E**nlargement or **E**levation

12. **What are the types of melanoma and their incidence?**
    Superficial spreading: 75% of all cases; most common
    Nodular: 15% of cases; most malignant; well circumscribed; deeply invasive
    Lentigo maligna melanoma: 5% of cases; relatively good prognosis
    Acral lentiginous: 5% of cases; most common type in people of color; appears on the soles, palms, subungual sites

13. **Which moles should be considered for removal?**
    Growing and darkening nevi should be excised, especially in sun-sensitive patients. Itching is a sign of early malignant change. Ulceration is a late sign. Because melanoma may be familial in origin, children of patients with melanoma should be carefully screened for very dark nevi.

14. **How should suspicious nevi be biopsied?**
    Total excision of the lesion with a narrow (1-mm) margin of normal skin plus primary repair should be done. Partial incisional biopsy is acceptable if the lesion is large or if total excision would require reconstructive surgery. Punch biopsy, incisional biopsy, or saucerization are all appropriate as long as a **full-thickness** specimen is obtained. Thorough pathologic study is essential.

15. **Do melanomas spontaneously regress or even disappear?**
    Rarely melanomas can regress or even disappear. Remarkably, such patients have a poor prognosis despite the fact that the primary lesion has regressed or even sloughed off because metastatic disease to the lymph nodes and viscera may have already occurred.

16. **What are the Breslow and Clark classifications of melanoma invasion?**
    Clark selected five levels of melanoma thickness in the skin:
    - Level I—intradermal melanoma that does not metastasize; may be better termed atypical melanotic hyperplasia: a benign lesion
    - Level II—melanoma that penetrates the basement membrane into the papillary dermis

- Level III—melanoma that fills the papillary dermis and encroaches on the reticular dermis in a pushing fashion
- Level IV—melanoma that invades the reticular dermis
- Level V—melanoma that works its way into the subcutaneous fat

The **Breslow method** requires an optical micrometer fitted to the ocular position of a standard microscope. This technique is a more exact determination of tumor invasion. Lesions are classified as follows:

≤ 0.75 mm
0.76–1.5 mm
1.51–3.99 mm
≥ 4.0 mm

Lesions < 1 mm include melanoma in situ and thin invasive tumors. The cure rate in the latter is over 95% with excision. Tumors of 1.0–4.0 mm are called intermediate but involve risk of metastasis. Lesions > 4.0 mm are high-risk lesions with a poor cure rate.

All melanomas should be checked by both methods because some tumors may show a low Breslow measurement with a deeper Clark level, indicating a great risk of recurrence and spread. Measurement of thickness is important, and the tumor should be measured from the total height of the lesion vertically at the point of maximal thickness. In addition, if ulceration is present, the measurement should be from the bottom of the ulcer crater down to the deepest margin of the lesion. (See Figure 64-1.)

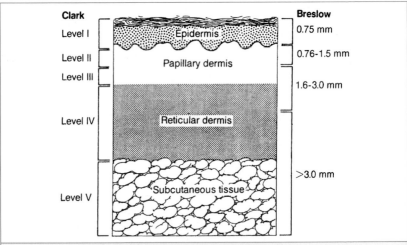

Figure 64-1. The Clark and Breslow classifications of melanoma invasion. (From Young OM, Mathes ST: In Schwartz SI (ed): Principles of Surgery, 6th ed. New York, McGraw-Hill, 1994, with permission.)

17. **What is the TNM staging system for melamoma?**

The TNM (primary tumor, regional nodes, metastasis) staging system is the most comprehensive classification of melanoma. Using established risk factors for advanced disease, it stratifies patients based on the thickness of the melanoma, ulceration, micrometastases or nodal metastastes, and distant metastatic disease. Recently revised, it more accurately predicts prognosis and the need for further treatment.

18. **What are the chances of nodal and systemic spread of the various degrees of melanoma invasion?**
Regional node metastases occur in about 2% of melanomas < 0.76 mm in depth; the distant spread approaches 0%. In tumors 0.76–1.5 mm thick, nodes are cancerous in 25% and distant spread is 8%. In tumors 1.5–4.0 mm thick, node metastasis occurs in 57% and distant spread in 15%. In tumors > 4 mm, node metastasis occurs in ≤ 62% and distant spread is about 72%.

19. **What are the characteristics of a subungual melanoma?**
Subungual lesions are often mistaken for a chronic inflammatory process; therefore, most patients present quite late. They are usually older than patients with other forms of cutaneous melanoma. The great toe is the most common site of origin. Amputation at or proximal to the metatarsal phalangeal joint and regional sentinel lymph node biopsy are advised by most authors. The primary lesions are usually deeply invasive, and the lymph nodes are positive for cancer in the majority of cases, either at the time of the original diagnosis or at subsequent follow-up.

20. **Describe the technique of sentinal lymph node (SLN) biopsy.**
The SLN biopsy is based on the theory that lymph from a solid neoplasm initially drains to a central, culprit sentinel node (SN). These SNs are the first nodes at risk for metastatic disease. The nodes can be biopsied and examined with serial sectioning and immunohistochemical staining. The SLN identification technique requires the cooperation of a surgeon, radiologist, and pathologist. Lymphoscintigraphy with the injection of radioactive technetium sulfur colloid (99mTeSC) is performed around the site of the primary melanoma. Scans are then performed in 15 minutes. The SLN is located and the overlying skin is marked. Four hours later, the patient is taken to the operating room for intradermal injection of blue contrast dye (lymphazurin 1%) around the primary site. A hand-held gamma probe identifies the hot spot, and a small incision is made over this area for removal of the SLN. A combination of blue contrast dye and radiocolloid provides the highest yield of SN identification

KEY POINTS: MELANOMA

1. The term *melanoma* implies a malignant tumor.

2. Melanoma is the sixth most common cancer in the United States and the fastest rising cancer in men.

3. The warning signs of melanoma are skin lesions that display asymmetry, irregular borders, color changes, diameter > 5–6 cm, and enlargement or elevation.

21. **How is SLN biopsy changing the treatment of melanoma?**
An SN is now recognized as an independent predictor of survival. SLN biopsy also selctively, with minimal morbidity, identifies patients who might benefit from complete lymphadenectomy or who might benefit from biochemotherapy (see question 32). There may also be a significant psychological benefit for patients whose biopsies are found to be benign.

22. **Does elective lymph node dissection (ELND) improve cure rates in patients with melanoma?**
The Mayo Clinic trial and World Health Organization melanoma group trial have not shown a benefit for ELND for stage I and II melanoma involving the extremities and trunk. The Intergroup Melanoma Trial demonstrated that for patients younger than 60 years with tumors 1.1–2.0 mm thick, there was a significant improvement in 5-year survival (96% versus 84%). However, beginning with the work of Morton et al., who used lymphoscintigraphy to identify routes of lymph drainage and SLN identification, SLN biopsy has come to the fore. In this approach, the

first-echelon node is removed. If it is negative for metastasis, further node dissection is not per-formed. (If the SLN is positive for metastasis, surgical lymph node dissection is completed at a separate time.)

23. **Do routine histologic studies miss micrometastases? What newer methods help to identify such spread?**
   Routine sectioning of a lymph node exposes only 1% of the total volume of tissue. Cell cultures were originally used to identify micrometastases. This technique has been abandoned in favor of an assay with a combination of reverse transcriptase (RT) plus polymerase chain reaction (PCR). In one study, histologically and RT/PCR–positive patients had a recurrence rate of 42% at 3 years. If both assays were negative for cancer, the rate was 6.6% at 3 years. Histologically negative and RT/PCR–positive patients had a 3-year recurrence rate of 22%.

24. **What are the results of lymph node studies in patients undergoing SLN biopsy and node dissection?**
   Brobeil and associates found 13.9% micrometastases in SLNs. In lesions > 4.0 mm, 30% of nodes were cancerous. From 1.5–4.0 mm, 18% of nodes were cancerous, and in lesions of 1.0–1.5 mm, 7% of nodes contained melanoma. In lesions < 0.76 mm, no melanoma was found. In patients who underwent node dissection after the SLN-positive report, 8% had further posi-tive nodes. All patients with cancerous lymph nodes in the dissections had tumors > 3.0 mm.

25. **What features of melanoma are unfavorable for prognosis and metastatic risk?**
   Tumor thickness (Breslow), anatomic invasion of dermis (Clark), nodal status, angiolymphatic invasion, regression, microsatellitosis, neurotropism, mitotic index (> 6/mm^2), trunk versus extremities, ulceration, and male gender are unfavorable.

26. **Does ulceration of a melanoma make a difference in outcome?**
   Yes, it is worse. In the new American Joint Committee on Cancer (AJCC) staging system, ulcera-tion decreases survival in every stage.

27. **If indicated, which types of node dissection should be performed?**
   If there is no evidence of gross involvement of nodes except for the histologically positive SLN, a functional type dissection is preferred by most authorities because it preserves vital nerves and vessels.

28. **Is in-continuity removal of primary site and nodes ever indicated?**
   Only if the primary lesion is near the regional lymph node areas and if the SLNs are positive.

29. **How much normal skin should be removed around a melanoma?**
   Whereas melanoma in situ can be cured with an excisional margin of 0.5 mm, a thin melanoma of < 1.0 mm can be excised with a 1.0-cm margin of normal skin and underlying subcutaneous tissue (down to the fascia). For thicker lesions, a 2-cm margin is now advised.

30. **Does pregnancy worsen the prognosis of melanoma?**
   No.

31. **Does melanoma respond to chemotherapy?**
   Dacarbazine (DTIC) is the most active single agent cytotoxic drug against metastatic melanoma. The response rate is 20%, and the average duration of response is a 6-month period free of dis-ease. Multidrug regimens are not much more effective.

32. **What is biochemotherapy?**
This term refers to a combination of cytotoxic therapy and immunotherapy with interleukin-2 (IL-2) and interferon alpha (IFN). The Eastern Cooperative Oncology Group (ECOG) trial 1684 has shown increased disease-free and overall survival rates with high-dose interferon therapy for patients with melanomas > 4 mm and surgically resected nodal metastases.

33. **Can radiotherapy be helpful in melanoma treatment?**
Radiotherapy is quite helpful as palliative treatment of metastatic disease.

34. **Should amputation be used in the management of locally advanced melanoma?**
With the development of isolation perfusion, the indications for major limb amputation are rare. Patients who might benefit from amputation are those who have experienced recurrences after isolation limb perfusion and those with severe comorbidities who are not candidates for limb perfusion. Partial digital amputation is the recommended therapy for subungual melanoma.

35. **What is isolation perfusion? How is it used in melanoma?**
Although studies have not shown that isolation perfusion conveys a survival advantage in primary melanoma, this technique is often used in setting of multiple or recurrent intransit metastases of an extremity. Melphalan (commonly used) or other chemotherapy preparations (e.g., interferon, tumor necrosis factor) are circulated through an isolated extremity using a pump oxygenator at mild hyperthermic temperatures. Successful isolation perfusion preserves a functional extremity, has a superior response rate, and incurs less morbidity than systemic therapy.

36. **What is the treatment of a patient with metastatic nodes confined to a single area when the primary site is unknown?**
If careful workup reveals no other foci of melanoma, radical lymph node dissection should be carried out. Cure rates as high as 15% have been reported in these unusual situations.

37. **How do you manage postlymphadenectomy edema of an extremity, especially the leg?**
Custom-made support stockings should be placed immediately after surgery.

38. **What should you do in the follow-up care of patients undergoing curative surgery for melanoma?**
Besides frequent physical examinations, chest radiographs and liver function tests are important.

39. **Is cure possible in a patient with a single, isolated, distant metastasis of melanoma?**
Absolutely yes. In a series reported by Overett and Shiu, a survival rate of 33% was achieved in a large series of patients undergoing resection of single, isolated, distant metastases. Such patients, of course, must be carefully studied to rule out other evidence of spread.

WEB SITE

http://www.acssurgery.com

BIBLIOGRAPHY

1. Albertini JJ, Cruse CW, Rapaport D, et al: Intraoperative radiolymphoscintigraphy improves sentinel lymph node identification for patients with melanoma. Ann Surg 223:217–224, 1996.

2. Balch CM, Buzaid AC, Soong SJ, et al: Final version of the American Joint Committee on Cancer staging system for cutaneous melanoma. J Clin Oncol 19:3635–3648, 2001.

3. Balch CM, Houghton AN, Sober AJ, Soong S: Cutaneous Melanoma. St. Louis, Quality Medical Publishing, 1998.

4. Brobeil TE, Glass F: Results of complete lymph node dissection in 83 melanoma patients with positive sentinel nodes. Ann Surg Oncol 5:119–125, 1998.

5. Gershenwald JE, Colome MI, et al: Patterns of recurrence following negative sentinel lymph node biopsy in 243 patients with stage I or II melanoma. J Clin Oncol 16:2253–2260, 1998.

6. Morton DL, Wen DR, Wong JH, et al: Technical details of intraoperative lymphatic mapping for early stage melanoma. Arch Surg 127:392–399, 1992.

7. Overett TK, Shiu MH: Surgical treatment of distant metastatic melanoma: Indications and results. Cancer 56:1222–1230, 1985.

8. Reintgen D, Balch CM, Kirkwood J, Ross M: Recent advances in the care of the patient with malignant melanoma. Ann Surg 225:1–14, 1997.

9. Rineborg U, Anderson R, et al: Resection margins of 2 versus 5 cm for cutaneous malignant melanoma with a tumor thickness of 0.8 to 2.0 mm—Swedish Melanoma Study Group. Cancer 77:1809–1814, 1996.

10. Shapiro R: Surgical approaches to malignant melanoma: Practical guidelines. Dermatol Clin 20:681, 2002.

11. Sharpless SM, Das Gupta TK: Surgery for metastatic melanoma. Semin Surg Oncol 14:311–318, 1998.

12. Vrouenraets BC, Nieweg OE, Kroon BBR: 35 years of isolated limb perfusion for melanoma: Indications and results. Br J Surg 83:1319–1328, 1996.

13. Wagner, JD, Gordon, MS, et al: Current therapy of cutaneous melanoma. Plast Reconstr Surg 105:1774–1801, 2000.

CHAPTER 65

PAROTID TUMORS

Joyesh K. Raj, M.D., and William R. Nelson, M.D.

1. **What is the differential diagnosis of a mass located in front of the ear in a patient of any age?**

   If the mass is painless, discrete, nontender, and located just anterior or just beneath the ear lobe, a parotid tumor is the first choice. The differential diagnosis for other isolated masses include parotitis, primary salivary neoplasm, upper jugular chain node enlargement, tumor of the tail of the submandibular gland, enlarged preauricular or parotid lymph node, branchial cleft cyst, epithelial inclusion cyst, or any mesenchymal neoplasm. Diffuse unilateral enlargement of the parotid gland indicates parotid duct obstruction that can either be persistent or intermittent because of calculi in the main duct. Bilateral diffuse enlargement may be caused by systemic conditions such as mumps, starch-eaters disease, and fatty infiltration.

2. **What is the most likely diagnosis of a mass found high in the gland in front of the tragus of the ear?**

   An enlarged lymph node is the most likely diagnosis, although parotid tumors are occasionally found in this location. In older patients who exhibit solar irradiated facial skin and numerous skin keratoses or have a history of skin cancer around the upper face, metastatic skin cancer in the node must be ruled out.

3. **What is the likelihood that a parotid mass is malignant?**

   Sixty percent of all salivary gland tumors are benign, and 40% are variably malignant. The most common benign tumor (80%) is the mixed salivary gland tumor, or pleomorphic adenoma. Although "benign," this mixed salivary gland tumor can recur locally and behave in a locally malignant manner.

4. **List the types of benign parotid tumors and their frequency.**
   - Mixed tumor (pleomorphic adenoma) is most common (80%) and, although benign, has some local malignant potential.
   - Warthin's tumor: 14%
   - Benign lymphoepithelial lesion: 1%
   - Oxyphil adenoma, oncocytoma, and other rare lesions: < 1% each

5. **In addition to the parotid, name two other locations for salivary gland tumors. What is the frequency of malignant tumors in these locations?**
   - Submandibular glands: 50% malignant
   - Minor salivary glands (oral cavity): 75% malignant

6. **Do mixed tumors spread systemically?**

   Very rarely. There have been 43 reported cases. Typically, these rare metastatic events are found in cervical lymph nodes. The lung and brain were the most common distant sites of metastatic disease, all with classical microscopic findings of mixed tumor.

7. **Describe the types of malignant tumors and list their frequency.**

   In the parotid region, the presence of pain, rapid enlargement of a nodule, skin involvement, or facial nerve paralysis is highly suggestive of a malignancy.

- Mucoepidermoid carcinoma: 44% (the low-grade variety of this tumor is "almost benign")
- Malignant mixed tumor: 17%
- Acinic cell carcinoma: 17%
- Adenocarcinoma: 10%
- Adenoid cystic carcinoma: 9%
- Epidermoid carcinoma: 7%

8. **Describe the characteristic behavior of adenoid cystic carcinoma.**
It is uncommon in the parotid but does recur locally with perineural invasion. It may recur 15 years or more after treatment.

9. **How should a parotid mass be evaluated and treated? Should a biopsy be performed?**
A moveable, rubbery-feeling mass should not be biopsied preoperatively. A parotid lobectomy is normally carried out with dissection of the facial nerve (cranial nerve [CN] VII), followed by frozen section of the tumor. If a tumor is found to be malignant preoperatively by needle aspiration biopsy (which is obtained secondary to nerve involvement), a complete lobectomy should be performed, keeping in mind that cancer may involve one or more nerve branches. The decision about nerve branch resection can only be determined surgically with actual evidence of neural invasion. Most authorities also advocate removal of adjacent upper neck nodes. With histologic evidence of node involvement, a modified neck dissection is indicated.

10. **What is the surgical treatment of a deep lobe parotid tumor?**
These are quite uncommon because the lobe is only one fifth of the size of the entire gland and lies completely beneath the facial nerve (CN VII). Typically, a superficial parotidectomy is performed first followed by dissection and preservation of the facial nerve. Then the tumor in the deep lobe is removed along with any residual deep lobe tissue.

11. **What does a partial or temporary facial nerve (CN VII) paralysis in the presence of an untreated parotid mass suggest?**
With gradual paralysis, cancer is the likely diagnosis (> 95%). Sudden onset of unilateral CN VII weakness suggests Bell's palsy, which is typically the result of an inflammatory process and thus may be reversible. Mixed tumors rarely present with nerve paralysis. Facial nerve paralysis has an ominous prognosis. Radical surgery plus radiotherapy may help control cancer in rare cases.

12. **What is the best imaging modality that can be used to identify parotid lesions?**
Deep lobe tumors occasionally extend into the oral pharynx and oral cavity, and the margins of infiltration as well as the extent of tumor are best delineated by magnetic resonance imaging (MRI). This, however, cannot differentiate between malignant and benign lesions. Routine MRI is not necessary when treating a freely moveable superficial parotid tumor.

13. **Can children develop parotid tumors?**
Parotid tumors are uncommon in children, and a greater proportion of their tumors are malignant (50%).

14. **What is the cause of parotid tumors?**
The cause is not clear. Inflammatory disease or stones in the parotid duct have been incriminated, and smoking may play a part in the production of Warthin's tumors.

15. **What is the recommended treatment of benign-appearing parotid tumors?**
As a rule, it is safer to remove all parotid masses. The only exceptions are long-standing parotid lesions of apparently benign type in older or infirm patients. Aspiration biopsies can be useful

here to confirm the diagnosis of mixed tumors or other benign lesions in situations in which surgery would be high risk.

16. **What is the most likely diagnosis of a recently enlarging parotid mass in a patient who is HIV positive?**
A benign lymphoepithelial lesion is most likely. If needle biopsy confirms this diagnosis, surgery is not necessary because of the benign nature of the process in the face of eventual AIDS development. If a cyst is present, fluid aspiration can decrease or temporarily eliminate the swelling.

17. **If a malignancy is identified on a frozen section of the superficial lobe of the gland, is further surgery necessary?**
Removal of the remaining salivary tissue, including the deep lobe, is usually advocated. Low-grade mucoepidermoid carcinoma does not require radical removal. Careful histologic study, of course, is absolutely essential in determining the type of malignant neoplasm. If cancer is confirmed, a limited upper neck dissection is advised. A classical neck dissection is not performed in patients with parotid cancer unless there is evidence of nodal disease.

18. **Is further surgery necessary when a mixed tumor is identified in the superficial lobe?**
Few, if any, cases recur if the resection margins are grossly clean, there is no spillage at surgery, and there is no microscopic penetration of the capsule.

19. **When is the appropriate time for nerve grafting after parotid cancer resection?**
Interposition grafting can be performed after noncancerous frozen sections of the nerve ends have been confirmed. A nerve graft from the contralateral greater auricular nerve is usually preferred.

20. **Is it necessary to dissect the facial nerve (CN VII) when performing a parotid tumor resection?**
Yes. For a Warthin's tumor, which usually develops in the lower part of the parotid, careful local excision (without identifying the nerve) is permissable because local recurrence is uncommon. Mixed tumors arising in rare anterior locations may also be excised locally without nerve dissection.

KEY POINTS: PAROTID TUMORS

1. The most common benign tumor is a mixed tumor or pleomorphic adenoma.

2. The most common malignant tumor is mucoepidermoid carcinoma.

3. The facial nerve branch most commonly injured during a parotidectomy is the ramus marginalis mandibularis.

21. **Which facial nerve branch is most commonly injured during a parotidectomy?**
Most commonly injured is the ramus marginalis mandibularis, the lowest branch of the nerve that innervates the depressor muscles of the lower lip. This nerve must be preserved. If weakness of the lower lip does occur because of neuropraxia (a common complication even of careful surgery), it will with resolve within 8 weeks.

22. **What are the most common causes of postparotidectomy facial nerve paresis?**
Postoperative palsy is rare. Neuropraxia is typically caused by rough handling of the facial nerve and branches. Coagulation of bleeding vessels, which leads to temporary thermal injury of the nerve; careless suctioning around the nerve itself; and excessive traction of the nerve may result in several weeks of distressing palsy. Despite the greatest care, some patients may still develop temporary paralysis, but most should resolve in weeks.

23. **Why do some patients complain of anesthesia of the ear lobe after surgery?**
They have temporary or permanent injury to the posterior branch of the greater auricular nerve. This nerve can be preserved if it is not involved with tumor and not adherent to the tumor itself.

24. **When is a lymph node dissection indicated?**
Only for clinically positive (palpable) nodes and high-grade cancers.

25. **When should postoperative radiation therapy be used after parotidectomy?**
In all except very low-grade cancers. A radical neck dissection is not performed without evidence of nodal involvement.

26. **What are the cure rates with surgery for parotid cancer?**
In low-grade cancers, cure rates may approach 90%. In one large series of all types of cancers, survival rates at 5, 10, and 15 years were approximately 62%, 54%, and 47%, respectively.

27. **Is the stage or histologic grade of the tumor more important in determining the prognosis of adenoid cystic carcinoma?**
Multivariate analysis shows that tumor stage is more prognostic than tumor grade. Early-stage tumors, even in the face of high-grade histology, enjoy a good prognosis.

28. **How common is a salivary fistula after superficial parotidectomy?**
Rare. If all except a few fragments of the superficial lobe are removed cleanly, fistulas should not occur. The deep lobe itself is rarely, if ever, the source of salivary leak after removal of the superficial lobe.

29. **What is Frey's syndrome?**
Gustatory sweating, also known as auriculotemporal nerve syndrome, is a well-known sequela after parotidectomy. Patients become socially debilitated by episodes of unilateral hyperhidrosis, pain, and flushing in the cutaneous distribution of the auriculotemporal nerve when they eat. The most widely accepted theory of the pathophysiology is the aberrant regeneration theory. In this theory, autonomic fibers from the parotid gland, when damaged by surgery or trauma, regrow into the sheath of the severed auriculotemporal nerve, causing the syndrome. Nonsurgical treatment includes medications such as topical anticholinergics and systemic atropine. Surgical treatments include neurectomy with or without the insertion of a graft to provide a barrier to reinnervation.

30. **When is chemotherapy used after parotidectomy in the face of malignancy?**
Total gross excision of parotid cancer, sparing facial nerve if possible and followed by regional radiotherapy, provides excellent rates of control and survival with only moderate toxicity. Patients presenting postoperatively with gross residual tumor or recurrence after surgery should be considered for trials of more aggressive treatment with combined chemotherapy or altered fractionation schemes of irradiation.

31. **Can a mixed tumor metamorphose into a true malignancy?**
Possibly, but it is rare.

32. **Can facial nerve (CN VII) function be preserved despite the sacrifice of facial branches?**
Occasionally, lip elevator function can be maintained by preserved branches from the zygomatic or buccal branches of the facial nerve that cross over and accomplish similar function as the cut nerve branch.

33. **Which tumor suppressor gene is most often associated with parotid cancer?**
p53 has been found in some parotid cancers. These lesions are usually advanced and larger than those without p53.

WEB SITE

http://www.acssurgery.com

BIBLIOGRAPHY

1. Blevins NH, Jackler RK, Kaplan MJ, Boles R: Facial paralysis due to benign parotid tumors. Arch Otol Head Neck Surg 118:427–430, 1992.

2. Christensen NR, Jacobsen SD: Parotidectomy: Preserving the posterior branch of the great auricular nerve. J Laryngol Otol 111:556–559, 1997.

3. Goldwyn RM, Cohen MN: The Unfavorable Result in Plastic Surgery. Philadelphia, Lippincott Williams & Wilkins, 2001.

4. Ismail Y, McLean NR, Chippindale AJ: MRI and malignant melanoma of the parotid gland. Br J Plast Surg 54:636–637, 2001.

5. Kelley DJ, Spiro RH: Management of the neck in parotid carcinoma. Am J Surg 172:695–697, 1996.

6. Malata CM, Camilleri IG, McLean NR, et al: Malignant tumors of the parotid gland: A 12-year review. Br J Plast Surg 50:600–608, 1997.

7. Ogata H, Ebihara S, Mukai K: Salivary gland neoplasms in children. Jpn J Clin Oncol 24:88–93, 1994.

8. Spiro RH, Huvos AG: Stage means more than grade in adenoid cystic carcinoma. Am J Surg 164:623–638, 1992.

9. Teymoortash A, Werner JA: Value of neck dissection in patients with cancer of the parotid gland and a clinical N0 neck. Onkologie 25:122–126, 2002.

10. Toonkel LM, Guha S, Foster P, Dembow V: Radiotherapy for parotid cancer. Ann Surg Oncol 1:468–472, 1994.

11. Tullio A, Marchetti C, Sesenna E, et al: Treatment of carcinoma of the parotid gland: The result of a multicenter study. J Oral Maxillofac Surg 59:263–270, 2001.

12. Yugueros P, Loellner JR, Petty PM: Treating recurrence of benign parotid pleomorphic adenomas. Ann Plast Surg 40:573–576, 1998.

CHAPTER 66

HODGKIN'S DISEASE AND MALIGNANT LYMPHOMAS

Christina A. Finlayson, M.D.

1. **What is the differential diagnosis of lymphadenopathy?**

   The significance of cervical, axillary, or inguinal lymphadenopathy depends on the characteristics of the lymph nodes and associated symptoms. Infection, autoimmune disease, and malignancy are all included in the differential diagnosis.

2. **What historical information helps to direct the diagnostic investigation of lymphadenopathy?**

   It is unusual for a patient older than 40 years to have nonspecific lymphadenopathy; over 70% of enlarged cervical lymph nodes in this age group are malignant. Patients younger than 40 years are more likely to have a nonspecific or infectious cause, although the mean age of Hodgkin's lymphoma diagnosis is 32 years.

   The duration of adenopathy helps with the diagnosis. A newly enlarged lymph node is more suggestive of infection, although an enlarging lymph node can undergo internal hemorrhage with a rapid increase in size. Travel and occupation history, exposure to pets, geographic area of residence, and sexual history provide clues to infectious agents. A history of smoking is associated with lung, upper gastrointestinal, and head and neck malignancy.

   Systemic symptoms, including fever, weight loss, night sweats, and pruritus, are present in 30% of patients with Hodgkin's and 10% of patients with non-Hodgkin's lymphoma.

3. **A 25-year-old man presents for evaluation of a 1-cm, soft inguinal lymph node that has been present for 1 month. How should the diagnostic evaluation proceed?**

   Examine all draining lymph node basins including cervical, submandibular, auricular, occipital, supraclavicular, axillary, epitrochlear, inguinal, and popliteal. Supraclavicular adenopathy is virtually always associated with malignant or granulomatous disease. Peripheral adenopathy in the groin and axilla is often a response to trauma, frequently occult. The limb should be examined thoroughly.

   A lymph node < 1 cm in size is usually not significant. Nodes > 2 cm are often malignant or granulomatous. Whereas hard nodes are typical of metastatic malignancy, soft nodes could be anything.

   Reexamine the patient in 1 month. If regression has not occurred, biopsy the node.

4. **A 48-year-old woman presents with a 3-cm, firm lymph node in the left supraclavicular area. How may her evaluation differ from that of the previous patient?**

   The age of the patient, the size and consistency of the lymph node, and its location virtually mandate fine-needle aspiration (FNA) or open biopsy. Malignancy must be excluded. Hodgkin's and non-Hodgkin's lymphomas as well as metastatic disease from a primary intraabdominal, genital, lung, or breast primary frequently present this way. Head and neck tumors rarely metastasize to this location but tend to spread first to cervical lymph nodes.

   A period of observation is not appropriate.

5. **Should antibiotics be used during a "watch-and-wait" period when a specific site of infection has not been identified?**

Lymph nodes are rarely the target of invading organisms. When infected nodes are present, other signs of inflammation, including warmth, erythema, and pain, accompany the swelling. If a specific infection is not identified, the empiric use of "shot-in-the-dark" antibiotics does not have therapeutic or diagnostic benefit.

6. **Can FNA be used if lymphoma is in the differential diagnosis?**

FNA is an established diagnostic tool used in the evaluation of breast, thyroid, and metastatic disease. When a patient presents with lymphadenopathy, often a diagnosis can be established from a lymph node aspirate that implicates a cancer other than lymphoma.

Establishing a definitive diagnosis of lymphoma by FNA is not reliable. The pathologist often requires intact lymph node architecture to reach a diagnosis and to provide accurate tumor typing. The recent addition of flow cytometry evaluation of the aspirate sample has increased the diagnostic yield of FNA for lymphoma. However, many aspirates appear normal and cannot be processed by flow cytometry. In this setting, most patients require surgical biopsy to obtain adequate tissue for histology as well as immunohistochemical evaluation.

7. **How should a surgeon do a lymph node biopsy for suspected lymphoma?**

The primary role of the surgeon in lymphoma is to diagnose and stage the disease. The cervical lymph nodes are usually the site of involvement (75%), followed by the axillary (15%) and inguinal lymph nodes (9%). It is common for a primary node involved with a tumor to be accompanied by smaller reactive lymph nodes. Therefore, it is important to select the largest, most suspicious lymph node for biopsy. Because the architecture of the lymph node is important for the pathologist, the node should be removed in one piece. Do not crush, clamp, or cauterize the node. The node must go to the laboratory fresh, wrapped in saline-soaked gauze. Soaking the node in water or formalin distorts the cellular architecture.

Talk to your pathologist. A frozen section can determine whether you have enough tissue.

8. **What are the clinical differences between Hodgkin's and non-Hodgkin's lymphoma?**

Hodgkin's lymphoma usually presents with either a neck or a mediastinal mass. It arises first in the lymph nodes and rarely involves extranodal sites initially. It tends to spread contiguously to adjacent nodal stations rather than "skipping" to distant sites. Most patients present with early stage I or II disease. Epitrochlear, popliteal, or mesenteric nodal involvement is unusual. There is a bimodal age distribution with an early peak in the 20s and a later peak in the 60s.

Non-Hodgkin's lymphomas originate from lymphocytes and also are called *lymphocytic lymphomas*. The incidence of these tumors has increased over the past 20 years. Some of this increase has occurred because of an association with AIDS, but this is not the whole story.

In contrast to Hodgkin's lymphoma, non-Hodgkin's lymphomas are often extranodal and spread noncontiguously. They rarely present as localized disease; bone marrow and liver involvement is common. Non-Hodgkin's lymphoma involves epitrochlear, popliteal, and mesenteric lymph nodes as well as Waldeyer's ring. It accounts for almost all gastrointestinal lymphomas. Most patients present with advanced-stage disease.

9. **What is Waldeyer's ring?**

This is the mucosa of the posterior oropharynx covering a bed of lymphatic tissue that aggregates to form the palatine, lingual, pharyngeal, and tubal tonsils. These structures form a ring around the pharyngeal wall. This may be the site of primary or metastatic tumor.

10. **Why are tumors staged?**

Quantifying the size of the tumor, the presence of nodal disease, and presence or absence of distant metastasis (TNM staging) provides an estimate of tumor burden. Because the primary tumor burden of lymphoma arises in nodal tissue, the usual TNM staging system is not used. Measuring the extent of disease helps to determine therapy and to predict prognosis.

KEY POINTS: HODGKIN'S DISEASE

1. The primary role of the surgeon is to diagnose and stage the disease.

2. The cervical lymph nodes are the usual site of involvement (75%), followed by the axillary (15%) and inguinal (9%) lymph nodes.

3. The node should be removed in one piece and not crushed, clamped, or cauterized.

4. The node should go to the pathologist fresh wrapped in saline-soaked gauze.

11. **How is lymphoma staged?**
    History and physical examination elicit systemic symptoms and identify involved lymph node stations. Obtain a complete blood count, creatinine, liver function tests, erythrocyte sedimentation rate, lactate dehydrogenase, and alkaline phosphatase. If a chest radiograph is abnormal, a computed tomography (CT) scan of the chest is required. A computed tomography (CT) scan of the abdomen and pelvis and bilateral bone marrow aspiration and biopsy are required in all cases. Lymphangiography and staging laparotomy are controversial.

12. **What staging system is used for Hodgkin's and low-grade non-Hodgkin's lymphomas?**
    Because lymphoma is a malignancy of the lymph nodes and the initial site of disease is rarely identifiable, the TNM staging system does not apply. Staging, therefore, is based on the distribution of the disease and systemic symptoms. Hodgkin's and low-grade non-Hodgkin's lymphomas use the Ann Arbor Staging Classification:

Stage I	Involvement of a single lymph node region or localized involvement of a single extralymphatic organ or site
Stage II	Involvement of two or more lymph node regions on the same side of the diaphragm *or* Localized involvement of a single extralymphatic organ or site and its regional lymph nodes
Stage III	Involvement of lymph node regions on both sides of the diaphragm, which may include localized involvement of an associated extralymphatic organ or site, involvement of the spleen, or both
Stage IV	Disseminated involvement of one or more extralymphatic organs (including bone marrow) with or without associated lymph node involvement *or* Isolated extralymphatic organ involvement with distant nodal involvement

    The subscript E denotes extralymphatic organ involvement, and the subscript S denotes splenic involvement in stage III or IV disease. E and S may be combined with involvement of both an extralymphatic site and the spleen.

    Each stage is subdivided into either A or B. Patients without systemic symptoms are As. Patients with weight loss of more than 10% in the preceding 6 months, unexplained temperatures > 38°C, or drenching night sweats are classified as Bs. Pruritus is often included in the description of B symptoms but does not qualify for B classification when it is the only presenting systemic symptom.

For example, a 24-year-old man who presents with an asymptomatic mass in the neck, no systemic symptoms, and no other sites of disease on staging is classified as stage IA. A 70-year-old woman who presents with a localized small bowel lymphoma (low-grade) that involves the mesenteric (regional) lymph nodes and has had a temperature of 38.5°C over the past 6 weeks is classified as stage II$_E$B.

13. **What staging system is used for intermediate- and high-grade non-Hodgkin's lymphomas?**
The National Cancer Institute Modified Staging System is used:
Stage I   Localized nodal or extranodal disease
Stage II   Two or more nodal sites of disease or one localized extranodal site plus
             draining lymph nodes with no poor prognostic features
Stage III   Stage II plus one or more poor prognostic features
Poor prognostic features include Karnofsky performance status < 70, B symptoms, any mass > 10 cm in diameter, serum lactate dehydrogenase > 500, or ≥ 3 extranodal sites of disease.

14. **What is Karnofsky performance status?**
This is a scale used to quantify a patient's activity level, which reflects the impact of the disease. If a patient has a disease but it does not interfere with activities, the performance status is 100%. As disease progresses, activity decreases and performance status falls. A bed-bound patient is at 10%.

15. **What is the difference between clinical and pathologic staging?**
Clinical staging is based on history, physical examination, and radiographic evaluation. Abnormal lymph nodes identified by abdominal CT scan or lymphangiography imply clinical subdiaphragmatic disease. **Pathologic staging** requires the histologic conformation of all potentially involved tissues. Pathologic staging of abnormal lymph nodes identified by abdominal CT scan or lymphangiography requires staging laparotomy with biopsies. To identify the method of staging, a lower-case *c* for clinical staging or *p* for pathologic staging precedes the staging nomenclature. For example, cIII indicates a tumor staged clinically with abnormal lymph nodes identified by abdominal CT scan or lymphangiography. If a staging laparotomy is performed and pathologic confirmation identifies involved lymph nodes, the tumor is stage pIII.

16. **What is a staging laparotomy?**
This is a midline incision that permits attention to lymph node–bearing areas. Splenectomy is performed first, followed by wedge and core biopsies of each lobe of the liver. Lymph nodes are obtained from the celiac, mesenteric, portal, paraaortic, and paracaval areas. In premenopausal women, an oophoropexy secures the ovaries behind the uterus and preserves fertility in approximately 50% of women who require pelvic radiation. When the abdomen is closed, bone marrow biopsies are performed bilaterally.

17. **What are the indications for staging laparotomy?**
A staging laparotomy should be performed only when the results may change the clinical stage and when a change in stage will alter the planned treatment. Pathologic staging of surgically removed tissue is more accurate than clinical staging. In the Stanford experience, 43% of patients had a change in stage after laparotomy. Approximately 30% of patients in clinical stages (CS) I and II are "upstaged" to pathologic stage III or IV disease after surgery. Conversely, 20% of patients with clinical stage III or IV disease are "downstaged." In some subgroups of patients, however, the risk of subdiaphragmatic disease is so low (< 10%) that staging laparotomy rarely adds information. These subgroups include all CSIA women and CSIA men with a high neck presentation, lymphocyte-predominant histology, or mediastinal-only disease.
Obscuring the role of staging laparotomy in treating Hodgkin's disease is its lack of effect on survival because of the highly effective salvage chemotherapy available for patients who relapse.

Evidence indicates, however, that patients staged surgically have a lower incidence of recurrence and, therefore, are less likely to require a second course of treatment.

Staging laparotomy is not performed for non-Hodgkin's lymphoma.

18. **How is Hodgkin's lymphoma treated?**
Stage I and IIA disease may be treated with radiation alone if the tumor is not bulky and the prognostic factors are favorable. More advanced disease requires adjuvant chemotherapy. Combinations include three or more of the following: mechlorethamine, vincristine, procarbazine, prednisone (MOPP), doxorubicin, bleomycin, vinblastine, and dacarbazine (ABVD).

19. **What is the Working Formulation for non-Hodgkin's lymphoma?**
Non-Hodgkin's lymphoma includes many diverse histologic patterns, each with its own natural history and prognosis. Early attempts to classify these subtypes resulted in six chaotic classification schemes. The Working Formulation was created to standardize the nomenclature for non-Hodgkin's lymphomas. It categorizes each cytologic description into three general categories: low, immediate, and high grade. Each category has a similar natural history, treatment plan, and prognosis.

20. **Does the natural history for each category of non-Hodgkin's lymphoma differ?**
Yes. Low histologic grades grow slowly, with waxing and waning symptoms over a long period. High histologic grades progress rapidly and, if left untreated, are fatal in a short period. Ironically, chemotherapy has been most successful in the intermediate and aggressive subtypes. Intermediate-grade lymphomas often respond to standard combination chemotherapy. Aggressive lymphoma, when treated promptly with combination chemotherapy, has a 75% complete response rate and 50% chance of long-term survival.

21. **Is there a role for the surgical treatment of lymphoma?**
Yes. Localized non-Hodgkin's lymphoma of the gastrointestinal (GI) tract most commonly arises from the stomach. It originates in the lymphoid tissue of the submucosa. Surgery has been the mainstay of treatment, and complete resection of early-stage disease is frequently curative. Patients with more advanced disease may benefit from adjuvant radiation and chemotherapy.

Lymphoma at other locations within the GI tract often presents as a surgical emergency. The diagnosis is often made at the time of the operation, and attention is focused on treating perforation, obstruction, or hemorrhage. Resection of the tumor is indicated if the disease appears localized.

22. **What is the risk of a second cancer in patients successfully treated for Hodgkin's lymphoma?**
It is higher. The more common of these second cancers are lung, breast, sarcoma, leukemia, and non-Hodgkin's lymphoma. Patients who received radiation therapy to the cervical area require annual thyroid function testing to detect radiation-induced hypothyroidism. Young women who received thoracic radiation require screening for breast cancer. Annual mammography should be started 10 years after treatment but no later than age 40 years.

WEB SITES

1. http://www.lymphoma.org

2. www.cancer.gov

3. www.cancer.org

BIBLIOGRAPHY

1. Bazemore AW, Smucker DR: Lymphadenopathy and malignancy. Am Fam Physician 66:2103–2110, 2002.

2. Fleming I (ed): The Surgeon and Malignant Lymphoma. Surgical Oncology Clinics of North America. Philadelphia, W.B. Saunders, 1993.

3. Hoppe RT: NCCN practice guidelines for Hodgkin's disease. Oncology 13:18–25, 1999.

4. Nynadoto P, Muhonen T, Joensu H: Second cancer among long-term survivors from Hodgkin's disease. Int J Radiat Oncol Biol Phys 42:373–378, 1998.

5. Patient Care Committee of the Society for Surgery of the Alimentary Tract (SSAT): Splenectomy. J Gastrointest Surg 3:218–219, 1999.

6. Walsh RM, Heniford BT: Role of laparoscopy for Hodgkin's and non-Hodgkin's lymphoma. Semin Surg Oncol 16:284–292, 1999.

7. Young NA, Al-Saleem TI, Ehya H, Smith MR: Utilization of fine-needle aspiration cytology and flow cytometry in the diagnosis and subclassification of primary and recurrent lymphoma. Cancer 84:252–261, 1998.

8. Zelenetz AD, Hoppe RT: NCCN: Non-Hodgkin's lymphoma. Cancer Contrl 8(suppl 2):102–113, 2001.

CHAPTER 67

NECK MASSES

Nathan W. Pearlman, M.D.

1. **What causes lumps in the neck?**
   Enlarged lymph nodes, benign or malignant tumors, congenital abnormalities, and normal anatomy.

2. **Can neck masses be part of normal anatomy?**
   Yes. In some patients, the neck mass is nothing more than a submaxillary gland or omohyoid muscle that has become prominent with aging and loss of surrounding fat. This finding usually is apparent if the other side of the neck is carefully examined.

3. **A 34-year-old man presents with a 2–3-cm mass just below the angle of the mandible. What are the likely causes?**

Nonspecific lymphadenopathy	Branchial cleft cyst
Infectious mononucleosis	Submaxillary or parotid gland tumor
Intraoral infection	Lymphoma
Carotid body tumor	Metastatic carcinoma

4. **Doesn't this patient seem awfully young for metastatic cancer?**
   Yes, but it still occurs in this age group, particularly thyroid, tongue, and nasopharyngeal cancer.

5. **This is a long list. Is there any way to narrow it?**
   - Inflammatory nodes and nodes of mononucleosis are mildly tender, relatively soft, bilateral (one side may be more symptomatic than the other) of recent onset. They generally are < 3 cm in diameter, the patient usually reports a history of a systemic illness, and the skin over the tender nodes is normal.
   - Lymphadenopathy caused by intraoral infection is also of recent onset but exquisitely painful, indurated, and unilateral; the overlying skin is often erythematous.
   - Carotid body tumors may be tender and unilateral but are long standing, more rubbery than infectious nodes, and cannot be separated from the carotid pulse.
   - A branchial cleft cyst is unilateral, relatively soft, nontender, and long standing; it also trans-illuminates.
   - Nodes of lymphoma are nontender and have the consistency of the submaxillary gland. They may be unilateral or bilateral and of recent onset or several months' duration. In addition, signs of systemic illness may or may not be present.
   - Submaxillary or parotid tumors are rubbery and nontender and occupy the position of the contralateral gland.
   - Lymphadenopathy caused by metastatic cancer is hard, nontender, and often larger than 3–4 cm.
   - Tuberculosis can mimic all of these conditions.

6. **Why not just remove the mass or lymph node and see what it is?**
   Open biopsy can unduly complicate further management when it is the *initial* diagnostic maneuver. If lymphoma or an unusual infection is present but not suspected, the node may be mishandled when sent to the pathology or microbiology departments. If metastatic cancer is the problem, the scar tissue created by the biopsy may be difficult to distinguish from

tumor on computed tomography (CT) or magnetic resonance imaging (MRI), leading to inaccurate staging. The scar also may resemble cancer at subsequent surgery, potentially resulting in a larger operation than originally needed. A better choice for histologic diagnosis is fine-needle aspiration (FNA), which is 95% accurate and avoids the problems of open biopsy.

7. **A complete head and neck examination shows nothing abnormal, but FNA of the node reveals squamous cancer. What should be done next?**
Examination of mouth, pharynx, larynx, esophagus, and tracheobronchial tree under anesthesia (triple endoscopy) should be done. If nothing is seen, blind biopsy of the nasopharynx, tonsils, base of tongue, and pyriform sinuses should be done at the same sitting.

KEY POINTS: DIFFERENTIAL DIAGNOSIS OF NECK MASSES

1. Enlarged lymph nodes

2. Benign or malignant tumors

3. Congenital abnormalities

4. Normal anatomy (e.g., submaxillary gland or omohyoid muscle that has become prominent with age)

8. **Isn't this a bit much?**
No. The squamous cancer came from somewhere, and the most likely site is somewhere in the region (e.g., mouth, pharynx). In approximately 15% of patients, the primary tumor is detected at triple endoscopy when it cannot be found on office examination, and another 10% of patients are found to have a synchronous second primary tumor elsewhere in the aerodigestive tract.

9. **Why not just start with triple endoscopy and skip all the other folderol?**
Examination with the patient awake provides information about tongue and laryngeal function that cannot be obtained when the patient is asleep, and treatment planning depends on such knowledge. In addition, examination under anesthesia may be a blind search because of collapse of the tongue and pharynx, unless directed by findings while the patient is awake.

10. **Should CT scan or MRI be used?**
Both modalities may provide information about areas difficult to evaluate by physical examination, such as the base of the skull, and are helpful in staging if cancer is present. However, they do not replace the measures already outlined.

11. **We do all that and still can't find a primary tumor. What now?**
Two options exist. Most surgeons would treat the patient with a functional or modified radical neck dissection and postoperative irradiation to the neck and likely site of the primary tumor. Alternatively, one may proceed with irradiation alone to the neck and likely primary site, with neck dissection at a later date if the enlarged node or nodes persist after treatment.

12. **What if the primary tumor never shows up? Does this influence prognosis?**
No. Prognosis is determined by the presence of metastatic neck disease, not by whether a small primary tumor is or is not found.

13. **If the mass or enlarged node is in the posterior triangle of the neck, is the work-up still the same?**

Yes. Although most oral or pharyngeal tumors spread first to nodes in the anterior triangle, it is not uncommon for naso- or hypopharyngeal tumors, thyroid cancers, and lymphomas to present as enlarged nodes in the posterior triangle.

14. **What if FNA of the node reveals only lymphocytes or shows adenocarcinoma?**

The presence of lymphocytes most likely represents inflammation or lymphoma; however, if the "node" is just below the ear lobe, it may be a Warthin's tumor (cystadenoma-lymphomatosa) of the parotid. Adenocarcinoma found on FNA usually indicates metastases from thyroid cancer or a primary site below the clavicles, but it may mean salivary gland cancer if the "node" lies high in the anterior triangle. If only lymphocytes are present, excision of the node may be reasonable, as long as it was clearly not in the parotid or submaxillary gland. In the latter case, one should proceed with a parotidectomy or submaxillary gland excision.

15. **Lumps in the neck are common, and relatively few patients have cancer. Isn't this a cost-ineffective approach?**

No. Most patients with lumps in the neck have benign, self-limiting conditions, which should be apparent on the initial history and physical examination. If there is a question, FNA can be done. Only rarely is removal of the mass indicated for diagnosis or treatment.

On the other hand, if neck lumps are routinely excised to facilitate the work-up (or to see what they are), the physician will constantly be surprised by what is found (e.g., metastatic cancer, lymphoma, tuberculosis). The work-up outlined above will then have to be undertaken anyway— and in a field dirtied by the biopsy. Such a course is not cost effective but, in fact, is a waste of time and resources.

WEB SITE

http://www.acssurgery.com

BIBLIOGRAPHY

1. Attie JN, Setzon M, Klein I: Thyroid cancer presenting as an enlarged cervical lymph node. Am J Surg 166:428–430, 1993.
2. Lee NK, Byers RM, Abbruzzese JL, Wolfe P: Metastatic adenocarcinoma to the neck from an unknown primary source. Am J Surg 162:306–309, 1991.
3. Rice DH, Spiro RH: Metastatic carcinoma of the neck, primary unknown. In Current Concepts in Head and Neck Cancer. Atlanta, American Cancer Society, 1989, pp 126–133.
4. Tarantino DR, McHenry CR, Strickland T, Khiyami A: The role of the fine-needle aspiration biopsy and flow cytometry in the evaluation of persistent neck adenopathy. Am J Surg 176:413–417, 1998.

WHAT IS ATHEROSCLEROSIS?

Craig H. Selzman, M.D.

CHAPTER 68

1. **Are elderly individuals the only ones who have atherosclerosis?**
   No. The initial (or type I) lesion, consisting of lipid deposits in the intima, has been well charac-terized in infants and children.

2. **What is a fatty streak?**
   Fatty streaks or type II lesions are visible as yellow-colored streaks, patches, or spots on the inti-mal surface of arteries. Microscopically, they are characterized by the intracellular accumulation of lipid.

3. **What is a foam cell?**
   A foam cell is any cell that has ingested lipids, thus giving the histologic appearance of a sudsy vacuole. In general, a foam cell refers to a lipid-laden macrophage; however, other cells that uptake lipids, particularly vascular smooth muscle cells, also may be considered foam cells.

4. **Describe the progression of atherosclerosis.**
   Although the sequence of events is not always consistent, fatty streaks progress to type III or intermediate lesions. This growth is characterized by extracellular pools of lipid, which are gen-erally clinically occult. However, when the pools coalesce to create a core of extracellular lipid (type IV lesion or atheroma), the blood vessel architecture has been altered sufficiently to become clinically overt. With smooth muscle cell (SMC) proliferation and collagen deposition, the atheroma becomes a fibroatheroma (type V). The fibroatheroma is characterized by throm-bogenic surface defects that provoke intramural hemorrhage or intraluminal thrombus (type V lesion), resulting in vessel occlusion, which, in the case of a coronary artery, results in myocar-dial infarction.

5. **Of the 100 medical students in your class, how many have significant atherosclerosis?**
   In 1953, Enos reported autopsy findings from 300 American male battle casualties in Korea (average age, 22 years). He noted that 77% of the hearts had some gross evidence of coronary atherosclerosis. About 39% of the men had luminal narrowing, estimated at 10–90%, and 3% had plaques causing complete occlusion of one or more coronary vessels. However, a subse-quent study evaluating 105 combat casualties in Vietnam demonstrated that only 45% exhibited atherosclerosis, and fewer than 5% were considered severe. Finally, a recent study looking at 105 trauma victims corroborated the Korean War study by demonstrating a 78% incidence of atherosclerosis, with left main or significant two- and three-vessel involvement in 20%.

6. **What are the classic risk factors for atherosclerotic cardiovascular disease?**
   Tobacco use, hyperlipidemia, hypertension, diabetes mellitus, and family history of cardiovas-cular disease.

7. **How do such diverse risk factors produce similar disease?**
   That is the million-dollar question. Do parallel pathways lead to a final atherosclerotic lesion, or do the apparently dissimilar risk factors activate signals that converge to a few dominant events,

promoting the development of atherosclerosis? Certainly, this question has broad therapeutic implications. It would be a lot easier to inhibit a single proximal point in this process rather than to treat multiple divergent, more distal cellular pathologic events.

8. **What is the response to injury?**
The premise that atherogenesis represents an exaggerated inflammatory, fibroproliferative response to injury has evolved into an attractive unifying hypothesis of vascular disease and repair. Mechanical, metabolic, and toxic insults may injure the vessel wall. The common denominator is endothelial injury. Disruption of the endothelium not only results in endothelial cell dysfunction but also allows adhesion and transmigration of circulating monocytes, platelets, and T lymphocytes. Within the developing lesion, the activated cells release potent growth-regulatory molecules that may act in both a paracrine and autocrine manner. Under the influence of cytokines and growth factors, vascular smooth muscle cells (VSMCs) adapt to a synthetic phenotype and begin proliferation and migration across the internal elastic lamina into the intimal layer. Stimulated VSMCs allow the deposition of extracellular matrix, thus converting the initial lesion to a fibrous plaque.

9. **What is C-reactive protein? Is it just another random, nonclinically relevant marker of inflammation?**
C-reactive protein (CRP) is one of many acute phase proteins elaborated from hepatocytes upon inflammatory stimulation. Originally isolated from the serum of patients with pneumonia, it has a high binding affinity for pneumococcal C-polysaccharide. Although CRP is best known as an active peptide by neutralizing foreign antigens, controlling tissue damage, and promoting tissue repair, it is increasingly considered a sensitive marker of inflammation.

   Unlike other markers of inflammation, CRP levels are stable over long periods of time, have no diurnal variation, can be measured inexpensively with available high-sensitivity assays, and have shown specificity in predicting risk of cardiovascular events. Indeed, elevation of CRP levels might be more predictive of cardiac events than elevation of low-density lipoprotein (LDL) levels. These observations may influence therapy because nonhyperlipidemic patients with elevated CRP levels might benefit from aggressive statin (HMG-reductase inhibitors) therapy.

10. **Does vascular injury mean only direct physical injury, as with an angioplasty catheter?**
No. Injury is a catch-all word that includes physical injury such as angioplasty, hypertension, and shear forces (atherosclerotic lesions typically occur at bifurcations) as well as other diverse insults, including viruses, bacteria, nicotine, homocysteine, and oxidized LDLs.

11. **Are lipids important?**
The lipid hypothesis of atherosclerosis suggests that the cellular changes in atherosclerosis are reactive events in response to lipid infiltration. Indeed, antilipid therapy is one of the few strategies that has induced regression of atherosclerosis in randomized, prospective clinical trials. Strong evidence also derives from patients with genetic hyperlipidemias; homozygotes rarely live beyond age 26 years.

12. **What is syndrome X?**
Syndrome X is a metabolic phenomenon in healthy, nonobese, nondiabetic people who have hyperinsulinemia associated with elevated blood sugar, high blood pressure, and increased triglycerides with decreased high-density lipoprotein (HDL) cholesterol levels. Clinically, such patients develop premature cardiovascular disease. Insulin resistance with elevated insulin levels, with or without overt diabetes, fuels important aspects of atherogenesis, including dyslipidemias, endothelial dysfunction, hypertension, and SMC proliferation.

13. **Why would vitamin E be (even theoretically) protective against cardiovascular disease?**
Antioxidant therapy with vitamins C and E as well as beta-carotene is intuitively sound. In vitro, these agents afford resistance of LDL to oxidation and reduce elaboration of vessel-injuring reactive oxygen species. Reactive oxygen metabolites (as much as 5% of oxygen), such as superoxide and hydrogen peroxide, directly injure vascular cells, impair endothelial vasomotor function, promote platelet aggregation and leukocyte adhesion, and stimulate vascular SMC proliferation. Although descriptive, case-control, and prospective cohort studies have found inverse associations between the frequency of coronary artery disease and dietary intake of antioxidant vitamins, randomized therapeutic trials thus far have exhibited no benefit of doing so.

14. **What is homocysteine?**
This amino acid intermediate in the metabolism of methionine is an essential amino acid in the synthesis of both animal and plant proteins. Excessive homocysteine in the vessel wall reacts with LDPs to create damaging reactive oxygen species. Epidemiologic evidence correlates elevated levels of homocysteine and decreased levels of folate with cardiovascular disease.

15. **How does homocysteine rank as a risk factor for atherosclerosis?**
It is estimated that 10% of the risk of coronary artery disease in the general population is attributable to homocysteine. An increase in 5 µmol/L in plasma homocysteine concentration (normal, 5–15 µmol/L) raises the risk of coronary disease by as much as an increase of 20 mg/dL in the cholesterol concentration.

16. **Should everyone take folate supplements?**
Folic acid, vitamins B_{12} and B_6, and pyridoxine are important cofactors for the enzymatic processing of homocysteine. Indeed, the reduction in mortality from cardiovascular causes since 1960 has been correlated with the increase in vitamin B_6 supplementation in the food supply. Furthermore, the Food and Drug Administration recently mandated folic acid fortification in flour and cereal products as a method of preventing atherosclerotic-related death. Although these supplements may decrease homocysteine levels, the expected decrease in cardiovascular events has not yet been documented in prospective, randomized clinical trials.

17. **What microorganisms have been implicated in atherosclerosis?**
Bacteria include *Chlamydia pneumoniae, Helicobacter pylori*, streptococci, and *B. typhosus*. Viruses include influenza, herpes virus, adenovirus, and cytomegalovirus.

KEY POINTS: ATHEROSCLEROSIS

1. The classic risk factors for atherosclerotic cardiovascular disease include tobacco use, hyperlipidemia, hypertension, diabetes mellitus, and family history of cardiovascular disease.

2. It is estimated that 10% of the coronary artery disease in the general population is attributable to homocysteine.

3. The bacteria implicated in atherosclerosis include *Chlamydia pneumoniae, Heliobacter pylori*, streptococci, and *B. typhosus.*

18. **Are individuals with sexually transmitted diseases (STDs) at greater risk for cardiovascular disease?**
The initial epidemiologic description linking *Chlamydia* species to atherosclerosis was reported by venerologists in South America in the 1940s. *Chlamydia pneumoniae*, a ubiquitous

respiratory organism, is the predominant species subsequently identified in cardiovascular lesions. More than 50% of the population has antichlamydial antibodies (ACAs) by age 50 years; yet this 50% of the population does not have this STD.

19. **Is there an *Helicobacter pylori* peptic ulcer equivalent in atherosclerosis? Should we all take a macrolide a day?**
     The jury is still out. It is unlikely that eradication of *Chlamydia* species will have the same profound effect on disease as eradication of *H. pylori*. However, *C. pneumoniae* may be another factor, exacerbating the response to injury. Evidence suggests that antibiotic therapy decreases the number of cardiovascular events in patients with elevated antichlamydial antibody titers.

20. **What is the role of the endothelium?**
     A healthy blood vessel wall is lined by a monolayer of phenomenally metabolically active endothelial cells. The surface area of the endothelium is approximately 5000 m^2 but comprises only 1% of the total body weight. While acting as a physical barrier to protect the underlying vessel and allowing formed blood elements to flow freely, thus preventing thrombosis, this seemingly bucolic layer is a central control center of vascular physiology. The endothelium is a key docking point for monocytes, neutrophils, and lymphocytes by virtue of its ability to express sticky, cell-specific adhesion molecules. The endothelium is a source for cytokines and peptide growth factors that act in both autocrine and paracrine fashion to promote atherogenesis.

21. **What are some of the products of endothelial cells that govern vasomotor tone?**
     Factors that favor vascular relaxation include nitric oxide and prostacyclin. Conversely, factors favoring vascular constriction include thromboxane, leukotrienes, free radicals, endothelins, and cytokines (e.g., tumor necrosis factor and interleukin-1).

22. **What is the importance of vascular thrombosis?**
     Thrombosis is central to the pathogenesis of acute arterial insufficiency and acute coronary or cerebrovascular syndromes, including unstable angina, non–Q-wave myocardial infarction, acute (ST-elevation) myocardial infarction, and vessel occlusion after vascular intervention (angioplasty).

23. **Describe the three main phases of platelet activation involved with thrombus formation.**
     The three main phases of platelet activation include adhesion, aggregation, and secretion. With exposure of the subendothelial space after vascular injury, platelets adhere to basement membrane proteins, especially collagen. This adhesion depends on binding of endothelial or circulating von Willebrand factor (vWF) to the platelet membrane glycoprotein 1b receptor. Platelet aggregation is an energy-dependent process that requires adenosine triphosphate (ATP). The predominant mechanism of aggregation involves binding of fibrinogen to the platelet glycoprotein IIb/IIIa receptor. Platelet secretion usually follows aggregation. Released products include the contents of dense bodies (serotonin, calcium, ATP) and alpha granules (vWF, fibrinogen, growth factors, platelet factor 4, and coagulation factors).

24. **Is atherosclerosis an inflammatory disease?**
     Yes.

25. **Would taking an aspirin a day help?**
     Maybe. Strategies aimed at limiting the inflammatory cascade offer promise as antiatherosclerosis therapy. Examples in daily use include aspirin, fibrinolytics, 3-hydroxyl-3-methylglutaryl

(HMG)-reductase inhibitors, and estrogens. Others in the preclinical arena include gene therapy, anticytokine therapy, and antigrowth factor therapy. Certainly, primary prevention is important in limiting the initial injury stimulus. However, the smoldering inflammation involved with atherosclerosis may best be attacked by modifying the vascular cells' response to these insults.

WEB SITE

http://www.acssurgery.com

BIBLIOGRAPHY

1. Boushey CJ, Beresford SA, Omenn GS, et al: A quantitative assessment of plasma homocysteine as a risk factor for vascular disease: Probable benefits of increasing folic acid intakes. JAMA 274:1049–1057, 1995.

2. Cain BS, Meldrum DR, Selzman CH, et al: Surgical implications of vascular endothelial physiology. Surgery 122:516–526, 1997.

3. Diaz MN, Frei B, Vita JA, et al: Antioxidants and atherosclerotic heart disease. N Engl J Med 337:408–416, 1997.

4. Enos WF, Holmes RH, Beyer J: Coronary disease among United States soldiers killed in action in Korea. JAMA 152:1090–1093, 1953.

5. Gupta S, Leatham EW, Carrington D, et al: Elevated *Chlamydia pneumoniae* antibodies, cardiovascular events, and azithromycin in male survivors of myocardial infarction. Circulation 97:633–636, 1997.

6. Ross R: Atherosclerosis—an inflammatory disease. N Engl J Med 340:115–126, 1999.

7. Stary HC, Chandler AB, Dinsmore RE, et al: A definition of advanced types of atherosclerotic lesions and a histological classification of atherosclerosis. Circulation 92:1355–1374, 1995.

CHAPTER 69

ARTERIAL INSUFFICIENCY

Mark Nehler, M.D., and William C. Krupski, M.D.

1. **Describe claudication and its physiology.**

   Intermittent claudication consists of reproducible lower extremity muscular pain induced by exercise and relieved by short periods of rest. It is caused by arterial obstruction to affected muscular beds, which restricts the normal exercise-induced increase in blood flow, producing transient muscle ischemia. Studies have shown that more than half of patients with intermittent claudication have never complained of this symptom to their physicians, assuming that difficulty with walking is a normal consequence of aging.

2. **List the different nonoperative therapies for intermittent claudication.**

   Risk factor modification, exercise, and pharmacologic therapies. Smoking cessation reliably doubles walking distances, and the need for eventual amputation in patient's with lower extremity arterial occlusive disease decreases after smoking cessation. Exercise (defined as walking until onset of leg pain, resting, and then resuming walking) for 30–60 minutes, 3 days per week for 6 months has also been demonstrated in multiple randomized trials to increase walking distance by more than 100%. Currently, the only Food and Drug Administration (FDA)–approved drugs for the treatment of claudication are pentoxifylline (minimally effective) and cilostazol (appears more effective).

3. **Define critical limb ischemia.**

   Critical limb ischemia potentially threatens the viability of the limb. Symptoms include rest pain (e.g., foot pain at rest) typically occurring at night when the patient is supine and the gravity contribution to foot arterial pressure is no longer present. This pain is relieved with foot dependency or short periods of ambulation. Poor tissue circulation does not heal minor skin breakdown caused by incidental trauma. These ischemic ulcers are frequently painful and can progress to gangrene.

4. **What is the ankle brachial index (ABI)?**

   ABI is the highest ankle pressure (anterior tibial or posterior tibial artery) divided by the higher of the two brachial pressures. The normal ABI is slightly > 1 (1.10). An ABI of 1.0–0.5 is typical of patients with claudication. Patients with rest pain have an ABI < 0.5, and patients with tissue necrosis have an ABI much lower.

5. **Describe the natural history of claudication.**

   Multiple natural history studies have documented the benign nature of claudication. The cumulative 10-year amputation rate is 10%. One third of patients experience symptom deterioration, and half of these patients require some sort of revascularization. Continued smoking and diabetes are major risk factors for progression.

6. **Describe the natural history of critical limb ischemia.**

   In the past, it was commonly believed that chronic ischemic rest pain or necrosis inevitably led to either reconstruction or major amputation. This is both simplistic and inaccurate. Clearly, continuous ischemic rest pain or progressive gangrenous changes are unstable conditions that require therapy. However, the control groups from several pharmacologic trials for critical limb ischemia noted improvement over time in 40%. Vascular disease is a systemic disease, and 50% of patients with critical limb ischemia succumb to cardiac disease within 5 years.

7. **What are segmental limb pressures? How are they used?**
    Just as the ABI is recorded at the ankle, cuffs at the high thigh, above knee, and below knee level can record pressures. Noting the location of decreases in arterial pressure can determine the level of the vascular obstruction.

8. **Describe the natural history of graft occlusions.**
    Although bypass grafts can dramatically improve lower extremity circulation, they have a limited life expectancy. When these grafts fail, the limb involved is frequently in worse circulatory trouble than before the bypass. This is because of division of major arterial collateral pathways during the operation and thrombus propagation or embolization to occlude distal arteries at the time of graft occlusion.

9. **What is the prognosis of young patients with vascular disease?**
    Significant atherosclerosis in young patients (age < 40 years) is infrequent. These patients are almost exclusively heavy smokers with a high incidence of hypercoaguable states (defective fibrinolysis, anticardiolipin antibodies, homocysteinemia, or deficiencies in natural anticoagulants). Those with limb-threatening conditions frequently progress to limb loss despite attempts at revascularization. Reconstructive procedures have limited longevity and require frequent revision in this population.

10. **Describe the anatomic distribution of vascular disease in diabetes.**
    Diabetic patients are unique. They have a predilection for calcification of the arterial wall, rendering diagnostic studies (ankle pressure, ABI) unreliable because of false elevation. The digital arteries are usually spared, and the great toe pressure can be used to approximate the ankle pressure. The inflow arteries (i.e., aorta, iliacs, common femorals) are usually spared. Intermittent disease is often present in the superficial femoral and popliteal arteries. Significant occlusive disease most commonly affects the profunda femoris, posterior and anterior tibials, and pedal arteries, with relative sparing of the peroneal artery.

11. **What are the implications of renal failure on outcomes?**
    Patients with end-stage renal failure who have critical limb ischemia are at the end of life, with 3 year survival rates < 30%, similar to patients with metastatic cancer. In addition, the healing potential for partial foot amputations after successful revascularization is limited.
    Reconstructions in these patients are technically difficult because of calcified distal targets. The combination of these problems has caused many vascular surgeons to discourage vascular reconstructions in these patients.

12. **Discuss the concept of inflow versus outflow.**
    The limb is thought of as a separate circulation network when planning revascularization procedures. Adequate leg circulation requires blood to enter the leg from the heart (inflow) and reach the foot from the thigh (outflow). In the normal limb, the inflow to the leg is via the aorta and iliacs, and common and deep femoral arteries. The normal outflow to the foot is the popliteal and three tibial arteries (anterior, posterior, and peroneal). For bypasses to work, they need adequate inflow (i.e., blood coming into them) and outflow (i.e., a vascular bed to supply).

13. **What are the choices for autogenous conduits?**
    The success of infrainguinal bypass is highly dependent on the conduit (what the graft is made of). The best choices for conduit in order of preference would be a single segment greater saphenous vein, spliced pieces of saphenous vein, spliced lesser saphenous veins, arm veins, spliced arm veins, and prosthetic material with a distal vein cuff. Cryopreserved cadaver veins

are expensive and are generally of limited durability. Prosthetic grafts are best used for above-the-knee popliteal targets, because the bend at the knee joint and the size mismatch at more distal arteries decrease their longevity in these positions markedly.

14. **What are the indications for arteriography?**
Arteriography is only performed in order to plan future operations or interventions. Diagnostic arteriography without intervention is rarely used in lower extremity occlusive disease. Arteriography is expensive and carries a finite risk of bleeding, arterial injury with thrombosis, and renal failure from contrast agent toxicity (combined 3%).

15. **What are the patency rates of inflow procedures?**
The durability of vascular reconstructions is measured by patency. Patency has three types, all measured via a life table method, which accounts for the moderate number of deaths (primarily cardiac origin) occurring in vascular patients over time. Patency can be **primary** (the graft has remained functioning without any intervention), **assisted primary** (the graft has never thrombosed but has required some intervention to keep it functioning), or **secondary patency** (the graft has thrombosed, but an intervention has reopened it and it is again functioning). The four most common procedures to improve inflow are iliac angioplasty, aortofemoral bypass, femoro-femoral bypass, and axillofemoral bypass. The most durable is the aortofemoral bypass, which has a 10-year primary patency of 80%. Five-year primary patency rates for iliac angioplasty, axillofemoral, and femorofemoral bypass are 65%, 70%, and 70%, respectively.

16. **What are the patency rates of infrainguinal bypass procedures?**
Infrainguinal bypasses include grafts to the above-knee popliteal, below-knee popliteal, the tibials, and the pedal arteries. Five-year primary patency rates for above-knee popliteal grafts with saphenous vein and prosthetic are 80% and 65%, respectively. Five-year primary patency rates for below-knee saphenous vein popliteal grafts are 75%. Five-year primary patency rates for tibial bypasses are 65%. Five-year primary patency rate for pedal bypass is 50%.

17. **Name the primary cause of perioperative mortality.**
The majority (> 90%) of all peripheral vascular disease patients have underlying coronary artery disease. Because of the ambulatory limitations of their peripheral vascular disease, most of these patients have no overt coronary symptoms. The most common cause of perioperative mortality in vascular surgery is myocardial infarction. The decision to work-up and revascularize (surgically or with angioplasty and stenting) coronary artery disease in these patients before the vascular operation is an area of ongoing controversy.

18. **Name the primary cause of perioperative morbidity.**
Wound complications occur in ≤ 25% of patients undergoing lower extremity bypass for critical limb ischemia. Postoperative lymphedema, ischemic neuropathy, and prolonged (often measured in months rather than weeks) wound healing are all important issues for these patients.

19. **What are the causes of graft failure?**
Early failure (within 30 days) is caused by technical problems with the operation (graft kinking or twisting, narrowing of the anastomosis, bleeding, infection, intimal flaps, or embolization). Graft failure at months 2 through 18 is most often caused by fibrointimal hyperplasia at distal anastomoses or venous valve sites within the graft. Late graft failure (> 18 months) is most frequently caused by recurrent atherosclerosis. Hypercoaguable states are an unusual cause of graft failure.

20. **What therapeutic options are available for graft failure?**
If a vein graft fails immediately postoperatively, the correct approach is to explore the distal anastomosis and to fix the presumed technical problem. If a graft fails weeks to months after

implantation, the correct course is somewhat controversial. Exploring the graft to mechanically remove thrombus and repair any stenoses has a poor success rate and is not recommended. Using thrombolytic therapy to open the graft and then repair any underlying stenoses seems attractive, but the longevity of grafts treated in this manner has been poor, with < 50% remaining patent at 1 year. Replacing the vein graft with a new bypass provides the most durable alternative providing it is technically possible and the patient is an operative candidate. Inflow grafts that occlude are usually managed with operative thrombectomy and revision of the distal anastomotic stenosis.

KEY POINTS: ARTERIAL INSUFFICIENCY

1. Ankle-brachial index (ABI) is the highest ankle pressure divided by the higher of the two brachial pressures.

2. Critical limb ischemia potentially threatens the viability of the limb.

3. Patients with end-stage renal failure who have critical limb ischemia are at the end of life, with 3-year survival rates < 30%.

4. If a vein graft fails immediately postoperatively, the correct approach is to explore the distal anastomosis and to fix the presumed technical problem.

21. **What method of graft surveillance should be used?**
Because of the limited options for occluded vein bypass grafts, ultrasound studies are used to detect stenoses within the graft before occlusion. Various criteria have been championed to accurately detect > 50% narrowing within the graft or native inflow and outflow arteries. Natural history data indicate that grafts with > 50% stenoses left untreated have high intermediate-term failure rates. Recurrent symptoms and changes in the ABI are too insensitive to detect these lesions.

22. **What therapeutic options are available for graft stenoses?**
The majority of vein graft stenoses are caused by fibrointimal hyperplasia of sclerotic portions of the graft or valve sites. These lesions are a firm rubber consistency and less amenable to long-term success with percutaneous angioplasty. Open techniques (resection and interposition vein grafting or vein patch angioplasty) are more durable but also cause more patient morbidity.

23. **What is the role of iliac angioplasty and stenting?**
Iliac artery atherosclerotic lesions that respond best to balloon angioplasty are of short length (< 3 cm) and are confined to the common iliac artery. Nondiabetic patients fare better than diabetic patients. Current reports of initial success is > 90%, which has improved with the usage of stents to treat iatrogenic arterial dissections (splitting the arterial wall at the intima or media layers), but their effect on long-term success is still unproven.

24. **How is viability determined in cases of acute ischemia?**
The five P's of acute ischemia are **p**ain, **p**allor, **p**ulselessness, **p**aresthesia, and **p**aralysis. Early findings with acute ischemia include absent pulse, pain, and pallor. Paresthesia and paralysis are later findings. Classical teaching states irreversible muscle ischemia after 6 hours. However, in clinical practice, there are many overlaps. Perhaps the most sensitive finding that indicates limb nonviability is muscle rigor in the calf. The vast majority of ischemic limbs can be managed with initial heparin therapy followed by angiography and surgery or thrombolysis the next day(s).

25. **How is thrombus distinguished from embolus in acute ischemia?**
The diagnosis of acute thrombotic versus embolic lower extremity arterial occlusion is complicated. Findings suggestive of embolus include no history of vascular disease, normal contralateral leg circulation, no history of cardiac arrhythmia or recent myocardial infarction, and no
known cardiac thrombus. Patients with embolus frequently have rather profound leg ischemia
because of the proximal nature of the occlusion (aortic or femoral bifurcation) and the absence of
any developed collaterals. Occasionally, arteriography is required to differentiate between the two.

26. **When is thrombolysis indicated?**
Thrombolytic therapy requires a patient without contraindications (bleeding risks) and a thrombus that can be crossed with a guidewire. The lytic medication (urokinase, streptokinase, or tissue plasminogen activator) needs to be placed directly within the thrombus. Acute native arterial
occlusions should not have evidence of patent outflow arteries (e.g., a thrombosed popliteal
artery aneurysm). Arterial embolus in an extremity that is not severely ischemic and can tolerate
the time course of successful thrombolysis (frequently multiple hours of intra-arterial infusion
and repeat trips to the angiography suite for angiograms to help determine optimal catheter
repositioning for complete thrombus lysis). The use of thrombolytic therapy for graft occlusions
is more controversial because of the relatively poor long-term durability of these grafts after
flow is restored.

27. **What is compartment syndrome?**
Reperfusion after acute ischemia can lead to profound tissue swelling in the involved extremity.
Edema of the involved muscle can increase the pressure within the fascia bound muscle compartments (i.e., anterior, lateral, deep posterior, and superficial posterior) to a level that exceeds
the capillary perfusion pressure (> 30 mmHg). Muscle death is then inevitable unless the pressure is relieved by opening the compartments surgically, a procedure known as fasciotomy.
Patients complain of intense pain and swelling, with associated paresthesia. Pedal pulses can
remain palpable.

WEB SITE

http://www.acssurgery.com

BIBLIOGRAPHY

1. Carter SA: The challenge and importance of defining critical limb ischemia. Vasc Med 2:126–131, 1997.

2. Faries P, Morrissey NJ, Teodorescu V, et al: Recent advances in peripheral angioplasty and stenting. Angiology 52:617–626, 2002.

3. Gahtan V: The noninvasive vascular laboratory. Surg Clin North Am 78:507–518, 1998.

4. Lau H, Cheng SW, Hui J: Eighteen-year experience with femoro-femoral bypass. Aust N Z J Surg 70:275–278, 2000.

5. Nehler MR, Hiatt WR: Exercise therapy for claudication. Ann Vasc Surg 13:109–114, 1999.

6. Nehler MR, Taylor LM Jr, Moneta GL, Porter JM: Natural history, nonoperative treatment, and functional assessment in chronic lower extremity ischemia. In Moore W (ed): Vascular Surgery: A Comprehensive Review.
Philadelphia, W.B. Saunders, 1998, pp 251–265.

7. Ouriel K, Veith F: Acute lower limb ischemia: Determinants of outcome. Surgery 124:336–342, 1998.

8. Pomposelli FB Jr, Arora S, Gibbons GW, et al: Lower extremity arterial reconstruction in the very elderly:
Successful outcome preserves not only the limb but also residential status and ambulatory function. J Vasc
Surg 28:215–225, 1998.

CHAPTER 70

CAROTID DISEASE

Rao Gutta, M.D., and B. Timothy Baxter, M.D.

1. **What diseases affect the carotid arteries?**
   Atherosclerosis is by far the most common (accounting for 90% of lesions in the Western world). The carotid also can be affected by fibromuscular dysplasia, inflammatory arteriopathies (e.g., Takayasu's arteritis), extrinsic compression (e.g., neoplasm), and trauma.

2. **What are the most common symptoms of carotid artery disease?**
   - Transient ischemic attack (TIA)
   - Reversible ischemic neurologic deficit (RIND)
   - Cerebrovascular accident (CVA)
   - Amaurosis fugax

3. **Define TIA, RIND, and CVA.**
   These clinical terms describe a spectrum of cerebral ischemic syndromes. A **TIA** is a neurologic deficit that lasts < 24 hours. Most TIAs last only 15–30 seconds. **RIND** lasts longer than 24 hours and completely resolves within 1 week (usually within 3 days). **CVA**, or acute stroke, is a stable neurologic deficit that may show gradual improvement over a long period.

4. **Define amaurosis fugax.**
   It is an episode of transient (minutes to hours) monocular blindness, often likened to a window shade pulled across the eye. It is caused by decreased blood flow through or embolization into the ophthalmic artery.

5. **What are Hollenhorst plaques?**
   They are bright yellow plaques of cholesterol, usually at a branch point in the retinal vessels, that have embolized from the carotid bifurcation. Clinically, this finding indicates that the atheromatous plaque in the carotid is quite friable. Further embolization may occur with manipulation at the time of surgery.

6. **What mechanisms produce neurologic deficits?**
   - Embolization from atherosclerotic arteries or the heart
   - Reduced blood flow
   - Occlusive disease with thrombosis
   - Intracranial hemorrhage

7. **What is the natural history of a TIA?**
   The natural history of a TIA is defined by the pathology of the ipsilateral carotid artery. In patients with severe stenosis (> 70%), the risk of ipsilateral stroke within 24 months is 26%. For those with moderate disease (50–69%), the risk is 22% at 5 years. With minimal stenosis (< 30%), the risk is 1% at 3 years (see Required Reading in Chapter 1).

8. **What is the effect of aspirin on TIAs?**
   Acetylsalicylic acid is a cyclooxygenase inhibitor that decreases platelet stickiness and lowers the incidence of both TIAs and stroke.

9. **What does a carotid bruit signify?**
   Unfortunately, a carotid bruit is a general marker for atherosclerosis and is specific for very little; it is more predictive of a cardiac event than a neurologic event. Although a carotid bruit indicates increased risk of neurologic events, it is just as likely to occur on the contralateral side as on the side of the bruit.

10. **Does the sound of a bruit correlate with the degree of stenosis?**
    No. As a stenosis progresses, the bruit should actually diminish and disappear as flow decreases.

11. **What test should be ordered to evaluate a cervical bruit?**
    Duplex scanning.

12. **When is surgery indicated for symptomatic carotid artery disease?**
    Surgery is strongly indicated for symptomatic carotid artery disease associated with > 70% stenosis. The absolute risk reduction of stroke is 17% at 2 years. Recent data also suggest a smaller benefit in patients with symptomatic stenoses of 50–69% (6.5% risk reduction at 5 years). Patients with stenosis of < 50% do not benefit from surgery.

KEY POINTS: CAROTID DISEASE

1. The symptoms of carotid disease include transient ischemic attack, reversible ischemic neurologic deficit, cerebrovascular accident, and amaurosis fugax.

2. A carotid bruit is a general marker for atherosclerosis and is specific for very little; it is more predictive of a cardiac event than a neurologic event.

3. Surgery is strongly indicated for symptomatic carotid artery disease associated with > 70% stenosis.

13. **Should a patient with asymptomatic stenosis undergo surgery?**
    The absolute reduction in risk of stroke is 6% over a 5-year period in asymptomatic patients with > 60% stenosis who undergo carotid endarterectomy (CEA) plus aspirin versus patients treated with aspirin alone (5.1% versus 11%). Thus, CEA should be performed for asymptomatic carotid disease when the patient is expected to live at least 3 years and when the CEA can be performed with a combined stroke and mortality rate of < 3%.

14. **What are the complications of carotid endarterectomy?**
    TIA or stroke (approximately 2%)
    Hematoma
    Cranial nerve injury
    Hypertension
    Hypotension

15. **Which cranial nerves (CNs) may be injured during CEA? What are the clinical signs of injury?**
    Facial nerve (CN VII): injury to the marginal mandibular branch may cause droop of the ipsilateral corner of the mouth
    Glossopharyngeal nerve (CN IX): difficulty in swallowing both solids and liquids
    Vagus nerve (CN X): hoarseness, loss of effective cough
    Superior laryngeal nerve (branch of the vagus): voice fatigue, loss of high-pitch phonation
    Hypoglossal nerve (CN XII): deviation of the tongue to the ipsilateral side, difficulty with speech and chewing

16. **What is the danger of wound hematoma after surgery?**
The main danger is airway compromise, which may necessitate emergent decompression by opening of the wound. Whether vacuum drains prevent this complication is not clear.

17. **What are the possible causes of postoperative hypertension?**
   - Denervation of the carotid sinus
   - Cerebral rennin, norepinephrine production, or both
   - Preexisting hypertension
   - Central neurologic deficit

18. **When do neurologic events occur during CEA?**
   - Dissection: dislodgement of material from the arterial wall with embolization
   - Clamping: ischemic infarct
   - Postoperatively: intimal flap, reperfusion, external carotid artery clot

19. **What is a shunt? When is it used?**
A shunt is a small plastic tube that diverts blood flow around the surgically opened carotid artery while endarterectomy is performed. A shunt is used to ensure adequate cerebral blood flow and to avoid intraoperative cerebral ischemia. Many surgeons routinely use shunts, but others use them selectively, if at all. The decision to use a shunt is based on intraoperative assessment, including temporary clamping of the carotid under local anesthesia, measurement of stump pressure, intraoperative electroencephalography, or transcranial Doppler. None of these methods is 100% accurate.

20. **What is stump pressure?**
Stump pressure is the back pressure of the internal carotid artery after clamping. It is used to assess the adequacy of cerebral perfusion. The "safe" pressure varies from author to author, but is probably around 40 mmHg.

21. **Does stenosis recur after carotid endarterectomy?**
Yes. The reported incidence has been quite variable and ranges from < 2% to as much as 36%. During the first 24 months after operation, restenosis is thought to be secondary to myointimal hyperplasia. Beyond this time, it is caused by progression of disease (atherosclerosis). The incidence is lower when the arteriotomy is closed with a vein patch angioplasty.

22. **What is the most common complication associated with reoperation endarterectomy?**
Cranial nerve injury (reported incidence = 2–20%). Most injuries are transient, however.

23. **In which layer of the artery is the carotid endarterectomy performed?**
The outer layers of the tunica media.

24. **What anatomic landmark is useful in identifying the level of the carotid artery bifurcation?**
The facial vein.

25. **How many branches of the internal carotid artery are located in the neck?**
None.

26. **When the internal carotid artery is occluded, which branches of the external carotid artery form collaterals and reestablish circulation in the circle of Willis?**
The periorbital branches of the external carotid artery form communications with the ophthalmic artery, a branch of the internal carotid.

27. **What are the functions of the carotid sinus and the carotid body?**
Both are located at the carotid bifurcation and are innervated by the glossopharyngeal and vagus nerves, respectively. The function of the carotid sinus is regulation of blood pressure. Hypertension stimulates efferent impulses to the vasomotor center in the medulla, inhibiting sympathetic tone and increasing vagal tone. The carotid body regulates respiratory drive and acid–base status via chemoreceptors. It also induces bradycardia when manipulated (this is your target during carotid massage for cardiac dysrhythmias).

28. **When was the first successful surgical procedure of the extracranial carotid artery performed? Who is credited with it?**
In 1954 by Eastcott.

CONTROVERSY

29. **What is the role of CEA?**
Although CEA remains the standard of care for carotid artery disease, percutaneous angioplasty with stenting has been investigated as an alternative. The underlying rationale is to decrease morbidity, hospital costs, and anesthetic risks and to improve long-term patency. Reported rates of success, morbidity, and mortality run the gamut from stroke and death rates comparable to CEA (2.4%) to significantly higher neurologic risk (stroke rate, 8.8%) and higher cost. One randomized trial is currently under way in Great Britain, and applications for two other studies are being considered in the United States. Carotid angioplasty has no apparent benefit compared with CEA.

WEB SITE

http://www.acssurgery.com

BIBLIOGRAPHY

1. Barnett HJM, Taylor DW, Eliasziw M, et al, for the North American Symptomatic Carotid Endarterectomy Trial Collaborators: Benefit of carotid endarterectomy in patients with symptomatic moderate or severe stenosis. N Engl J Med 339:1415–1425, 1998.

2. Beebe HG: Scientific evidence demonstrating the safety of carotid angioplasty and stenting: Do we have enough to draw conclusions yet? J Vasc Surg 27:788–790, 1998.

3. Executive Committee for the Asymptomatic Carotid Atherosclerosis Study: Endarterectomy for asymptomatic carotid artery stenosis. JAMA 273:1421–1429, 1995.

4. Jordan WD, Voellinger DC, Fisher WS, et al: A comparison of carotid angioplasty with stenting versus endarterectomy with regional anesthesia. J Vasc Surg 28:397–402, 1998.

5. Mansour MA, Kang SS, Baker WH, et al: Carotid endarterectomy for recurrent stenosis. J Vasc Surg 25:877–883, 1997.

6. Moore WS, Kempszinski RF, Nelson JJ, Toole JF, for the ACAS Investigators: Recurrent carotid stenosis: Results of the asymptomatic carotid atherosclerosis study. Stroke 29:2018–2025, 1998.

7. North American Symptomatic Carotid Endarterectomy Trial Collaborators: Beneficial effect of carotid endarterectomy in symptomatic patients with high-grade stenosis. N Engl J Med 325:445–453, 1991.

8. Yadav JS, Roubin GS, Iyer S, et al: Elective stenting of the extracranial carotid arteries. Circulation 95:283–381, 1997.

CHAPTER 71

ABDOMINAL AORTIC ANEURYSM

Mark Nehler, M.D., and William C. Krupski, M.D.

1. **What is an abdominal aortic aneurysm (AAA)?**
   A ≥ 50% increase in normal aortic diameter. Normal infrarenal aortic diameter is 2.0 cm for men. A definition of AAA as an aorta ≥ 3.0 cm in diameter is appropriate.

2. **What is the incidence of AAA?**
   - 3% in unselected adult patients screened with ultrasound
   - 5% in patients with known coronary artery disease
   - 10% in patients with known peripheral vascular disease

3. **What is the etiology of AAA?**
   Elastin is the primary load-bearing element of the aorta. In the normal human aorta, there is a gradual reduction in the amount of elastin present in the distal compared with the proximal aorta. Elastin fragmentation and degeneration are observed histologically in AAA walls. These observations help explain the predilection of AAAs in the infrarenal aorta. Absence of vasa vasorum in the infrarenal aorta has led to the suggestion of a nutritive deficiency. The degradation of aortic media in aneurysmal disease implies a disrupted balance between proteolytic enzymes and their inhibitors.

4. **Do AAAs have a genetic component?**
   Multiple reports describe a familial subgroup of AAAs. Therefore, screening of AAA patients' first-degree relatives who are 50 years old and older makes sense. Two prospective studies demonstrated that approximately 30% of these relatives also harbor an AAA. The proposed genetic defect has been linked to abnormal type III collagen.

5. **Are patients with AAA prone to aneurysms in other vascular beds?**
   Yes. Forty percent of patients with a popliteal artery aneurysm harbor an AAA. Seventy-five percent of patients with a femoral artery aneurysm also have an AAA. Patients with thoracic aneurysms have a 20% chance of having a simultaneous AAA. Five percent of patients develop aortic aneurysms proximal to their graft at ≥ 5 years after infrarenal AAA repair.

6. **Can AAAs reliably be detected on physical examination?**
   No. The aortic bifurcation is at the level of the umbilicus. Therefore, the pulsatile mass of an AAA is located in the epigastrium. Thus, only relatively large AAAs can be detected in thin patients.

7. **Can AAAs be detected by radiography?**
   Plain abdominal or lumbar spine radiographs can detect occult AAA in about 20% of cases. A thin rim of calcification identifies the aneurysmal aortic wall. The majority of AAAs contain insufficient calcium to be visualized by radiography.

8. **Which imaging method is the best for screening patients for AAA?**
   Abdominal ultrasound (US) permits measurement accuracy within 0.3 cm and data in both cross-sectional and longitudinal dimensions.

9. **What is the best single imaging modality to plan AAA repair?**
    The contrast-enhanced computed tomography (CT) scan is the best one. Diameter measurements are accurate within 0.2 cm. Venous anomalies (i.e., retroaortic or circumaortic left renal vein, inferior vena cava duplication, and left-sided inferior vena cava) that dramatically alter the operative approach are well visualized on CT. Although CT is excellent at detecting aneurysmal rupture or leak (92% accuracy and 100% specificity), it is less useful for predicting suprarenal aneurysm involvement (sensitivity, 83%; specificity, 90%; positive predictive value, 48%).

10. **What is the manifestation of a symptomatic AAA?**
    Acute low back pain is the most common presenting symptom (82%), but only one third of AAAs are diagnosed before rupture. A hypotensive elderly man with acute onset of low back pain has a leaking AAA until proven otherwise.

11. **What is the appropriate management of a patient suspected of a ruptured AAA?**
    Just before emergent surgical exploration, patients who are hemodynamically unstable with a pulsatile abdominal mass should have an electrocardiogram to rule out myocardial infarction.

12. **Should all patients presenting with AAA rupture undergo repair?**
    Patients in profound shock or cardiac arrest at the time of presentation have little chance of survival. Extreme age, dementia, metastatic cancer, and other severe end-stage medical problems should force you to reassess this allocation of medical resources.

13. **Do all patients with ruptured AAAs make it to surgery?**
    Approximately half of patients with a ruptured AAA die before reaching the hospital. One fourth of those who make it to the hospital die before they can be brought to the operating room. Therefore, only 25% of patients make it to surgery.

14. **How is a ruptured AAA treated operatively?**
    The patient should not be anesthetized until completely prepped and draped and ready for immediate incision because the blood pressure may decrease dramatically upon induction of anesthesia. Rapid proximal aortic control is the key to successful outcome of operations for ruptured AAA. This can be at the diaphragm (in an unstable patient, with free intraperitoneal bleeding or a retroperitoneal hematoma that extends proximal to the left renal vein) or at the infrarenal aortic segment (in a stable patient with a lower retroperitoneal hematoma). Intraluminal balloon occlusion of the aorta is an option with free intraperitoneal rupture. As soon as control is obtained, the patient is resuscitated and clamps are moved to the more standard infrarenal location. Distal control can also be obtained with balloons or packs to prevent iliac venous injury.

KEY POINTS: ABDOMINAL AORTIC ANEURYSM

1. An AAA is defined as a ≥ 50% increase in normal aortic diameter.

2. Forty percent of patients with a popliteal artery aneurysm harbor an AAA.

3. CT is the single best imaging modality to plan an AAA repair.

4. AAA should be repaired electively when the size reaches 5.5 cm in diameter.

15. **How should patients with symptomatic nonruptured AAAs be managed?**
Symptomatic AAAs are rapidly expanding and at high risk for rupture. Therefore, most vascular surgeons agree that symptomatic but intact AAAs should be repaired expeditiously (as early as is conveniently possible).

16. **Are there any alternatives to open surgical repair for ruptured AAA?**
Endovascular prosthetic grafts have been successfully placed in high-risk patients with symptomatic AAAs or contained ruptures both in the aortic and aortoiliac position.

17. **What are the rupture rates of AAAs?**
A 5-cm diameter AAA has an annual rupture risk of < 1%. The risk of AAA rupture increases with size. Annual rupture risk is 10% for a 6-cm AAA and 30% for AAAs > 7 cm.

18. **How fast do AAAs enlarge?**
The average expansion rate of all AAAs is 0.4 cm/year. However, 20% of all AAAs demonstrate no change in size over time. Conversely, 20% expand at a rate > 0.5 cm/year. Rapid expansion (0.5 cm/6 months) is considered to be predictive of rupture and an indication for repair.

19. **When are angiograms helpful in the diagnostic workup for AAA?**
Traditionally, angiography has been indicated in patients when there is concern regarding the extent of the proximal neck, concomitant visceral occlusive disease, renal artery anomalies, a prior colectomy with need to visualize the visceral circulation, or lower extremity occlusive or aneurysmal disease.

20. **What is the difference between extraperitoneal and transabdominal approach?**
Elective aortic graft placement can be carried out equally well via a transperitoneal or extraperitoneal approach. The former provides better pelvic exposure. The extraperitoneal approach provides superior exposure of the suprarenal aorta and facilitates postoperative pulmonary management.

21. **What are endografts? Are they durable?**
Endovascular grafts are graft-covered stents that are placed via the femoral artery by interventional (i.e., radiographic) methods to exclude the aneurysm without the need for an abdominal incision or cross clamping the aorta. Multiple different series of successful endovascular AAA repair have been reported. Successful endograft placement has been reported in a wide variety of high-risk operative candidates. Many vascular surgeons and interventionalists are making aortic endograft placement their preferred treatment for patients with AAAs. The major drawbacks are late leaks or rupture from the graft, the cost of the procedure, and the need for long-term patient follow-up.

22. **At what size should asymptomatic AAAs be repaired electively?**
They should be repaired electively when the AAA reaches 5.5 cm in diameter. The only benefit for repair of an asymptomatic AAA is to prevent subsequent rupture and death. Therefore, all candidates for elective repair must expect to live at least 5 years.

23. **What are the technical aspects of AAA surgery?**
The two important decisions are the location of arterial clamps and the type of graft to place. The majority of cases can be managed by placing the arterial clamp below the renal arteries. This avoids prolonged ischemia to the kidneys. The aneurysm is opened after clamping proximally and distally. Lumbar artery orifices are oversewn to prevent bleeding from collateral arteries. The inferior mesenteric artery is often occluded, but when it is patent and not vigorously backbleeding, it may require reimplantation.

24. **What are the major noncardiac complications of AAA repair?**
    Renal failure (elevation in creatinine) and intestinal ischemia (bloody diarrhea).

WEB SITE

http://www.acssurgery.com

BIBLIOGRAPHY

1. Barry MC, Burke PE, Sheehan S, et al: An "all comers" policy for ruptured abdominal aortic aneurysms: How can results be improved? Eur J Surg 164:263–270, 1998.

2. Boyle JR, Thompson MM, Nasim A, et al: Endovascular abdominal aortic aneurysm repair in the "hostile abdomen." J Royal Coll Surg Edinb 43:283–285, 1998.

3. Hill BB, Wolf YG, Lee WA, et al: Open versus endovascular AAA repair in patients who are morphological candidates for endovascular treatment. J Endovasc Ther 9:255–261, 2002.

4. Holzenbein TJ, Kretschmer G, Dorffner R, et al: Endovascular management of "endoleaks" after transluminal infrarenal abdominal aneurysm repair. Eur J Vasc Endovasc Surg 16:208–217, 1998.

5. Killen DA, Reed WA, Gorton ME, et al: 25-year trends in resection of abdominal aortic aneurysms. Ann Vasc Surg 12:436–444, 1998.

6. Lawrence PF, Wallis C, Dobrin PB, et al: Peripheral aneurysms and arteriomegaly: Is there a familial pattern? J Vasc Surg 28:599–605, 1998.

7. Lederle FA, Johnson GR, Wilson SE, et al: Rupture rate of large abdominal aortic aneurysms in patients refusing or unfit for elective repair. JAMA 287:2968–2972, 2002.

8. Lederle FA, Wilson SE, Johnson GR, et al: Immediate repair compared with surveillance of small abdominal aortic aneurysms. N Engl J Med 346:1437–1444, 2002.

CHAPTER 72

VENOUS DISEASE

Thomas A. Whitehill, M.D., and Mark Nehler, M.D.

1. **Where does deep venous thrombosis (DVT) originate?**
   More than 95% of DVTs develop in the deep veins of the lower extremities; the majority originate in the valve sinuses of the calf veins.

2. **What is the usual source of a pulmonary embolus?**
   Calf vein thrombosis may propagate proximally into the deep venous system to involve the popliteal, femoral, or iliac veins (or a combination of veins). These proximal DVTs are the culprits in > 90% of pulmonary emboli.

3. **What is Virchow's triad?**
   (1) Hypercoagulability, (2) disruption of an intact venous intimal lining, and (3) stasis of venous blood flow. In most patients with DVT, at least two of these three components are operative.

4. **What are the major hypercoagulable syndromes (thrombophilia)?**
   Factor V Leiden mutation, antithrombin III deficiency, protein C deficiency, protein S deficiency, dysfibrinogenemia, lupus anticoagulant, antiphospholipid syndrome, prothrombin 20210A mutation, and abnormalities of fibrinolysis are the major examples. The most common is the factor V Leiden mutation (i.e., activated protein C resistance).

5. **What causes venous intimal injury?**
   Venous intimal changes may be secondary to vein wall trauma, infection, inflammation, indwelling catheters, or surgery. Venodilation during anesthesia and surgery may produce microscopic intimal tears as well as stasis. The injured venous intima initiates the release of thromboplastic substances that can activate the coagulation cascade.

6. **What causes stasis of venous blood flow?**
   Venostasis is common in surgical patients; it occurs during anesthesia, after certain types of trauma, and with perioperative immobility.

7. **What are the usual clinical risk factors for DVT?**
   Risk factors include malignancy (especially pancreatic, genitourinary, stomach, lung, colon, and breast cancer), age older than 40 years, female gender, obesity, history of venous thrombosis or pulmonary embolism, major surgical procedures, pregnancy, limited mobility, hypercoagulable state, and trauma.

8. **What signs and symptoms suggest DVT? How can DVT be accurately diagnosed?**
   The signs and symptoms are calf or thigh pain, tenderness, increased skin temperature, swelling, or superficial venous dilatation. None of these signs is specific for DVT. Even the well-known Homan's sign (i.e., calf pain with dorsiflexion of the foot) is unreliable; its accuracy is only 50%. Doppler ultrasound examination (duplex scanning) detects DVT proximal to the calf veins with > 95% accuracy; unfortunately, it is not as sensitive in detecting calf vein DVT. Ascending venography is still the reference standard.

9. **Is there any value to D-dimer testing?**
Measurement of D-dimer cross-linked fibrin degradation products (FDPs), formed by the action of plasmin on cross-linked fibrin, has been proposed as an alternative to initial noninvasive testing. A sensitivity of 96.8% and a specificity of 35.2% have been reported for the enzyme-linked immunosorbent assay (ELISA) test, making it theoretically possible to limit noninvasive testing to those with positive D-dimer testing. Unfortunately, the ELISA test is time consuming and impractical as a screening test. More rapid (1 hour) ELISA assays are now available. Prospective evaluation of the safety of withholding anticoagulation therapy in patients who are D-dimer negative has been limited. False-positive results are a problem in patients with malignancy, infection, or recent surgery.

10. **What methods of perioperative DVT prophylaxis should be used? In which surgical patients?**
Perioperative DVT prophylaxis is strongly recommended in all high-risk patients who are older than age 40 years and undergoing major general or orthopedic procedures. In general surgical patients, well-applied prophylactic measures decrease the relative risk of DVT by 67%. The best prophylaxis for DVT includes pre- and postoperative walking. Intermittent pneumatic compression stockings and some form of heparin therapy (low-dose unfractionated heparin [LDUH] or low molecular weight heparin [LMWH]) are recommended as the patient's risk profile increases.

KEY POINTS: VENOUS DISEASE

1. More than 95% of deep vein thromboses (DVTs) develop in the deep veins of the lower extremities; the majority originate in the valve sinuses of the calf veins.

2. Virchow's triad consists of hypercoagulability, disruption of an intact venous intimal lining, and stasis of venous blood flow.

3. The best prophylaxis for DVT includes pre- and postoperative walking.

11. **How does heparin work?**
Heparin binds to antithrombin III (ATIII), rendering it more active. Low-dose heparin (5000 U administered subcutaneously every 8–12 hours until the patient is fully ambulatory) activates ATIII, inhibits platelet aggregation, and decreases the availability of thrombin.

12. **What is LMWH?**
LMWH is a fragment of heparin produced by chemical breakdown. It exerts its anticoagulation effect by binding with ATIII and inhibiting several coagulation enzymes, principally factor Xa. It has a longer half-life than standard preparation heparin and can be administered once daily. LMWH gives a more predictable anticoagulant response at high doses and thus can be administered without monitoring (it is not necessary to follow the partial thromboplastin time).

13. **Should the placement of an inferior vena cava (IVC) filter ever be considered?**
In patients with a documented, recurrent pulmonary embolism while taking adequate anticoagulation therapy or with an absolute contraindication to anticoagulation, an IVC filter can be placed to prevent embolization or propagation of clot to the lungs. A significant rate of recurrent DVT has been associated with IVC filters.

14. **What are the characteristics of chronic venous insufficiency and postphlebitic syndrome?**

The primary characteristic is venous valvular incompetence with distal ambulatory venous hypertension. After DVT, involved venous segments eventually recanalize to some degree. However, their delicate valves remain scarred or trapped by residual organized thrombus. The loss of valvular function disables the venomotor pump. The vein walls become thicker and less compliant, increasing resistance to proximal blood flow. These factors result in distal venous hypertension. Protein-rich fluids, fibrin, and red blood cells are extravasated and deposited through large pores in the distended microcirculation during periods of venous hypertension. This process leads to inflammation, scarring, fibrosis of the subcutaneous tissues, and discoloration by hemosiderin deposition ("brawny" edema). The resultant inflammatory reaction, scarring, and interstitial edema create a further barrier to capillary flow and diffusion of oxygen; adequate nutrition to the skin is inhibited. These changes may lead to tissue atrophy and ulceration (i.e., venous stasis ulcer).

15. **Do all patients with DVT develop postphlebitic syndrome?**

No. Recent epidemiologic studies suggest that the incidence of venous ulceration is about 5%. As many as one in five post-DVT patients have absolutely no symptoms and maintain normal noninvasive vascular test data. The median time for the appearance of a first venous stasis ulcer is 2.5 years. Of interest, 50% of patients with venous ulcers have no history of DVT (probably because of previous asymptomatic calf vein DVT).

16. **How are patients with postphlebitic syndrome treated?**

With proper patient education and compliance, postphlebitic stasis sequelae can be controlled by nonoperative means in well over 90% of patients, particularly if no residual venous outflow obstruction complicates valvular incompetence. Nonoperative treatment consists of graded elastic compression stockings (or Unna boots) to retard swelling *and* periodic leg elevation during the day. Patients must be taught to elevate their legs above the heart ("toes above your nose") at regular intervals (e.g., 10–15 minutes every 2 hours). Compliance is critical.

17. **Distinguish between phlegmasia alba dolens and phlegmasia cerulea dolens.**

Iliofemoral venous thrombosis is characterized by unilateral pain and edema of an entire lower extremity, discoloration, and groin tenderness. A total of 75% of the cases of iliofemoral venous thrombosis occur on the left side, presumably because of compression of the *left* common iliac vein by the overlying right common iliac artery (May-Thurner syndrome). In **phlegmasia alba dolens** (literally, painful white swelling), the leg becomes pale and white. Arterial pulses remain normal. Progressive thrombosis may occur with propagation proximally or distally and into neighboring tributaries. The entire leg becomes both edematous and mottled or cyanotic. This stage is called **phlegmasia cerulea dolens** (literally, painful purple swelling). When venous outflow is seriously impeded, arterial inflow may be reduced secondarily by as much as 30%. Limb loss is a serious concern; aggressive management (i.e., venous thrombectomy, catheter-directed lytic therapy, or both) is necessary.

18. **What is venous claudication?**

When venous recanalization fails to occur after iliofemoral venous thrombosis, venous collaterals develop to bypass the obstruction to venous outflow. These collaterals usually suffice while the patient is at rest. However, leg exercise induces increased arterial inflow, which may exceed the capacity of the venous collateral bed and result in progressive venous hypertension. The pressure buildup in the venous system results in calf pain commonly described as tight, heavy, or bursting (venous claudication). Relief is obtained with rest and elevation but is not as prompt as with arterial claudication.

19. **How can one distinguish primary varicose veins from secondary varicose veins?**

Primary varicose veins result from uncomplicated saphenofemoral venous valvular incompetence and have a greater saphenous distribution, positive tourniquet test result, no stasis sequelae (dermatitis or ulceration), and no morning ankle edema (lymphedema).

Secondary varicose veins are most commonly a consequence of deep and perforator venous incompetence secondary to postphlebitic syndrome.

20. **Why do people develop primary varicose veins?**

The most common cause is congenital absence of venous valves proximal to the saphenofemoral junction. There are normally no valves in the vena cava or common iliac veins and only an occasional valve in the external iliac veins. Thus, the sentinel valve in the common femoral vein just above the saphenofemoral junction is of critical importance. However, anatomic studies reveal that this valve is absent on one or the other side in 30% of patients.

21. **How, when, and in whom should varicose veins be treated?**

Varicose veins that cause discomfort or serious cosmetic embarrassment require treatment. Better results are obtained with early treatment before continuous retrograde pressure and flow down the superficial system and into communicating perforating veins (whenever the patient is standing) cause secondary, irreversible perforator incompetence. High saphenous vein ligation at an early stage can arrest progression of this gravitational process. The distal varicosities can be managed by selective surgical stripping, sclerotherapy, or both.

WEB SITE

http://www.acssurgery.com

BIBLIOGRAPHY

1. Clarke-Pearson DL, Dodge RK, Synan I, et al: Venous thromboembolism prophylaxis: Patients at high risk to fail intermittent pneumatic compression. Obstet Gynecol 101:157–163, 2003.

2. Franks PJ, Sharp EJ, Moffatt CJ: Risk factors for leg ulcer recurrence: A randomized trial of two types of compression stockings. Age Ageing 24:490–494, 1995.

3. Gallix BP, Achard-Lichere C, Dauzat M, et al: Flow-independent magnetic resonance venography of the calf. J Magn Reson Imaging 17:421–426, 2003.

4. Geerts W, Heit JA, Clagett GP, et al: Prevention of venous thromboembolism. Chest 119:132s–175s, 2001.

5. Ginsberg JS: Management of venous thromboembolism. N Engl J Med 335:1816–1828, 1996.

6. Janssen MC, Wollersheim H, Verbruggen B, et al: Rapid D-dimer assays to exclude deep venous thrombosis and pulmonary embolism: Current status and new developments. Semin Thromb Hemost 24:393–400, 1998.

7. Philbrick JT, Heim S: The d-dimer test for deep venous thrombosis: Gold standards and bias in negative predictive value. Clin Chem 49:570–574, 2003.

8. Sorensen HT, Mellemkjaer L, Steffensen FH, et al: The risk of a diagnosis of cancer after primary deep venous thrombosis or pulmonary embolism. N Engl J Med 338:1169–1173, 1998.

NONINVASIVE VASCULAR DIAGNOSTIC LABORATORY

Darrell N. Jones, Ph.D.

CHAPTER 73

1. **What is the role of the vascular diagnostic laboratory (VDL) in the assessment and treatment of patients with suspected vascular disease?**

   Although traditional evaluation by an experienced clinician remains the foundation of vascular diagnosis, clinical assessment has its limitations. For example, only one third of cervical bruits are associated with significant carotid artery disease; conversely, as many as two thirds of patients with severe carotid disease present without a cervical bruit. Half of patients with extensive deep venous thrombosis (DVT) of the lower extremity lack signs and symptoms referable to the lower extremities, and more than half of patients presenting with clinical signs of DVT are venographically normal. As many as 40% of diabetic patients have no large-vessel peripheral arterial occlusive disease. The VDL provides objective, quantitative, and functional status data to delineate the severity of extracranial cerebrovascular disease, peripheral arterial occlusive disease, and acute and chronic venous disease.

2. **What differentiates the VDL from diagnostic radiology and ultrasound?**

   The VDL provides functional information rather than or in addition to the morphologic data provided by radiology tests and general ultrasound images. This information is particularly important for peripheral arterial occlusive disease, in which anatomic information about the site of stenosis or occlusion is of limited value without knowledge of the functional significance.

CEREBROVASCULAR DISEASE

3. **Which noninvasive tests should be used to diagnose extracranial carotid artery disease?**

   Duplex ultrasound has a sensitivity of 97% in detecting carotid artery disease and an accuracy of 95% in correctly classifying carotid stenoses as > 50% reduction in diameter. No other noninvasive test has comparable accuracy.

4. **What is duplex ultrasound?**

   Duplex ultrasound uses both image and velocity data (hence the name duplex) in a nearly simultaneous presentation of ultrasound echo images (B-mode ultrasound) and blood velocity waveforms obtained by Doppler ultrasound. The Doppler signals are obtained from a single small region of the blood vessel. Average velocities can be estimated for multiple such regions over a large area of the vessel. By assigning colors to the velocities, blood flow can be visually represented. Such a presentation, called colorflow duplex ultrasound, aids the duplex examination but cannot replace the information obtained from the Doppler velocity waveform.

5. **Why is blood velocity important in assessing the degree of carotid artery stenosis?**

   It is often difficult to measure accurately the arterial lumen on a B-mode ultrasound image because the acoustic properties (and hence the image) of noncalcified plaque, thrombus, and even blood may be similar. Arterial narrowing forces blood through a narrower channel, which increases the blood velocity. This velocity can characterize the degree of arterial narrowing.

Current practice classifies the degree of internal carotid stenosis based exclusively on the Doppler velocity data.

6. **What are the velocity criteria and categorical ranges of carotid artery stenosis?**
The criteria developed at the University of Washington (Table 73-1) are the most widely accepted. Note that progressive carotid stenosis *increases* the flow velocity signal as the volume of blood is squeezed through a smaller and smaller orifice. The category > 80% has been termed critical stenosis because of the high rate of disease progression and high incidence of neurologic symptoms for patients in this category.

TABLE 73-1. UNIVERSITY OF WASHINGTON CRITERIA

Stenosis	Criteria
0%	Peak systolic velocity < 125 cm/sec and no velocity disturbance
1–15%	Peak systolic velocity < 125 cm/sec with turbulence during systolic deceleration
16–49%	Peak systolic velocity < 125 cm/sec with turbulence in the entire cardiac cycle
50–79%	Peak systolic velocity > 125 cm/sec and diastolic velocity < 140 cm/sec
80–99%	Diastolic velocity > 140 cm/sec
100%	Absent flow velocity signal

VENOUS DISEASE

7. **What noninvasive test is used to diagnose acute DVT?**
Duplex ultrasound has replaced venous occlusion plethysmography as the accepted standard. Colorflow duplex is useful because it helps to identify small veins from the muscle and fascial layers. The ultrasound assessment involves the following steps:
1. Examine the vein for echogenic thrombus.
2. Compress the vein, using pressure on the ultrasound probe, looking for complete collapse. Inability to compress the vein suggests thrombosis. Partial compression suggests partial thrombosis.
3. A Doppler signal from the vein that is phasic with respiration suggests no proximal occlusive thrombus. A signal that is spontaneously present but nonphasic suggests flow around an occlusion via small collateral veins. Absence of a Doppler signal in the vein suggests absence of flow.

8. **Can duplex ultrasound be used for surveillance in patients at high risk for DVT?**
Diagnosis of DVT in asymptomatic patients presents a dilemma. The sensitivity of duplex ultrasound is reduced from the reported 95% to < 80% for above-knee detection of DVT in asymptomatic patients. Calf DVT detection is much worse, with sensitivities as low as 20% in many reported series. However, serial contrast venography, although more specific, is not a practical surveillance strategy.

9. **Does venous occlusion plethysmography still have a role in the assessment of DVT?**
Yes. Venous occlusion plethysmography or impedance plethysmography (IPG) has high sensitivity and specificity in detecting occlusive thrombi above the knee, particularly for iliofemoral occlusive thrombi (95%). Because IPG provides functional information about deep venous outflow from the legs, it provides diagnosis of nonvisualized caval or iliac thrombosis, diagnosis of recurrent acute proximal thrombosis superimposed on chronic thrombosis, and functional evaluation of residual or chronic outflow obstruction (venous claudication).

10. **What noninvasive tests are useful for evaluation of venous incompetence?**
Doppler ultrasound can detect venous reflux in the deep veins of the legs and in the greater and lesser saphenous veins. With experience, the test can be done using a simple Doppler (continuous wave versus pulsed Doppler), but duplex ultrasound is often used to facilitate identification of the vein segments and valves and to position a pulsed Doppler sample reliably. Some laboratories measure the duration of reflux during controlled proximal compression as an indicator of severity of valve incompetence, but unless a valvuloplasty or valve transposition is planned for the identified incompetent valve, such specific measures appear to have little clinical utility.

PERIPHERAL ARTERIAL OCCLUSIVE DISEASE

11. **What is the primary test for diagnosis of lower extremity ischemia?**
The ankle brachial index (ABI) or systolic pressure ratio is normally greater than or equal to 1.0. Typically, Doppler ultrasound is used (instead of a stethoscope) as the flow sensor distal to the pressure cuff, but plethysmographic instruments also may be used. Doppler signals are usually monitored at the posterior tibial artery or dorsalis pedis artery.

KEY POINTS: NONINVASIVE VASCULAR DIAGNOSTIC LABORATORY

1. Duplex ultrasound has a sensitivity of 97% in detecting carotid artery disease and an accuracy of 95% in correctly classifying carotid stenoses as > 50% reduction in diameter.

2. The primary test for diagnosis of lower extremity ischemia is the ankle branchial index.

3. The noninvasive test used to diagnose acute DVT is duplex ultrasound.

12. **What is gained by measuring pressures at limb levels other than the ankle?**
Segmental limb pressure (SLP) measurements, performed at the upper thigh, lower thigh, calf, and ankle, localize the arterial segment(s) involved in peripheral arterial occlusive disease.

13. **What tests are used for assessing peripheral artery disease in diabetic patients who may have incompressible arteries caused by medial calcification?**
Pulse volume recording (PVR) is a pneumoplethysmographic technique that tracks the limb volume changes over the cardiac cycle. It measures the segmental pressure changes with pneumatic cuffs as a function of the limb volume changes. The relative PVR amplitudes identify the presence of peripheral artery disease and localize the arterial segment involved. The PVR is unaffected by medial calcification. Great-toe pressure also may be used to diagnose and assess disease severity in diabetic patients because medial calcification rarely affects the digital arteries.

14. **How should the patient with suspected intermittent claudication be evaluated?**
The patient first should be evaluated by obtaining ABIs or segmental limb pressures at rest. The patient with ischemia at rest does not normally need further evaluation. The patient with mild arterial insufficiency at rest or even normal resting pressures should perform an exercise stress test (treadmill walking using either fixed or variable load protocols) followed by ABIs. The distance that the patient is able to walk allows assessment of functional disability, and the postexercise reduction in ankle pressure, or lack thereof, allows assessment of whether the disability is caused by arterial insufficiency rather than musculoskeletal or neurologic pain.

CONTROVERSIES

15. **Can carotid endarterectomy be performed on the basis of duplex study alone?**
     The argument for elimination of arteriography in selected cases is persuasive because the carotid arteriogram alone has a morbidity rate > 1%. This rate may represent 25% of the usual total morbidity associated with carotid endarterectomy. However, to realize the benefit of surgery based on duplex ultrasound, the duplex study must have a high positive predictive value (PPV). Fortunately, the PPV is high for severe lesions that meet suitably strict criteria (e.g., peak systolic velocities > 290 cm/sec and end-diastolic velocities > 80 cm/sec).

16. **Does duplex ultrasound have a role in the diagnosis of peripheral arterial disease?**
     Its role is limited. Peripheral arterial disease must be assessed functionally, not anatomically. Duplex ultrasound can be used to localize disease that has already been assessed for its functional significance (exercise, not surgery, is typically prescribed for claudication alone).

17. **Does transcranial Doppler have a role in the noninvasive diagnosis of cerebrovascular disease?**
     No. Although the technique is widely touted, recent large studies emphasize that the Doppler evaluation of the intracranial arteries does not change the clinical management of any patient.

18. **Should D-dimer blood tests be required before patients are evaluated by ultrasound for DVT?**
     D-dimer is a degradation product of cross-linked fibrin. Blood plasma levels of D-dimer are often elevated in patients with DVT. However, DVT is not the only cause of elevated D-dimers and cannot be used instead of ultrasound to diagnose the presence of DVT. Conversely, in selected patient subgroups, a low D-dimer level has a very high negative predictive value and can prevent unnecessary ultrasound testing. The test should be restricted to nonsurgical patients, patients who are not anticoagulated, patients in the outpatient setting, and patients in whom there is a low clinical suspicion of DVT such as a painful limb without swelling or bilateral ankle swelling.

WEB SITE

http://www.acssurgery.com

BIBLIOGRAPHY

1. Baker WF: Diagnosis of deep venous thrombosis and pulmonary embolism. Med Clin North Am 82:459–476, 1998.
2. Gerlock AJ, Giyanani VL, Krebs C: Applications of Noninvasive Vascular Techniques. Philadelphia, W.B. Saunders, 1988.
3. Moneta GL, Edwards JM, Papanicolaou G, et al: Screening for asymptomatic internal carotid artery stenosis: Duplex criteria for discriminating 60% to 99% stenosis. J Vasc Surg 21:989–997, 1995.
4. Shirit D, et al: Appropriate indications for venous duplex scanning based on D-dimer assay. Ann Vasc Surg 16:304–308, 2002.
5. Zierler RE, Sumner DS: Physiologic assessment of peripheral arterial occlusive disease. In Rutherford RB (ed): Vascular Surgery, 5th ed. Philadelphia, W.B. Saunders, 2000, pp 140–165.

CORONARY ARTERY DISEASE

Joseph C. Cleveland, Jr., M.D.

CHAPTER 74

1. **What is angina, and what causes it?**
   Angina pectoris reflects myocardial ischemia. Patients often describe the sensation as pressure, choking, or tightness. Angina is typically produced by an imbalance between myocardial oxygen supply and myocardial oxygen demand. The classic presentation is a man (male-to-female ratio = 4:1) out shoveling snow on a cold night after a big meal after having a fight with his wife.

2. **How is angina treated?**
   The treatment options for angina include medical therapy or myocardial revascularization. Medical treatment is directed toward decreasing myocardial oxygen demand. Strategies include nitrates (nitroglycerin, isosorbide), which dilate coronary arteries minimally but also decrease blood pressure (afterload) and therefore myocardial oxygen demand; **beta receptor antagonists**, which decrease heart rate, contractility, and afterload; and **calcium channel antagonists**, which decrease afterload and may prevent coronary vasoconstriction. **Aspirin** (antiplatelet therapy) is also important. Newer antiplatelet agents such as clopidogrel (Plavix) and eptifibatide (Integrilin) are promoted in the management of acute coronary syndromes. Plavix, however, is a very potent, efficacious agent, and operation (i.e., coronary artery bypass grafting [CABG]) within 1 week of Plavix exposure increases the risk of postoperative bleeding by threefold.

   If medical therapy is unsuccessful in alleviating angina, myocardial revascularization with either percutaneous transluminal coronary angioplasty (PTCA), with or without placement of a stent, or CABG may be appropriate.

3. **What are the indications for CABG?**
   1. **Left main coronary artery stenosis:** Stenosis > 50% involving the left main coronary artery is a robust predictor of poor long-term outcome in medically treated patients. A substantial portion of the myocardium is supplied by this artery; thus, PTCA is too hazardous. Even if the patient is asymptomatic, survival is markedly improved with CABG.
   2. **Three-vessel coronary artery disease (70% stenosis) with depressed left ventricular (LV) function or two-vessel coronary artery disease (CAD) with proximal left anterior descending (LAD) involvement:** In randomized trials, patients with three-vessel disease and depressed LV function showed a survival benefit with CABG compared with medical therapy. CABG also confers survival benefit in patients with two-vessel CAD and ≥ 95% LAD stenosis. An important caveat, however, in managing patients with depressed LV function is that operative mortality increases when the ejection fraction (EF) falls below 30%.
   3. **Angina despite aggressive medical therapy:** Patients who have lifestyle limitations because of CAD are appropriate candidates for CABG. Data from the Coronary Artery Surgery Study (CASS) suggest that patients treated with surgery have less angina, fewer activity limitations, and an objective increase in exercise tolerance compared with medically treated patients.

4. **What is done during a "traditional" CABG procedure?**
   CABG is an arterial bypass procedure that can be done both on bypass and off bypass. The left internal mammary artery (LIMA) is harvested as a pedicled graft. Cardiopulmonary bypass (CPB) is established by cannulating the ascending aorta and the right atrium, and the heart is

arrested with cold blood cardioplegia. Segments of the greater saphenous vein are then reversed and sewn with the proximal (inflow) portion of the bypass graft originating from the ascending aorta and the distal (outflow) portion of the bypass graft anastomosed to the coronary artery distal to the obstructing lesion. The LIMA is typically sewn to the LAD. When the anastomoses are finished, the patient is weaned from CPB, and the chest is closed. Typically, one to six bypass grafts are constructed (hence the terms *triple* or *quadruple bypass*).

5. **What is an off-pump CABG (OPCAB)?**

CABG can be performed without cardiopulmonary bypass and arrest of the heart. When done with the heart beating through a median sternotomy, CABG is then called an OPCAB. The heart is positioned with commercially available stabilization devices, and the vessel to be bypassed is immobilized and snared to provide temporary occlusion. The venous or arterial conduit is then sewn to the immobilized coronary artery, and the occlusion of the vessel is released.

6. **Why would one choose an OPCAB instead of a traditional CABG?**

CABG with cardiopulmonary bypass is the gold standard. However, cardiopulmonary bypass is associated with several adverse clinical consequences such as acute lung dysfunction, stroke, renal failure, liver failure, bleeding, and the promotion of a proinflammatory state. It is thought, although not yet well delineated, that performing CABG without CPB may reduce these complications. Patients with comorbidities of lung disease, cerebrovascular disease, renal disease, or severe peripheral vascular disease may have improved outcomes when CABG is performed without the use of cardiopulmonary bypass.

7. **Does CABG improve myocardial function?**

Yes. Hibernating myocardium is improved by CABG. Myocardial hibernation refers to the reversible myocardial contractile function associated with a decrease in coronary flow in the setting of preserved myocardial viability. Some patients with global systolic dysfunction exhibit dramatic improvement in myocardial contractility after CABG.

8. **Is CABG helpful in patients with congestive heart failure (CHF)?**

Possibly. CABG improves CHF symptoms that are related to ischemic myocardial dysfunction. Conversely, if heart failure is secondary to long-standing irreversibly infarcted muscle (i.e., scar), CABG does not prove beneficial. The critical preoperative evaluation must assess the viability of nonfunctional myocardium. A rest–redistribution thallium scan is useful to determine the segments of myocardium that are still viable.

9. **Is CABG valuable in preventing ventricular arrhythmias?**

No. Most ventricular arrhythmias in patients with CAD originate from the border of irritable myocardium that surrounds infarcted muscle. Implantation of an automated implantable cardiac defibrillator (AICD) is indicated for patients with life-threatening ventricular tachyarrhythmias.

10. **What is the difference between PTCA and CABG?**

Six randomized, controlled clinical trials have compared PTCA with CABG. Although collectively they analyzed data from more than 4700 patients, 75% of patients who originally met inclusion criteria were excluded from participation because they had multivessel CAD, which was not deemed suitable for PTCA.

Several important features emerged from these trials. Overall mortality and myocardial infarction rates were no different for CABG and PTCA in five of the six studies. Only the German Angioplasty Bypass Surgery Investigational Study showed a higher short-term combined incidence of death and myocardial infarction (MI) in the CABG group.

The major difference between the two treatment strategies was freedom from angina and reintervention. Overall, whereas 40% of PTCA-treated patients required repeat PTCA or CABG, roughly 5% of CABG-treated patients required reintervention. The CABG-treated patients also experienced fewer episodes of angina compared with the PTCA-treated patients.

A more recent trial comparing PTCA with stent (percutaneous coronary intervention [PCI]) implantation also showed no difference in the composite endpoint of death or Q-wave MI between the CABG or PCI groups. In this investigation, freedom from reintervention was 80% at 1 year in the PCI group.

The unavoidable conclusion is that the recommendation of PTCA with stenting or CABG should be individualized for each patient. The two therapies should not be viewed as exclusionary or competitive; some patients may benefit from a combination of PTCA and CABG. CABG results in a more durable revascularization, although with the inherent risk of perioperative complications.

KEY POINTS: CORONARY ARTERY DISEASE

1. Hibernating myocardium is improved by coronary artery bypass grafting (CABG).

2. CABG is not helpful in preventing ventricular arrhythmias.

3. The rule of thumb for vessel patency is 90% patency at 10 years for the internal mammary graft, 50% patency at 10 years for saphenous vein grafts, and 80% patency at 1 year for PTCA plus stent of stenotic vessel.

11. **What is the rule of thumb for vessel patency?**

Internal mammary graft:	90% patency at 10 years
Saphenous vein graft:	50% patency at 10 years
PTCA 1 stent of stenotic vessel:	80% patency at 1 year

12. **What operative and technical problems are associated with CABG?**
The operative complications broadly include technical problems with the bypass graft anastomosis, sternal complications, and incisional complications associated with the saphenous vein harvest incision. Technical problems with the coronary artery anastomosis usually lead to MI. Sternal complications predictably result in sepsis and multiple organ failure. Incisions for saphenous vein harvest also may result in problems with edema, infection, and pain postoperatively.

13. **What are the risks of CABG? Which comorbid factors increase the operative risk for CABG?**
Estimating operative risk is a critical component of counseling patients before surgical revascularization. The Society of Thoracic Surgeons (STS) and the Veterans' Administration have developed and promoted two large databases. Factors that increase the risk of CABG include depressed left ventricular EF (LVEF), previous cardiac surgery, priority of operation (emergency versus elective), New York Heart Association Classification, age, peripheral vascular disease, chronic obstructive pulmonary disease, and decompensated heart failure at the time of surgery. These comorbidities figure prominently in outcome. Quite simply, raw mortality data for CABG can be misleading. Different surgeons can perform identical operations but have different raw mortality rates if one surgeon operates on young triathletes with CAD and the other surgeon operates on old couch potatoes who smoke two packs of cigarettes per day. Through assessment of these comorbid factors, a fairer representation of predicted to observed outcome can be determined. In this manner, using observed to expected outcomes with risk-adjusted models represents an honest comparison of CABG mortality rates.

14. **What steps are taken if a patient cannot be weaned from CPB?**
   The surgeon is in fact treating shock. As in hypovolemic shock (e.g., a bullet transecting the aorta), the basic principles include the following:
   - Volume resuscitation until left- and right-sided filling pressures are optimized
   - When filling pressures are adequate, initiation of inotropic support
   - Push inotropic support to toxicity (usually ventricular tachyarrhythmias) and insert an intraaortic balloon pump (IABP). The ultimate extension of CPB includes the placement of an LV or right ventricular assist device (or both). These devices can support the circulation while allowing for myocardial recovery.

CONTROVERSIES

15. **Is there an advantage to surgical revascularization with all arterial conduits?**
   The logical extension of the observation that an internal mammary artery has superior patency to a saphenous vein has sparked an interest in total arterial revascularization. Instead of using saphenous veins as bypass conduits, some surgeons also use the right internal mammary artery, the gastroepiploic artery, and the radial artery as bypass conduits instead of vein. Convincing data suggest a survival benefit as well as freedom from angina when the LIM artery is used as a conduit. The data supporting total arterial revascularization are much less clear.

16. **What are the options for a patient with continued angina who is deemed not suitable for CABG?**
   For patients on optimized medical treatment who are not surgical candidates (because of prohibitive comorbidities or poor quality coronary artery targets for bypass), an alternative is a procedure called transmyocardial myocardial revascularization (TMR). TMR uses a laser to burn small holes from the endocardium to the epicardium. Although it was originally believed that the laser brought blood from the endocardial capillary network to the myocardium, it has been repeatedly observed that laser-created channels are filled with thrombus within 24 hours and subsequently occluded. Therefore, it is postulated that the laser energy invokes an inflammatory response with a resultant increase in angiogenic factors (vascular endothelial growth factor, tumor growth factor beta, fibroblast growth factor). Although promising experimental data and clinical trials support TMR as therapeutic, one wonders if a placebo effect is not operative in promoting anginal relief.

WEB SITE

http://www.acssurgery.com

BIBLIOGRAPHY

1. Bypass Angioplasty Revascularization Investigation (BARI) Investigators: Comparison of coronary artery bypass surgery with angioplasty in patients with multivessel disease. N Engl J Med 335:217–225, 1996.
2. CABRI Trial Participants: First year results of CABRI (Coronary Angioplasty versus Bypass Revascularization Investigation). Lancet 346:1179–1184, 1995.
3. Cleveland JC Jr, Shroyer ALW, Chen AY, et al: Off-pump coronary artery bypass grafting decreases risk-adjusted mortality and morbidity. Ann Thorac Surg 72:1282–1288, 2001.
4. Gundry SR, Romano MA, Shattuck OH, et al: Seven-year follow-up of coronary artery bypasses performed with and without cardiopulmonary bypass. J Thorac Cardiovasc Surg 115:1273–1277, 1998.

5. Hamm CW, Reimers J, Ischinger T, et al (for the German Angioplasty Bypass Surgery Investigation): A randomized study of coronary angioplasty compared with bypass surgery in patients with symptomatic multivessel coronary disease. N Engl J Med 331:1037–1043, 1994.

6. Henderson JA, Pocock SJ, Sharp SJ, et al: Long-term results of RITA-1 Trial: Clinical and cost comparisons of coronary angioplasty and coronary artery bypass grafting. Randomised intervention treatment of angina. Lancet 352:1419–1425, 1998.

7. Horvath KA, Aranki SF, Cohn LH, et al: Sustained angina relief 5 years after transmyocardial laser revascularization with a CO2 laser. Circulation 104(suppl I):I81-I84, 2001.

8. Rodriguez A, Mele E, Peyregne E, et al: Three-year follow-up of the Argentine Randomized Trial of Percutaneous Transluminal Coronary Angioplasty versus Coronary Artery Bypass Surgery in Multivessel Disease (ERACI). J Am Coll Cardiol 27:1178–1184, 1996.

9. SOS Investigators: Coronary artery bypass surgery versus percutaneous coronary intervention with stent implantation in patients with multivessel coronary artery disease (the Stent or Surgery Trial): A randomized controlled trial. Lancet 360:965–970, 2002.

CHAPTER 75

MITRAL STENOSIS

David A. Fullerton, M.D., and Glenn J.R. Whitman, M.D.

1. **What causes mitral stenosis?**
   Rheumatic fever.

2. **Which gender most commonly gets mitral stenosis?**
   Women by a ratio of 3:2.

3. **What are the physical findings of mitral stenosis?**
   On ascultation, an opening snap and a diastolic murmer are heard best at the apex.

4. **How is the diagnosis confirmed?**
   By echocardiography, preferably transesophageal echocardiography (TEE).

5. **What is the Gorlin formula?**
   A formula used to calculate the area of a heart valve. In simplified terms:

   Mitral valve area = cardiac output ÷ $\sqrt{\text{mean pressure gradient across the valve}}$

6. **What is the normal size of the mitral valve?**
   The normal cross-sectional area is 4–6 cm^2.
   Mild mitral stenosis is < 2 cm^2.
   Severe mitral stenosis is < 1 cm^2.

7. **What is the pathophysiology of mitral stenosis?**
   Increased left atrial pressure is necessary to push blood through a stenotic mitral valve from the left atrium into the left ventricle. Increased left atrial pressure is transmitted retrograde into the pulmonary veins and pulmonary capillaries and ultimately into the pulmonary arteries. It gives the patient a sensation of dyspnea. A left atrial pressure of approximately 25 mmHg increases pulmonary capillary pressure enough to produce pulmonary edema.
   Example: To maintain adequate left ventricular filling across a 1.5-cm^2 valve, a pressure gradient of 20 mmHg is required. With a normal left ventricular end-diastolic pressure of 5 mmHg, a 20-mmHg gradient produces a left atrial pressure of 25 mmHg. Left atrial pressure rises even further as flow across the valve increases (increased cardiac output). This high left atrial pressure backs up and floods the lungs (pulmonary edema).

8. **What is the main symptom of mitral stenosis?**
   Dyspnea on exertion (DOE).

9. **What hemodynamic conditions precipitate symptoms in patients with mitral stenosis?**
   Tachycardia: Because blood flows through the mitral valve during diastole, a shorter diastole (tachycardia) means less time for blood to move through the stenotic mitral valve, which decreases stroke volume.
   Loss of atrial kick: As left atrial pressure increases, the left atrium stretches bigger and the normally organized atrial impulse becomes chaotic (i.e., atrial fibrillation). Increased pressure

is required to move blood through the stenotic valve. Loss of presystolic atrial contraction may decrease left ventricular filling by as much as 30%.

10. **What complications may result from mitral stenosis?**
    1. Hemoptysis from severe pulmonary venous congestion
    2. Thromboembolism in patients in atrial fibrillation
    3. Endocarditis
    4. Pulmonary hypertension and right heart failure

KEY POINTS: MITRAL STENOSIS

1. Mitral stenosis is caused by rheumatic fever.

2. Physical findings include auscultation of an opening snap and a diastolic murmur, heard best at the apex.

3. Mitral commissurotomy and mitral valve replacement are the two operations that may be done for mitral valve stenosis.

11. **Why does mitral stenosis cause pulmonary hypertension?**
    - Retrograde transmission of increased left atrial pressure
    - Reflex pulmonary vasoconstriction initiated by left atrial distention
    - Hypertrophy of the pulmonary arteries, leading to remodeling of the pulmonary vasculature

12. **What is the medical therapy of mitral stenosis?**
    - Beta blockers slow the ventricular rate to about 60 bpm.
    - Digoxin slows the ventricular rate (by slowing atrioventricular nodal conduction) in patients with atrial fibrillation.
    - Diuretics (furosemide) relieves pulmonary edema.
    - Warfarin (Coumadin) is used if the patient is in atrial fibrillation.

13. **What is the natural history of mitral stenosis?**
    The survival with moderate mitral stenosis is approximately 50% at 10 years.

14. **What are the indications for mechanical intervention in mitral stenosis?**
    - Symptomatic patients with moderate-to-severe mitral stenosis
    - Asymptomatic patients with a mitral valve area < 1 cm^2

15. **What is the procedure of choice for mitral stenosis?**
    If the patient has mobile valve leaflets, no calcium in the valve leaflets, and minimal concurrent mitral regurgitation, then balloon valvuloplasty with a catheter may be an option.

16. **Which patients may be appropriate candidates for balloon valvuloplasty?**
    Again, this can be a tough call, but patients may be candidates if they are without calcification of the mitral annulus or leaflets, have little or no mitral regurgitation, and have little or no fusion of the mitral chordae tendineae.

17. **What are the results of balloon valvuloplasty?**
    - Mortality rate < 1%.
    - Initial success can be as high as 95% in properly selected patients.

- Valve area may increase to 2 cm^2.
- < 90% event-free (you and your patient do not want "events") survival at 7 years, again in properly selected patients.

18. **Which operations may be done for mitral stenosis?**
    - **Mitral commissurotomy:** The mortality rate is < 2%, and recurrence of mitral stenosis is 2% per year.
    - **Mitral valve replacement:** The mortality rate is 6%.

BONUS QUESTION

19. **What is the Lutembacher syndrome?**
    Mitral stenosis associated with an atrial septal defect. This results in a left-to-right shunt and overworks the right ventricle.

WEB SITE

http://www.acssurgery.com

BIBLIOGRAPHY

1. Bonow RO, Carabello B, de Leon AC Jr, et al: ACC/AHA guidelines for the management of patients with valvular heart disease. J Am Coll Cardiol 32:1486–1588, 1998.
2. Hammermeister K, Sethi GK, Henderson WG, et al: Outcomes 15 years after valve replacement with a mechanical versus bioprosthetic valve: Final report of the VA randomized trial. J Am Coll Cardiol 36:1152–1158, 2000.
3. Iung B, Garbarz E, Michand P, et al: Late results of percutaneous mitral commissurotomy in a series of 1024 patients: Analysis of late clinical deterioration: Frequency, anatomic findings and predictive factors. Circulation 99:3270–3278, 1999.
4. Palacios IF, Sanchez PL, Harrell LC, et al: Which patients benefit from percutaneous mitral balloon valvuloplasty? Prevalvuloplasty and post valvuloplasty variables that predict long-term outcome. Circulation 105:1465–1471, 2002.
5. Rahimtoola SH, Durairaj A, Mehra A, Nuno I: Current evaluation and management of patients with mitral stenosis. Circulation 106:1183–1188, 2002.

CHAPTER 76

MITRAL REGURGITATION

David A. Fullerton, M.D., and Glenn J.R. Whitman, M.D.

1. **List the causes of mitral regurgitation.**

   Rheumatic fever

   Endocarditis

   Ruptured chordae tendineae

   Senile mitral annular calcification

   Papillary muscle dysfunction from ischemia

   Annular dilatation from left ventricular dilation

2. **What is the pathophysiology of mitral regurgitation?**

   The left ventricle ejects blood via two routes: (1) antegrade, through the aortic valve, or (2) retrograde, through the mitral valve. The amount of each stroke volume ejected retrograde into the left atrium is the **regurgitant fraction**. To compensate for the regurgitant fraction, the left ventricle must increase its total stroke volume. This ultimately produces volume overload of the left ventricle and leads to ventricular dysfunction.

3. **What are the symptoms of mitral regurgitation?**

   Dyspnea on exertion and loss of exercise tolerance are the symptoms of heart failure.

4. **What determines left atrial pressure in mitral regurgitation?**

   The compliance of the left atrium.

5. **Why does acute mitral regurgitation cause severe symptoms?**

   With acute mitral regurgitation, the normal left atrium is noncompliant. Hence, left atrial pressure increases rapidly, flooding the lungs (i.e., congestive heart failure) and causing severe symptoms. Conversely, chronic mitral regurgitation is associated with progressive dilatation of the left atrium. With increased left atrial compliance, the left atrial pressure may not increase.

6. **What hemodynamic conditions exacerbate mitral regurgitation?**

   Increased left ventricular afterload: Increased systemic arterial blood pressure increases the impedance against which the left ventricle must pump to eject blood antegrade. The regurgitant fraction is therefore increased (more blood goes backwards through the mitral valve).

   Tachycardia: Because mitral regurgitation occurs during systole, tachycardia (i.e., more systoles per minute) increases the regurgitant fraction.

   Volume overload: Left ventricular distension secondary to volume overload stretches the mitral anulus, impairs coaptation of the mitral valve leaflets, and increases mitral regurgitation.

7. **What is the murmur of mitral regurgitation?**

   A holosystolic murmur is best heard at the apex with radiation to the left axilla.

8. **How is the diagnosis confirmed?**

   By color Doppler echocardiography, especially transesophageal echocardiography (TEE; the left atrium lies right on the esophagus). The regurgitant jet may be accurately visualized and quantitated. Echocardiography also allows determination of the anatomic abnormality of the mitral valve apparatus that is responsible for the regurgitation.

9. **What is the medical therapy for mitral regurgitation?**
   - Afterload reduction with **angiotensin-converting enzyme (ACE) inhibitors**
   - **Diuretics** (furosemide) for lower left ventricular preload
   - **Digoxin** provides ventricular rate control for patients in atrial fibrillation
   - **Warfarin** (Coumadin) is used for patients in atrial fibrillation

10. **What are the indications for surgery in patients with mitral regurgitation?**
    - Severe mitral regurgitation, especially with a ruptured chordae tendineae
    - Symptoms despite medical therapy
    - Progressive mitral regurgitation by echocardiography
    - Deteriorating left ventricular systolic function. Because mitral regurgitation lowers the total impedance of left ventricular ejection (much of each stroke volume escapes via the low resistance mitral valvular "back door"), the left ventricular ejection fraction (LVEF) should be greater than normal in the presence of mitral regurgitation. An LVEF < 55% in the presence of mitral regurgitation suggests left ventricular dysfunction.
    - Pulmonary artery pressure increases with exercise

KEY POINTS: MITRAL REGURGITATION

1. The symptoms are dyspnea on exertion and loss of exercise tolerance.

2. The murmur of mitral regurgitation is a holosystolic murmur heard best at the apex with radiation to the left axilla.

3. Mitral valve regurgitation is corrected with mitral valve repair or mitral valve replacement.

4. Mitral valve repair is preferable to replacement because of lower operative mortality rates, less risk of thromboembolism, less risk of endocarditis, better long-term left ventricular function, and less need (if any) for chronic anticoagulation.

5. Repair also avoids prosthetic valve-related complications.

11. **How is mitral regurgitation corrected?**
    Mitral valve repair. Mitral valve repair is the preferred surgical procedure. This preserves the mitral apparatus, maintaining the continuity between the left ventricular muscle and the mitral anulus via the chordae tendineae. Loss of this continuity by resection of the apparatus places the left ventricle at a mechanical disadvantage that over time leads to left ventricular dilatation and dysfunction.
    Mitral valve replacement. An inability to repair the regurgitant valve mandates replacement. If replacement is necessary, efforts should be made to preserve the posterior leaflet of the mitral valve. In most series, mitral valve replacement is required in < 30% of cases.

12. **Why is it preferable to repair rather than replace the mitral valve?**
    - Lower operative mortality
    - Less risk of thromboembolism
    - Less risk of endocarditis
    - Less need (if any) for chronic anticoagulation
    - Better long-term left ventricular function
    - Avoids valve-related complications

13. **How is the mitral valve repaired?**
    The redundant portion(s) of the valve leaflet(s) is resected, the leaflet is reapproximated, and the mitral anulus is plicated and reinforced with a prosthetic anuloplasty ring. The anuloplasty ring

is sewn around the perimeter of the anulus on the left atrial side of the valve. In so doing, the mitral leaflets are supported by competent chordae tendineae, and the circumference of the mitral anulus is decreased. Competency of the repaired valve is assessed intraoperatively using TEE.

14. **What is the operative mortality of mitral valve repair versus mitral valve replacement?**
Repair: 2%; replacement: 6%.

15. **How durable are mitral valve repairs?**
The risk of requiring another mitral valve operation is approximately 2% per year.

BONUS QUESTION

16. **What is systolic anterior motion (SAM) of the mitral valve?**
SAM is a complication of mitral valve repair. After mitral valve repair, the anterior leaflet of the mitral valve may billow into the left ventricular outflow tract during systole, creating two problems: (1) dynamic left ventricular outflow tract obstruction and (2) mitral regurgitation (anterior displacement of the anterior leaflet causes it to be foreshortened). SAM should be suspected if cardiac output is low after mitral valve repair and may be diagnosed by echocardiography. It is exacerbated by an increased contractile state of the myocardium, so inotropic agents should be avoided. Patients with SAM are treated by volume-loading and beta-blocking agents. If these measures fail, the valve should be replaced.

WEB SITE

http://www.acssurgery.com

BIBLIOGRAPHY

1. Bonow RO, Carabello B, de Leon AC Jr, et al: ACC/AHA guidelines for the management of patients with valvular heart disease. J Am Coll Cardiol 32:1486–1588, 1998.
2. Carabello BA: The ten most commonly asked questions about mitral regurgitation. Cardiol Rev 10:321–322, 2002.
3. Enruquez-Sarano M, Nkomo V, Mohty D, et al: Mitral regurgitation: Natural history in operated and nonoperated patients. Adv Cardiol 39:122–129, 2002.
4. Galloway AC, Grossi EA, Bizekis CS, et al: Evolving techniques for mitral valve reconstruction. Ann Thorac Surg 236:288–293, 2002.
5. Irvine T, Li XK, Sahn DJ, Kenny A: Assessment of mitral regurgitation. Heart 88(suppl 4):iv11–19, 2002.

CHAPTER 77

AORTIC VALVULAR DISEASE

Christopher D. Raeburn, M.D., and Alden H. Harken, M.D.

1. **What are the most common causes of aortic stenosis?**
   Rheumatic heart disease is now a rare cause of aortic stenosis, so the most common causes are now congenital anomalies and calcific (degenerative) disease.

2. **What is the most common anatomic anomaly in aortic stenosis?**
   Bicuspid aortic valve (normal valve is tricuspid) occurs in 2% of the general population. More than 50% of patients with aortic stenosis older than age 15 years have a bicuspid aortic valve.

3. **What are the most common symptoms of aortic stenosis in adults? Infants?**
   Most patients with aortic stenosis are asymptomatic. In adults, the development of angina, syncope, or dyspnea on exertion (congestive heart failure [CHF]) portends a poor prognosis unless valve replacement is performed. CHF is the most common presentation of aortic stenosis in infants.

4. **What is the expected survival of patients with aortic stenosis?**
   Asymptomatic patients with aortic stenosis have a near normal life expectancy. After symptoms occur, the 3-year mortality of patients who do not undergo valve surgery is 75%. Thus, it is important to catch patients before they are symptomatic.

5. **What is the most feared complication of aortic stenosis?**
   Sudden death.

6. **What physical findings suggest aortic stenosis?**
   Systolic crescendo-decrescendo (diamond-shaped) murmur, diminished peripheral pulses, or delayed pulse upstroke (call it *pulsus parvus et tardus* if you want to shine on medicine rounds).

7. **What are the typical findings of aortic stenosis on chest radiographs and electrocardiogram (ECG)?**
   Both chest radiographs and ECG may show normal results even with severe aortic stenosis; thus, these are not good screening tests. On chest radiograph, calcification of the aortic valve and an enlarged cardiac silhouette may be seen. ECG is fairly sensitive in detecting left ventricular hypertrophy (LVH) and may also reveal conduction defects (these occur secondary to extension of valvular calcification into the adjacent conduction tissue).

8. **How is the diagnosis of aortic stenosis confirmed?**
   Echocardiography with Doppler ultrasound is nearly 100% accurate in diagnosing hemodynamically significant aortic stenosis. This noninvasive test also accurately estimates aortic valve area and gradient and has all but replaced cardiac catheterization as the diagnostic test of choice for aortic stenosis.

9. **When is cardiac catheterization indicated in patients with echocardiography-confirmed aortic stenosis?**
Approximately 50% of patients with aortic stenosis will have some degree of associated coronary artery disease (CAD). Patients requiring aortic valve replacement who have surgically treatable CAD should have coronary artery bypass graft (CABG) performed at the time of the valve surgery. Thus, coronary angiography should precede aortic valve surgery in patients ≥ 40 years or in those with angina or significant risk factors for CAD.

10. **When is an operation indicated for aortic stenosis?**
Asymptomatic patients with aortic stenosis rarely require surgery; however, essentially all patients with symptomatic aortic stenosis should undergo aortic valve replacement. Indications for valve replacement in asymptomatic patients include progressive LVH, left ventricular dysfunction, or valve area < 0.6 cm^2.

11. **Can aortic valvotomy be used to treat aortic stenosis?**
Although valvotomy effectively palliates patients with congenital aortic stenosis, it is rarely curative. Most children with the condition will require aortic valve replacement later in life. Aortic valve replacement, not valvotomy, is the procedure of choice in adults.

12. **What is the Ross procedure?**
The patient's own pulmonary valve and proximal pulmonary artery are harvested (autograft) and used to replace the native, diseased aortic valve. A pulmonary allograft (harvested and frozen from a human cadaver) is then used to reconstruct the right ventricular outflow tract.

13. **What type of valvular prosthesis should be used in children requiring aortic valve replacement?**
In children younger than 15 years (as well as young adults between the ages of 15 and 30 years), rapid calcification occurs in porcine valves placed in the aortic position. Thus, mechanical valves (or the Ross procedure; see question 12) should be used.

14. **What type of valvular prosthesis should be used in adults requiring aortic valve replacement?**
Whether to use a mechanical or a bioprosthetic valve depends upon the patient's age and the risk of lifelong anticoagulation. Mechanical aortic valves afford excellent long-term relief of hemodynamically significant aortic stenosis but require lifelong anticoagulation. Bioprosthetic valves in the aortic position do not require anticoagulation; however, 30% of these valves exhibit structural deterioration at 10 years.

15. **What are the most common causes of aortic insufficiency?**
Infective valvular endocarditis, aortic dissection, connective tissue disease (e.g., Marfan syndrome), and prosthetic (mechanical) valve dysfunction.

16. **What physical findings suggest aortic insufficiency?**
A rapid rise and fall of the arterial pulse (refer to this as a water-hammer pulse or, better yet, a Corrigan's pulse to dazzle your chief medicine resident).

7. **What is a Quincke's pulse?**
Capillary pulsations secondary to aortic insufficiency that can be detected by transmitting a light through the patient's fingertip or by pressing a glass slide on his or her lip.

8. **How is the diagnosis of aortic insufficiency confirmed?**
As with aortic stenosis, echocardiography or Doppler ultrasound are the tests of choice.

KEY POINTS: AORTIC VALVULAR DISEASE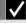

1. The most common causes are congenital anomalies and calcific (degenerative) disease.

2. The most feared complication is sudden death.

3. Surgical intervention is indicated for all patients with symptoms and for asymptomatic patients with left ventricular hypertrophy, left ventricular dysfunction, or valve area < 0.6 cm^2.

19. **When is an operation indicated for aortic insufficiency?**
    This depends on the cause of the aortic insufficiency and whether it is acute or chronic. Aortic insufficiency caused by an ascending aortic dissection is a surgical emergency. Aortic insufficiency secondary to infective endocarditis may or may not require aortic valve replacement (see question 20). Patients with chronic (mild to moderate) aortic insufficiency that does not progress enjoy a near-normal life expectancy. Patients with severe aortic insufficiency require valve surgery before they develop irreversible left ventricular dysfunction. Asymptomatic patients with severe aortic insufficiency benefit from aortic valve replacement when their left ventricle begins to fail or enlarges (end-systolic left ventricular diameter ≥ 55 mm or end-diastolic left ventricular diameter ≥ 75 mm).

20. **What are the indications for aortic valve replacement in patients with infective endocarditis?**
    Progressive CHF, recurrent septic emboli, infection uncontrolled by antibiotics (often fungal, gram-negative rods or *Staphylococcus aureus*) and a prolongation of the P-R interval. Although hard to believe, the junction of the left and noncoronary aortic valvular cusps is immediately adjacent to the atrioventricular (A-V) node. Thus, a perivalvular abscess can slow A-V conduction.

21. **What is the operative mortality of aortic valve replacement?**
    Thirty-day mortality is ≤ 4%. In low-risk patients, the mortality can approach 1%; however, the mortality skyrockets to 20% in patients with associated CAD and left ventricular dysfunction.

22. **What are the complications of aortic valve replacement?**
    - Bleeding requiring reexploration (2%)
    - Heart block (2%), again, caused by the proximity to the A-V node
    - Stroke (1%) caused by air or calcium left in the heart after closure of the aortotomy
    - Low cardiac output (≥ 5%) in patients with preoperative left ventricular failure

23. **What are the long-term results of aortic valve replacement?**
    Patients who survive the immediate perioperative period improve both symptomatically and functionally, and age-corrected survival returns to near normal (75% at 10 years). Aortic valve replacement partially reverses LVH and dilatation.

24. **Can balloon valvotomy be used for adult calcific aortic stenosis?**
    Initially, it was hoped that balloon valvotomy could replace surgery and provide long-term palliation in older patients who are at higher surgical risk because of decreased ventricular function. However, it is exactly this group who fare least well after balloon valvotomy; < 50% are alive at 1 year after surgery.

25. **What are the indications for balloon valvotomy?**
    Balloon valvotomy is effective in infants and young children with congenital aortic stenosis and a tiny aortic annulus. The intermediate results are similar to surgical valvotomy. In adults, bal-

loon valvotomy should be used primarily as a bridge to aortic valve replacement or transplantation in critically ill patients. Temporary improvement in ventricular function suggests that the patient will benefit from aortic valve replacement. Balloon valvotomy may also relieve the symptoms of women with severe aortic stenosis in the second trimester of pregnancy.

26. **Is percutaneous aortic valve replacement feasible?**
Although percutaneous transcatheter placement of a bioprosthetic aortic valve has been reported, this approach is still largely experimental.

CONTROVERSIES

27. **Should the Ross procedure ever be performed?**
For: The Ross procedure provides excellent, long-term (sometimes lifelong) hemodynamic relief of aortic stenosis and avoids the need for mechanical valves, thus avoiding the need for anticoagulation. An additional benefit is the regenerative capacity of the aortic autograft; it may actually increase in size as the patient grows.
Against: The Ross procedure is a technically demanding operation and has a significant learning curve with high associated morbidity. The procedure destroys a normal pulmonary valve, thus potentially giving the patient two (instead of one) valve diseases.

28. **Should a tissue valve be used in young adults between ages 15 and 30 years?**
For: Anticoagulation is not necessary for tissue valves placed in the aortic position; thus, the risk of significant bleeding complications in active patients is avoided. For women in the childbearing years, the advantages are very real.
Against: Early valve dysfunction secondary to valve calcification occurs more aggressively in younger patients; thus, valve replacement may be necessary before 10 years.

29. **Should minimally invasive approaches to aortic valve replacement be attempted?**
For: Aortic valve replacement can be performed via a ministernotomy. This approach avoids a complete sternotomy and may improve cosmesis and decrease blood loss.
Against: Aortic valve replacement via conventional sternotomy is surprisingly well tolerated and has excellent long-term results. Comparative studies have identified no difference in quality of life between minimally invasive and conventional aortic valve replacement. Furthermore, long-term results of the minimally invasive approach are not yet available.

WEB SITE

http://www.acssurgery.com

BLIOGRAPHY

. Akins CW, Hilgenberg AD, Vlahakes GJ, et al: Results of bioprosthetic versus mechanical aortic valve replacement performed with concomitant coronary artery bypass grafting. Ann Thorac Surg 74:1098–1106, 2002.
. Al-Halees Z, Pieters F, Qadoura F, et al: The Ross procedure is the procedure of choice for congenital aortic valve disease. J Thorac Cardiovasc Surg 123:437–441, 2002.

3. Bonow RO, Carabello B, de Leon AC, et al: ACC/AHA guidelines for the management of patients with valvular heart disease. Executive summary. A report of the American College of Cardiology/American Heart Association Task Force on Practice Guidelines (Committee on Management of Patients With Valvular Heart Disease). J Heart Valve Dis 7:672–707, 1998.

4. Borer JS: Aortic valve replacement for the asymptomatic patient with aortic regurgitation: A new piece of the strategic puzzle. Circulation 106:2637–2639, 2002.

5. Carabello BA: Evaluation and management of patients with aortic stenosis. Circulation 105:1746–1750, 2002.

6. Chaliki HP, Mohty D, Avierinos JF, et al: Outcomes after aortic valve replacement in patients with severe aortic regurgitation and markedly reduced left ventricular function. Circulation 106:2687–2693, 2002.

7. Cribier A, Eltchaninoff H, Bash A, et al: Percutaneous transcatheter implantation of an aortic valve prosthesis for calcific aortic stenosis: First human case description. Circulation 106:3006–3008, 2002.

8. Detter C, Deuse T, Boehm DH, et al: Midterm results and quality of life after minimally invasive versus conventional aortic valve replacement. Thorac Cardiovasc Surg 50:337–341, 2002.

9. Detter C, Fischlein T, Feldmeier C, et al: Aortic valvotomy for congenital valvular aortic stenosis: A 37-year experience. Ann Thorac Surg 71:1564–1571, 2001.

10. Lamb HJ, Beyerbacht HP, de Roos A, et al: Left ventricular remodeling early after aortic valve replacement: Differential effects on diastolic function in aortic valve stenosis and aortic regurgitation. J Am Coll Cardiol 40:2182–2188, 2002.

11. McCrindle BW, Blackstone EH, Williams WG, et al: Are outcomes of surgical versus transcatheter balloon valvotomy equivalent in neonatal critical aortic stenosis? Circulation 104(suppl I):I152-II58, 2001.

12. Paparella D, David TE, Armstrong S, Ivanov J: Mid-term results of the Ross procedure. J Card Surg 16:338–343, 2001.

13. Russo CF, Mazzetti S, Garatti A, et al: Aortic complications after bicuspid aortic valve replacement: long-term results. Ann Thorac Surg 74:S1773–S1776, 2002.

14. Yener N, Oktar GL, Erer D, et al: Bicuspid aortic valve. Ann Thorac Cardiovasc Surg 8:264–267, 2002.

CHAPTER 78

THORACIC SURGERY FOR NON-NEOPLASTIC DISEASE

J. Timothy Sherwood, M.D., and Marvin Pomerantz, M.D.

TUBERCULOSIS

1. **What are the clinical manifestations of pulmonary tuberculosis?**
   They can be almost anything or nothing (it has been stated that if you know tuberculosis, you know all of medicine), but the most common symptoms and signs are chronic fever; weight loss; night sweats; and cough, sometimes with hemoptysis. Chest radiograph typically shows upper lobe infiltrates, with or without cavitation, and can be misdiagnosed as a neoplastic process. HIV-positive or immunocompromised patients usually have mediastinal adenopathy, pleural effusions, and a miliary pattern.

2. **How is the diagnosis of pulmonary tuberculosis made?**
   Positive acid-fast bacilli (AFB; "red snappers") smear in sputum sample; sensitivity improves with bronchoalveolar lavage (BAL) specimens. Culture growth will identify specific organism (i.e., atypicals) as well as drug sensitivity (watch out for multidrug resistance [MDR]).

3. **What is the current medical treatment for active tuberculosis?**
   Initial therapy consists of a 6-month regimen with isoniazid, rifampin, and pyrazinamide for the first 2 months, and then isoniazid and rifampin for another 4 months. With this schedule, 95% of patients have tuberculosis-negative sputum at the end of therapy. Partial responders should receive therapy for longer than 6 months, and those with MDR-TB may receive ethambutol or streptomycin.

4. **What are the indications for surgery in patients with tuberculosis?**
   Surgery is indicated for complications of the disease. The most common surgical indication in the United States is MDR-TB with destroyed lung and persistent cavitary disease. This lung tissue is resistant to drug penetration and can also "spill" organsims into healthy lung tissue. Other indications include hemoptysis, exclusion of lung cancer, bronchial stenosis, bronchopleural fistula, middle lobe syndrome, or mycobacterium other than tubercle bacilli (MOTT).

5. **What is MOTT, and what is the role of surgery with this disease?**
   Atypical mycobacterial infections, nontuberculosis mycobacterial infections, and infection with mycobacteria other than tuberculosis are synonyms. The most common of these organisms is the *Mycobacterium avium* complex (MAC). Others include *M. chelonae* and abscesses, *M. kansaii*, *M. fortuitum*, and *M. xenopi*. MAC typically produces fibrocavitary disease of the upper lobes or the middle lobe or lingula of thin, white women. Surgery is indicated for localized disease, and in combination with drug therapy, it results in sputum conversion in ≥ 95% of patients with relapse rates of < 5%. Other indications for surgery are the same as for regular tuberculosis.

PLEURAL EFFUSION

6. **What is a pleural effusion?**
   Pleural fluid is generated in normal adults at a rate of 5–10 L per 24 hours in the combined hemithoraces, but normal adults have only 20 mL of pleural fluid present at any time. Pleural

effusions develop when there is either increased production or decreased resorption. Pathologic conditions leading to effusions include increased capillary permeability (inflammation, tumor), increased hydrostatic pressure (e.g., in congestive heart failure [CHF]), decreased lymphatic drainage (tumor, radiation fibrosis), decreased oncotic pressure (hypoalbuminemia), or combinations of these.

7. **How does one determine the cause of a pleural effusion?**
History and physical examination, chest radiograph (upright and decubitus), and thoracentesis are used. Thoracentesis should be used to evaluate the pleural fluid. Bloody fluid is typical of trauma, pulmonary embolism, malignancy, milky fluid with chylothorax (triglyceride > 110), and purulent fluid with empyema. Fluid should be checked for cell count; cytology; pH; Gram stain; culture; and glucose, protein, lactate dehydrogenase (LDH), amylase, and triglyceride level. Exudates have a protein ratio > 0.5 and an LDH ratio > 0.6. The most common cause of transudate is CHF; the most common cause of exudate is malignancy and infection. Glucose < 60 mg/dL is seen in only parapneumonic effusions, rheumatoid effusion, tuberculous pleuritis, and malignancy.

8. **What is the management of a pleural effusion?**
Thoracentesis or a tube thoracostomy should be used to evacuate the effusion completely. The underlying problem (e.g., CHF) should be corrected if possible. If the effusion is persistent (e.g., malignancy), then pleurodesis (stick the parietal and visceral pleurae together) can be performed with sclerosants (talc) or mechanical abrasion. Pleural symphysis (stuck pleura) results in decreased surface area for production, eliminates the pleural space for accumulation, and prevents lung collapse and compression. Chest tubes are generally removed when output is < 75 mL per 24 hours.

9. **What does an air-fluid level on an initial chest radiograph indicate?**
An air-fluid level before any drainage procedure may represent a bronchopleural fistula. These fistulas may resolve with chest tube drainage or require open thoracotomy for definitive repair.

EMPYEMA

10. **What is an empyema, and what causes it?**
An empyema is a purulent (infected) effusion. Fluid or blood in the pleural space can be directly innoculated (with bugs) during surgery or trauma (33%) or by contamination from contiguous sites (50%) such as bronchopulmonary infection (most common). Most empyemas are parapneumonic, and the most commonly involved organisms are *Staphylococcus aureus*, enteric gram-negative bacilli, and anaerobes. Many times, infections are polymicrobial. Often there is no growth of an empyema culture because of effective antibiotic therapy or inadequate culture techniques, particularly with anaerobes.

11. **What are the three stages of empyema development?**
They are the **exudative** stage (low viscosity fluid), **fibrinopurulent** stage (transitional phase with heavy fibrinous deposits and turbid fluid), and **organizing** stage (capillary ingrowth with lung trapping by collagen). This process usually evolves over 6 weeks.

12. **How is an empyema diagnosed?**
Characteristic clinical and radiographic findings are used. Computed tomography (CT) scan is very helpful in defining loculations. Thoracentesis may reveal frank pus, and Gram stain shows many white blood cells (WBCs) and organisms. Biochemical analysis varies, but it is generally an exudate with a low pH (< 7), high LDH (> 1000 IU/L), and low glucose (< 50 mg/dL).

KEY POINTS: THORACIC SURGERY FOR NON-NEOPLASTIC DISEASE

1. Surgery is indicated for complications of tuberculosis, with the most common indication in the United States being multiple drug-resistant tuberculosis with destroyed lung and persistent cavitary disease.

2. An empyema is a purulent (infected) effusion.

3. The three stages of empyema are the exudative stage (low viscosity fluid), fibrinopurulent stage (transitional phase with heavy fibrinous deposits and turbid fluid), and organizing stage (capillary ingrowth with lung trappng by collagen).

13. **How should an empyema be treated?**
    Antibiotic therapy directed by Gram stain and culture. If early, tube thoracostomy may be curative. Conversion to open tube drainage (empyema tube) may be necessary if persistent purulent drainage occurs. Instillation of fibrinolytic enzymes (e.g., streptokinase or TPA) may be helpful. An infected loculated (lots of discontinuous cystic pockets) effusion <14 days old should undergo video-assisted thoracoscopic surgery (VATS) decortication (i.e., resection of the thickened, adherent peel). The probability of conversion to open thoracotomy increases with the age of the effusion or empyema.

14. **What is a decortication?**
    The cortex is the outside wall or peel of the empyema (like an orange). Thus, decortication is the surgical release and removal of the abscess cavity walls. Successful decortication allows the lung to expand and fill the entire pleural space; if complete expansion does not occur, then the effusion may recur, and continued lung trapping is likely.

15. **What are the complications of an empyema left untreated?**
    The most common is pulmonary fibrosis with lung trapping and resultant dyspnea. Others include contraction and deformity of the chest wall, spontaneous drainage through the chest wall (empyema necessitans), bronchopleural fistula, osteomyelitis, pericarditis, mediastinal or subphrenic abscess, sepsis, and death. None of these outcomes is particularly appealing, so in the absence of overwhelming contraindications, all empyemas warrant therapy.

WEB SITE

http://www.acssurgery.com

BIBLIOGRAPHY

1. American Thoracic Society: Diagnosis and treatment of disease caused by nontuberculous mycobacteria. Am J Respir Crit Care Med 156(suppl 2 pt 2):S1–S25, 1997.

2. Colice GL, Curtis A, Deslauriers J, et al: Medical and surgical treatment of parapneumonic effusions: An evidence-based guideline. Chest 118:1158–1171, 2000.

3. de Hoyos A, Sundaresan S: Thoracic empyema.Surg Clin North Am 82:643–671, 2002.

4. Mault JR, Pomerantz M: Mycobacterium tuberculosis and other mycobacteria. Chest Surg Clin North Am 9:227–238, 1999.

5. Pomerantz M, Brown J: Surgery of pulmonary mycobacterial disease. In Kaiser LR, Kron IL, Spray TL (eds): Mastery of Cardiothoracic Surgery. Philadelphia, Lippincott-Raven, 1998, pp 265–271.

6. Wiedeman HP, Rice TW: Lung abscess and empyema. Semin Thorac Cardiovasc Surg 7:119–128, 1995.

CHAPTER 79

LUNG CANCER

Jamie M. Brown, M.D.

1. **How common is lung cancer?**

   The incidence of lung cancer is approximately 180,000 new cases annually or 54.2 per 100,000 patients. More than 162,000 patients die annually, so the overall survival rate is 10%. This number has not improved over the past 35 years despite some treatment advances because of:

   1. Teenage smoking and smoking in general
   2. Increased incidence in nonsmokers
   3. Presentation of lung cancer in advanced stage in most patients

2. **What risk factors are thought to be important in the development of lung cancer?**

   - 90% of patients have a smoking history
   - Chemicals (aromatic hydrocarbons, vinyl chloride)
   - Radiation (radon gas and uranium)
   - Asbestos
   - Metals (chromium, nickel, lead, and arsenic)
   - Environmental factors (air pollution, coal tar, petroleum products)

3. **Do genes and heredity play a role in lung cancer?**

   Yes. A family history of lung cancer probably increases the risk of getting lung cancer. Furthermore, a large array of important biomarkers that influence prognosis have been identified in lung cancer cells and lung cancer tissue.

   Past:
   - Light microscopic evidence of vascular invasion
   - Lymphatic invasion
   - Cellular pleomorphism and mitotic figures

   Present:
   - Proto-oncogenes, growth factors, growth factor receptors
     - Insulin-like growth factor (IGF)
     - Epidermal growth factor receptor (EGFR)
     - K-*ras* mutation (cell growth regulation)
     - C-*myc* overexpression (cell growth)
     - *bcl*-2 underexpression (loss of apoptosis regulation)
   - Loss of tumor suppressor genes
     - p53
     - Retinoblastoma (RB gene)
     - Chromosomal allele loss
     - Fragile histidine triad gene (FHit)
     - Retinoic acid receptor α (RARα)
   - Overactivation of angiogenesis
     - Platelet-derived growth factor (PDGF)
     - Vascular endothelial-derived growth factor (VEGF)

Future:
- Gene therapy directed at above
- Antiangiogensis therapy
- Immunopotentiation
    Adoptive immunotherapy: isolation, expansion, and reinfusion of tumor-infiltrating lymphocytes
    Nonspecific immunostimulation
    Tumor vaccines
No single marker yet has a clear meaning with respect to prognosis in a given patient.

4. **What are the major histologic types of lung cancer?**
   The most important distinction is between small cell and non–small cell carcinoma because of fundamental differences in tumor biology and clinical behavior (Table 79-1). Patients with small cell lung cancer are classified as having either limited or extensive disease. **Limited** means that all known disease is confined to one hemithorax and regional lymph nodes, including mediastinal, contralateral hilar, and ipsilateral supraclavicular nodes. **Extensive** describes disease beyond these limits, including brain, bone marrow, and intra-abdominal metastases.

   With small cell or neuroendocrine carcinoma, the small cell type is usually extensive at presentation, and 5-year survival is 5%. Neuroendocrine carcinoma, which is well differentiated, is known as *atypical carcinoid* and has a good prognosis but is not "benign."

TABLE 79-1. MAJOR HISTOLOGIC TYPES OF LUNG CANCER		
Type	Incidence	Comments
Non–small cell carcinomas	**80%**	
Adenocarcinoma	40%	Has increased in nonsmokers
Squamous cell carcinoma	40%	Referred to as epidermoid, is associated histologically with keratin pearls, and is promoted by smoking and other inhaled irritants
Large-cell carcinoma	15%	
Brochoalveolar carcinoma	5%	Single nodule, multiple nodules, or nonresolving infiltrate on chest x-ray
Small cell carcinoma	**20%**	Very poor prognosis

5. **Is lung cancer screening effective?**
   Old dogma: No.
   Current thinking: Yes. The thinking is as follows: lung cancer accounts for more cancer deaths than other cancers. Eighty-five percent of patients present with advanced uncurable lung cancer. We have not changed survival for lung cancer. Early-stage cancers that are asymptomatic can be found by chest radiograph and helical computed tomography (CT). Unfortunately, public health policy does not endorse screening for lung cancer.

6. **How do patients with lung cancer present?**
   Cough   70%
   Weight loss   10%

Bone pain	30%
Paraneoplastic syndrome	10%
Asymptomatic	10%

7. **What is a paraneoplastic syndrome?**
   Paraneoplastic syndromes of lung cancer may be **metabolic** (e.g., hypercalcemia, Cushing's syndrome), **neurologic** (e.g., peripheral neuropathy; polymyositis; or Lambert-Eaton syndrome, which is similar to myasthenia gravis), **skeletal** (e.g., clubbing, hypertrophic osteoarthropathy), **hematologic** (e.g., anemia, thrombocytosis, disseminated intravascular coagulation), or **cutaneous** (e.g., hyperkeratosis, acanthosis nigricans, dermatomyositis). Of interest, the presence of a paraneoplastic syndrome does not influence the ultimate curability of the lung cancer.

8. **Does the staging system for lung cancer have prognostic and therapeutic importance?**
   Yes. The patient's survival is related to the stage at presentation (Table 79-2).

TABLE 79-2. STAGING OF LUNG CANCER		
Stage	Subset	Description
I	Ia	Intraparenchymal tumor with or without extension to the visceral pleura, 2 cm from the carina, and no lymph node metastatic spread
	Ib	Tumor > 3 cm or through parietal pleura, no positive nodes
II	IIa	Primary tumor is similar to that of stage I with extension to interbronchial lymph nodes (N_1)
	IIb	Tumor invades chest wall without nodal involvement (T_3N_0)
III	IIIa	Extension of tumor into hilar or mediastinal lymph nodes (N_2) or chest wall with N_1 nodes
	IIIb	All elements of IIIa plus extension of tumor to mediastinal structures (heart or great vessels) or contralateral hilar, paratracheal, or supraclavicular lymph nodes (N_3)
IV		Malignant pleural effusion or metastatic disease (M_1)

9. **Describe the work-up of a patient with a mass on chest radiograph.**
   The work-up should be directed toward diagnosis, staging, and risk assessment.
   1. **Diagnosis**
      - Sputum cytology—low diagnostic yield
      - Brochoscopy—low diagnostic yield if tumor not visible
      - CT-guided fine-needle aspiration
      - Thoracoscopy and biopsy; wedge excision
   2. **Staging**
      - CT scan (chest)—tumor, mediastinal lymph node assessment
      - Positron emission tomography (PET)—90% sensitive and 80% specific for nodes, mets
      - Bronchoscopy—endobronchial invasion
      - Thoracoscopy—lymph node sampling
      - Mediastinoscopy—sample N2 and N3 nodes

3. **Risk assessment**
   - Pulmonary
     Spirometry—V/Q screening; if borderline, must leave patient with ≥ of 800 mL FEV_1 after resection
     Arterial blood gas analysis
   - Cardiac
     Electrocardiogram
     History of myocardial infarction, prior intervention
   - Cardiopulmonary
     Able to walk a flight of stairs; if yes, will tolerate lobectomy
     Maximal oxygen (O_2) consumption < 15 mL/kg/min

10. **How are patients with lung cancer treated?**
    The most effective treatment for lung cancer is surgical resection. Unfortunately, 75% of patients present with advanced disease and are not candidates for resection. Fortunately, preoperative chemotherapy with a cisplatinum-containing regimen has increased the number of stage III patients who are candidates for resection. This recent innovative therapy may translate into improved survival rates. For stage III lung cancer, several clinical trials have shown an advantage to preoperative chemotherapy and radiation treatment called neoadjuvant therapy. Even lower-stage disease or tumors at high risk of recurrence may benefit from newer chemotherapeutic regimens.

KEY POINTS: LUNG CANCER

1. The overall survival rate for patients with lung cancer is 10%.

2. Ninety percent of patients have a smoking history.

3. The most effective treatment for lung cancer is surgical resection.

11. **Does radiation therapy have a place in the therapy of lung cancer?**
    Radiation therapy is effective palliative but not curative therapy for lung cancer. Specifically, patients who present with a superior vena cava syndrome or a blocked bronchus with distal pneumonia frequently can be "opened up" with radiation therapy. Radiation is also excellent for the palliation of pathologic bone pain. Some—but not all—clinical trials have shown some benefit from preoperative chemoradiation treatment in advanced-stage lung cancer.

12. **What is the survival rate of patients treated for non–small cell lung cancer at 5 years?**

Stage I:	Ia	70%
	Ib	50%
Stage II:	IIa	40%
	IIb	30%
Stage III:	IIIa	20%
	IIIb	10%
Stage IV:		2%

Note that for chest wall invasion with no lymph nodes, survival is 50% at 5 years, although this is still called stage IIb. Also, if stage Ia (small tumor, no positive nodes) cancer is not resected, survival decreases from 70% to 7%.

13. **What is mediastinoscopy?**

Mediastinoscopy is a staging procedure in which the paratracheal, subcarinal, and proximal peribronchial lymph nodes are sampled from a small incision made in the suprasternal notch.

14. **What are the indications for mediastinoscopy?**

Mediastinal staging is indicated in patients with either apparent or documented lung cancer who have:

- Known lung cancer with mediastinal lymph nodes > 1 cm accessible by cervical mediastinal exploration, as assessed by CT scan
- Adenocarcinoma of the lung and multiple mediastinal lymph nodes < 1 cm
- Central or large (> 5 cm) lung cancers with mediastinal lymph nodes < 1 cm
- Lung cancer and are at high risk of thoracotomy and lung resection

If the mediastinoscopy has negative results, the surgeon should proceed with thoracotomy, biopsy, and curative lung resection.

15. **Is malignant pleural effusion or recurrent nerve involvement with tumor an absolute contraindication to surgical resection for lung cancer?**

A malignant pleural effusion is an absolute contraindication to surgical resective therapy. Conversely, both King George V and Arthur Godfrey had successful surgical resections in the face of recurrent nerve involvement with tumor.

WEB SITE

http://www.acssurgery.com

BIBLIOGRAPHY

1. Ginsberg RJ, Ruckdeschel JC (eds): Lung Cancer: Past, Present, and Future. Part I. Chest Surgery Clinics of North America, vol. 10. Philadelphia, W.B. Saunders, 2000.

2. Mountain EF: Revision in the international system for staging lung cancer. Chest 111:1710, 1997.

3. Pass HI: Adjunctive and alternate treatment of bronchogenic lung cancer. Chest Surg Clin North Am 1:1–20, 1991.

4. Saunders CA, Dussek JE, O'Doherty MJ, Maisey MN: Evaluation of fluorine 18-fluorodeoxyglucose: Whole body positron emission tomography imaging in staging lung cancer. Ann Thorac Surg 67:790–797, 1999.

5. Sonett JR, Krasna MJ, Suntharalingam M, et al: Safe pulmonary resection after chemotherapy and high-dose thoracic radiation. Ann Thorac Surg 68:316–320, 1999.

6. Strauss GM: Prognostic markers in resectable non-small-cell lung cancer. Hematol Oncol Clin North Am 11:409–434, 1997.

CHAPTER 80

SOLITARY PULMONARY NODULE

Jamie M. Brown, M.D., and Marvin Pomerantz, M.D.

1. **What is a solitary pulmonary nodule?**
   A solitary pulmonary nodule or "coin lesion" is < 3 cm and is discrete on chest radiograph. It is usually surrounded by lung parenchyma.

2. **What causes a solitary pulmonary nodule?**
   The most common causes of a pulmonary nodule are either neoplastic (carcinoma) or infectious (granuloma). Pulmonary nodules may also represent lung abscess, pulmonary infarction, arteriovenous malformations, resolving pneumonia, pulmonary sequestration, hamartoma, and others. As a general rule of thumb, likelihood of malignancy is proportionate to the patient's age. Thus, whereas lung cancer is rare (although it does occur) in 30-year-old individuals, in 50-year-old smokers, the chances of malignancy may be as high as 50–60%.

3. **How does a solitary pulmonary nodule present?**
   Typically, a solitary nodule is picked up incidentally on routine chest radiograph. In several large series, more than 75% of lesions were surprise findings on routine chest radiograph. Fewer than 25% of patients had symptoms referable to the lung. Solitary nodules are now seen on other sensitive imaging tests such as helical computed tomography (CT).

4. **How frequently does a solitary pulmonary nodule represent metastatic disease?**
   Fewer than 10% of solitary nodules represent metastatic disease. Accordingly, an extensive workup for a primary site of cancer other than the lung is not indicated.

5. **Can a tissue sample be obtained by fluoroscopic or CT-guided needle biopsy?**
   Yes, but the results do not change the treatment. If the needle biopsy tissue indicates cancer, the nodule must be removed. If the needle biopsy is negative for cancer, the nodule must still be removed. Positron emission tomography (PET) is 90% sensitive in identifying malignant tumors.

6. **Are radiographic findings important?**
   Only relatively. The resolution of modern CT scanners allows the best identification of characteristics that suggest cancer:
   1. Indistinct or irregular spiculated borders of the nodule.
   2. The larger the nodule, the more likely it is to be malignant.
   3. Calcification in the nodule generally is associated with benign disease (the opposite of breast cancer). Specifically, whereas central, diffuse, or laminated calcifications are typical of a granuloma, calcifications with more dense and irregular "popcorn" patterns are associated with hamartomas. Unfortunately, eccentric foci of calcium or small flecks of calcium may be found in malignant lesions.
   4. Nodules can be studied using a CT scanner by measuring their change in relative radiodensity after injection of contrast. This information improves the accuracy of predicting the presence of malignancy.

KEY POINTS: SOLITARY PULMONARY NODULE

1. A solitary pulmonary nodule or "coin lesion" is < 3 cm and is discrete on chest radiograph.

2. The most common causes of a pulmonary nodule are either neoplastic or infectious.

3. If the lesion proves to be cancer, anatomic lobectomy is the procedure of choice.

7. **What social or clinical findings suggest that a nodule is malignant rather than benign?**
Unfortunately, none of the findings is sufficiently sensitive or specific to influence the work-up. Both increasing age and a long smoking history predispose patients to lung cancer. Winston Churchill should have had lung cancer, but he did not. Thus, the fact that the patient is the president of the spelunking club (histoplasmosis), has a sister who raises pigeons (cryptococcosis), grew up in the Ohio River Valley (histoplasmosis), works as sexton for a dog cemetery (blastomycosis), or just took a hiking trip through the San Joaquin Valley (coccidioidomycosis) is interesting associated history but does not affect the work-up of a solitary pulmonary nodule.

8. **What is the most valuable bit of historic data?**
The most valuable is an old chest radiograph. If the nodule is new, it is more likely to be malignant, whereas if the nodule has not changed in the past 2 years, it is less likely to be malignant. Unfortunately, even this observation is not absolute.

9. **If a patient presents with a treated prior malignancy and a new solitary pulmonary nodule, is it safe to assume that the new nodule represents metastatic disease?**
No. Even in patients with known prior malignancies, < 50% of new pulmonary nodules are metastatic. Thus, the work-up should proceed exactly as for any other patient with a new solitary pulmonary nodule.

10. **How should a solitary pulmonary nodule be evaluated?**
A complete travel and occupational history is interesting but does not affect the evaluation. Because of the peripheral location of most nodules, bronchoscopy has a diagnostic yield of < 50%. Even in the best hands, sputum cytology has a low yield. CT scanning is recommended because it can identify other potentially metastatic nodules and delineate the status of mediastinal lymph nodes. As indicated previously, percutaneous needle biopsy has a diagnostic yield of approximately 80% but rarely alters the subsequent management. PET scanning may suggest cancer with accuracy.
The mainstay of management in patients who can tolerate surgery is resection of the nodule, usually by lobectomy if cancer is suspected, for diagnosis by either a minimally invasive thoracoscopy approach or a limited thoracotomy.

11. **If the lesion proves to be cancer, what is the appropriate surgical therapy?**
Although several series have suggested that wedge excision of the nodule is sufficient, an anatomic lobectomy remains the procedure of choice. This can often be accomplished by a video-assisted approach. A solitary nodule that turns out to be cancer should be early-stage disease and has a 65% 5-year survival rate if there are no notable metastases. Unfortunately, the recurrence rate even for stage I tumors or a small nodule is 30% over 5 years. Recurrences are split between local and distant.

BIBLIOGRAPHY

1. Dewey TM, Mack MJ: Lung cancer: Surgical approaches and incisions. Chest Surg Clin North Am 10:803–820, 2000.

2. Ginsberg RJ, Rubinstein LV: Randomized trial of lobectomy versus limited resection for T1 N0 non–small cell lung cancer. Lung Cancer Study Group. Ann Thorac Surg 60:615–622, 1995.

3. Khouri NF, Meziane MA, Zerhouni EA, et al: The solitary pulmonary nodule: Assessment, diagnosis and management. Chest 91:128–133, 1987.

4. Miller DL, Rowland CM, Deschamps C, et al: Surgical treatment of non–small cell lung cancer 1 cm or less in diameter. Ann Thorac Surg 73:1541–1545, 2002.

5. Nesbitt J, Putnam JB Jr, Walsh GL, et al: Survival in early stage non–small cell lung cancer. Ann Thorac Surg 60:466–472, 1995.

6. Walsh GL, Pisters KM, Stevens C: Treatment of stage I lung cancer. Chest Surg Clin North Am 10:17–38, 2001.

CHAPTER 81

DISSECTING AORTIC ANEURYSM

Laurence H. Brinckerhoff, M.D., and David N. Campbell, M.D.

1. **Why is the term *dissecting aortic aneurysm* really incorrect?**
   The correct term should be **dissecting aortic hematoma** because the lesion is not an aneurysm. Blood dissects between the middle and outer layers of the media and adventitia of the aorta (specifically, there does not need to be an intimal tear, although there usually is).

2. **When should the diagnosis be entertained?**
   Suspicion is the most important factor because no one feature is common to patients presenting with aortic dissections. In any patient who presents with severe knifelike, ripping chest and back pain, the diagnosis of aortic dissection should be considered.

3. **After the diagnosis is entertained, how should the patient be managed?**
   Two thirds of patients are hypertensive, so blood pressure must be controlled. The other diagnosis to be strongly considered is acute myocardial infarction (MI). An electrocardiogram often rules out MI, but some aortic dissections tear off a coronary artery; thus, both acute infarction and aortic dissection occur concurrently (this patient group is in big trouble).

4. **What is the most significant diagnostic clue on physical examination?**
   A new aortic valvular diastolic murmur, indicating aortic valvular regurgitation caused by distortion of the valve structure by the mural hemotoma. In addition, the dissecting hematoma can encircle the lumen or actually cleave the takeoff of the subclavian or femoral vessels, resulting in the loss of pulses. Neurologic findings, including paraplegia and hemiplegia, may also be present because of similar flap occlusion of the great vessels.

5. **Which chest radiograph findings are helpful in diagnosis?**
   Widened mediastinum and loss of aortic knob silhouette—a hematoma surrounding the aorta makes the aortic outline blurry—are helpful findings.

6. **How is the diagnosis confirmed? What are the best diagnostic studies?**
   The literature reports the high accuracy of transesophageal echocardiography (TEE) and computed tomography angiography (CTA) in the diagnosis of aortic dissections. Some institutions rely solely on one of these diagnostic tool (both studies are operator dependent). However, the aortogram is still the gold standard, but it requires more time. If time allows and the patient is stable, an aortogram should be obtained to confirm the diagnosis, type of dissection (ascending versus descending), status of the aortic valve, and status of the coronary arteries. In fact, the modalities may be complementary: whereas the TEE or CTA confirms the diagnosis, the aortogram defines location and evaluates the status of the aortic valve and coronary arteries.

7. **What are the types of dissection?**
   The following classification has both therapeutic and prognostic value:
   Ascending (type A) involves only the ascending or both the ascending and descending aorta.
   Descending (type B) involves only the descending aorta.

8. **Who cares whether a dissection involves the ascending (type A) or descending (type B) aorta?**

Ascending dissections require early surgical correction to avoid extension into the coronary or carotid arteries, rupture into the pericardium (tamponade), or both.

Descending dissections do not involve the ascending aorta and may be managed medically or surgically (see Controversies).

9. **What is the key to medical management?**

The blood pressure (BP) should be lowered to 100–110 mmHg (systolic) with a combination of sodium nitroprusside and propranolol. Propranolol is particularly important because it decreases the contractility of the myocardium (dp/dt), thereby decreasing the shearing force that prevents propagation of the dissection down the aorta. Conceptually, the BP should be lowered as much as possible, but the patient must continue to perfuse the end organs (i.e., make urine).

10. **What are the principles and advantages of surgical management?**

Ascending dissection
1. To close off the hematoma by obliterating the most proximal intimal tear
2. To restore competency of the aortic valve
3. To restore flow to any branches of the aorta that have been sheared off and receive blood flow from a false lumen
4. To protect the heart during these maneuvers and to restore coronary blood flow if a coronary artery has been sheared off
5. To look for tears in the transverse aortic arch

Technique: Use of deep hypothermia circulatory arrest with or without retrograde cerebral perfusion is in vogue at present. This technique allows the arch to be inspected and the distal anastomosis of the Dacron graft to be sewn accurately to the distal ascending aorta in an open fashion. Whether to replace or repair the aortic valve is controversial.

Descending dissection
1. To close off the hematoma by obliterating the most proximal intimal tear
2. To restore blood flow to branches of the aorta fed by the false channel

Technique: Surgery is performed using partial cardiopulmonary bypass, or the "clamp and run" technique, in which the aorta is cross-clamped and the graft is sewn in as fast as possible (see Controversies).

KEY POINTS: DISSECTING AORTIC ANEURYSM

1. The correct term should be *dissecting aortic hematoma* because the lesion is not an aneurysm.

2. A new aortic valvular diastolic murmur, indicating aortic valvular regurgitation caused by distortion of the valve structure by the mural hematoma.

3. Ascending dissections require early surgical correction to avoid extension into the coronary or carotid arteries, rupture into the pericardium, or both.

4. Descending dissections may be managed medically; blood pressure should be lowered to 100–110 mmHg with a combination of sodium nitroprusside and propranolol.

11. **What are the operative complications?**
- Hemorrhage (20%): very common because of the use of heparin and the poor quality of aortic tissue (like wet Kleenex)
- Renal failure (20%)
- Pulmonary insufficiency (30% higher in repair of descending dissections)

- Paraplegia: often presents before operation; as a surgical complication, it usually occurs only with descending dissections (11%)
- Acute MI or low cardiac output (30%)
- Bowel infarction (5%)
- Death (15%): higher for acute than chronic dissections and higher for repair of ascending dissections

12. **What are the long-term results?**
Of patients who survive the operation, two thirds die within 7 years because of comorbid cardiac and cerebrovascular disease.

CONTROVERSIES

13. **Which is preferred: surgical or medical management of descending dissections?**
Initial surgical management
- Approximately 25% of patients initially treated medically need an operation eventually.
- Operative mortality is much lower today (20%) than in the past.
- Medical management has the same in-hospital mortality (20%).
Initial medical management
- This avoids unnecessary operation and its attendant cost and complication rate.

14. **What is the preferred management of aortic insufficiency in ascending dissections?**
Replacement of aortic valve
- Easy (valved conduits now available)
- Eliminates aortic insufficiency completely
- Should be done in patients with Marfan syndrome
Repair of aortic valve
- With native valve reconstruction, when done correctly, the need to replace the valve at a later time Is only 10%.
- Avoids need for anticoagulation, which is necessary when a mechanical valve is used to replace the aortic valve.

15. **What is the preferred repair of descending dissections?**
1. **Partial left atrial-to-femoral artery bypass**
For:
- Allows unloading of the heart
- Allows distal perfusion to avoid visceral ischemia
- Allows as much time as needed to complete anastomosis
Against: requires heparinization
2. **Simple aortic cross-clamping**
For: Fast
Against: Placement of the graft has to be done in < 30 minutes or the complication rate, particularly paraplegia, increases significantly.

16. **Are there any other alternatives for the treatment of patients with acute aortic dissection?**
Although in the early stages of development, the use of endovascular stents may prove to be a useful treatment option. The use of these stents is still considered experimental, and the long-term results are not known.

WEB SITE

http://www.acssurgery.com

BIBLIOGRAPHY

1. Barron DJ, Livesey SA, Brown IW, et al: Twenty-year follow-up of acute type A dissection: The incidence and extent of distal aortic disease using magnetic resonance imaging. J Card Surg 12:147–159, 1997.

2. Cigarroa JE, Isselbacher EM, DeSanctis RW, Eagle KA: Diagnostic imaging in the evaluation of suspected aortic dissection. Old standards and new directions. N Engl J Med 328:35–43, 1993.

3. Glower DD, Fann JI, Speier RH, et al: Comparison of medical and surgical therapy for uncomplicated descending aortic dissection. Circulation 82(suppl IV):39–46, 1990.

4. Khan IA, Nair CK: Clinical, diagnostic, and management perspectives of aortic dissection. Chest 112:311–328, 2002.

5. Nienaber CA, von Kodolitsch Y, Nicolas V, et al: The diagnosis of thoracic aortic dissection by noninvasive imaging procedures. N Engl J Med 328:1–9, 1993.

6. Okita Y, Takamoto S, Ando M, et al: Mortality and cerebral outcome in patients who underwent aortic arch operations using deep hypothermic circulatory arrest with retrograde cerebral perfusion: No relation of early death, stroke, and delirium to the duration of circulatory arrest. J Thorac Cardiovasc Surg 115:129–138, 1998.

7. Safi HJ, Miller CC, Reardon MJ, et al: Operation for acute and chronic aortic dissection: Recent outcome with regard to neurologic deficit and early death. Ann Thorac Surg 66:402–411, 1998.

8. Wheat MW Jr, Palmer RF, Bartley TB, Seelman RC: Treatment of dissecting aneurysms of the aorta without surgery. J Thorac Cardiovasc Surg 50:364–373, 1995.

HYPERTROPHIC PYLORIC STENOSIS

CHAPTER 82

Denis D. Bensard, M.D.

1. **What is pyloric stenosis?**

   Hypertrophic pyloric stenosis (HPS) is idiopathic thickening and elongation of the pylorus that produces gastric outlet obstruction. HPS is the most common surgical cause of *nonbilious* vomiting in infants. Offspring of an affected parent have an increased incidence of HPS (10%); the highest rate (20%) occurs in boys born to affected mothers.

2. **Describe the typical presentation of HPS.**

   The typical presentation is a healthy infant who initially fed normally but who presents at age 2–6 weeks with a history of "projectile" vomiting. The emesis is nonbilious. After vomiting, the infant appears hungry and will refeed immediately. With time, the infant becomes dehydrated and, if allowed to progress, malnutrition follows.

3. **What are the physical findings?**

   Affected infants suffer some degree of dehydration. The abdomen is nondistended and soft. A palpable pyloric tumor, known as the "olive," confirms the diagnosis. An olive is palpable in 50% of patients. Associated findings are rare, but mild jaundice occurs in 5% of infants because of reduced glucuronyl transferase activity.

4. **How is the diagnosis confirmed?**

   Ultrasonographic criteria include pyloric diameter > 1.4 cm, wall width > 4 mm, and pyloric channel length > 1.6 cm. Alternatively, a barium upper gastrointestinal (UGI) examination may be used to confirm the diagnosis (gastric outlet obstruction, pyloric channel narrowing). Current analyses suggest that UGI is the most cost-effective initial radiologic diagnostic test because, unlike ultrasound, alternative causes of nonbilious vomiting (e.g., gastroesophageal reflux, malrotation, duodenal stenosis) can be identified.

5. **Describe the likely electrolyte abnormalities.**

   Electrolyte levels are often normal, but long-standing vomiting will eventually result in hypokalemic, hypochloremic metabolic alkalosis because of the loss of gastric acid (HCl). Earlier consideration of the diagnosis has led to a significant reduction in this classic electrolyte abnormality at presentation. Dehydration is corrected with either 0.9% NaCl or, in less severe cases, 0.5% NaCl with 30 mEq/L KCl. After dehydration and electrolytes are corrected, pyloromyotomy is performed.

6. **What procedure is recommended for the correction of HPS?**

   The Fredet-Ramstedt pyloromyotomy is recommended. A superficial incision is made longitudinally over the pyloric muscle in an avascular area, and the muscle fibers are fractured to expose the underlying mucosa. At the conclusion of the pyloromyotomy, the gastric mucosa should bulge upward into the cleft, and the pyloric muscle walls should move independently of one another. Air is injected into the stomach via the nasogastric tube to identify inadvertent mucosal perforation. Pyloromyotomy may be performed either via a transverse incision in the right upper quadrant (i.e., an open procedure) or via three small (3-mm) incisions in the epigastrium (i.e., a laparoscopic procedure). The results of open and laparoscopic pyloromyotomy appear equivalent.

7. **What should be done if a perforation is identified?**
The mucosa should be closed with several fine sutures and covered with an omental patch. If the mucosal injury is too extensive, the myotomy should be closed with sutures and a second, parallel myotomy should be made at 45–180° from the original myotomy.

8. **When can postoperative feeding begin?**
Small-volume feedings are started after the infant has recovered from anesthesia (2–3 hours) and advanced to goal. Small amounts of vomiting are common (20%), but most infants achieve full feeds within 24 hours postoperatively. Incomplete pyloromyotomy is uncommon (< 1%) and is not considered unless symptoms of gastric outlet obstruction persist for 7–10 days after surgery.

9. **Describe several hypotheses about the pathogenesis of HPS.**
Recent studies of the abnormal pyloric complex demonstrate improper innervation of pyloric smooth muscle, excessive contraction of circular pyloric smooth muscle (decreased nitric oxide synthase), increased extracellular matrix proteins (collagen), and increased expression or local synthesis of growth hormones (i.e., insulin-like growth factor-1, transforming growth factor beta-1, platelet derived growth factor).

BIBLIOGRAPHY

1. Campbell BT, McLean K, Barnhart DC, et al: A comparison of laparoscopic and open pyloromyotomy at a teaching hospital. J Pediatr Surg 37:1068–1071, 2002.
2. Chen EA, Luks FI, Gilchrist BF, et al: Pyloric stenosis in the age of ultrasonography: Fading skills, better patients? J Pediatr Surg 31:829–830, 1996.
3. Garza JJ, Morash D, Dzakovic A, et al: Ad libitum feeding decreases hospital stay for neonates after pyloromyotomy. J Pediatr Surg 37:493–495, 2002.
4. Hulka F, Campbell JR, Harrison MW, et al: Cost-effectiveness in diagnosing infantile hypertrophic pyloric stenosis. J Pediatr Surg 32:1604–1608, 1997.
5. Miozzari HH, Tonz M, von Vigier RO, et al: Fluid resuscitation in infantile hypertrophic pyloric stenosis. Acta Paediatr 90:511–514, 2001.
6. Ohshiro K, Puri P: Pathogenesis of infantile hypertrophic pyloric stenosis: Recent progress. Pediatr Surg Int 13:243–252,1998.

CHAPTER 83

INTESTINAL OBSTRUCTION OF NEONATES AND INFANTS

Richard J. Hendrickson, M.D., and Denis D. Bensard, M.D.

1. **What signs or symptoms suggest intestinal obstruction in the neonate?**
   Signs and symptoms vary according to the level of obstruction. Proximal intestinal obstruction leads to the early onset of bilious emesis, generally with minimal abdominal distention. In contrast, neonates with distal intestinal obstruction present after the first day of life with bilious vomiting and pronounced abdominal distention. Bilious emesis should always be interrogated further in infants and children.

2. **What is the differential diagnosis of intestinal obstruction in neonates?**
   Look for an anal opening, which eliminates the diagnosis of imperforate anus. Next obtain an abdominal radiograph. The extent of gaseous distention of the bowel implicates a proximal or distal bowel obstruction. No attempts should be made to distinguish small from large bowel obstruction.

Proximal (minimal bowel gas)	**Distal** (significant bowel gas)
Duodenal atresia, stenosis	Ileal atresia
Malrotation with midgut volvulus	Meconium ileus or plug
Jejunal atresia	Hirschsprung's disease

3. **When are contrast studies of the gastrointestinal (GI) tract indicated?**
   If peritonitis or pneumoperitoneum is present, proceed to exploratory laparotomy without delay. Malrotation with volvulus must be distinguished from the other cause of congenital duodenal obstruction (duodenal atresia). In this setting, upper GI is the study of choice. In volvulus, the upper GI demonstrates distention of the proximal duodenum, corkscrewing of the distal duodenum, and limited or no progression of contrast into the distal bowel. Conversely, duodenal atresia appears as a blind ending pouch in the first or second portion of the duodenum. Contrast enema is generally the preferred study in all other forms of neonatal intestinal obstruction.

Disorder	**Barium Enema**
Ileal atresia	Microcolon; no reflux into terminal ileum
Meconium ileus	Microcolon; reflux into terminal ileum with filling defects
Meconium plug	Normal colon; large filling defect of left colon
Hirschsprung's disease	Narrowed rectosigmoid; dilated proximal colon

4. **Describe intestinal atresia.**
   Atresia can occur anywhere in the GI tract: duodenal (50%), jejunoileal (45%), or colonic (5%). Duodenal atresia arises from a failure of recanalization during the 8th–10th week of gestation; jejunoileal and colonic atresia are caused by an in utero mesenteric vascular accident.

5. **Distinguish duodenal atresia from other forms of intestinal atresia.**
   Duodenal atresia is characterized by the onset of bilious vomiting (85% of atresia distal to the ampulla of Vater) within the first day of life; significant abdominal distention is absent. Approximately 25% of affected infants have trisomy 21. The abdominal radiograph demonstrates a "double bubble" caused by the distended stomach and first or second portions of duodenum. Surgical correction is performed by duodenoduodenostomy.

Jejunoileal atresia produces bilious vomiting at 2–3 days of life with moderate to severe abdominal distention. The abdominal radiograph shows dilated loops of bowel with air–fluid levels. Barium enema reveals a microcolon and no reflux of contrast into the dilated bowel. Associated anomalies are uncommon. Surgical correction involves end-to-end anastomosis with or without limited intestinal resection.

Colonic atresia, similar to jejunalileal atresia, is associated with the late onset of bilious vomiting, no passage of meconium, and moderate to severe abdominal distention. The abdominal radiograph reveals dilated loops of bowel with air–fluid levels suggesting distal intestinal obstruction. Barium enema demonstrates a microcolon with a cutoff observed in a proximal colonic segment. Twenty percent of affected infants suffer an associated anomaly of the heart, musculoskeletal system, abdominal wall, or GI tract. Surgical management includes limited colonic resection with primary anastomosis.

6. **Describe malrotation with midgut volvulus.**

    During the 6th–12th week of gestation, the intestine undergoes evisceration, growth, return to the abdominal cavity, and counterclockwise rotation with fixation. Malrotation is an error in both rotation and fixation. Abnormal fixation and a narrow-based mesentery predispose to twisting of the midgut on its blood supply (superior mesenteric artery), vascular occlusion (strangulation), and obstruction (malrotation with midgut volvulus). Typically, a previously well neonate or child without a history of surgery presents with bilious vomiting, abdominal distention, and variable degrees of shock. If the infant is acutely ill, no further studies are needed and surgical exploration is indicated. If the diagnosis is in question and the infant is stable, an upper GI study, not a barium enema, is performed. Surgical treatment entails four parts: (1) division of abnormal peritoneal bands, (2) correction of malrotation, (3) restoration of a broad-based mesentery, and (4) appendectomy because of the location of the cecum in the right upper quadrant.

7. **Is midgut volvulus a surgical emergency?**

    Yes! The risk of strangulation caused by the rotational anomaly and abnormal peritoneal bands implies a surgical emergency. Delay places the infant at risk of losing the entire midgut and potentially dying.

8. **What is meconium ileus (MI)?**

    MI is the obstruction of the terminal ileum by highly viscid, tenacious meconium. MI is a complication of cystic fibrosis (CF). Fifteen percent of neonates with CF present with MI. The combination of hyperviscous mucus secreted by the abnormal intestinal glands and pancreatic insufficiency leads to abnormal meconium and obstructs the lumen of the terminal ileum. Symptoms of feeding intolerance, bilious emesis, and abdominal distention begin in the second to third days of life. Unlike most forms of neonatal intestinal obstruction, surgery is reserved for patients refractory to nonoperative treatment or complex MI (atresia, volvulus, perforation). Sixty percent of infants with simple MI can be treated successfully with Gastrografin enemas and rectal irrigation. If an operation is indicated, the objective is to remove the obstructing meconium by limited resection or enterostomy with evacuation of the meconium and irrigation of the distal bowel.

9. **What is Hirschsprung's disease?**

    In this disease, the intestine is innervated by cells originating in the neural crest. During the 5th–12th week of gestation, neural crest cells migrate in a craniocaudal direction and disperse within the wall of the intestine (intermuscular, to Auerbach's plexus; submucosal, to Meissner's plexus). Hirschsprung's disease arises from the failure of normal enteric innervation. The bowel remains in a contracted, spastic state and produces a functional rather than a true mechanical obstruction. Abdominal distention, feeding intolerance, and delayed or absent meconium within the first 48 hours of life are the presenting findings in infants. Older patients suffer chronic constipation, abdominal distention, and failure to thrive. Because the disease always affects the most distal bowel (80–85% rectosigmoid) with a variable involvement of proximal bowel, barium enema demonstrates the characteristic radiographic appearance of a spastic, contracted rectum with dilated proximal bowel. Suction rectal biopsy documenting the absence of ganglion cells and presence of nerve hypertrophy confirms the diagnosis. Surgical correction is performed by excision of the aganglionic (distal colorectal) segment and coloanal anastomosis.

10. **What is intussusception? What are the therapeutic options?**

Intussusception is the invagination of proximal bowel (intussusceptum) into the distal bowel (intussuscipien). Swelling, vascular compromise, and obstruction follow. Nearly two thirds of cases occur in the first 2 years of life. The cause is thought to be a result of lymphoid hyperplasia in the terminal ileum after viral infection. The diagnosis should be suspected in previously well infants, 6–9 months of age, with vomiting, crampy abdominal pain, and bloody stools. Barium or air enema is both diagnostic and therapeutic. Injection of contrast demonstrates colonic obstruction with no reflux into the proximal bowel. Controlled hydrostatic reduction with barium or air is successful in 90% of cases. If hydrostatic reduction is unsuccessful or in children with peritonitis, operative reduction is indicated. The risk of recurrent intussusception is 5% for either radiographic or surgical reduction.

11. **What examples of neonatal obstruction can escape early detection and present later in life?**

Although most conditions are identified within the first week to month of life, lesions other than atresia may be identified in children and even adults.

Duodenal stenosis. Unlike duodenal atresia, stenosis results in narrowing but not complete obstruction of the duodenum. Thus, infants fed formula or pureed foods may not become symptomatic until childhood. Children with intermittent abdominal pain and symptoms of gastric outlet obstruction require an upper GI study, particularly if they have trisomy 21.

Malrotation. One third of patients with malrotation are identified after the first month of life. Children present with bilious emesis and intermittent abdominal pain, and malrotation is generally identified by an upper GI series. Malrotation with midgut volvulus should be suspected in any ill child with signs of intestinal obstruction and no history of abdominal surgery.

Hirschsprung's disease. One third of patients are diagnosed after the first year of life. A long history of constipation refractory to therapy mandates rectal biopsy, particularly in patients with trisomy 21.

Intussusception. One third of cases occur after age 2 years. A pathologic lead point (i.e., polyp, tumor, hematoma, Meckel's diverticulum) is present in one third of older patients.

BIBLIOGRAPHY

1. Aquino A, Domini M, Rossi C, et al: Correlation between Down's syndrome and malformation of pediatric surgical interest. J Pediatr Surg 33:1380–1382, 1998.

2. Daneman A, Alton DJ, Ein S, et al: Perforation during attempted intussusception reduction in children—a comparison of perforation with barium and air. Pediatr Radiol 25:81–88, 1995.

3. Godbole P, Stringer MD: Bilious vomiting in the newborn: How often is it pathologic? J Pediatr Surg 37:909–911, 2002.

4. Long FR, Kramer SS, Markowitz RI, Taylor GE: Radiographic patterns of intestinal malrotation in children. Radiographics 16:547–560, 1996.

5. Maxson RT, Franklin PA, Wagner CW: Malrotation in the older child: Surgical management, treatment, and outcome. Am Surg 61:135–138, 1995.

6. Reding R, de Ville de Goyet J, Gosseye S, et al: Hirschsprung's disease: A 20 year experience. J Pediatr Surg 32:1221–1225, 1997.

CHAPTER 84

IMPERFORATE ANUS

Frederick M. Karrer, M.D., and Denis D. Bensard, M.D.

1. **What is imperforate anus?**

   It is a congenital defect in which the opening of the anus is absent or misplaced, usually fistulizing anteriorly to the perineum or genitourinary (GU) tract. Anorectal malformations range from slight anterior malpositioning of the anus to complex cloacal deformities. Children with anorectal malformations commonly have other congenital anomalies, such as the VACTERL association.

2. **What is the VACTERL association?**

   V = **V**ertebral defects
   A = **A**norectal malformations
   C = **C**ardiac anomalies
   T = **T**racheoesophageal fistula
   E = **E**sophageal atresia
   R = **R**enal anomalies
   L = **L**imb defects

   The incidence of renal anomalies increases with the severity of the imperforate anus—from 10% with low lesions to 75% with high lesions.

3. **How do you determine the severity of the defect in boys?**

   The key is whether the boy has a high or low lesion. Low lesions are characterized by a fistula to the perineum somewhere along the midline raphe between the anus and the urethral meatus. After 24 hours, most infants with low lesions demonstrate meconium at the fistula. Other signs of a low lesion include white "pearls" along the raphe or a raised loop of skin, the so-called bucket-handle deformity. Boys with high lesions typically have flat buttocks without a good buttocks crease and may have meconium at the urethral meatus or apparent on urinalysis.

4. **How is the lesion assessed in girls?**

   Most affected girls (> 90%) have a rectovestibular or rectovaginal fistula, which usually can be determined by careful perineal examination. Girls with cloacal deformities (i.e., one orifice) have a high incidence of GU obstruction such as hydrocolpos or bladder obstruction. In low lesions, the anal opening is displaced anteriorly on the perineum. The normal location of the anus is halfway between the vaginal orifice and the coccyx.

5. **How are infants with anorectal malformations treated?**

   Infants with high lesions should be managed initially with a sigmoid colostomy and later with a pull-through procedure called posterior sagittal anorectoplasty. Infants with low lesions usually can be managed with immediate anoplasty or dilatation and delayed repair.

6. **What is a posterior sagittal anorectoplasty (PSARP)?**

   PSARP is a procedure performed through a longitudinal incision in the midline of the perineum, which permits visualization of the pelvic musculature and sphincters and clear exposure of the rectum and fistula. After closure of the fistula, the rectum is repositioned within the sphincteric muscle complex, and a neoanus is created.

7. **What are the results after surgical reconstruction?**

Continence, defined as voluntary bowel movements with no soiling, depends on the type of lesion. Continence approaches 100% for low lesions but is rare with the highest lesions such as cloaca deformities in girls or bladder-neck fistulas in boys. Constipation is present in almost 50% of patients but is more frequent with the simpler defects.

KEY POINTS: IMPERFORATE ANUS

1. Imperforate anus is a congenital defect in which the opening of the anus is absent or misplaced, usually fistulizing anteriorly to the perineum or genitourinary tract.

2. Infants with high lesions should be managed initially with a sigmoid colostomy and later with a pull-through procedure called posterior sagittal anorectoplasty.

3. Infants with low lesions usually can be managed with immediate anoplasty or dilatation and delayed repair.

BIBLIOGRAPHY

1. deVries PA, Pena A: Posterior sagittal anorectoplasty. J Pediatr Surg 17:638–643, 1982.

2. Jones NM, Humphreys MS, Goodman TR, et al: The value of anal endosonography compared with magnetic resonance imaging following the repair of anorectal malformations. Pediatr Radiol 33:183, 2003.

3. Kluth D, Lambrecht W: Current concepts in the embryology of anorectal malformations. Semin Pediatr Surg 6:180–186, 1997.

4. Pena A: Anorectal malformations. Semin Pediatr Surg 4:35–37, 1995.

5. Pena A, Hong A: Advances in the managemant of anorectal malformations. Am J Surg 180:370–376, 2000.

6. Sarin YK, Sinha A, Gupta A: High anorectal malformation in boys: Need for clarity of definition and management. J Pediatr Surg 37:1637, 2002.

CHAPTER 85

TRACHEOESOPHAGEAL MALFORMATIONS

Denis D. Bensard, M.D., and David A. Partrick, M.D.

1. **What are tracheoesophageal fistula (TEF) and esophageal atresia (EA)?**
   The trachea and esophagus appear as a ventral diverticulum arising from the primitive foregut during the third week of gestation. The trachea and esophagus undergo separation by the ingrowth of ectodermal ridges during the fourth week of gestation. Failure of separation results in anomalous connection of the trachea to the esophagus (i.e., TEF) with or without incomplete formation of the esophagus (i.e., EA).

2. **Describe the three most common variants and the relative incidence of each type.**
   - Proximal EA with distal TEF ("proximal pouch with distal fistula"): 85%
   - Isolated EA: 10%
   - TEF without EA ("H fistula"): 5%

3. **What other anomalies occur with tracheoesophageal malformations?**
   TEF and EA result from an insult during the critical phase of embryogenesis (3–8 weeks' gestation). Up to 70% of infants with tracheoesophageal malformations suffer one or more concomitant anomalies. Cardiovascular anomalies are the most prevalent (35%), followed by anomalies of the gastrointestinal (24%), genitourinary (20%), skeletal (13%), and central nervous (10%) systems. Twenty-five percent of infants born with tracheoesophageal malformation have one or more components of the VACTERL association (see question 2 in chapter 84).

4. **Does the presence of other anomalies alter management and outcome?**
   Healthy infants without concomitant anomalies generally undergo early repair with a nearly 100% survival rate, whereas infants who are severely premature or have life-threatening anomalies typically undergo delayed repair. Infants with lethal anomalies, such as trisomy 18, receive palliative care only.

5. **Describe the clinical presentation, diagnosis, and preoperative management of patients with EA with distal TEF.**
   Early in the newborn period, affected infants demonstrate excessive salivation (i.e., inability to swallow secretions), choking, or regurgitation with feeding (i.e., inability to swallow feeds). Respiratory distress quickly ensues because of aspiration of secretions or feeds from the esophageal pouch and reflux of gastric acid into the airways and lungs via the distal TEF. A nasogastric tube cannot be advanced into the stomach. The radiograph demonstrates a blind-ending proximal esophageal pouch and an air-filled stomach caused by the anomalous connection of the distal esophagus to the airway. The infant is maintained in a semi-upright position with sump catheter drainage of the proximal esophageal pouch to minimize contamination of the lungs either because of aspiration or reflux.

6. **Describe the clinical presentation, diagnosis, and preoperative management of isolated EA.**
   Isolated EA is associated with excessive salivation, choking, and regurgitation of feeds. The inability to pass a nasogastric tube into the stomach and a gasless abdomen apparent on

radiograph suggests the diagnosis. Preoperative management is directed to the identification of associated anomalies and determination of gap length. Sump catheter drainage of the proximal esophageal pouch is maintained to minimize aspiration. Gastrostomy is generally performed within the first 24 hours of life to permit feeding and assessment of the distal esophageal length. Typically, infants with EA undergo delayed repair to permit growth of the distal esophagus and reduction of gap distance.

7. **Describe the clinical presentation, diagnosis, and preoperative management of TEF without EA.**
These infants demonstrate repeated choking or cyanotic spells with feeding caused by the reflux of feeds from the esophagus to the lungs via the anomalous tracheoesophageal connection. Older infants and children may present with recurrent bouts of pneumonia or unexplained reactive airway disease resulting from the intermittent contamination of the lungs via the fistula. Video esophagography and bronchoscopy are used to demonstrate the fistula.

8. **How are tracheoesophageal malformations corrected surgically?**
Surgical treatment entails restoration of esophageal continuity and elimination of the pathologic connection of the esophagus to the airway. Correction of EA with or without TEF requires thoracotomy, with or without ligation of TEF, and end-to-end esophageal anastomosis. The first successful procedure was performed by Cameron Haight in 1941. At 5–7 days after surgery, an esophagogram is performed; if no leak is visualized, oral feedings are started and the pleural drain is removed.

TEF without EA is approached via a cervical incision, avoiding thoracotomy. The fistulous tract is divided and healthy tissue is interposed to prevent recurrence.

9. **What are the early and late complications of surgical repair?**
Early complications

Anastomotic disruption	5%
Recurrent TEF	5%
Anastomotic leak	15%
Tracheomalacia	15%

Early complications are related to the basic surgical principles of wound healing. Anastomotic disruption generally results from poor blood supply and tension.
Late complications

Anastomotic stricture	25%
Gastroesophageal reflux	50%
Esophageal dysmotility	100%

Most strictures (50%) respond to one to three dilatations performed in the first 6 months of life. Refractory strictures require identification of associated gastroesophageal reflux (GER), which may worsen stricture formation. The frequency of GER appears related to gap length (i.e., the greater the gap distance, the greater the risk of significant GER).

KEY POINTS: TRACHEOESOPHAGEAL MALFORMATIONS

1. The three most common variants are proximal esophageal atresia (EA) with distal tracheoesophageal fistula (TEE), isolated EA, and TEF without EA.

2. Early in the newborn period, affected infants demonstrate excessive salivation, choking, or regurgitation with feeding.

3. Surgical treatment entails restoration of esophageal continuity and elimination of the pathologic connection of the esophagus to the airway.

BIBLIOGRAPHY

1. Brown AK, Tam PK: Measurements of gap length in esophageal atresia: A simple predictor of outcome. J Am Coll Surg 182:41–45, 1996.

2. Dunn JC, Fonkalsrud EW, Atkinson JB: Simplifying the Waterston's stratification of infants with tracheo-esophageal fistula. Am Surg 65:908–910, 1999.

3. Saing H, Mya GH, Cheng W: The involvement of two or more systems and the severity of associated anomalies significantly influence mortality in esophageal atresia. J Pediatr Surg 33:1596–1598, 1998.

4. Somppi E, Tammela O, Ruuska T, et al: Outcome of patients operated on for esophageal atresia: 30 years' experience. J Pediatr Surg 33:1341–1346, 1998.

5. Spitz L: Esophageal atresia: Past, present, and future. J Pediatr Surg 31:19–25, 1996.

6. Torfs CP, Curry CJ, Bateson TF: Population-based study of tracheoesophageal fistula and esophageal atresia. Teratology 52:220–232, 1995.

7. Tovar JA, Diez Pardo JA, Murcia J, et al: Ambulatory 24-hour manometric and pH metric evidence of permanent impairment of clearance capacity in patients with esophageal atresia. J Pediatr Surg 30:1224–1231, 1995.

CHAPTER 86

CONGENITAL DIAPHRAGMATIC HERNIA

Denis D. Bensard, M.D., and Richard J. Hendrickson, M.D.

1. **What is the most common type of congenital diaphragmatic hernia (CDH)?**
   Congenital abnormalities of the diaphragm include a posterolateral defect (Bochdalek hernia), an anteromedial defect (Morgagni hernia), or the eventration (central weakening) of the diaphragm. The Bochdalek hernia is the most common variant and generally occurs on the left (80%). Approximately 20% occur on the right, and < 1% are bilateral.

2. **What signs and symptoms suggest CDH?**
   Neonatal respiratory distress is the most common manifestation of CDH caused by associated lung maldevelopment. At birth or shortly thereafter, the infant develops severe dyspnea, retractions, and cyanosis. On physical examination, breath sounds are diminished on the ipsilateral side, heart sounds can be heard more easily in the contralateral chest, and the abdomen is scaphoid because of the herniation of abdominal viscera into the chest. Mediastinal shift may result impairing venous return and cardiac output.

3. **How is the diagnosis confirmed?**
   A chest radiograph demonstrates multiple loops of air-filled intestine in the ipsilateral thorax. If a chest radiograph is obtained before entry of significant amounts of air into the bowel, a confusing pattern of mediastinal shift, cardiac displacement, and opacification of the hemithorax may be observed. Insertion of a nasogastric tube followed by repeat chest radiograph often demonstrates the tube (i.e., stomach) in the chest and confirms the diagnosis.

4. **Are other anomalies associated with CDH?**
   Fifty percent of infants with CDH have associated anomalies. Fewer than 10% of patients with multiple major concurrent anomalies survive. Excluding intestinal malrotation and pulmonary hypoplasia, cardiac anomalies (63%) are the most frequent, followed by genitourinary (23%), gastrointestinal (17%), central nervous system (14%), and other pulmonary (5%) anomalies.

5. **What therapeutic measures should be initiated before transport or operation?**
   Perhaps the easiest and most effective palliative intervention is decompression of the stomach with a nasogastric tube, which prevents further distention of the bowel and lung compression. Endotracheal intubation permits adequate ventilation and oxygenation. Ventilatory pressures are kept low (< 30 mmHg), and the infant is ventilated at a rapid rate (40–60 breaths/min) to avoid barotrauma. Venous access and fluid resuscitation complete preliminary resuscitation.

6. **What is the "honeymoon period"?**
   The honeymoon period describes the interval of time in which a neonate demonstrates adequate oxygenation and ventilation in the absence of maximal medical therapy. Regardless of subsequent deterioration, a honeymoon period suggests that pulmonary function is compatible with survival.

7. **Describe the operative approach.**
   CDH results in a physiologic derangement of the lungs that is not reversed by surgical reconstruction of the diaphragm. Thus, repair of CDH is not a surgical emergency. The infant must be stabilized

before surgical repair is attempted. A transabdominal approach allows reduction of the herniated abdominal viscera from the chest, repair of the diaphgramatic defect without obstructed vision or tension, correction of malrotation, and stretching of the abdominal cavity or creation of a ventral hernia with a prosthetic patch if the reduced viscera are not easily accomodated in the abdomen.

8. **What is the most feared complication of diaphragmatic hernia?**
The most feared complication is persistent fetal circulation (PFC). In CDH, one or both lungs are hypoplastic, the pulmonary vascular bed is reduced, and the pulmonary arteries exhibit thickened muscular walls that are hyperreactive. Newborns with CDH are particularly prone to the development of pulmonary hypertension. PFC arises from a sustained increase in pulmonary artery pressure. Blood is shunted away from the lungs, and the unoxygenated blood is diverted to the systemic circulation (right-to-left shunt) through the patent ductus arteriosus and patent foramen ovale. PFC results in hypoxemia, profound acidosis, and shock. PFC is triggered by acidosis, hypercarbia, and hypoxia, all potent vasoconstrictors of the pulmonary circulation.

9. **Is PFC correctable? If so, how?**
Yes. Various strategies are used to prevent or reverse PFC:
    1. **Monitoring:** Oximetry or arterial sampling (preductal in the right upper extremity; postductal in the lower extremity) permits early detection of shunting of unoxygenated blood to the systemic circulation.
    2. **Ventilation:** Hypercarbia is corrected by mechanical ventilation; adequate sedation; and, if necessary, pharmacologic paralysis.
    3. **Oxygenation:** Hypoxemia is corrected by adequate ventilation and high concentrations of inspired oxygen (generally $FiO_2 = 100\%$).
    4. **Resuscitation:** Metabolic acidosis is managed by restoring adequate tissue perfusion (intravenous fluids or blood, inotropes, and sodium bicarbonate).
    5. **Rescue:** Salvage therapies include administration of pulmonary vasodilators via the ventilatory circuit (nitric oxide) or systemic circulation (priscoline, prostaglandin E_2), high-frequency ventilation, and extracorporeal membrane oxygenation (ECMO).

10. **What is the survival rate for patients with CDH?**
The overall survival rate is 60%. The major determinants of survival are the degree of pulmonary hypoplasia and associated major congenital anomalies. Among infants surviving the early newborn period without significant lung dysfunction, the survival rate approaches 100%.

11. **Does in utero intervention have a role in the treatment of patients with CDH?**
To date, fetal surgery for CDH remains experimental. In a prospective trial reported in 1997, the results of intrauterine repair of CDH were compared with conventional postnatal surgery with similar outcome. The investigators concluded that because open fetal surgery does not improve survival or outcome, prenatally diagnosed CDH should be treated postnatally.

BIBLIOGRAPHY

1. Clark RH, Hardin WD, Hirschl RB, et al: Current surgical management of congenital diaphragmatic hernia: A report from the congenital diaphragmatic hernia study group. J Pediatr Surg 33:1004–1009, 1998.
2. Fauza DO, Wilson JM: Congenital diaphragmatic hernia and associated anomalies: Their incidence, identification, and impact on prognosis. J Pediatr Surg 29:1113–1117, 1994.
3. Harrison MR, Adzick NS, Bullard KM, et al: Correction of congenital diaphragmatic hernia in utero VII: A prospective trial. J Pediatr Surg 32:1637–1642, 1997.
4. Nobuhara KK, Lund DP, Mitchell J, et al: Long-term outlook for survivors of congenital diaphragmatic hernia. Clin Perinatol 23:873–887, 1996.
5. Weber TR, Kountzman B, Dillon PA, et al: Improved survival in congenital diaphragmatic hernia with evolving therapeutic strategies. Arch Surg 133:498–503, 1998.

ABDOMINAL TUMORS

Frederick M. Karrer, M.D., and Denis D. Bensard, M.D.

CHAPTER 87

1. **What are the most common malignant solid abdominal tumors in children?**
   Neuroblastomas, Wilms' tumors, and hepatoblastomas, in that order. Neuroblastomas are derived from neural crest tissue; in the abdomen, they originate from the adrenal glands and paraspinal sympathetic ganglia. Wilms' tumor (nephroblastoma) derives from the kidney, and hepatoblastomas originate in the liver.

2. **Is it tough to differentiate Wilms' tumor from neuroblastomas clinically?**
   Yes. Both tumors present as an asymptomatic abdominal mass. The differences are summarized in Table 87-1. In addition, because neuroblastomas produce hormones, affected children may exhibit flushing, hypertension (catecholamine release), watery diarrhea, periorbital ecchymosis, and abnormal ocular movements.

TABLE 87-1. DIFFERENTIATION BETWEEN WILMS' TUMOR AND NEUROBLASTOMA		
	Wilms' Tumor	Neuroblastoma
Age at presentation	3–4 yr	1–2 yr
Extend across midline	Rare	Common
Surface on palpation	Smooth	Knobby
X-ray calcifications	No	Yes

3. **How are Wilms' tumors and neuroblastomas treated?**
   See Table 87-2.

TABLE 87-2. TREATMENT OF WILMS' TUMOR AND NEUROBLASTOMA		
	Wilms' Tumor	Neuroblastoma
Primary surgical excision	Important (likely)	Important (less likely)
Chemotherapy	Enormous impact	Less responsive

4. **What are the major prognostic factors in neuroblastomas and Wilms' tumor?**
   In **neuroblastomas**, age at presentation is the major prognostic factor. Children younger than 1 year have an overall survival rate > 70%, whereas the survival rate for children older than 1 year is < 35%. Shimada proposed a prognostic classification based on evaluation of histologic parameters (tumor differentiation, mitosis-karyorrhexis index [MKI]) as well as age. Aneuploid tumors, tumors with low MKI, and tumors with < 10 copies of the n-myc gene also have better outcomes.

Age is also important in children with **Wilms' tumors**, but the prognosis is better because the tumors are more readily excised and much more sensitive to chemotherapy.

5. **What are the differences between hepatoblastomas and hepatocellular carcinomas? How are the tumors treated?**
    Hepatoblastomas usually occur in infants and young children, whereas hepatocellular carcinoma usually occurs in children older than 10 years. Hepatocellular carcinoma usually is associated with cirrhosis and hepatitis B and is histologically identical to the adult form. Surgical resection is the primary therapy for both tumors. Hepatoblastomas often have a good response to adjunctive chemotherapy, whereas hepatocellular carcinoma rarely responds to chemotherapy.

CONTROVERSY

6. **Should patients with hepatoblastoma receive preoperative chemotherapy to shrink the tumors?**
    Preoperative chemotherapy does shrink tumors, resulting in easier hepatic resection and lower surgical morbidity. This benefit must be weighed against the considerable toxicity of chemotherapeutic agents.

KEY POINTS: ABDOMINAL TUMORS

1. The most common malignant solid abdominal tumors in children are neuroblastomas, Wilms' tumor, and hepatoblastomas.

2. In neuroblastomas, age at presentation is the major prognostic factor.

3. Hepatoblastomas usually occur in infants and young children, whereas hepatocellular carcinomas usually occur in children older than 10 years.

BIBLIOGRAPHY

1. Caty MG, Shamberger RC: Abdominal tumors in infancy and childhood. Pediatr Clin North Am 40:1253–1271, 1993.
2. Herrera JM, Krebs A, Harris P, Barriga F: Childhood tumors. Surg Clin North Am 80:747–760, 2000.
3. Reynolds M: Pediatric liver tumors. Semin Surg Oncol 16:159–172, 1999.
4. Shamberger RC, Guthrie KA, Ritchey ML, et al: Surgery related factors and local recurrence of Wilms' tumor in National Wilms' Tumor Study 4. Ann Surg 229:292–297, 1999.
5. Shimada M: Tumors of the neuroblastoma group. Pathology 2:43–59, 1993.
6. Stocker JT: Hepatic tumors in children. Clin Liver Dis 5:259–281, 2001.

CHAPTER 88

CONGENITAL CYSTS AND SINUSES OF THE NECK

Frederick M. Karrer, M.D., and Denis D. Bensard, M.D.

1. **What are branchial cleft anomalies?**

   Cysts, sinuses, and fistulas that result from incomplete obliteration of the first, second, or third branchial clefts, and are present in early fetal development.

2. **Which anomaly is the most common?**

   Second branchial cleft anomalies are by far the most common, presenting near the mid- to upper border of the sternocleidomastoid (SCM) muscle. First branchial remnants are less common and third clefts are quite rare. (See Table 88-1.)

TABLE 88-1.	BRANCHIAL CLEFT ANOMALIES		
Branchial Cleft	**Internal Opening**	**Exterior Opening**	**Frequency**
First	External auditory canal	Angle of the jaw	8%
Second	Tonsillar fossa	Anterior border of the SCM	> 90%
Third	Piriform sinus	Suprasternal notch	< 1%

3. **How do patients with branchial cleft anomalies present?**

   Those with complete fistulas or sinuses present with intermittent drainage of a mucoid fluid on the neck. Patients with cysts usually present later with a mass (sterile or infected). Complete surgical excision is the treatment of choice.

4. **What are the major operative hazards of branchial cleft remnant excision?**

   The second branchial cleft tracts through the bifurcation of the carotid artery. The facial nerve is in close proximity to the first branchial cleft fistula. The superior laryngeal nerve and the recurrent laryngeal nerve are both at risk in dissection of a third branchial cleft.

5. **What is a thyroglossal duct cyst?**

   A thyroglossal duct cyst is the most common congenital cyst found in the neck. It is caused by failure of normal obliteration of the migration tract of the thyroid gland. Embryologically, the thyroid descends from the base of the tongue (foramen caecum) to its normal location in the low anterior neck.

6. **How do patients with thyroglossal duct cysts present?**

   They present with a paramidline mass in the upper neck; if infected, they may present with fever, tenderness, and erythema.

KEY POINTS: CONGENITAL CYSTS AND SINUSES OF THE NECK

1. The most common brachial cleft anomaly is the second brachial cleft anomaly presenting near the mid- to upper border or the sternocleidomastoid muscle.

2. A thyroglossal duct cyst is the most common congenital cyst found in the neck.

3. A cystic hygroma is a congenital lymphatic malformation that is benign an usually presents as a soft mass in the lateral neck.

7. **How are thyroglossal duct cysts treated?**
The best treatment is complete excision of the cyst, along with the tract. Because embryologically the thyroid descends before formation of the hyoid cartilage, the tract may pass right through the hyoid. Therefore, complete tract removal requires excision of the central portion of the hyoid and dissection up to the base of the tongue (i.e., the Sistrunk procedure).

8. **What is a cystic hygroma?**
A cystic hygroma is a congenital lymphatic malformation with a predilection for the neck. It is a benign lesion that usually presents as a soft mass in the lateral neck. Excision is often challenging because the lymph cysts do not respect the fascial planes and often intertwine with the neurovascular structures in the neck. Near-total excision is the treatment of choice.

BIBLIOGRAPHY

1. Alqahtani A, Nguyen LT, Flageole H, et al: 25 years experience with lymphangioma in children. J Pediatr Surg 34:1164–1168, 1999.

2. Brown RL, Azizkhan RG: Pediatric head and neck lesions. Pediatr Clin North Am 45:889–905, 1998.

3. Kang L, Chang CH, Yu CH, et al: Prenatal detection of cystic hygroma using three-dimensional ultrasound. Ultrasound Med Biol 28:719, 2002.

4. Organ GM, Organ CH Jr: Thyroid gland and surgery of the thyroglossal duct: Exercise in applied embryology. World J Surg 24:886–890, 2000.

5. Smith CD: Cysts and sinuses of the neck. In O'Neill JA, Rowe MI, Grosfeld JL, et al (eds): Pediatric Surgery, 5th ed. St. Louis, Mosby, 1998, pp 757–771.

6. Telander RL, Filston HC: Review of head and neck lesions in infancy and childhood. Surg Clin North Am 72:1429–1447, 1992.

CHAPTER 89

LIVER TRANSPLANTATION

Thomas E. Bak, M.D., Michael E. Wachs, M.D., and Igal Kam, M.D.

1. **When and where was the first liver transplant performed?**
   Dr. Thomas Starzl performed the first operation on March 1, 1963, at the University of Colorado in Denver.

2. **Is liver transplantation considered a safe and effective operation?**
   Yes. Although still a major operation with significant risks, patient and graft survival have continuously improved. One-year survival should be well over 90% in major centers.

3. **What are the most common indications for liver transplantation in the United States?**
   Noncholestatic cirrhosis characterizes > 50% of the recipients. This group includes those with viral hepatitis, alcoholic cirrhosis (Laennec's), and Budd-Chiari syndrome. Cholestatic cirrhosis makes up an additional 15%, with primary sclerosing cholangitis (PSC) and primary biliary cirrhosis heading this group. Other indications include biliary atresia, acute hepatic necrosis, malignant neoplasms, and metabolic disease.

4. **Has the most common disease requiring transplantation shifted over the years?**
   Yes. The largest percentage of people now being transplanted have hepatitis C. There are also more retransplants performed because some diseases such as hepatits C and PSC can recur in transplanted livers.

5. **How is the waiting list run?**
   Changes have been made to the list so that the sickest patients get transplanted first. New scoring systems (Mayo End-stage Liver Disease [MELD] score) have been devised to give more weight to objective markers of illness rather than the more subjective medical criteria used in the past. This point system has also minimized the importance of time spent on the waiting list. The goal of these changes is to reduce waiting list mortality.

6. **What are some of the recent advances in liver transplant surgery?**
   Operative techniques have improved such that some liver transplant recipients do not require a stay in the intensive care unit, venovenous bypass, or external biliary drainage, and operative times are shorter (4–5 hours). Improved immunosuppression medications have reduced rejection rates and side effects.

7. **How long can a liver be kept "on ice"?**
   Optimal cold ischemia should be < 12 hours.

8. **What are some common postoperative complications of liver transplantation?**
   Postoperative bleeding, infection, and biliary complications are the most common. Primary nonfunction (< 5%) and early hepatic artery thrombosis (5%) are less common, but they usually require an urgent retransplant.

9. **What is the "piggy-back" technique?**
   This is a technique in which the recipient's sick liver is carefully resected off of his or her vena cava, which is left in situ. The upper donor cava is then sewn to a common cuff of native hepatic veins. The donor's lower cava is ligated. Using this method, it is possible to do the complete transplant with minimal if any vena caval occlusion, resulting in less intraoperative hemodynamic instability.

10. **Is living-donor liver transplantation an option?**
    Yes. Initially used in the pediatric population using an adult left lateral segment graft, this procedure has evolved into fairly common practice. The Far East has had a large number of adult-to-adult left lobe graft series. Elsewhere, this has been replaced with a right lobe donor operation. Both the donor and recipient liver lobes quickly regenerate to normal size. Results in experienced centers mimic those of cadaveric transplant with similar patient survival, albeit at higher complication and retransplant rates.

KEY POINTS: LIVER TRANSPLANTATION

1. The most common indication for liver transplantation in the United States is noncholestatic cirrhosis.

2. Optimal cold ischemia time for the liver is < 12 hours.

3. Transjugular intrahepatic portosystemic shunts can be used in potential transplant recipients as a bridge to transplantation.

11. **How have transjugular intrahepatic portosystemic shunts (TIPS) improved this field of surgery?**
    TIPS can be used in potential transplant recipients as a bridge to transplantation. This procedure is very effective in controlling portal hypertension without the need for a major abdominal operative shunt. A prior portocaval shunt does complicate a liver transplant, but it is not a contraindication to liver transplantation.

CONTROVERSIES

12. **Should liver transplants be performed in individuals with alcoholic liver disease?**
    Transplant centers have strict criteria that alcohol-induced liver transplant recipients must undergo extensive psychological testing and abstain from alcohol before being placed on the waiting list. The recidivism rate (i.e., transplant patients who start drinking again) remains low. Financially, the cost is comparable, if not lower, than continued medical management of end-stage liver disease. We currently do provide care for other self-inflicted medical problems, such as cigarette smokers. The public must realize that people are not being pulled off bar stools and taken to the hospital for their transplant.

13. **Should patients with hepatic malignances have liver transplants?**
    Patients with hepatocellular carcinoma have had successful transplants, although their survival is considerably lower than recipients transplanted for other causes. Other hepatic malignancies, including cholangiocarcinoma, are generally considered contraindications to transplantation. Whether scarce donor livers should be allocated to these patients continues to be a complex issue

14.   **Should adult-to-adult living donors be used?**
The evolving field of adult-to-adult living donor liver transplant (ALDLTx) requires a healthy donor to undergo a major, potentially life-threatening operation. The benefits include a timely, life-saving procedure for a loved one, reducing the recipient's risk of not having a cadaveric liver available in time. The ethics of whether to subject the donor to major liver resective surgery remains debatable. Even more debatable is whether it is permissible to accept a donor liver for a recipient with liver cancer who already has a poor outlook.

WEB SITE

http://www.transplantation-soc.org

BIBLIOGRAPHY

1. Bak T, Wachs M, Trotter JF, et al: Adult-to-adult living donor liver transplant using right lobe grafts: Results and lessons learned from a single center experience. Liver Transpl 7:680–686, 2001.

2. Barker CF, Brayman KL, Markmann JF, et al: Transplantation of abdominal organs. In Townsend CM, Beauchamp RD, Evers BM, et al (eds): Sabiston Textbook of Surgery: The Biological Basis of Modern Surgical Practice, 16th ed. Philadelphia, W.B. Saunders, 2001.

3. Ginns LC, Cosimi AB, Morris PJ: Transplantation. Malden, MA, Blackwell Science, 1999.

4. Lok ASF, Villamil FG, McDiarmid SV (eds): Liver Transplantation for Viral Hepatitis [entire volume]. Liver Transpl 8(suppl 1), 2002.

CHAPTER 90

KIDNEY AND PANCREAS TRANSPLANTATION

Thomas E. Bak, M.D., Michael E. Wachs, M.D., and Igal Kam, M.D.

1. **What are the most common indications for kidney transplantation?**
   End-stage renal disease (ESRD) caused by hypertension, diabetes, glomerulonephritis, and polycystic kidney disease.

2. **Why should patients be taken off dialysis and have kidney transplants?**
   Although not a life-saving transplant like liver or heart transplantation, kidney transplantation will improve patients' quality of life. Patient 5-year survival is higher posttransplant when compared with continued dialysis. Finally, there is a cost savings with kidney transplantation compared with long-term dialysis.

3. **How long is kidney graft survival?**
   Cadaveric kidney transplant survival rates have steadily improved over the years. Currently, 1-year graft survival is 90%, with a 10-year graft survival of > 50%.

4. **How long can kidneys be kept "on ice"?**
   Kidneys can survive and function after longer cold ischemia time than other solid organs. Function can be maintained up to 72 hours, although optimal function is achieved if cold ischemia is kept under 24 hours. Patients on the waiting list frequently continue to work and travel and still have plenty of time to get to the hospital for tranplant. Also, United Network of Organ Sharing (UNOS) kidneys are frequently sent via commercial airlines all across the country.

5. **Where is the transplanted kidney placed?**
   Most commonly, the kidney is placed in the right iliac fossa. The peritoneal cavity is reflected superiorly, and the external iliac vessels are exposed. The renal artery and vein are then anastomosed end-to-side to the iliac vessels.

6. **What are the indications for nephrectomy?**
   Indications for nephrectomy include chronic infection, symptomatic polycystic kidney disease, intractable hypertension, and heavy proteinurea. The majority of transplant recipients do not need to undergo native nephrectomies.

7. **Are living-donor kidney transplants recommended?**
   There are definite advantages to receiving a living-donor kidney. The average survival times of these kidneys are significantly better. Also, the long cadaveric kidney waiting time (usually measured in years) can be avoided. Donors are carefully screened to ensure health and lack of any coercion.

8. **Is donating a kidney a major operation for living donors?**
   The standard of care for donor operations has become a laparoscopic donor nephrectomy. This technique has proven to be safe, with no negative effects on the kidney. The benefits of this modification over the open technique are much quicker recovery and shorter return-to-work time. This has generally increased the number of people interested in being living donors.

9. **What are the indications for kidney-pancreas (K-P) transplantation?**
In general, all type 1 diabetics who have poorly controlled diabetes despite optimal medical manage-ment should be considered for K-P transplantation as long as they are acceptable surgical risks. Unfortunately, many older patients have significant, even prohibitive, comorbidities. A pancreas transplant adds significant morbidity and mortality risks over a kidney-only transplant.

10. **Can a patient undergo pancreas transplantation before or after a kidney transplant?**
Yes. Patients can receive a simultaneous K-P transplant. This is the most common course, and the operation is done through a midline abdominal incision with the pancreas and kidney placed on opposite iliac vessels. Patients can also receive a pancreas-only transplant or pancreas-after-kidney transplant. The survival for these grafts is similar. Some centers are now shifting to portal drainage of the pancreas, with the venous outflow established to the superior mesenteric vein.

KEY POINTS: KIDNEY AND PANCREAS TRANSPLANTATION

1. The most common indication for kidney transplantation is end-stage renal disease caused by hypertension, diabetes, glomerulonephritis, and polycystic kidney disease.

2. Cadaveric kidney transplant survival rates have steadily improved over the years, with current 1-year graft survival rates of 90% and a 10-year graft survival rate of > 50%.

3. In general, all type 1 diabetics with poorly controlled diabetes despite optimal medical management should be considered for kidney-pancreas transplantation as long as they are acceptable surgical risks.

11. **How are digestive enzymes drained in a pancreas transplant?**
The donor pancreas is procured with a duodenal cuff still attached, with enzymatic drainage from the graft into this cuff intact. The duodenal cuff is then drained into a piece of recipient's small intestine with an enteric anastomosis. An alternative is to attach the duodenal cuff to the bladder. This allows amylase levels to be followed in the urine, but metabolic and infectious complications frequently require a conversion to enteric drainage.

12. **What are some complications commonly seen with pancreas transplant?**
Leakage from the duodenal cuff, graft venous thrombosis, infection, rejection, and graft pancre-atitis are all potential complications. The incidence of these is decreasing as more experience is gained, and pancreas graft survival now approaches kidney graft survival.

CONTROVERSIES

13. **Is HLA (human leukocyte) matching still important?**
It is somewhat important. Historically, HLA matching was an important consideration when matching cadaver kidneys to recipients. With today's improved immunosuppressive agents, many transplant surgeons believe that HLA matching is no longer critical. Six antigen match kid-neys are still shared nationally and do enjoy some improvement in long-term graft survival. Donor organ quality remains the primary determinant in how well the transplanted organ func-tions. For example, a poorly matched living-donor kidney will still usually outlast a well-matched cadaveric kidney.

14. **Does pancreas transplantation halt the progression of diabetic disease?**
    This is still unproven. Logically, we would expect it to. Regression of neuropathy and eye dysfunction has been reported. Recently, long-term recipients have exhibited some regression of microscopic nephropathy.

15. **Are islet cell transplants the answer in the future?**
    Probably, although this has been frustratingly slow to achieve. Recent protocols using new immunosuppressive regimens and new islet cell isolation techniques have shown promise, but long-term data are still not widely available. The process requires that isolated islet cells be extracted from a donor pancreas. These cells are then injected into the portal vein, lodge in the liver, and produce insulin. Theoretically, patients achieve the benefit of a pancreas transplant without the surgical risk.

WEB SITE

http://www.transplantation-soc.org

BIBLIOGRAPHY

1. Bartlett ST: Laparoscopic donor nephrectomy after seven years. Am J Transpl 2:896–897, 2002.
2. Donovitch G: Handbook of Kidney Transplantation, 3rd ed. Philadelphia, Lippincott Williams & Wilkins, 2001.
3. Fioretto P, Steffes MW, Sutherland DER, et al: Reversal of lesions of diabetic nephropathy after pancreas transplantation. N Engl J Med 339:69–75, 1998.
4. Morris JP: Kidney Transplantation: Principles and Practice, 5th ed. Philadelphia, W.B. Saunders, 2001.

CHAPTER 91

HEART TRANSPLANTATION

Daniel R. Meldrum, M.D., Azad Raiesdana, M.D., Jeffrey A. Breall, M.D., and John W. Brown, M.D.

1. **Who performed the first experimental heart–lung transplant?**
   Alexis Carrel, a French-born American surgeon, developed the vascular techniques required for heart–lung transplantation and performed the first experimental heart–lung transplant in 1907. He transplanted the lungs, heart, aorta, and vena cava of a 1-week-old cat into the neck of a large adult cat. For devising the technique of vascular anastomosis and other outstanding accomplishments, Carrel received the Nobel Prize in 1912 (the first Nobel Prize awarded to a scientist working in an American laboratory).

2. **Who performed the first successful experimental heart–lung transplant?**
   V.P. Demikhov performed the first successful heart–lung transplant in a dog in 1962.

3. **Who developed the surgical strategy required for human heart transplantation?**
   Norman Shumway.

4. **Who performed the first human heart transplant? When?**
   C.N. Bernard performed the first human heart transplant in December, 1967 (in Capetown, South Africa, after visiting Dr. Shumway), although Dr. Shumway set the stage by developing the technique in animals. Shumway and the Stanford group performed the first heart transplant in the United States and accomplished the first successful clinical series.

5. **Who performed the first successful heart–lung transplant? When?**
   Dr. Bruce Reitz at Stanford in 1981 on a 21-year-old woman with pulmonary hypertension secondary to an atrial septal defect.

6. **How many heart transplants are performed annually? Is the number increasing or decreasing?**
   In 1983 approximately 300 heart transplants were performed worldwide. By 1988, the number had rapidly increased to approximately 3000 and remains relatively stable between 3500 and 4000.

7. **What anastomoses (surgical connections) must be performed for a combined heart and lungs transplant?**
   The operation requires only a right atrial-to-cava (inflow) anastomosis and an aortic (outflow) anastomosis with a connection at the trachea. Heart–lung transplant is less complicated (fewer anastomoses) than heart transplant alone, which may explain why heart–lung transplant was attempted first.

8. **What anastomoses must be performed for a heart transplant?**
   Left atrial, right atrial, aortic, and pulmonary arterial.

9. **Who is an acceptable cardiac donor?**
   Acceptable cardiac donors meet the following criteria:

1. Requirements for brain death
2. Consent from next of kin
3. ABO blood group compatibility with recipient
4. Within 20% of the same size as recipient
5. Absence of history of cardiac disease
6. Normal echocardiogram (ventricular wall motion)
7. Normal heart by inspection during organ recovery

10. **Who is an acceptable cardiac recipient?**
Although selection criteria are evolving as a result of improved techniques and outcomes, the following criteria are standard: age between newborn and 65 years; irremediable New York Heart Association Functional Class IV cardiac disease; normal renal, hepatic, pulmonary, and central nervous system function; pulmonary vascular resistance < 6–8 Wood units; and absence of malignancy, infection, recent pulmonary infarction, and severe peripheral vascular or cerebrovascular disease. Diabetes is a relative contraindication; the steroids used in post-transplant immunosuppression make diabetes difficult to manage. Also, normal psychological status has proven to be important.

11. **What are the most common indications for heart transplant in adults and in children?**
In adults, coronary artery disease (ischemic cardiomyopathy) and idiopathic cardiomyopathy each account for approximately 45% of transplants.
In children, congenital heart disease and cardiomyopathy are most common, with hypoplastic left heart being the most common congenital malformation requiring heart transplantation.

12. **What percentage of potential recipients (on the transplant list) die while waiting for a heart transplant?**
20%.

13. **At what point does donor heart ischemic time influence mortality?**
Donor heart ischemic time > 6 hours definitely increases mortality. Ischemic times between 4 and 6 hours stun the donor heart. Most transplant teams try to keep ischemic times (from donor harvest to perfusion in the recipient) to < 4 hours.

14. **Who pioneered hypothermic myocardial preservation?**
Henry Swan at the University of Colorado. He submerged anesthetized children in a bathtub of ice water before cardiac procedures.

15. **How is cardiac allograft rejection prevented?**
Pharmacologically induced immunosuppression is performed by using one of two protocols. The first is triple therapy, which combines cyclosporine, azathioprine, and prednisone. The second major protocol incorporates the monoclonal antibody OKT3 into the triple therapy protocol. OKT3 is substituted for cyclosporine for the first 2 weeks after transplant.

16. **What is OKT3?**
OKT3 is a mouse monoclonal antibody that binds to and blocks the T-cell CD3 receptor. A monoclonal antibody is an antibody generated from the clones of a single cell. For instance, a single B cell, which recognizes the CD3 receptor as an antigen (foreign), is immortalized in cell culture and produces the monoclonal antibody in limitless supply. The CD3 receptor, which is common to all T cells, is important for antigen recognition and T-cell activation; therefore, OKT3 is highly immunosuppressive.

KEY POINTS: CRITERIA FOR ACCEPTABLE HEART DONORS

1. Donors must meet the criteria for brain death.

2. Consent from donor's next of kin.

3. ABO blood group compatibility with recipient.

4. Donor must be within 20% of same size as recipient.

5. Donor must have no history of cardiac disease and a normal echocardiogram.

6. Donor heart must appear normal by inspection during organ recovery.

17. **What complications are associated with the use of OKT3?**
OKT3 may have severe side effects, including pulmonary edema and high fevers, that result from transient cytokine release, which may occur when OKT3 binds to the T-cell activation site. Because OKT3 is an antigen (an antibody from a different species [i.e., a mouse]), patients develop anti-OKT3 antibodies fairly quickly; the result is that OKT3 can only be used to treat one rejection episode. Severe side effects occur in < 5% of patients.

18. **Does HLA mismatch influence the incidence of rejection after heart transplantation? Is HLA typing routinely performed before heart transplantation?**
Yes and no. In a multi-institutional, multivariate analysis of 1719 cardiac transplant recipients by Jarcho et al., HLA mismatch increased the incidence of rejection. However, HLA typing is not routinely done before heart transplantation because it takes too long. In addition, with three of six mismatches, there was still only a trend toward increased rejection-related deaths ($P = 0.14$). If longer organ preservation times can be achieved, donor/recipient HLA matching will become feasible and should improve survival rates. Again, ABO blood group compatibility does influence graft survival.

19. **What are the major complications of heart transplantation?**
   - Allograft rejection (days to weeks)
   - Infection (months)
   - Transplant coronary artery disease (years)

20. **What is the incidence of transplant coronary artery disease? What are the risk factors?**
Nearly 50% of patients have angiographic evidence of coronary artery disease by 5 years after transplant. However, only approximately 10% develop at least 70% stenosis (hemodynamically significant stenosis). Severe stenosis is highly predictive of the need for retransplantation. Risk factors for transplant coronary artery disease include male gender of the donor or recipient, older donor age, and donor hypertension.

21. **How is cardiac allograft rejection diagnosed?**
Clinical suspicion is raised by new-onset cardiac arrhythmia, fever, or hypotension. Diagnosis depends on endomyocardial biopsy, which is performed at regular intervals to detect histologic evidence of rejection before signs or symptoms occur. Radionuclide ventriculography and echocardiography are useful adjuncts in following the hemodynamic manifestations of rejection. Electrocardiography itself is not very sensitive in the diagnosis of rejection.

22. **Are 3-hydroxy-3-methylglutaryl coenzyme A (HMG-CoA) reductase inhibitors ("statin" drugs) generally recommended for post-cardiac transplant patients?**
Yes. Hypercholesterolemia is common after transplantation, and HMG-CoA reductase inhibitors reduce the development of the diffuse atherosclerosis that tends to occur in transplanted hearts. In addition, statins have an early effect on mortality, which suggests that these drugs may also have immunosuppressive effects.

23. **What are ventricular assist devices (VADs)?**
These devices are designed to unload either the right (RVAD) or left (LVAD) ventricle while supporting the pulmonary or systemic circulation. Patients with these VADs may be ambulatory, and the devices may be worn for weeks to months. VADs may be used as a bridge to transplant (when the patient is listed for transplantation) or as destination therapy (when no transplant is planned).

24. **What is the most serious complication of transvenous endomyocardial biopsy?**
Cardiac perforation occurs in 0.5% of cases. This can rapidly lead to tamponade and circulatory collapse.

25. **What is the typical infection pattern for a posttransplant patient?**
First postoperative month: conventional bacterial pathogens encountered in surgical patients
1–4 months: opportunistic pathogens, especially cytomegalovirus
>4 months: both conventional and opportunistic infections

26. **Is the transplanted heart denervated?**
Initially, yes, but it is believed that partial reinnervation begins within 1 year. Because of this, the heart's anatomically mediated reflexes are blunted (e.g., higher resting heart rate because of decreased or absent vagal tone).

27. **Can one heart be successfully transplanted twice?**
Yes. Meiser et al. transplanted the same heart a second time on March 19, 1991, 42 hours after the initial transplantation. Second transplant of the same heart has since been reported by others.

28. **What is "domino heart transplant"?**
The good heart from a heart–lung recipient is transplanted into a patient requiring a heart transplant. Some patients with primary lung dysfunction have secondary irreversible cardiac dysfunction (i.e., Eisenmenger's syndrome); others, however, such as patients with cystic fibrosis, have good cardiac function. Patients with good cardiac function may serve as donors and increase the donor pool.

29. **Is the heart capable of making tumor necrosis factor (TNF)? What does TNF have to do with heart transplantation?**
TNF, typically described as a macrophage- or monocyte-derived inflammatory cytokine, is also produced in large quantities by the heart. TNF released by the heart after ischemia-reperfusion probably contributes to immediate injury (dysfunction) and possibly to later rejection. Anti-TNF strategies are intuitively promising (but undocumented) therapeutic strategies.

30. **What is the overall 30-day mortality rate after heart transplant? What is the breakdown in mortality between adult and pediatric patients?**
The registry of the International Society for Heart and Lung Transplantation, which has data for approximately 45,000 heart transplants, has recorded a 30-day mortality rate of 10%. The 30-day mortality rate for adult recipients is about 8%; for pediatric recipients, it is slightly higher.

31. **What are the 5- and 10-year actuarial survival rates for heart transplant recipients?**
75% and 50%, respectively (and the quality of life is dramatically improved).

32. **What work remains to be done in heart transplantation?**
The future of heart transplantation is bright. Knowledge gained in experimental myocardial ischemia-reperfusion injury and protection is accelerating. New, exciting ways to manipulate myocardial immunology (e.g., signal transduction, gene therapy, chimerism) will further extend donor ischemic times and improve postoperative myocardial function and graft tolerance. Ultimately, genetic alteration of donor hearts will increase the donor pool.

WEB SITE

http://www.transplantation-soc.org

BIBLIOGRAPHY

1. Hosenpud JD, Bennett LE, Keck BM, et al: The Registry of the International Society for Heart and Lung Transplantation: Eighteenth official report—2001. J Heart Lung Transplant 20:805–815, 2001.

2. Kobashigawa JA: Advances in immunosuppression for heart transplantation. Adv Card Surg 10:155–174, 1998.

3. Kupiec-Weglinski JW: Graft rejection in sensitized recipients. Ann Transplant 1:34–40, 1996.

4. Kuvin JT, Kimmelstiel CD: Infectious causes of atherosclerosis. Am Heart J 137:216–226, 1999.

5. Leier CV, Binkley PF: Parenteral inotropic support for advanced congestive heart failure. Prog Cardiovasc Dis 41:207–224, 1998.

6. Meldrum DR: Tumor necrosis factor in the heart [review]. Am J Physiol 274:R577, 1998.

7. Meldrum DR, Dinarello CA, Meng X, et al: Ischemic preconditioning decreases post-ischemic myocardial TNF: Potential ultimate effector mechanism of preconditioning. Circulation 98:II214-II218, 1998.

8. Mindan JP, Panizo A: Pathology of heart transplant. Curr Top Pathol 92:137–165, 1999.

9. Orbaek Andersen H: Heart allograft vascular disease: An obliterative vascular disease in transplanted hearts. Atherosclerosis 142:243–263, 1999.

10. Pillai R, Bando K, Schueler S, et al: Leukocyte depletion results in excellent heart-lung function after 12 hours of storage. Ann Thorac Surg 50:211–214, 1990.

11. Reardon MJ, Letsou GV, Anderson JE, et al: Orthotopic cardiac transplantation after minimally invasive direct coronary artery bypass. J Thorac Cardiovasc Surg 117:390–391, 1999.

12. Spann JC, Van Meter C: Cardiac transplantation. Surg Clin North Am 78:679–690, 1998.

CHAPTER 92

LUNG TRANSPLANTATION

Daniel R. Meldrum, M.D., Azad Raiesdana, M.D., Jeffrey A. Breall, M.D., and John W. Brown, M.D.

1. **What are the general types of lung transplants?**
   Single, double (bilateral), and heart–lung.

2. **Which human organ transplant was performed first, the heart or the lung?**
   Although heart transplantation has progressed more rapidly, the first lung transplant preceded the first heart transplant.

3. **Who performed the first human lung transplant? When?**
   James Hardy performed the first human lung transplant in 1963; however, more than 20 years passed before lung transplantation was performed routinely in clinical practice (during that 20 year period, only 1 patient did well enough to leave the hospital). This delay was caused by initial graft failure secondary to inadequate organ preservation, long ischemic times, lack of good immunosuppressive agents, and technical difficulties (primarily with the bronchial—not the vascular—anastomoses).

4. **Who is a candidate for a lung transplant?**
   Candidates include patients with no other medical or surgical alternative who are likely to die of pulmonary disease within 18 months, are younger than 65 years, are not ventilator dependent, and do not have a history of malignancy. Psychological stability in the recipient is also important.

5. **What are the most common indications for single lung transplant?**
   - Emphysema (40%)
   - Idiopathic pulmonary fibrosis (20%)
   - Alpha-1 antitrypsin deficiency (11%)
   - Primary pulmonary hypertension and pulmonary hypertension secondary to correctable congenital heart disease (10%)

6. **What are the most common indications for a double-lung transplant?**
   - Cystic fibrosis (35%)
   - Emphysema (20%)
   - Alpha-1 antitrypsin deficiency (11%)
   - Primary pulmonary hypertension and pulmonary hypertension secondary to correctable congenital heart disease (20%)
   - Idiopathic pulmonary fibrosis (8%)

7. **What are the most common indications for heart–lung transplant?**
   Primary pulmonary hypertension (30%) and cystic fibrosis (16%) are instances in which bad lungs have ruined a good heart. Conversely, with congenital heart disease (27%), a bad heart has destroyed good lungs.

8. **What is sewn to what during a single-lung transplant? A double-lung transplant?**
During a single-lung transplant, recipient-to-graft bronchial, pulmonary artery, and pulmonary vein (atrial cuff) anastomoses are required. Anastomoses for double transplant are the same; however, cardiopulmonary bypass is required more often during double-lung transplant. During implantation of the second lung, diversion of the entire cardiac output to the freshly ischemic lung often results in reperfusion lung edema and hypoxemia.

9. **Which diagnoses carry the best results for single-lung transplants?**
Patients with emphysema and alpha-1 antitrypsin deficiency do significantly better, with 1-year survival rates of 80%.

10. **Why is the number of combined heart–lung transplants performed annually decreasing?**
Approximately 250 heart–lung transplants were performed in 1990; the number has decreased to approximately 150 in 1999. As the results of single- and double-lung transplants have improved, the need to perform heart–lung transplants in patients with isolated pulmonary disease has been obviated.

11. **What are the most common complications after lung transplant?**
   - Airway surgical healing defects (early)
   - Rejection (early)
   - Bacterial and cytomegalovirus infections (weeks to months)
   - Bronchiolitis obliterans (months to years)

12. **What is bronchiolitis obliterans?**
Bronchiolitis obliterans, a major cause of long-term morbidity after lung transplantation, is a process in which membranous and respiratory bronchioles demonstrate histologic evidence of subepithelial scarring that eventually progresses to occlusion of the bronchiolar lumen. Clinically, it is characterized by dyspnea and airflow obstruction.

13. **What are the risk factors for the development of bronchiolitis obliterans after lung transplant?**
Donor age > 40 years and donor ischemic times > 6 hours.

14. **How is lung transplant rejection diagnosed?**
Unlike heart transplants, the diagnosis of rejection in transplanted lungs is imprecise and based on a collection of symptoms and signs. Decreased oxygen saturation, fever, decreased exercise tolerance, and radiologic infiltrate suggest rejection. Sequential quantitative lung perfusion scans that demonstrate a decrease in perfusion are helpful in the diagnosis of rejection after single-lung transplants. Transbronchial biopsy is useful after single- and double-lung transplants.

15. **Describe the phenomenon of chimerism in transplantation.**
Chimerism is leukocyte sharing between the graft and the recipient so that the graft becomes a genetic composite of both the donor and recipient. Chimerism enhances the host's tolerance of the graft because the recipient does not recognize the donor organ as foreign. The first evidence of chimerism was observed in 1969 when female recipients of male livers developed entirely female Kupffer cell (liver macrophage) systems (as demonstrated by the Barr bodies in the macrophage). In 1992, the concept of immune cell *sharing* became clinically evident when it was discovered that leukocytes from donor kidneys occupied remote lymph nodes.

16. **Do resident macrophages exist in the heart and lungs?**
    Absolutely yes. Resident myocardial macrophages and resident alveolar macrophages are incredibly active cellular components of the heart and lungs.

17. **Does chimerism develop in the heart and the lungs?**
    Yes. Because the heart and lungs each have leukocytes to share, they participate in chimerism.

18. **Why is chimerism exciting?**
    Nature is trying to teach us how to perform transplantation without the use of immunosuppression. Our job is to learn why chimerism is induced in some recipients and not in others. That is, we should dissect the mechanisms of chimerism induction so that we may therapeutically induce chimerism in all recipients.

19. **What are the major types of preservation solutions for heart and lung grafts?**
    Euro-Collins (EC) solution and University of Wisconsin (UW) solution for lung and crystalloid cardioplegia and UW solution for hearts.

20. **What percentage of pulmonary blood flow goes to the transplanted lung after single-lung transplant?**
    Predictably, almost all of the pulmonary blood flow passes through the lower resistance circuit of the transplanted lung (depending on the pulmonary vascular resistance of the contralateral native—i.e., sick—lung). If a preoperative perfusion scan exists, other factors being equal, the lung with the best perfusion is preserved and the bad lung is replaced.

KEY POINTS: LUNG TRANSPLANTATION

1. The most common indication for single lung transplant is emphysema.

2. The most common indication for double lung transplant is cystic fibrosis.

3. Chimerism is leukocyte sharing between the graft and the recipient so that the graft becomes a genetic composite of both donor and recipient.

4. Bronchiolitis obliterans, a major cause of long-term morbidity after lung transplantation, is a process in which membranous and respiratory bronchioles demonstrate histologic evidence of subepithelial scarring that eventually progresses to occlusion of the bronchiolar lumen.

21. **Is cardiopulmonary bypass required for lung transplantation?**
    No. However, for patients with pulmonary hypertension (primary or secondary), cardiopulmonary bypass is routinely used before removal of the recipient's lung. Cardiopulmonary bypass is always on standby. This is tricky anesthesia. One lung is transiently excised from a patient who is living (barely) on two bad lungs.

22. **Is living-related lung transplant possible?**
    Yes. Living-related lung transplants are an innovative approach to increasing the donor pool. Typically, only one lobe from the donor is used to replace a whole lung in the recipient.

23. **What is lung volume reduction surgery? How may it be important to patients on the lung transplant waiting list?**
    Lung volume reduction surgery offers a therapeutic option for patients who are either not candidates to receive a lung transplant or on a long waiting list. Lung volume reduction surgery

removes nonfunctional or destroyed lung. Removal of defunctionalized lung makes more room for airflow in the functional lung, thereby decompressing the distended chest.

24. **Who is the best candidate for lung volume reduction surgery?**
The best candidates are patients without contraindication who have absent or reduced perfusion of approximately one third of the lung (usually caused by a big cyst or emphysematous region), with good flow distribution in the remainder of the lung. Thus, quantitative lung perfusion scans provide essential information for patient selection.

25. **What are the contraindications to lung reduction surgery?**
    - Pulmonary hypertension (mean pulmonary artery pressure [PAP] > 35 mmHg or systolic PAP > 45 mmHg)
    - Significant coronary artery disease
    - Previous thoracotomy or pleurodesis (visceral and parietal pleural fusion)
    - Long-standing history of asthma, bronchiectasis, or chronic bronchitis with purulent sputum
    - Severe kyphoscoliosis

26. **What is the most common nonbacterial cause of pneumonia in lung transplant patients?**
Cytomegalovirus (CMV), usually occurring 4–8 weeks postoperatively. Primary CMV infection usually results in more serious illness than reactivation disease. CMV-seronegative recipients should receive only blood products that are serologically negative.

27. **In addition to immune suppressive therapy, what other factors put transplanted lungs at risk for infection?**
Lung denervation, interruption of lymphatic clearance and bronchial circulation, and impaired mucociliary clearance.

28. **What are the main differences in composition between EC and UW solutions?**
EC solution is a glucose-based solution with an ionic composition that approximates that of the intracellular environment.
UW solution does not contain glucose but does contain the following components not found in EC solution: hydroxy-ethyl starch (prevents expansion of the interstitial space), lactobionate and raffinose (suppress hypothermia-induced cell swelling), glutathione and allopurinol (reduce cytotoxic injury from oxygen free radicals), and adenosine (substrate for adenosine triphosphate formation, vasodilation, and activation of the protective mechanisms of "protective preconditioning").

29. **How many lung transplants are performed annually? Is the number increasing or decreasing?**
Of interest, although the first human lung transplant was performed in 1963, significant numbers were not performed until the late 1980s (in 1986, 1 lung transplant; in 1989, 132 lung transplants). This number rapidly increased to 700 per year in 1994 and has since declined to approximately 625 per year worldwide.

30. **Are the survival rates different for single- and double-lung transplants?**
No. The 3-year actuarial survival rate is about 50% for each.

31. **What are the 1-year, 2-year, and 3-year actuarial survival rates for single-lung retransplants?**
Actuarial survival rates are 45%, 40%, and 30%, respectively. Predictably, such patients do significantly worse.

BIBLIOGRAPHY

1. Baumgartner WA: Myocardial and pulmonary protection: Long-distance transport. Prog Cardiovasc Dis 33:85–96, 1990.

2. Christie JD, Bavaria JE, Palevsky HI, et al: Primary graft failure following lung transplantation. Chest 114:51–60, 1998.

3. Cooper JD, Patterson GA: Lung transplantation. In Sabiston D, Spencer F (eds): Surgery of the Chest, 7th ed. Philadelphia, W.B. Saunders, 1995, pp 2117–2134.

4. Gaynor JW, Bridges ND, Clark BJ, et al: Update on lung transplantation in children. Curr Opin Pediatr 10:256–261, 1998.

5. Hosenpud JD, Bennett LE, Keck BM, et al: The Registry of the International Society for Heart and Lung Transplantation: Eighteenth official report—2001. J Heart Lung Transplant 20:805–815, 2001.

6. Keller CA: The donor lung: Conservation of a precious resource. Thorax 53:506–513, 1998.

7. Meyers BF, Patterson GA: Technical aspects of adult lung transplantation. Semin Thorac Cardiovasc Surg 10:213–220, 1998.

8. Nunley DR, Grgurich W, Iacono AT, et al: Allograft colonization and infections with pseudomonas in cystic fibrosis lung transplant recipients. Chest 113:1235–1243, 1998.

9. Rich S, McLaughlin VV: Lung transplantation for pulmonary hypertension: Patient selection and maintenance therapy while awaiting transplantation. Semin Thorac Cardiovasc Surg 10:135–138, 1998.

10. Sundaresan S: The impact of bronchiolitis obliterans on late morbidity and mortality after single and bilateral lung transplantation for pulmonary hypertension. Semin Thorac Cardiovasc Surg 10:152–159, 1998.

11. Waddell TK, Keshavjee S: Lung transplantation for chronic obstructive pulmonary disease. Semin Thorac Cardiovasc Surg 10:191–201, 1998.

12. Zenati M, Keenan RJ, Courcoulas AP, et al: Lung volume reduction or lung transplanation for end-stage pulmonary emphysema? Eur J Cardiothorac Surg 14:27–31, 1998.

XI. UROLOGY

THE SURGICAL APPROACH TO INFERTILITY

Randall B. Meacham, M.D., and Alex J. Vanni

CHAPTER 93

1. **How common a problem is infertility?**
   Infertility is the inability to establish a pregnancy during 1 year of well-timed intercourse. This affects 15% of all couples in the United States. In 50% of such couples, the woman is responsible; in 30% of couples, a male factor prevents pregnancy; and in 20% of couples, it is a combination of both.

2. **What are the odds that a fertile couple will become pregnant after a single episode of well-timed intercourse?**
   During a given ovulatory cycle, 18% of fertile couples become pregnant after well-timed intercourse.

3. **What is the best timing for intercourse if a couple is trying to conceive?**
   Sperm can survive in the cervical mucus for 48 hours. To achieve pregnancy, therefore, the most effective timing of intercourse is every other day, starting a few days before ovulation.

4. **What environmental factors may play a role in male infertility?**
   Although reproductive function is relatively durable, various toxins have a negative impact on male fertility. Cigarette smoke and alcohol have been implicated as dose-dependent gonadotoxins, as have recreational drugs, including marijuana, cocaine, and heroin. Radiation (in amounts as low as 200 rads) can influence spermatogenesis, as can chemotherapeutic agents. Calcium channel blockers may interfere with the ability of sperm to fertilize eggs.

5. **Can a vasectomy be successfully reversed?**
   Yes, but the success rate is affected by the amount of time since the original vasectomy. Among patients who are less than 3 years from vasectomy, the conception rate after reversal is roughly 75%. This success rate declines to about 50% when the reversal is performed 3–8 years after vasectomy and further declines to 30% when 15 or more years have passed.

6. **What is in vitro fertilization (IVF)?**
   With IVF, eggs are harvested from a woman and combined with sperm in a laboratory setting. The resulting embryos are then transferred to the uterine cavity, where they mature into a fetus. In a specialized version of this technology (i.e., intracytoplasmic sperm injection), an individual sperm is injected into each egg, thus facilitating fertilization and allowing pregnancy even in the presence of small numbers of motile sperm.

7. **What is the role of IVF in male infertility?**
   Because use of IVF greatly reduces the number of motile sperm needed to generate a pregnancy, it can be quite helpful in men with poor semen quality. The IVF team needs only as many motile sperm as there are oocytes (eggs) to be fertilized.

8. **Can sperm obtained directly from the testicle be used to generate a pregnancy?**
   For the past several years, it has been recognized that incubation of testicular tissue generally yields small numbers of motile sperm. Through the use of IVF, such sperm can generate

pregnancies. Even among men suffering from severe testicular failure, it may be possible to retrieve adequate sperm for use in IVF.

9. **What is the role of sperm freezing in the treatment of infertility?**
Sperm can be frozen (cryopreserved) with relative ease. After they are cryopreserved, sperm remain viable for extended periods (years). Cryopreservation can be helpful among men planning to undergo treatment with chemotherapy or radiation therapy.

10. **Does wearing boxer shorts versus tight underwear affect male fertility?**
No.

KEY POINTS: SURGICAL APPROACH TO INFERTILITY

1. Infertility is defined as the inability to establish pregnancy during 1 year of well-timed intercourse.

2. In 50% of infertile couples a female factor prevents pregnancy, in 30% of couples a male factor prevents pregnancy, and in 20% of couples infertility is due to a combination of both female and male factors.

3. The most common cause of male infertility is varicocele.

11. **Because normal levels of testosterone are necessary for sperm production, is it helpful to give subfertile men additional testosterone?**
Although decreased levels of testosterone can cause impaired male fertility, giving additional testosterone to men with normal testosterone levels can actually cause a dramatic decline in semen quality. Administration of exogenous testosterone causes the patient to cease production of native testosterone within the testes. The resultant decrease in intratesticular testosterone actually results in a decline in sperm production.

12. **What is the most common cause of male infertility?**
Varicocele, a collection of dilated veins above one or both testes. Among men presenting for treatment of infertility, 40% have a varicocele. Correction of varicocele leads to improvement in semen quality in 70% of patients.

13. **If we can clone Dolly (a sheep derived from cloning a fully differentiated mammary cell), can we clone humans?**
Although for a number of critical ethical reasons cloning technology is not currently used in human reproduction, it theoretically allows the cloning of any individual, creating a genetic duplicate. However, cloning probably will not play a role in the treatment of human infertility.

14. **Is IVF associated with an increase in genetic abnormalities?**
This issue is controversial, but probably no. At least one recent publication suggested that infants conceived by either intracytoplasmic sperm injection or IVF have twice the risk of major birth defects compared with naturally conceived infants.

15. **Will giving supplemental testosterone improve male fertility?**
No. Exogenous testosterone induces a profound decrease in spermatogenesis and has been explored as a means of male contraception.

16. **What is cloning as it pertains to humans?**
Just like Dolly the sheep, human cloning involves nuclear transplantation of the desired clone into an egg devoid of its nucleus. Rather than creating whole human beings, the more controversial ethical dilemma is whether to permit cloning of cells or organs for subsequent transplantation in order to cure human disease.

17. **Are undescended testes associated with male infertility?**
Yes. Cryptorchidism is associated with male infertility. The decreased fertility correlates with severely reduced total germ cell counts in prepubertal undescended testes. Bilateral testicular maldescent does decrease semen quality. Interestingly, unilateral cryptorchidism may impair semen quality as well. This suggests that both the abnormally descended testis and its normally positioned counterpart are adversely affected. Surgical repositioning of the testis improves semen quality; the earlier it is done, the better.

WEB SITE

http://www.auanet.org

BIBLIOGRAPHY

1. Cortes D, Thorp JM, Visfeldt J: Cryptorchidism: Aspects of fertility and neoplasms. A study of 1,335 consecutive boys who underwent testicular biopsy simultaneously with surgery for cryptorchidism. Horm Res 55:21–27, 2001.
2. Hansen M, Kurinczuk JJ, Bower C, Webb S: The risk of major birth defects after intracytoplasmic sperm injection and in vitro fertilization. N Engl J Med 346:725–730, 2002.
3. Hargreave T, Ghosh C: Male fertility disorders. Endocrinol Metab Clin North Am 27:765–782, 1998.
4. Ismail MT, Sedor J, Hirsch IH: Are sperm motion parameters influenced by varicocele ligation? Fertil Steril 71:886–890, 1999.
5. Johnson MD: Genetic risks of intracytoplasmic sperm injection in the treatment of male infertility: Recommendations for genetic counseling and screening. Fertil Steril 70:397–411, 1998.
6. Kim ED, Winkel E, Orejuela F, et al: Pathological epididymal obstruction unrelated to vasectomy: Results with microsurgical reconstruction. J Urol 160(6 pt 1):2078–2080, 1998.
7. Meriggiola MC, Costantino A, Cerpolini S: Recent advances in hormonal male contraception. Contraception 64:269–272, 2002.
8. Naysmith TE, Blake DA, Harvey VJ, et al: Do men undergoing sterilizing cancer treatments have a fertile future? Hum Reprod 13:3250–3255, 1998.
9. Palermo GD, Schlegel PN, Hariprashad JJ, et al: Fertilization and pregnancy outcome with intracytoplasmic sperm injection for azoospermic men. Hum Reprod 14:741–748, 1999.
10. Pellegrino ED, Kilner JF, Fitzgerald KT, et al: Therapeutic cloning. N Engl J Med 347:1619–1622, 2002.
11. Rutkowski SB, Geraghty TJ, Hagen DL, et al: A comprehensive approach to the management of male infertility following spinal cord injury. Spinal Cord 37:508–514, 1999.
12. Scherr D, Goldstein M: Comparison of bilateral versus unilateral varicocelectomy in men with palpable bilateral varicoceles. J Urol 162:85–88, 1999.
13. Wilmut I: Cloning for medicine. Sci Am 279:58–63, 1998.

CHAPTER 94

URINARY CALCULUS DISEASE

Brett B. Abernathy, M.D.

1. **What are the most common types of urinary stones found in North America?**
   - Calcium stones (calcium oxalate, calcium phosphate, or mixed calcium stones): 70%.
   - Struvite or magnesium ammonium phosphate stones, often associated with infection: 20%.
   - Uric acid stones (radiolucent): 5%
   - Cystine stones, often with a genetic association: 5%

2. **What are the typical presenting symptoms of a patient with an obstructing stone?**
   - Pain, usually colicky in the flank or radiating to the groin; patients are usually agitated and cannot get in a comfortable position
   - Hematuria, gross or microscopic
   - Nausea and vomiting caused by obstruction and pressure on the renal capsule

3. **What studies are best to diagnose stones?**
   1. **Excretory urogram**, or **intravenous pyelogram (IVP).** Ninety percent of stones are radiopaque and can be seen on a plain radiograph of the kidney, ureter, and bladder (KUB). The IVP serves as a functional study to determine the degree of obstruction, level of obstruction, and presence of a contralateral kidney.
   2. Currently, **rapid-sequence helical computed tomography (CT)** scan has gained popularity. Helical CT can accurately identify both renal and ureteral stones. Its advantages include no need for contrast; speed; and ability to identify calcium, uric acid, and cystine stones. Disadvantages include increased cost compared with IVP and inability to distinguish between radiolucent (uric acid) stones and radiopaque (calcium-containing) stones. A KUB should be obtained if the CT has positive results, to distinguish between radiolucent and radiopaque stones.
   3. **Ultrasound** is particularly advantageous in pregnant women.

4. **When should a patient with an obstructing stone be admitted to the hospital?**
   - Any sign of infection (e.g., fever, leukocytosis, bacteriuria); infection behind an obstructing stone may result in urosepsis and death
   - Intractable vomiting requiring intravenous (IV) fluids
   - Pain requiring parenteral analgesics
   - Bilateral obstructing stones or obstruction in a solitary kidney

5. **What are the treatment options for ureteral calculi?**
   - Wait and watch to see if the stone passes; it usually does. Approximately 90% of stones, 3 mm in size in the distal ureter, will pass. Fifty percent of 5-mm stones will pass, and 20% of stones larger than 6 mm will pass.
   - Ureteroscopy and stone basketing or intraureteral lithotripsy (stone blasting) with a laser (holmium, pulsed dye) or electrohydraulic lithotripsy (EHL)
   - Extracorporeal lithotripsy (ESWL), or shock waves directed at the stone to break it into small pieces that can then pass spontaneously
   - Open ureterolithotomy, now rarely used because of the success of the less invasive techniques listed above

KEY POINTS: URINARY CALCULUS DISEASE

1. The most common stones in patients in the United States are calcium stones.

2. Excretory urogram or intravenous pyelogram, rapid-sequence helical CT, and ultrasound are the imaging studies used to diagnose stones.

3. Steinstrasse is a collection of small calculi that pile up together in the ureter and cause obstruction or symptoms.

6. **What are the treatment options for renal calculi?**
   - Expectant management in asymptomatic noninfectious stones
   - ESWL
   - Ureteropyeloscopy with lithotripsy using a laser. This has become more popular with smaller, flexible, deflectable ureteroscopes, but it is still a challenging procedure for large stones.
   - Percutaneous nephrostolithotomy (particularly for stone burden > 2 cm)
   - Combination of ESWL and percutaneous nephrostolithotomy
   - Open lithotomy (less common because of the success of less invasive treatment options)

7. **What is a steinstrasse?**
   Steinstrasse (German for "stone street") is a collection of small calculi that pile up together in the ureter and cause obstruction or symptoms. This problem may occur after lithotripsy treatment.

8. **What is a stent?**
   A stent is a small plastic catheter that coils in the renal pelvis, traverses the ureter, and coils in the bladder. Stents are useful to relieve ureteral obstruction temporarily and possibly facilitate stone passage after the stent is removed. Stents often cause some degree of ureteral dilatation after they have been removed.

9. **What is a metabolic evaluation? Who needs one?**
   A metabolic evaluation involves examining both serum and 24-hour urine specimens for factors that contribute to stone formation. The goals are to identify an abnormality and to treat it medically to prevent further stone formation. Indications for metabolic evaluation include recurrent stones, multiple stones, bilateral stones, stones in children, and non–calcium-containing stones.

10. **Can stones be dissolved?**
    - Uric acid stones often can be dissolved by alkalinizing the urine and with hydration therapy.
    - Cystine, struvite, and apatite stones sometimes can be dissolved.
    - Calcium stones cannot be dissolved.

BONUS QUESTIONS

11. **Is there any type of stone that cannot be seen on helical CT scan?**
    Patients taking indinavir sulfate (Crixivan) for HIV infection can form stones from the crystals of the medication; these stones are not seen on CT scan.

12. **What toxic substance can be produced by using the holmium:YAG laser on uric acid stones?**
    Cyanide is produced from the uric acid. Although this sounds frightening, it is never a problem.

WEB SITE

http://www.transplantation-soc.org

BIBLIOGRAPHY

1. Menon M, Resnick M: Urinary lithiasis: Etiology, diagnosis and medical management. In Walsh PC, Retik AB, Vaughan ED, Wein AJ et al (eds): Campbell's Urology, 8th ed. Philadelphia, W.B. Saunders, 2002, pp 3229–3305.
2. Teichman JM, Vassar GJ, Glickman RD: Holmium: YAG lithotripsy photothermal mechanism converts uric acid calculi to cyanide. J Urol 160:320–324, 1998.

CHAPTER 95

RENAL CELL CARCINOMA

Brett B. Abernathy, M.D.

1. **How common is renal cell carcinoma?**
   In the United States, 30,000 new cases of renal cell carcinoma are predicted for 2004 and 2005, about 3% of all adult malignancies.

2. **How is kidney cancer detected?**
   The classic triad of hematuria, flank pain, and an abdominal mass is used; however, this triad is found in only about 10% of cases. About 20% of renal cell carcinomas are associated with a paraneoplastic syndrome. Many solid renal tumors are detected incidentally by a computed tomography (CT) scan of the abdomen performed for another reason.

3. **Are all solid masses in the kidney renal cell carcinoma?**
   No. Other solid masses include angiomyolipomas, oncocytomas, sarcomas, and metastatic lesions. However, all solid masses should be presumed to be renal cell carcinoma until proven otherwise.

4. **What is the unique relationship between renal cell carcinoma and its vasculature?**
   Renal cell carcinoma has a tendency to invade its own venous drainage. Tumor thrombus may extend along the renal vein into the inferior vana cava and even to the right atrium.

5. **How should suspected involvement of the vena cava be evaluated?**
   Magnetic resonance imaging or venacavography.

6. **How is renal cell carcinoma treated?**
   Surgery is the optimal treatment for localized renal cell carcinoma. The standard operation is a radical nephrectomy, including everything within Gerota's fascia. Radical nephrectomy can also be performed laparoscopically or with hand-assisted laparoscopic techniques.

7. **Does the whole kidney have to be removed in all cases of renal cell carcinoma?**
   No. Nephron-sparing surgery can be performed in cases of bilateral renal cell carcinoma or renal cell carcinoma in a solitary kidney. Because of the risk of postoperative tumor recurrence, nephron-sparing surgery in the presence of a normal contralateral kidney is, at best, controversial.

8. **How is metastatic renal cell carcinoma treated?**
   Chemotherapy has been disappointing. The most encouraging results to date are with interleukin-2 (IL-2) treatment; some evidence of definite durable responses has been noted. Research is ongoing using IL-2 with other forms of immune-enhancing strategies. Some forms of adoptive immunothcrapy have been encouraging.

KEY POINTS: RENAL CELL CARCINOMA

1. The classic triad is hematuria, flank pain, and an abdominal mass; however, this traid is found in only 10% of cases.

2. Surgery is the optimal treatment for localized renal cell carcinoma.

3. Stauffer's syndrome is diagnosed with elevated liver function tests in the presence of renal cell carcinoma that normalize after nephrectomy and tumor removal; it is thought to be a type of paraneoplastic syndrome.

BONUS QUESTION

9. **What is Stauffer's syndrome?**
   It is diagnosed with elevated liver function tests (LFTs) in the presence of renal cell carcinoma that normalize after nephrectomy and tumor removal. It is thought to be a type of paraneoplastic syndrome.

WEB SITE

http://www.transplantjournal.com

BIBLIOGRAPHY

1. Figlin RA: Renal cell carcinoma: Management of advanced disease. J Urol 161:391, 1999.

2. Greenlee RT, Hill-Harmon MB, Murray T, Thun M: Cancer statistics 2001. CA Cancer J Clin 51:15–36, 2001.

3. Novick AC, Campbell SC: Renal tumors. In Walsh RC, Retik AB, Vaughan ED, et al (eds): Campbell's Urology, 8th ed. Philadelphia, W.B. Saunders, 2002, pp 2672–2731.

4. Resnick MI, Novick AC: Urology Secrets, 2nd ed. Philadelphia, Hanley & Belfus, 1999.

CHAPTER 96

BLADDER CANCER

Brett B. Abernathy, M.D.

1. **How common is bladder cancer?**
   Approximately 54,300 new cases of bladder cancer were diagnosed in 2001 in the United States, and 12,400 patients died. The male-to-female ratio is almost 3:1.

2. **What are the risk factors for bladder cancer?**
   Cigarette smoking, exposure to aniline dyes or aromatic amines, phenacetin abuse, and chemotherapy (cyclophosphamide).

3. **How does bladder cancer present?**
   Painless hematuria (gross or microscopic). Frequency, urgency, and dysuria also may be presenting symptoms, especially for carcinoma in situ (CIS).

4. **What is the most common histologic type of bladder cancer?**
   Transitional cell carcinoma (TCC) makes up > 90% of bladder cancers. Other histologic types include adenocarcinoma, squamous cell carcinoma, and urachal carcinoma.

5. **How is TCC of the bladder treated?**
   With transurethral resection of the bladder tumor. Further treatment is determined by the pathologic stage of the disease.

6. **Is CIS a less aggressive type of bladder cancer?**
   No. TCC in situ is a flat but poorly differentiated tumor. It can metastasize and should be treated as an aggressive form of bladder cancer.

7. **How is CIS treated?**
   Immunotherapy with intravesical bacillus Calmette-Guérin (BCG) is currently the first-line treatment. Response rates to BCG approach 70%. Other intravesical agents, such as mitomycin C, are generally less effective than BCG.

8. **What are the side effects of BCG?**
   Mild symptoms of urinary frequency, urgency, and dysuria are common. Myalgias and low-grade fever (flulike symptoms) also occur. High or persistent fever suggests a more serious problem requiring antituberculous therapy. Rarely, death from BCG has been reported.

9. **How is muscle-invasive bladder cancer treated?**
   Radical cystectomy (or cystoprostatectomy in men) with some form of urinary diversion.

10. **What types of urinary diversion are used with radical cystectomy?**
    Diversion techniques require either a conduit or a continent reservoir. The most common is an ileal conduit. An external collection device must be worn with a conduit. Continent reservoirs are made of combinations of large and small bowel and must be emptied via the urethra or a continent stoma.

KEY POINTS: BLADDER CANCER

1. Bladder cancer presents as painless hematuria.

2. The most common histologic type is transitional cell carcinoma.

3. Carcinoma in situ of the bladder is treated with intravesical bacillus Calmette-Guérin.

11. **How is metastatic bladder cancer treated?**
    Metastatic bladder cancer requires chemotherapy. Most regimens include a platinum-based agent.

12. **Can invasive bladder cancer be cured without removal of the entire bladder?**
    This issue is controversial. Some cancers may be suitable for partial cystectomy (i.e., tumors isolated in the dome of the bladder). Investigations are ongoing to evaluate transurethral resection of bladder tumor plus radiation and chemotherapy to try to preserve the bladder in invasive TCC.

BONUS QUESTIONS

13. **In certain countries, TCC is not the predominant form of bladder cancer. What is the predominant histologic type? Why?**
    In countries such as Egypt, where schistosomiasis is endemic, squamous cell carcinoma of the bladder is common.

14. **Can any markers be used to help predict the prognosis of TCC?**
    The p53 tumor suppressor protein may be helpful in assessing the biologic behavior of the tumor and can assist with treatment option decisions. Monoclonal antibody MIB-1 may also be useful in predicting outcome for stage T2 or grade 2 tumors.

WEB SITE

http://www.transplantation-soc.org

BIBLIOGRAPHY

1. Greenlee RT, Hill-Harmon MB, Murray T, Thun M: Cancer statistics 2001. CA Cancer J Clin 51:15–36, 2001.

2. Herr HW, Bajorn DF, Scher HL: Can p53 help select patients with invasive bladder cancer for bladder preservation? J Urol 161:20, 1999.

3. Messing EM: Urothelial tumors of the urinary tract. In Walsh PC, Retik AB, Vaughan ED, et al (eds): Campbell's Urology, 8th ed. Philadelphia, W.B. Saunders, 2002, pp 2732–2784.

4. Resnick MI, Novick AC: Urology Secrets, 2nd ed. Philadelphia, Hanley & Belfus, 1999.

CHAPTER 97

PROSTATE CANCER

Brett B. Abernathy, M.D.

1. **How common is prostate cancer?**
   It is the most common malignancy diagnosed in men in the United States; almost 200,000 new cases were diagnosed in 2001.

2. **Do most men die with prostate cancer, rather than from it?**
   Yes, but approximately 31,500 men died of prostate cancer in 2001 in the United States. Thus, it should not be treated as benign.

3. **What are the early symptoms of prostate cancer?**
   There are none. By the time significant symptoms develop, the disease is likely to be advanced. This is an argument for screening to detect prostate cancer.

4. **What is the best screening method for prostate cancer?**
   Digital rectal examination (DRE) combined with serum prostate-specific antigen (PSA). Since PSA testing was introduced, there has been a stage migration with less metastatic disease and more local-regional disease being detected.

5. **How is prostate cancer diagnosed?**
   It is diagnosed with prostate biopsy, which is a biopsy using transrectal ultrasound for guidance. Many cancers are discovered incidentally at transurethral resection of the prostate (TURP) for benign prostatic hyperplasia (BPH).

6. **When is prostate biopsy indicated?**
   When either the PSA or DRE result is abnormal.

KEY POINTS: PROSTATE CANCER

1. Prostate cancer is the most common malignancy diagnosed in men in the United States.

2. The best screening method is a combination of digital rectal exam and serum prostate-specific antigen.

3. Clinically localized prostate cancer is treated with surgery, radiation, cryotherapy, or watchful waiting.

7. **Does an elevated PSA level mean a man has prostate cancer?**
   No. PSA can be elevated with BPH, prostatitis, or after prostate trauma. It is prostate specific, not prostate cancer specific.

8. **What is a free PSA?**
   Free PSA is the percentage of PSA that is not bound to a serum protein carrier. The ratio of free to total PSA is helpful in determining when to do a prostate biopsy. "Free"

is good because a higher ratio of free to total PSA is less likely to represent a prostate cancer.

9. **Are there any known risk factors for prostate cancer?**
   Yes. African-American men and men with a family history of prostate cancer are at an increased risk. A high-fat diet may play a role in increasing risk of many cancers, including prostate cancer.

10. **What is Gleason's sum?**
    It's a score that the pathologist gives prostate cancer to estimate its aggressiveness. The two predominant patterns of cancer are scored 1 to 5, and the sum is, therefore, between 2 and 10. Tumors can be well differentiated (2, 3, 4), moderately differentiated (5, 6, 7), or poorly differentiated (8, 9, 10).

11. **How is clinically localized prostate cancer treated?**
    Surgery (radical prostatectomy), radiation therapy by external beam or interstitial seed implant, cryotherapy, or watchful waiting.

12. **How is advanced metastatic prostate cancer treated?**
    Hormonal ablation therapy (orchiectomy or luteinizing hormone-releasing hormone agonist drugs) or chemotherapy, but these treatments are palliative and not curative.

13. **What is the best treatment for prostate cancer?**
    This is highly controversial. Patients must weigh factors such as age, overall health, grade and stage of the disease, and risk of side effects versus complications from the various treatment options.

WEB SITE

http://www.transplantation-soc.org

BIBLIOGRAPHY

1. Catalona WJ: Clinical utility of free and total prostate specific antigen. Rev Prostate 7(suppl):64–69, 1996.
2. D'Amico AV, Whittington R, Malkowicz SB, et al: Biochemical outcome after radical prostatectomy, external beam radiation therapy, or interstitial radiation therapy for clinically localized prostate cancer. JAMA 280:969, 1998.
3. Greenlee RT, Hill-Harmon MB, Murray T, Thun M: Cancer statistics 2001. CA Cancer J Clin 51:15–36, 2001.
4. Keetch DW, Humphrey PA, et al: Clinical and pathological features of hereditary prostate cancer. J Urol 155:1841–1842, 1996.
5. Polascik TJ, Pound CR, et al: Comparison of radical prostatectomy and iodine-125 interstitial radiotherapy for the treatment of clinically localized prostate cancer: A 7-year biochemical (PSA) progression analysis. Urology 51:884–890, 1998.
6. Resnick MI, Novick AC: Urology Secrets, 2nd ed. Philadelphia, Hanley & Belfus, 1999.
7. Reiter RE, deKernion JB: Epidemiology, etiology, and prevention of prostate cancer. In Walsh PC, Retik AB, Vaughan ED, et al (eds): Campbell's Urology, 8th ed. Philadelphia, W.B. Saunders, 2002, pp 3003–3024.

URODYNAMICS AND VOIDING DYSFUNCTION

Firouz Daneshgari, M.D.

CHAPTER 98

1. **What is urodynamics?**
   Urodynamic studies assess the functional aspects of the storage and emptying ability of the lower urinary tract (LUT). The principles of urodynamic studies originated from hydrodynamics. The components of urodynamic studies are cystometrogram, leak point pressures, urethral profile pressures, pressure-flow studies, uroflowmetry, and electromyography. These studies have evolved into videourodynamics with the addition of fluoroscopy (i.e., video).

2. **What is uroflowmetry?**
   Uroflowmetry is the measurement of voided urine (in milliliters) per unit of time (in seconds). The important elements of the test are voided volume (which should be > 150 mL), maximum flow rate (Q_{max}), and the curve of the flow (which should be bell shaped). The normal Q_{max} is > 20 mL/sec in men and > 25 mL/sec in women.

3. **What is benign prostatic hyperplasia (BPH)?**
   BPH is benign enlargement of the prostate gland that may lead to bladder outlet obstructive symptoms in men. These symptoms have recently been termed lower urinary tract symptoms (LUTS).

4. **What is an American Urological Association (AUA) symptom score?**
   It is a self-reported questionnaire developed and popularized by the AUA for the assessment of bothersome LUTS in men. This questionnaire has seven questions with a maximum score of 35. The higher the score, the more severe and bothersome the symptoms. The AUA symptom score has become an index for both the diagnosis and evaluation of treatment outcome in patients with LUTS.

5. **What are the main functions of the LUT?**
   Storage and emptying of urine are the main functions. For practical purposes, all symptoms of LUT dysfunction can be categorized into the malfunction of either storing or emptying ability.

6. **What are the control mechanisms for LUT function?**
   The control mechanisms for LUT function are recognized as central and peripheral. The central control mechanisms consist of the cortical portion of the frontal lobe of the brain and pontine micturition center. The peripheral control mechanisms include the thoracic sympathetic and lumbar parasympathetic innervation and neuromuscular apparatus of the LUT organs.

7. **What is the role of the autonomic nervous system in the function of the LUT?**
   Sympathetic fibers, which originate from the T10–L2 portion of the spinal cord, innervate the bladder neck and proximal urethra. These fibers mostly control the contraction of the proximal urethra or bladder neck and relaxation of the bladder, which results in storage of urine. The parasympathetic fibers, which originate primarily from the S2–S4 portion of the spinal cord, innervate the bladder body. The parasympathetic innervation allows contraction of the bladder smooth muscle, leading to bladder emptying.

8. **What is the role of the somatic nervous system in the function of the LUT?**
Voluntary control of the striated muscle of the external urinary sphincter is controlled by the somatic nervous system. Somatic fibers are conveyed to the sphincter by the pudendal nerve.

9. **What is bulbocavernosal reflex?**
Bulbocavernosal reflex tests the integrity of peripheral neurologic control of the LUT. This reflex is elicited by stimulation of the glans penis in men or the clitoris in women, which causes contraction of the external anal sphincter or bulbocavernosus muscle. Alternatively, the reflex may be stimulated by pulling the balloon of a Foley catheter against the bladder neck. This reflex is present in all normal men and in approximately 70% of normal women. Absence of this reflex in a man is strongly suggestive of a sacral neurologic lesion.

10. **What is the most common cause of incontinence in the geriatric population?**
The most common are transient causes, mostly external, that disrupt the fragile balance of LUT function in elderly patients and cause urinary incontinence. These causes can be recalled with the mnemonic **DIAPPERS**:
Delirium
Infections
Atrophic urethritis or vaginitis
Pharmaceuticals
Psychological (depression)
Endocrine (hypercalcemia, hyperglycemia)
Restricted mobility
Stool impaction

KEY POINTS: URODYNAMICS AND VOIDING FUNCTION

1. Uroflowmetry is the measurement of voided urine (in milliliters) per unit of time (in seconds).

2. Benign prostatic hypertrophy is benign enlargement of the prostate gland that may lead to bladder outlet obstructive symptoms in men.

3. The sacral roots involved in micturition physiology are S2-S4.

11. **What is spinal shock? What type of urinary dysfunction does it cause?**
Spinal shock is the loss of contractility of the smooth muscle below the level of spinal cord injury, leading to difficulty in bladder emptying or urinary retention. This phenomenon may last from hours to several months with a high chance of reversibility if the spinal cord injury is not permanent.

12. **What is autonomic dysreflexia? How is it treated?**
Autonomic dysreflexia results from systematic outpouring of sympathetic discharge, as in patients with spinal cord lesions at or above the T6 level. This dysreflexia is triggered by distention of the bladder or other stimulus of the bowel or LUT. It is manifested by hypertension, bradycardia, hot flush, sweating, and headache. Initial treatment consists of removal of the stimulus, such as emptying the bladder and placing the patient in a sitting position. Nifedipine or nitroprusside may be used as either prophylaxis or treatment of severe episodes. This condition may lead to significant cerebrovascular complication if untreated.

13. **What type of bladder dysfunction is seen in diabetic patients?**
Diabetic cystopathy is manifested primarily as atonic bladder with difficulty in emptying caused by impaired contractility of the bladder or detrusor muscle.

14. **What type of bladder dysfunction is seen in patients with multiple sclerosis (MS)?**
Urgency (83%), urge incontinence (75%), detrusor hyperreflexia (62%), and detrusor sphincter dyssynergia (25%) are among the most common LUT symptoms in patients with MS. Variation in symptoms depends on the site of involvement by MS. Involvement of pontine pathways (tegmentum) is associated with a much higher rate of urinary symptoms.

15. **Which sacral roots control the micturition physiology?**
S2–S4.

16. **What are the causes of urinary retention after abdominal or pelvic surgery?**
They are injuries or disruption of pelvic plexus innervation to the LUT.

17. **What is Ogilvie's syndrome?**
Acute massive dilatation of the cecum and ascending and transverse colon without organic obstruction is known as Ogilvie's syndrome. This syndrome can be seen in pelvic urologic surgeries, possibly as a result of an imbalance in parasympathetic stimulation of the colon.

18. **What is reflex versus psychic erection?**
Erection after local stimulation is termed reflex erection. The afferent nerves for reflex erection run in the pudendal nerves, and the efferent fibers are found in the S2–S4 parasympathetic outflow. The psychic erection is caused by stimulation of cerebral erotic centers. The afferent stimuli for psychic erection travel through the thoracolumbar sympathetic outflow and sacral parasympathetic fibers.

WEB SITE

http://www.transplantation-soc.org

BIBLIOGRAPHY

1. Bross S, Braun PM, Michel MS, et al: Preoperatively evaluated bladder wall tension as a prognostic parameter for postoperative success after surgery for bladder outlet obstruction. Urol 61:562–566, 2003.

2. Holtgrewe HL: Current trends in management of men with lower urinary tract symptoms and benign prostatic hyperplasia. Urology 51(suppl 4A):1–7, 1998.

3. Litwiller SE, Forhman EM, Zimmern PE: Multiple sclerosis and the urologist. J Urol 161:743–757, 1999.

4. Mochrer B, Carey M, Wilson D: Laparoscopic colposuspension: A systematic review. Br J Obstet Gynaecol 110:230–235, 2003.

5. Resnick NM, Yalla SV: Geriatric incontinence and voiding dysfunction. In Walsh PC, Retik AB, Vaughan ED, et al (eds): Campbell's Urology, 7th ed. Philadelphia, W.B. Saunders, 1998.

6. Steers WD, Barrett DM, Wein AJ: Voiding dysfunction, diagnosis, classification and management. In Gillenwater JY, Grayhack JT, Howards SS, Duckett JW (eds): Adult and Pediatric Urology, 3rd ed. St. Louis, Mosby, 1996.

7. Wang CC, Yang SS, Chen YT, Hsieh JH: Videourodynamics identifies the causes of young men with lower urinary tract symptoms and low uroflow. Eur Urol 43:386–390, 2003.

CHAPTER 99

PEDIATRIC UROLOGY

Kirstan K. Meldrum, M.D., and Mark P. Cain, M.D.

1. **A healthy 3-year-old girl develops a urinary tract infection (UTI). How should she be evaluated?**

   After treatment of the infection, the patient should undergo a urinary tract evaluation (this recommendation stands even in a little girl after only one UTI). Evaluation includes a renal-bladder sonogram and voiding cystourethrogram (VCUG). Approximately 50% of children younger than age 12 years who present with a UTI are found to have abnormalities of the genitourinary tract. The most common abnormalities identified are vesicoureteral reflux, obstructive uropathies, and neurogenic bladder.

2. **What is vesicoureteral reflux (VUR) disease?**

   With VUR, urine refluxes from the bladder into the upper urinary tract. Primary VUR is caused by an inadequate valvular mechanism at the ureterovesical junction, presumably related to a shortened submucosal ureteral tunnel. One half of children with culture-documented UTIs have VUR.

3. **Is VUR bad?**

   Sterile reflux is unlikely to cause renal damage; however, persistent reflux of infected urine leads to pyelonephritis and progressive renal scarring. Currently, renal scarring is the fourth leading cause for renal transplantation in children. The combination of VUR and elevated bladder storage pressures (e.g., neuropathic bladder or bladder outlet obstruction) is particularly harmful to the kidney.

4. **What are the indications for surgical correction of VUR?**

   Reflux disappears spontaneously in many children; however, high-grade reflux, especially when bilateral, is unlikely to resolve spontaneously. Children with high-grade reflux or breakthrough UTIs despite antibiotic prophylaxis should be managed surgically. Surgical management is also appropriate in children with reflux persisting into late childhood or adolescence.

5. **What is the most common cause of antenatal hydronephrosis?**

   Ureteropelvic junction (UPJ) obstruction. Hydronephrosis is the most common abnormality detected on prenatal ultrasound and accounts for 50% of all prenatally detected lesions. Fifty percent of prenatal hydronephrosis, in turn, is caused by UPJ obstruction. UPJ obstruction is bilateral in approximately 20% of cases and is associated with VUR in 15% of cases.

6. **What is the most common cause of UPJ obstruction?**

   Intrinsic stenosis. Less common causes include lower pole (of the kidney) crossing vessels, anomalous ureteral insertions, and peripelvic fibrosis.

7. **Can UPJ obstruction resolve spontaneously? What are the indications for pyeloplasty?**

   Yes, it can resolve spontaneously. Ultimately, only about 25% of children with evidence of UPJ obstruction require pyeloplasty. The indications for surgical intervention include worsening hydronephrosis, poor or declining renal function, pain, and the presence of a solitary kidney or bilateral hydronephrosis.

8. **What is the Meyer-Weigert law?**
    This law refers to the position of the ureteral orifices in patients with complete ureteral duplication. Occasionally, two ureteral buds develop independently from the mesonephric duct. As the ureteral buds are absorbed into the developing bladder, the bud located in a lower position along the duct (draining the lower pole of the kidney) is carried to a more cranial and lateral position. The ureteral bud located in a higher position along the duct (draining the upper pole of the kidney) is carried to a more caudal and medial position within the bladder. Lower pole ureters are more likely to reflux because of their lateral position within the bladder; however, upper pole ureters are more frequently obstructed and are more often associated with a ureterocele.

9. **What is a ureterocele?**
    A ureterocele is a cystic dilatation of the distal portion of the ureter. Ureteroceles are usually associated with the upper pole ureter of a duplicated collecting system; however, they also may develop from single ureters. They are usually ectopic (i.e., some portion of the ureterocele is positioned at the bladder neck or urethra) and frequently cause ureteral obstruction.

10. **What is an ectopic ureter?**
    A ureter with an ectopic opening at the level of the bladder neck or more caudally.

KEY POINTS: PEDIATRIC UROLOGY

1. The most common cause of antenatal hydronephrosis is ureteropelvic junction obstruction.

2. A ureterocele is a cystic dilatation of the distal portion of the ureter.

3. The most common location of an undescended testicle is the inguinal canal.

4. The most common cause of ambiguous genitalia in newborns is congenital adrenal hyperplasia, most commonly due to 21-hydroxylase deficiency.

11. **What is the most common presenting symptom in a girl with an ectopic ureter?**
    Incontinence. In females, an ectopic ureter will usually drain into the bladder neck, proximal urethra, or vestibule. The orifice also may be located in the vagina (25%) and, occasionally, the uterus. When the ectopic ureteral orifice is positioned below the external sphincter or within the female genital tract, incontinence can develop.

12. **Do boys with ectopic ureters present with incontinence?**
    No. The ectopic pathway in boys extends from the bladder neck through the posterior urethra to the mesonephric duct derivatives (i.e., vas deferens, epididymis, and seminal vesicle). Therefore, the ectopic ureteral orifice is always positioned above the continence mechanism.

13. **What percentage of full-term male infants have an undescended testicle?**
    Three percent. This number decreases to 0.8% by age 1 year.

14. **What is the most common location of an undescended testicle?**
    The inguinal canal (72% of undescended testicles). The testicle also may be located in the abdomen (8%) or prescrotal area (20%). Twenty percent of undescended testicles are nonpalpable at presentation; of these, 50% are absent completely.

15. **Why should the testicle be brought back into the scrotum?**
    Patients with cryptorchidism have a 40-fold increased risk of germ cell cancer compared with the normal population. Although positioning of the testicle within the scrotum does not

alleviate this risk, it does permit routine, thorough testicular examination. Patients with cryptorchidism also are at risk for infertility. Histologic studies have demonstrated progressive germ cell loss in the undescended testicle beginning at age 18 months. Early orchiopexy can minimize the extent of germ cell loss and thereby decrease the chance of future infertility. In general, the higher the testicle (i.e., within the abdomen), the greater the risk of cancer and infertility.

16. **What is the most common cause of bladder outlet obstruction in boys? In girls?**
Posterior urethral valves and ureterocele, respectively.

17. **What are the urinary manifestations of posterior urethral valves?**
Posterior urethral valves are congenital leaflets of tissue that extend from the verumontanum to the anterior urethra in boys. They occur at an incidence of 1 in 8000 live male births. Posterior urethral valves cause bladder outlet obstruction, which, in turn, leads to variable degrees of bladder and renal injury. Severe obstruction may result in oligohydramnios, pulmonary hypoplasia, bladder hypertrophy, vesicoureteral reflux, hydroureteronephrosis, and renal dysplasia. Fifty percent of affected children have reflux, and 33% of them progress to end-stage renal disease.

18. **What is a myelomeningocele? What are its urologic consequences?**
A myelomeningocele is a hernial protrusion of the spinal cord and its meninges through a defect in the vertebral column. The resulting neurologic injury causes, among other problems, bladder dysfunction. Patients with myelomeningocele usually are incontinent because of detrusor hyperactivity, detrusor hypoactivity, poor bladder compliance, inadequate outlet resistance, detrusor-outlet dyssynergy, or a combination of these factors. More importantly, patients with hyperactive, high-pressure bladders may develop upper urinary tract deterioration. Life-long follow-up is necessary because the neurologic lesion can change with time. Treatment goals include maintenance of a low-pressure urinary reservoir, prevention of urinary tract infections, prevention of upper urinary tract deterioration, and the achievement of continence.

19. **What is the most common cause of ambiguous genitalia in newborns?**
Congenital adrenal hyperplasia, most commonly caused by a 21-hydroxylase deficiency.

20. **What diagnostic evaluation should be performed in any male infant presenting with hypospadias and cryptorchidism?**
The presence of cryptorchidism and hypospadias should alert the physician to the possibility of an androgenized female. A karyotype should always be obtained before urogenital reconstruction.

21. **What is the most common solid renal mass in infancy? In childhood?**
In **infancy**, it is congential mesoblastic nephroma. This is a benign tumor of the kidney that can be managed with surgical excision alone.

In **childhood**, it is a Wilms' tumor. Wilms' tumor is associated with Beckwith-Wiedemann syndrome, isolated hemihypertrophy, and congenital aniridia. The most important prognostic factors are tumor stage and histology. Treatment is multimodal, consisting of surgery, chemotherapy, and radiation.

WEB SITE

http://www.transplantation-soc.org

BIBLIOGRAPHY

1. Baker LA, Silver RI, Docimo SG: Cryptorchidism. In Gearhart JP, Rink RC, Mouriquand PDE (eds): Pediatric Urology. Philadelphia, W.B. Saunders, 2001, pp 738–753.

2. Cooper CS, Snyder HM: Ureteral duplication, ectopy, and ureteroceles. In Gearhart JP, Rink RC, Mouriquand PDE (eds): Pediatric Urology. Philadelphia, W.B. Saunders, 2001, pp 430–452.

3. Dinneen MD, Duffy PG: Posterior urethral valves. Br J Urol 78:275–281, 1996.

4. Docimo SG: The results of surgical therapy for cryptorchidism: A literature review and analysis. J Urol 154:1148, 1995.

5. Elder JS, Peters CA, Arant BS Jr, et al: Pediatric vesicoureteral reflux guidelines panel summary report on the management of primary vesicoureteral reflux in children. J Urol 157:1846–1851, 1997.

6. Gill B, Kogan S: Cryptorchidism. Current concepts. Pediatr Clin North Am 44:1211–1227, 1997.

7. Gunther DF, Bukowski TP: Congenital adrenal hyperplasia: A spectrum of disorders. Contemp Urol 11:52–69, 1999.

8. Kirsch AJ, Escala J, Duckett JW, et al: Surgical management of the nonpalpable testis: The Children's Hospital of Philadelphia experience. J Urol 159:1340–1343, 1998.

9. Pohl HG, Rushton HG: The diagnosis and management of urinary tract infection in children. AUA Update Series 17:242–247, 1998.

10. Poppas DP, Bauer SB: Urologic evaluation of the myelodysplastic child. AUA Update Series 16:282–287, 1997.

11. Reddy PR, Mandell J: Ureteropelvic junction obstruction: Prenatal diagnosis; therapeutic implications. Urol Clin North Am 25:171–195, 1998.

12. Snyder HM: Anomalies of the ureter. In Gillenwater JY, Grayhack JT, Howards SS, Duckett JW (eds): Adult and Pediatric Urology, 3rd ed. St. Louis, Mosby, 1996, pp 2197–2228.

13. Strand WR: Urinary infection in children: Pathogenesis, bacterial virulence, and host resistance. In Gonzales ET, Bauer SB (eds): Pediatric Urology Practice. Baltimore, Lippincott Williams & Wilkins, 1999, pp 433–462.

CAN HEALTH CARE BE REFORMED?

Alden H. Harken, M.D.

CHAPTER 100

1. **Is health care reform an oxymoron?**
   Yes.

2. **What is fee for service?**
   The doctor establishes the price, and the patient agrees to pay it. This traditional system of exchange has great merit if both parties understand the value of the service provided. If either party (usually the patient) cannot estimate the service value, it is possible (even likely) that the doctor will honestly escalate the service value in a fashion unchecked by the patient's perceptions. Thus, in a fee-for-service system, medical prices tend to increase.

3. **What is discounted fee for service?**
   The patient gets together with a group of friends, and they come to the doctor with the following proposition: "Hey, Doc, you can dazzle us with your fancy medical talk, but we still think that your prices are too high. How about my pals and me will pay you 80% of what you charge us?"

4. **Is there a difference between hospital costs and hospital charges?**
   Absolutely. Hospital cost is the sum of the expenses (e.g., sutures, nurses' salaries, electricity, instrumentation sterilization, Band-Aids) that are expended in suturing a laceration, for example. The hospital typically charges about twice the cost (100% markup) for repairing a cut finger. This markup is highly industry specific. Thus, whereas intensely competitive food chains may make a profit of only 1 penny on a loaf of bread, hospitals and liquor stores usually charge twice the cost.

5. **What are fixed costs?**
   After accounting for light, heat, and staff (nurses, housekeepers, administrators) at a hospital but before seeing a single patient, doctors and the hospital have already spent a huge amount of money. Doctors and hospitals must pay fixed costs whether or not they provide any medical services at all.

6. **What are actual costs?**
   These are the incremental costs of actually providing a service in a hospital (in addition to the fixed costs of light and heat). For example, a patient shows up in the emergency department at midnight complaining of a lump on the tip of his nose. The doctor, with characteristic erudition, says, "Yep, you have a wart on your nose," and sends the patient home with a bill for $500. The actual cost of this encounter is obviously negligible. The patient is really paying for the fixed costs of nurses and emergency resuscitative equipment should he have a cardiac arrest.

7. **Is hospital accounting a precisely scientific and objective analysis of financial data?**
   No.

8. **What is health insurance?**
   Traditionally, people can purchase insurance that may pay either all or a portion of their hospital and physician charges if they become ill. Insurance companies make a profit, therefore, only

if the patient stays healthy. Insurance companies have elaborate tables to predict who will get sick, and they prefer to sell policies exclusively to young, healthy individuals. This practice is termed "skimming." The insurance company takes all of the risk—and they like to keep it low. Conversely, hospitals must cover fixed costs—and the more expensive (and more frequent) the health care that physicians provide, the better it is for the hospitals.

9. **What are health maintenance organizations (HMOs)?**
    HMOs are complex systems composed, in their most comprehensive form, of hospitals, doctors plus offices, and an insurance company. HMOs contract with large groups of people (potential patients) to maintain their health. Enrollees pay a monthly fee (just like health insurance) so that all hospital and physician charges are covered if the enrollees become ill. Unlike health insurance, however, in the HMO model, hospitals and physicians get paid whether or not the enrollee gets sick. So, it is better for everyone if enrollees stay healthy—and out of the hospital.

10. **Initially, a lot of physicians did not like HMOs. Why?**
    Because physicians are fiercely independent. They did not want a bunch of business managers telling them how to manage patients.

11. **Why are physicians fiercely independent?**
    We were probably born that way.

12. **Is that good?**
    Probably not. Eventually, everyone will need to work together and not hit each other when they are mad.

13. **Do HMO administrators really dictate how physicians manage their patients?**
    Yes and no. Physicians have developed medically effective and optimally efficient strategies—termed clinical pathways—for caring for many common illnesses. Although physicians must treat each patient individually, when we adhere to predetermined treatment guidelines (as encouraged by HMO administrators), patients usually get better faster and cheaper.

14. **Do physicians follow these clinical pathways?**
    Traditionally, no.

15. **What do HMO managers do?**
    They evaluate each physician's utilization of expensive resources (within the predetermined clinical pathways) relative to the health of the physician's patients.

16. **Do physicians welcome this kind of scrutiny?**
    No.

17. **What is a preferred provider organization (PPO)?**
    A PPO is a group of doctors who have elected to remain legally independent of a hospital and insurance company (if they joined together, they would be an HMO) and, most of all, patients. But PPOs maintain their independence as physicians, even though most PPOs require administrators to coordinate programs, keep the books, and keep the doctors from hitting each other. PPOs have the perception of independence, however.

18. **Is health care expensive?**
    Unfortunately, yes. Physicians argue that patients pay a lot but also get a lot. In the United States, patients expect unlimited access to liver transplantation and magnetic resonance imaging (MRI) for every headache. Americans believe that fancy, expensive health care is not just a privilege—it is a right.

19. **So what is the problem?**
The chief executive officers (CEOs) of big American corporations argue that the obligatory expense of health care is driving up the cost of U.S. products and making American companies less competitive in the global market—there is more health care than steel in a new Chevrolet.

20. **Does big business have a solution?**
They think so. The CEOs still want unlimited access to the most modern health care for themselves and their families. Without sounding cynical, the CEOs want to save health care dollars spent on their employees and "other people's families." They want to limit access to health care, but they do not want to wield the ax personally. So they developed the idea of capitation.

21. **What is capitation?**
The CEOs of large businesses come to hospitals, HMOs, or PPOs and say: "Why don't you provide all health care for all my employees at a fixed price, say, $180 per month per head?" (hence, capitation). In this model, physicians make the decisions about who gets how much medical care (satisfying their urge for independence), but they also promise to provide all necessary medical care for a prearranged price. Thus, they take all of the risk. CEOs like this model because they can still offer health care as an employee benefit and budget the cost in advance.

22. **Why do physicians not like capitation?**
All of a sudden physicians may have acquired a little more independence than they bargained for. Now they are paid in advance so that all costs of patients' health care are subtracted from the money they negotiated up front. Now they must advise against an MRI for every headache and break the news to Granny that she will not think better if they dialyze her blood urea nitrogen down to 50. This is the reverse of the good old days when physicians were rewarded if their patients got sick and stayed sick. Physicians could ply them with a smorgasbord of drugs and technologies. Now physicians are trying to control health care costs.

23. **Is all this change good?**
Absolutely. Medicine has always changed—and the faster, the better. Physicians were initially attracted to medicine as an intellectually stimulating discipline because medicine and surgery evolve rapidly.

24. **Can physicians keep up with all this change?**
Absolutely.

25. **Despite all of the medical Chicken Littles who sonorously declare that the sky is falling, is medicine (and even more clearly, surgery) still the most gratifying, stimulating, and rewarding profession?**
Absolutely.

BIBLIOGRAPHY

1. Blumenthal D: Controlling health care expenditures. N Engl J Med 344:766–769, 2001.
2. Dudley RA, Luft HS: Managed care in transition. N Engl J Med 344:1087–1092, 2001.
3. Fuchs VR: What's ahead for health insurance in the United States? N Engl J Med 346:1822–1824, 2002.
4. Iglehart JK: Changing health insurance trends. N Engl J Med 347:956–962, 2002.
5. Schroeder SA: Prospects for expanding health insurance coverage. N Engl J Med 344:847–852, 2001.
6. Wilensky GR: Medicare reform—now is the time. N Engl J Med 345:458–462, 2001.
7. Wood AJ: When increased therapeutic benefit comes at increased cost. N Engl J Med 346:1819–1821, 2002.
8. Wright JG: Hidden barriers to improvement in the quality of health care. N Engl J Med 346:1096, 2002.

CHAPTER 101

RISKS OF BLOODBORNE DISEASE

Caesar M. Ursic, M.D., and Doru I. E. Georgescu, M.D.

1. **What infectious diseases are transmissible via blood transfusion?**
   In developed nations with mature blood banking systems, by far the most common transfusion-acquired infections are hepatitis from the hepatitis B (HBV) and C (HCV) viruses. Other less commonly transmitted agents include the human immunodeficiency virus (HIV) and cytomegalovirus (CMV). Even rarer but still occasionally reported bloodborne infections are parasitic diseases such as malaria (genus, *Plasmodium*), babesiosis (genus, *Babesium*), Chagas disease (*Trypanosoma cruzi*), toxoplasmosis (*Toxoplasma gondii*), the lymphomas and leukemias caused by the human T-cell lymphotropic virus (HTLV-I), and infectious mononucleosis (Epstein-Barr virus). Bacterial contaminations are also rare but possible, especially in platelet preparations that are stored at room temperature. This may result in a toxic shock–like syndrome, the risk of which has been estimated as equivalent to the risk of HIV transmission.

2. **What are the estimated risks of HBV, HCV, and HIV transmission by blood transfusion in the United States?**
   Hepatitis B (HBV):   1 in 205,000
   Hepatitis C (HCV):   1 in 1,935,000
   HIV: 1 in 2,135,000 (expressed as the risk of seroconversion per transfused unit of allogenic blood)

3. **Which bloodborne pathogens pose a risk to surgeons?**
   Although the epidemic of HIV has increased general concern about bloodborne pathogens, the prevalence of hepatitis C virus (HCV) throughout North America has led to a shift of emphasis from HIV to hepatitis. Hepatitis B is an occupational risk in surgery, but vaccinations and a relatively efficient post-exposure protocol have reduced the consequences of contamination with HBV. Surgeons in the United States care for more patients with chronic hepatitis C than with chronic hepatitis B, and no vaccine is available for HCV infection. Although the rate of seroconversion for hepatitis C is 10% versus 30% for hepatitis B, when acute infection occurs, there is a much higher chance of developing chronic hepatitis (50% versus 10%) after HCV infection. Thus, HCV infection is the greatest threat to surgeons.

4. **What is the risk to health care workers of exposure to HBV?**
   The number of new infections in 2001 has dropped to approximately 78,000 from the estimated yearly incidence of 260,000 in the 1980s. At present, 1.25 million U.S. residents have chronic hepatitis B, with the highest prevalence occurring among 20–49-year-old individuals. Thirty percent of percutaneous hollow needle exposures are followed by acute infection. Thirty percent of hepatitis B cases are clinically occult, and ≤ 10% of infected people remain viral carriers for life. Many carriers are asymptomatic and suffer no active liver disease, although they are potentially infectious to others. Twenty-five percent of HBV-infected individuals eventually die from hepatic diseases.

5. **What is the risk to health care workers of exposure to HCV?**
   The number of new infections in 2001 was 25,000, down from 240,000 per year in the 1980s. Currently, 3.9 million (1.8%) U.S. residents have HCV infection, of whom 2.7 million are infected

chronically. The risk of seroconversion from a percutaneous hollow needle injury is 10%, but 90% of acute infections result in the chronic carrier state, which is typically asymptomatic. Although these data are still controversial, 50% of HCV infected patients will develop cirrhosis, and 50% of these patients will develop a hepatoma.

6. **What is the risk to health care workers of exposure to HIV?**
The risk of HIV seroconversion after percutaneous inoculation with HIV-contaminated blood is approximately 0.3%. Risk of infection also appears to be greater when the source of the blood is a terminally or severely ill patient. The U.S. Centers for Disease Control and Prevention (CDC) reports that 57 health care workers in the U.S. have been documented as seroconverting to HIV as a result of an occupational exposure to the virus. The majority of these individuals were either nurses (n = 24) or laboratory workers (n = 19); physicians accounted for only six of these cases. The routes of infection were percutaneous (puncture or cutting wounds) in 84% of the cases. Thus, the risk appears small relative to the large number of exposures that have probably occurred since the onset of the epidemic in the early 1980s. The CDC also reports that as of January 1, 1998, there has been no documented transmission of HIV infection from a patient to a surgeon secondary to occupational exposure.

7. **How well does hepatitis B vaccination protect against the disease?**
Effective protection against hepatitis B correlates positively with post-immunization anti-hepatitis B surface antibody (anti-HBs) serum titers of ≥ 10 mIU/mL. These titers are achieved in 95% of young, healthy recipients of the standard three-dose immunization regimen, and the actual protective efficacy (i.e., ability of the vaccine to prevent the disease) is estimated to approach 100% in these individuals. Although about 50% of successfully vaccinated adults demonstrate a decrease in their anti-HBs levels to nondetectable levels by 10 years, continued immunologic protection is thought to persist via the amnestic humoral response. Because of the persistence of this "immune memory" to the viral antigen, healthy individuals appear to enjoy lifelong protection after vaccination and do not require booster doses. A bivalent vaccine immunizing against both hepatitis A and B was approved in 2001 by the U.S. Food and Drug Administration for individuals 18 years of age and older, and it is as successful as the monovalent vaccine in conferring protection from the HBV infection with the added benefit of protecting against hepatitis A viral infection.

8. **Are patients at risk of infection from surgeons who are infected with HBV?**
Transmission of hepatitis B infection from surgeons to patients has been documented. Surgeons who are at risk for transmitting infection to patients are generally positive for the e-antigen of hepatitis B. The e-antigen is a degradation product of the nucleocapsid of the virus and represents active viral replication within the liver. People who test positive for the e-antigen have high viral titers and are quite infectious. The large number of documented transmissions of HBV to patients by surgical providers is particularly troublesome and may require restriction of clinical privileges. Furthermore, a recent report from England documented transmission of HBV infection from surgeons to patients even when the surgeon was negative for the e-antigen.

9. **What is the proper response after percutaneous exposure to a patient with known hepatitis B?**
This depends on the provider's vaccination status. Older individuals show a tendency to mount a weaker or delayed immunologic response as measured by peak serum titers of anti-HBs. If the provider has been vaccinated and has a positive antibody titer, no additional response is necessary. If the provider has not been vaccinated and is negative for antibodies to HBV or if the provider completed the series of vaccinations but exhibited a weak or absent antibody titer, then he or she should receive a dose of hepatitis B immunoglobulin and begin the hepatitis B vaccination series. For surgeons who were successfully immunized against HBV in the past, neither routine booster doses nor routine immunity status surveillance is recommended.

10. **What are the recommendations for hepatitis C immunization?**
There is currently no effective vaccine available against HCV. Immunoglobulin for HCV does not confer protection. Using universal barrier precautions remains the best strategy.

11. **Does laparoscopic surgery minimize the risk of HIV contamination?**
The laparoscopic technique reduces exposure to blood products and sharp instruments; however, the risks are different. The evacuation of the pneumoperitoneum during laparoscopic procedures releases aerosolized HIV-infected blood and peritoneal fluid into the operative suite. Evacuation of the pneumoperitoneum into a closed system diminishes this exposure.

12. **Is double gloving an effective method of protection?**
Although double gloving may not prevent percutaneous injury, it clearly reduces blood exposure. The contact rates between blood and the surgeon's skin are decreased by 70% when the surgeon wears two pairs of gloves. Whereas outer glove perforation occurs in 25% of cases, inner glove perforation occurs in only 10% of cases (surgeons, 8.7%; assistants, 3.7%). The longer the procedure, the more frequent are inner glove perforations. The nondominant index finger is the most common target.

13. **Are eye splash injuries a major threat to surgeons?**
A CDC study demonstrated that approximately 13% of documented HIV transmissions occurred by mucocutaneous contact. Eye splash injuries during surgery are often underestimated, although they are the easiest type of contact to prevent. A recent study examined 160 eye shields used by surgeons and assistants. All operations lasted ≥ 30 minutes. The shields were inspected for macroscopic splashes and then tested for microscopic splashes. Forty-four percent of the shields tested positive for blood. The surgeon was aware of a spray in only 8% of cases. The splashes were macroscopically visible in only 16% of cases. The risk of eye splashes was higher for surgeons than for assistants and increased with the length of the operation. The type of operation also proved to be a determining factor; vascular surgery and orthopedic surgery had the higher risks for eye splash injuries. Eye protection should be mandatory.

14. **What is the surgeons' rate of exposure to blood and body fluids?**
Percutaneous blood exposure occurs in 1.2–5.6% of surgical cases and mucocutaneous blood contact in 6.4–50.4%. The discrepancy among reported rates reflects differences in data collection, procedures performed, surgical technique, and degree of precautions. No health care worker has ever been infected through exposure of intact skin to blood and body fluids. However, transmission of HIV after mucocutaneous contact with HIV-infected blood has been reported. The risk of contamination is real for all personnel in the operating room, but it is much higher for surgeons and first assistants, who account for 80% of all body contamination and 65% of injuries.

15. **Again, what are the seroconversion rates for HIV and HBV exposure?**
Seroconversion rates from a hollow needle stick are 0.3% for HIV and 30% for HBV.

16. **What is the lifetime occupational risk of HIV infection for surgeons?**
The risk of HIV infection for a surgeon can be calculated by obtaining the product of HIV seroprevalence in surgical patients (0.32–50.00%), percutaneous injury rate (1.2–6.0%), and seroconversion rate (0.29–0.50%). The calculated risk per case of acquiring HIV ranges from 0.11 per million to 66 per million. Assuming that a surgeon performs 350 operations per year over a 30-year career, the estimated lifetime cumulative risk ranges from 0.12% to 50.0%, depending on the variables. Several assumptions are inherent in this calculation:
- The formula assumes a constant HIV prevalence, but it is estimated that the prevalence increases by 4.0–8.6% annually in the United States.
- The formula assumes that exposure to HIV-infected blood occurs only through percutaneous injuries, disregarding the risk caused by mucocutaneous exposure.

- The formula assumes that whereas every operation carries the same risk, the risk varies with the length of procedure and amount of blood loss.
- The formula assumes that the risk per case is the same for a trauma surgeon in center city Detroit and a plastic surgeon in Beverly Hills.

Clearly, these assumptions are imprecise.

17. **Are there effective methods to reduce the risk of transmission of bloodborne diseases to surgeons?**

For HBV infection, in addition to universal precautions, a highly effective vaccine is available, but it is not used as much as it should be. Most surgeons who are 45 years or older have not been vaccinated. A precisely defined postexposure protocol is also available. For HCV and HIV infections, the most pragmatic approach is to lower the rate of percutaneous and mucocutaneous injuries by observing barrier precautions and using safe surgical technique.

Finally, prompt response to blood exposure is required. Contamination of the hands or arms is best dealt with by immediate rescrubbing. If this is not practical, the area should be irrigated with povidone iodine, and rescrubbing should be accomplished soon thereafter.

BIBLIOGRAPHY

1. Barrie PS, Patchen Dellinger E, Dougherty SH, Fink MP: Assessment of hepatitis B virus immunization status among North American surgeons. Arch Surg 129:27–32, 1994.
2. Bell DM: Occupational risk of human immunodeficiency virus infection in healthcare workers: An overview. Am J Med 102(suppl 5B):81S–85S, 1997.
3. Cardo DM, Culver DH, Ciescielski CA, et al: A case-control study of HIV seroconversion in healthcare workers after percutaneous exposure. N Engl J Med 337:1485–1490, 1997.
4. Dodd RY, Notari EP, Stramer SL: Current prevalence and incidence of infectious disease markers and estimated window-period risk in the American Red Cross blood donor population. Transfusion 42:975–979, 2002.
5. Eubanks S, Newman L, Lucas G: Reduction of HIV transmission during laparoscopic procedures. Surg Laparosc Endosc 3:2–5, 1993.
6. Fry DE: Blood-borne diseases in 1998. Bull Am Coll Surg 83:13–18, 1998.
7. Gerberding JL: Reducing occupational risk of HIV infection. Hosp Pract 113–110, 115–118, 1991.
8. Klein HG: Allogenic transfusion risks in the surgical patient. Am J Surg 317:242–245, 1995.
9. Koff RS: Hepatitis A, hepatitis B, and combination hepatitis vaccines for immunoprophylaxis: An update. Digest Dis Sci 47:1183–1194, 2002.
10. Lin EY, Brunicardi C: HIV infection and surgeons. World J Surg 18:753–757, 1994.
11. Marasco S, Woods S: The risk of eye splash injuries in surgery. Aust N Z J Surg 68:785–787, 1998.
12. Megan J, Patterson M, Novak CB, et al: Surgeons' concern and practices of protection against bloodborne pathogens. Ann Surg 228:266–272, 1998.
13. Pietrabissa A, Merigliano S, Montorsi M, et al: Reducing the occupational risk of infections for the surgeons: Multicentric national survey on more than 15,000 surgical procedures. World J Surg 21:573–578, 1997.
14. Schreiber GB, Busch MP, Kleinman SH, et al: The risk of transfusion-transmitted viral infections: The retrovirus epidemiology donor study. N Engl J Med 334:1685–1690, 1996.
15. Szmuness W, Stevens CE, Harley EJ, et al: Hepatitis B vaccine: Demonstration of efficacy in a controlled clinical trial in a high-risk population in the United States. N Engl J Med 303:833–841, 1980.

CHAPTER 102

ETHICS IN THE SURGICAL INTENSIVE CARE UNIT

Ricardo J. Gonzalez, M.D.

1. **What are the four principles of medical ethics?**
   1. **Beneficence** describes the active role of doing good by intervention.
   2. **Nonmaleficence** is equivalent to saying, "First do no harm."
   3. **Autonomy** accounts for informed consent, competence, and the patient's right to refuse treatment and to know what's going on.
   4. **Justice** means that all patients should receive fair and equal care but that one patient's care should not squander limited resources for others.

2. **What is a do-not-resuscitate (DNR) order?**
   A DNR order instructs the surgeon not to resuscitate the patient if cardiopulmonary arrest occurs; however, a DNR order is much more involved and complicated than the acronym would have you believe. DNR is not absolute.

   The Joint Commission for the Accreditation of Healthcare Organizations mandates that hospitals have written guidelines that promote accountability for DNR orders. All DNR orders must be documented in writing, similar to all other orders, in the appropriate section of the patient's chart. They should specify the treatments to be withheld and treatments that the patient wishes to have implemented. Patients and families must participate in the DNR decision. Moreover, the DNR status should be discussed and reviewed with the other members of the health care team. Finally, a DNR order does not mean that the patient should be medically abandoned.

3. **What is the difference between withdrawing and withholding support?**
   A decision to withdraw should not be more problematic than a decision to withhold, because one cannot be sure that an intervention will work until you try it. There is no moral or ethical distinction between withdrawal and withholding of support. Either of the two allows natural progression of disease without the interface of medical technology. The decision to withdraw or withhold support does not equate with patient death, although the probability of death may be greater. After the decision has been made, appropriate management should focus on the patient's comfort and psychosocial support.

4. **What is an advance directive?**
   An advance directive is a method of delineating a competent patient's wishes for application at a time when he or she is no longer competent. Medical management or the lack thereof can be based on the patient's wishes rather than a perceived sense of what is best for the patient. Advance directives may be an informal document, such as a living will, or a formal legal document, such as medical durable power of attorney.

5. **What is durable power of attorney?**
   A durable power of attorney is a patient-appointed proxy decision maker. The proxy decision maker becomes active as soon as the patient is no longer able to make competent medical decisions. Hence, the durable power of attorney must have been established in advance of the cognitive decline of the patient.

6. **What is a living will?**

   A living will, much like a durable power of attorney, is a formal advanced directive in which a competent patient produces a pre-illness guideline for future care in accordance with his or her wishes.

7. **What is included in informed consent?**

   Information about the patient's condition as well as risks and benefits of the recommended treatment are included. Moreover, the operative and nonoperative alternatives (including no treatment) should be discussed with the patient. The patient's understanding of the information and alternatives should be assessed as part of the informed consent. Finally, informed consent is a voluntary decision made by the patient or on behalf of the patient by a proxy decision maker.

8. **What are futile care and medical futility?**

   Ultimately, old age and disease will conquer us all. The definition of medically futile or inappropriate treatment is still debated. Nonetheless, there are four main concepts of medical futility:
   1. Health care professionals are not required to provide **physiologically futile** treatment.
   2. **Imminent demise** argues against treatment if the patient has no likelihood of survival to discharge.
   3. Under the concept of **lethal condition**, medical care is considered futile if the patient will survive temporarily but ultimately expire as a result of the ongoing disease process.
   4. Quality of life or **qualitative futility** argues against treatment if the patient's quality of life is so poor that it would be unreasonable to prolong life.

   Care must be taken, however, in making medical decisions based on futility because these decisions may lead to self-fulfilling prophecies.

9. **What are the clinical determinants of brain death?**

   Many of the current concepts of brain death are based on the 1968 report from the ad hoc committee at Harvard Medical School, which called for a new neurologic definition of brain death. But it was not until 1981 that BEMAT justified the neurologic criteria of brain death by stressing the need for intact brainstem integrative function in order for a person to function as a whole. By definition, brain death requires loss of brainstem reflexes in an irreversibly comatose patient. Brain death includes loss of the pupillary, corneal, oculovestibular, oculocephalic, oropharyngeal, and respiratory reflexes for ≥ 6 hours. The patient also should undergo an apnea test, in which the pCO_2 is allowed to rise to at least 60 mmHg without coexistent hypoxia. The patient should be observed for the absence of spontaneous breathing. Other ancillary tests are not essential; for example, it is **not** necessary to perform an intravenous radioisotope cerebral angiogram or a four-vessel contrast cerebral angiogram or to document an isoelectric ("flat") electroencephalogram.

   Of note, all of the above criteria for brain death require the absence of central nervous system depression caused by barbiturates, narcotics, or hypothermia.

10. **What is a persistent vegetative state?**

    In a persistent vegetative state, typically seen after improvement of a comatose state, the patient lies motionless and without activity. The patient appears to be awake but does not have awareness of his or her surroundings or higher mental activity. Other names for this entity are *coma vigil* and *akinetic mutism*.

11. **What is euthanasia?**

    Euthanasia requires that the physician play an active role in assisting in the death of the patient. The concepts of physician-assisted suicide and active and passive euthanasia are highly controversial. In 1992, the Society of Critical Care Medicine published the results of a survey of critical care specialists; 87% had withdrawn life-prolonging support from patients. In addition, the most recent U.S. law pertaining to assisted suicide was passed in Oregon in 1994. This law makes it legal for a physician to prescribe medication to terminally ill patients for the purpose of committing suicide.

12. Who should approach patients' families about organ donation?

Some claim that the physician who has established good rapport with the patient's family should raise the issue of organ donation. Others believe that the local organ procurement personnel should approach the family because they have greater interest and training in the process. The best approach is probably a combined one.

13. What should patients' families be told when organ donation is feasible?

The surgeon should stress that the patient has died despite an actively beating heart. The family should be questioned about the patient's wishes regarding organ donation. All topics should be based on the concepts of informed consent. The family should be informed of the likelihood that several patients will benefit from the donated organs. The family needs to understand that there is no guarantee that the organs will be suitable for donation. They should be assured that they are not responsible for the cost of care provided after brain death is determined and that they may refuse organ donation without fear of prejudice.

14. What is the role of the hospital ethics committee?

The hospital ethics committee educates hospital staff members, creates policy, and provides a source of consultation.

The function of education is accomplished through grand rounds, seminars, special lectures, and journal clubs. The hospital ethics committee should be viewed as an intrinsic part of the hospital community. Developed policies should be reviewed by other committees and divisions of the hospital to foster a better sense of cohesiveness when ethical and moral dilemmas arise. The consultative function of the ethics committee produces the greatest amount of controversy. In fact, many hospitals negate this function by stating that it interferes with the physician–patient relationship. The hospital ethics committee can and should provide an arena for collaboration and general ethical education within the hospital.

BIBLIOGRAPHY

1. Ad Hoc Committee of the Harvard Medical School to Examine the Definition of Brain Death: A definition of irreversible coma. JAMA 205:337–340, 1968.
2. Aminoff MJ: The central nervous system. In Medical Diagnosis and Treatment. Norwalk, CT, Appleton & Lange, 1996.
3. Arnold RM, Siminoff LA, Frader JE: Ethical issues in organ procurement: A review for intensivists. Crit Care Med 12:29–48, 1996.
4. Bernat JL, Culver CM, Gert B: On the definition and criterion of death. Ann Intern Med 94:389–394, 1981.
5. Harken AH: Enough is enough. Arch Surg 10:1061–1063, 1999.
6. Kelley DF, Hoyt JW: Ethics consultation. Crit Care Med 12:49–70, 1996.
7. McCollough L, Jones J, Brody B: Surgical Ethics. Oxford, Oxford University Press, 1998.
8. Nyman DJ, Eidelman AL, Sprung CL: Euthanasia. Crit Care Clin 12:85–96, 1996.
9. Society of Critical Care Ethics Committee: Attitudes of critical care medicine professionals concerning foregoing life-sustaining treatments. Crit Care Med 20:320–326, 1992.
10. State of Oregon: ORS.251.215, The Oregon Death with Dignity Act. Official 1994 Oregon General Election Handbook, 1994, pp 121–124.
11. Younger SJ: Medical futility. Crit Care Clin 12:165–178, 1996.

INDEX

Page numbers in **boldface type** indicate complete chapters.